TEXTBOOK
OF
Orthodontics

TEXTBOOK
OF
Orthodontics

Samir E. Bishara, DDS, BDS, DOrtho, MS

Professor, Department of Orthodontics
University of Iowa
College of Dentistry
Iowa City, Iowa

W.B. SAUNDERS COMPANY
A Harcourt Health Sciences Company
Philadelphia London New York St. Louis Sydney Toronto

W.B. SAUNDERS COMPANY
A Harcourt Health Sciences Company

The Curtis Center
Independence Square West
Philadelphia, Pennsylvania 19106

Library of Congress Cataloging-in-Publication Data

Textbook of orthodontics / [edited by] Samir E. Bishara.

    p. ; cm.

Includes bibliographical references and index.

ISBN 0–7216–8289–8 (alk. paper)

    1. Orthodontics.   I. Bishara, Samir E.
[DNLM: 1. Orthodontics, Corrective—methods. 2. Malocclusion—therapy.
3. Maxillofacial Development. WU 400 T355 2001]

RK521 .T49 2001
617.6′43—dc21

                                              00-069695

Publishing Director: John Schrefer
Editor: Penny Rudolph
Developmental Editor: Jaime Pendill
Project Manager: Patricia Tannian
Project Specialist: Suzanne C. Fannin
Designer: Julia Ramirez

TEXTBOOK OF ORTHODONTICS   ISBN 0-7216-8289-8

Last digit is the print number: 9 8 7 6 5 4 3 2 1

Contributors

Athanasios E. Athanasiou, DDS, MSD, DrDent
Professor, Department of Orthodontics
School of Dentistry
Aristotle University of Thessaloniki
Greece

James J. Baldwin, DDS, MS
Associate Clinical Professor, Section of Orthodontics
Indiana University School of Dentistry
Indianapolis, Indiana

Robert L. Boyd, DDS, MEd
Professor and Chair, Department of Orthodontics
University of the Pacific
School of Dentistry
San Francisco, California

A. Denis Britto, BDS, MDS, DDS, MSD
Assistant Professor, Department of Orthodontics
Virginia Commonwealth University School
  of Dentistry
Richmond, Virginia

Donald J. Ferguson, DMD, MSD
Executive Director and Professor, Department of
  Orthodontics
Center for Advanced Dental Education
Associate Dean, Graduate School
St. Louis University
St. Louis, Missouri

Michael W. Finkelstein, DDS, MS
Professor, Department of Oral Pathology, Radiology,
  and Medicine
College of Dentistry
Department of Anatomy and Cell Biology
College of Medicine
University of Iowa
Iowa City, Iowa

**Thomas M. Graber, DMD, MSD, PhD, MD, DSc,
  ScD, OdontDr, FRCS**
Director, Kenilworth Dental Research Foundation
Clinical Professor, Department of Orthodontics
University of Illinois
Chicago, Illinois
Editor-in-Chief, World Orthodontic Journal, and
  Emeritus, American Journal of Orthodontics and
  Dentofacial Orthopedics

William F. Hohlt, DDS
Associate Professor, Section of Orthodontics
Indiana University School of Dentistry
Indianapolis, Indiana

Robert J. Isaacson, DDS, MSD, PhD
Professor, Department of Orthodontics
Virginia Commonwealth University School of
  Dentistry
Richmond, Virginia

David C. Johnsen, DDS, MS
Dean, College of Dentistry
Professor, Department of Pediatric Dentistry
University of Iowa
College of Dentistry
Iowa City, Iowa

Michael J. Kanellis, DDS, MS
Associate Professor, Department of Pediatric
  Dentistry
University of Iowa
College of Dentistry
Iowa City, Iowa

Robert G. Keim, DDS, EdD, PhD
Program Director, Assistant Chairman, Department
  of Orthodontics
Center for Craniofacial Molecular Biology
University of Southern California
Los Angeles, California

Andrew J. Kuhlberg, DMD, MDS
Assistant Professor, Department of Orthodontics
University of Connecticut
School of Dental Medicine
Farmington, Connecticut

Marla J. Magness, DDS, MS
Private Practice, Orthodontics
Houston, Texas

Ram S. Nanda, DDS, MS, PhD
Professor, The Endowed Chair, Department of
  Orthodontics
University of Oklahoma
College of Dentistry
Oklahoma City, Oklahoma

Peter Ngan, DMD
Professor and Chair, Department of Orthodontics
West Virginia University
Morgantown, West Virginia

Neil T. Reske, CDT, MA
Instructional Resource Associate, Department of
    Orthodontics
University of Iowa
College of Dentistry
Iowa City, Iowa

Bronwen Richards, DDS, MS
Private Practice
Rock Island, Illinois

W. Eugene Roberts, DDS, PhD
Professor and Head, Section of Orthodontics
Indiana University School of Dentistry
Indianapolis, Indiana

Shiva V. Shanker, DDS, MDS, MS
Clinical Assistant Professor, Department of
    Orthodontics
Ohio State University
Columbus, Ohio

Pramod K. Sinha, DDS, BDS, MS
Clinical Professor, Department of Orthodontics
St. Louis University
St. Louis, Missouri
Private Practice
Spokane, Washington

Peter M. Spalding, DDS, MS (Ped Dent), MS (Ortho)
Associate Professor and Chair, Department of Growth
    and Development
University of Nebraska Medical Center
College of Dentistry
Lincoln, Nebraska

Robert N. Staley, DDS, MA, MS
Professor, Department of Orthodontics
University of Iowa
College of Dentistry
Iowa City, Iowa

Katherine W. L. Vig, BDS, MS, DOrtho, FDS (RCS)
Professor and Chairman, Section of Orthodontics
Ohio State University
College of Dentistry
Columbus, Ohio

Vickie Vlaskalic, BDSc, MDSc
Assistant Professor, Department of Orthodontics
University of the Pacific
School of Dentistry
San Francisco, California

Deborah L. Zeitler, DDS, MS
Professor and Vice Chair, Department of Hospital
    Dentistry
University of Iowa
College of Dentistry
Iowa City, Iowa

This book is dedicated to my family and my friends for their unfailing and selfless love, support, and care, for which I will forever be grateful.

Foreword

This beautifully coordinated team effort of world class scientists and clinicians appropriately brings in the new millennium with a fine opus that will provide both the student and clinician with the very latest and best information on orthodontics.

There has been considerable change in this specialty since I published my first orthodontics textbook for Saunders in 1961. Orthodontics is the oldest and largest specialty in dentistry. It has attracted superb clinicians and has fostered more research via advanced training of specialists in the field than any other dental specialty. Scientifically based, evidence-based clinical practice is now a reality. There has been major progress on all fronts; i.e, growth and development, diagnosis, mechanotherapy and interdisciplinary teamwork with maxillofacial surgery, periodontics, prosthodontics, and other dental areas. Obviously, orthodontics as a specialty has been successful in attracting the largest group of residents in training, despite the rigorous 3-year graduate degree requirements. Competition for some 275 slots each year is keen. The academic qualifications of those chosen are outstanding. These residents expect to be challenged and properly trained.

Orthodontic indoctrination at the undergraduate dental level has been largely based on existing textbooks, and it has been successful in contributing to this abundance of riches of bright, eager, motivated residents. Expectations of proper indoctrination are high. Properly written texts are a major challenge because of rapidly changing technical material and basic scientific advances. Yesterday's information is not good enough. Unfortunately, the supply of orthodontic faculty has not kept pace with the demand. There is a faculty crisis today. The plain fact is that the textbook has assumed a more important role in the indoctrination of the would-be orthodontist. This book accepts that challenge and goes beyond it.

There are six major sections and a total of 30 chapters, written by 27 outstanding authors. Iowa-based Samir Bishara has called upon prominent faculty members from his own institution, one of the oldest and best in the world. (John J. Ravenscroft Patrick gave intensive 6-week orthodontic courses at the University of Iowa long before Edward H. Angle gave his 4-week courses in St. Louis. Angle used much of Patrick's material in his own courses, not always giving credit.) In addition to the Iowa faculty, leaders from around the world have joined the team, giving an impressive source of information that would not be available from any one school. It can be called, in modern technological parlance, a virtual faculty—a tour de force!

This extremely comprehensive text can serve as a fundamental information source for undergraduate and graduate orthodontic students and, of course, for all other dental specialties. It is a veritable gold mine of information. Read and learn; read and enjoy!

T.M. Graber,
Professor of Orthodontics,
University of Illinois, College of Dentistry

Preface

Over the last 150 years many substantial contributions to the science and art of orthodontics in the form of scientific articles, textbooks, and master's and PhD dissertations have been accomplished and published. Collectively, this body of knowledge that is now available is a product of hard work and great imagination of many individuals. These accomplishments helped bring orthodontics and orthodontists to a reasonable level of sophistication both diagnostically and technically. Metallurgical innovations of orthodontic wires, bonding of brackets, new bracket designs, and new imaging techniques have made orthodontics more efficient, as well as more patient friendly.

Although such technical advances have had a significant impact on the practice of orthodontics, the clinician still must develop the same time-honored skills to be able to properly diagnose and plan treatment for each patient. In other words, the clinician still must acquire certain basic tools that enable him or her to synthesize relevant information. The clinician must then apply this information to the individual patient in a systematic and consistent way.

This book is a modest attempt to provide such information in a logical format that helps students of orthodontics both understand and apply the basic concepts of diagnosis and treatment. Without such a basic foundation, diagnosis and treatment planning for a malocclusion becomes a difficult and misguided exercise for which prospective patients will bear the consequences.

The contributors to this text have worked hard to present their ideas in a format that is both clear as well as scientific. Reading the works of all of these authors has been an education as well as a revelation of the depth of their understanding and their abilities. To each one, I owe a debt of gratitude!

The text is organized into six sections:

Section I: Growth and Development. This section describes the overall physical changes that occur between the embryonic stage and adulthood. Special emphasis is given to the normal and abnormal development of the facial structures as well as to the development of the dentition and the occlusal relationships from the primary to the permanent dentitions.

Section II: Diagnosis. The systematic evaluation of the various dentofacial relationships is essential for the proper diagnosis of malocclusions. This section discusses the details of how each parameter needs to be evaluated for the clinician to be able to differentiate between relatively simple and more complex problems involving the dentition and skeletal and soft tissue structures.

Section III: Appliances. The principles that govern the construction and the use of fixed appliances are provided. The emphasis is on biomechanical concepts rather than on details of various techniques.

Section IV: Treatment and Treatment Considerations. The treatment approaches to different malocclusions that the clinician faces in the primary, mixed, and permanent dentitions are discussed. The complexities of the orthodontic treatment are outlined as they relate to specific malocclusions.

Section V: Other Aspects Related to Treatment. In addition to the proper diagnosis of the malocclusion and the choice of the appliance to be used, other parameters exist that need to be considered by the clinician, the patient, and the parents to successfully accomplish the desired treatment objectives.

Section VI: Orthodontics and Adjunct Treatment. A number of areas are considered to be an intricate part of the overall evaluation and management of the orthodontic patient. Some of these problems need either a special consideration from the orthodontist or the expertise and intervention of other specialists to provide the patient with the optimal treatment for a given malocclusion.

This text is not meant to provide a definitive approach to all types of malocclusion. On the other hand, I hope that it provides sufficient information to enable the clinician to properly diagnose the complexities of a given problem while also giving an overview of various treatment approaches to some of these problems.

Samir E. Bishara

Contents

SECTION VI   ORTHODONTICS AND ADJUNCT TREATMENT

SECTION I

Growth and Development

CHAPTER 1

Overview of General Embryology and Head and Neck Development

Michael W. Finkelstein

KEY TERMS

embryonic period
fetal period
zygote
cleavage
blastomeres
morula
blastocyst cavity
blastocele
blastocyst
trophoblast
inner cell mass
syncytiotrophoblast
cytotrophoblast
uteroplacental circulation
bilaminar disk
hypoblast
primitive yolk sac
exocoelomic cavity
epiblast
amniotic cavity
extraembryonic mesoderm
chorionic cavity
extraembryonic coelom
connecting stalk
chorion

secondary or definitive
 yolk sac
gastrulation
primitive streak
primitive pit
primitive node
invagination
endoderm
mesoderm
ectoderm
notochordal process
notochordal canal
notochord
prochordal plate
neurulation
neural plate
neuroectoderm
neural folds
neural groove
neural tube
anterior neuropores
posterior neuropores
rhombomeres
neural crest cells
homeobox (HOX) genes

paraxial mesoderm
somites
somitocoele
somitomeres
sclerotome
dermatome
myotome
intermediate mesoderm
visceral (splanchnic)
 mesoderm
parietal (somatic) mesoderm
buccopharyngeal membrane
stomodeum
arches
grooves
pouches
membranes
mesenchyme
ectomesenchyme
frontonasal prominence
maxillary prominences
mandibular prominences
nasal placodes
medial nasal prominences
lateral nasal prominences

nasal pits
intermaxillary segment
nasolacrimal ducts
primary palate
secondary palate
lateral palatine shelves
body
base
tuberculum impar
lateral lingual swellings
hypobranchial eminence
copula
terminal sulcus
thyroid diverticulum
thyroglossal duct
foramen cecum
neurocranium
viscerocranium
cartilaginous neurocranium
 (chondrocranium)
membranous neurocranium
sutures
fontanelles
cartilaginous viscerocranium
membranous viscerocranium

OVERVIEW OF GENERAL EMBRYOLOGY

Understanding embryologic development is a complex process requiring an ability to visualize and conceptualize structures in three dimensions. Embryology has been traditionally considered part of anatomy and consequently, requires learning numerous anatomic terms. Learning embryology is critical to understanding normal postnatal growth as well as the development of various craniofacial abnormalities. The purpose of this chapter is to provide a general overview of the first 8 weeks of human development and a more

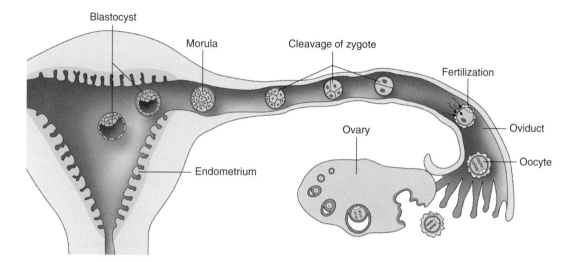

Figure 1-1 Summary of the first week showing development and migration of the zygote, morula, and blastocyst in the uterine tube and uterus. (From Moore KL, Persaud TVN: *The developing human: clinically oriented embryology,* ed 6, Philadelphia, 1998, WB Saunders.)

detailed description of the development of the head and neck.

Phases of Development

Prenatal human development is traditionally divided into the **embryonic period,** occurring from fertilization through the eighth week of development, and the **fetal period,** lasting from week 9 to term. Weeks 4 through 8 are especially important because the tissues and organ systems are developing rapidly from the original three germ layers. Exposure of embryos to teratogens, such as viruses and drugs, during these weeks may result in congenital abnormalities.

Weeks 1 and 2 of Development Human development begins when a spermatozoon fertilizes an oocyte resulting in the formation of a **zygote** (Figure 1-1). Fertilization typically occurs in the ampulla of the uterine tube (oviduct). The zygote undergoes **cleavage,** a series of mitotic divisions, as it moves along the uterine tube toward the uterus. The cells resulting from cleavage are called **blastomeres.** They adhere to one another and form a ball of cells called a **morula,** which enters the uterus about three days after fertilization.

A fluid-filled space called the **blastocyst cavity** or **blastocele,** develops within the morula, and the entire structure is now called the **blastocyst** (Figure 1-2). Six days after fertilization, two distinct cell types comprise the blastocyst. The **trophoblast** forms a single layer of cells covering the outside of the blastocyst. The **inner cell mass** (embryoblast) is the cluster of cells located inside the trophoblast. The inner cell mass develops into the embryo whereas the trophoblast forms the

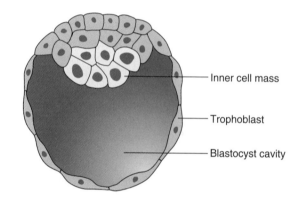

Figure 1-2 The blastocyst at approximately 6 days has two distinct cell populations surrounding the fluid-filled blastocyst cavity. The trophoblast forms the embryonic portion of the placenta, and the inner cell mass (embryoblast) develops into the embryo.

embryonic part of the placenta and other peripheral structures associated with the embryo.

Two important events occur in the blastocyst at the end of the first week and beginning of the second week after fertilization. First, the blastocyst adheres to the surface of the endometrium and implantation begins. Second, the inner cell mass forms a bilaminar disk, and, consequently, the second week of development is sometimes called the *bilaminar disk stage.*

The trophoblast differentiates into two layers— an outer multinucleated cellular syncytium called the **syncytiotrophoblast** and an inner **cytotrophoblast** (Figure 1-3). The syncytiotrophoblast invades endometrial connective tissue and erodes capillaries. Erosion of endometrial blood vessels causes maternal blood to flow into cavities, or lacunae, within the syncytiotrophoblast. This blood flow represents a

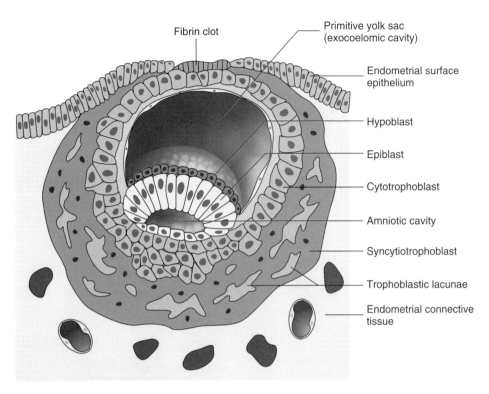

Fibrin clot

Primitive yolk sac
(exocoelomic cavity)

Endometrial surface
epithelium

Hypoblast

Epiblast

Cytotrophoblast

Amniotic cavity

Syncytiotrophoblast

Trophoblastic lacunae

Endometrial connective
tissue

Figure 1-3 The blastocyst, approximately 9 days after fertilization, is embedded within the endometrium. The trophoblast has differentiated into the cytotrophoblast and syncytiotrophoblast. Cavities called *trophoblastic lacunae* develop within the syncytiotrophoblast. The inner cell mass is now a bilaminar disk consisting of epiblast and hypoblast. The amniotic cavity is located between the epiblast and cytotrophoblast, and the blastocyst cavity has become the primitive yolk sac.

primitive circulation between the endometrium and the placenta known as the **uteroplacental circulation.** Meanwhile the blastocyst becomes embedded within the connective tissue of the endometrium. Endometrial epithelium then covers the blastocyst and the surface defect created by invasion of the blastocyst.[1]

While the blastocyst is becoming embedded in the endometrium, the inner cell mass, as stated earlier, differentiates into a two-layered, or **bilaminar, disk** comprised of epiblast and hypoblast (see Figure 1-3). The **hypoblast** consists of squamous or cuboidal cells adjacent to the blastocyst cavity, later known as the **primitive yolk sac (exocoelomic cavity).** The **epiblast** is made of columnar cells and is separated from the cytotrophoblast by a space called the **amniotic cavity.**

The primitive yolk sac is lined in some areas by hypoblast and in other areas by squamous epithelial cells (Figure 1-4). The **extraembryonic mesoderm** consists of loose connective tissue located between the outer surface of the primitive yolk sac and the inner surface of the cytotrophoblast. Lacunae filled with fluid develop in the extraembryonic mesoderm. The lacunae fuse and form a new space called the **chorionic cavity (extraembryonic coelom)** (Figure 1-5). The chorionic

cavity surrounds the yolk sac and amniotic cavity except where the bilaminar disk attaches to the trophoblast by the **connecting stalk.** Later in development the connecting stalk develops blood vessels and becomes the umbilical cord. The **chorion** is comprised of the chorionic cavity, extraembryonic mesoderm, cytotrophoblast, and syncytiotrophoblast.[1] Meanwhile, the hypoblast produces additional cells that migrate along the inside of the primitive yolk sac. The primitive yolk sac is squeezed off, and its remnants form the **secondary, or definitive, yolk sac** (see Figure 1-5). By the end of the second week of development the hypoblast has formed a localized area of thickening called the *prochordal plate* at the cranial end of the bilaminar disk.

Gastrulation: Week 3 During **gastrulation** the bilaminar embryonic disk is converted into a trilaminar disk. Gastrulation occurs during the third week after fertilization. This time period is sometimes called the trilaminar disk stage. At the beginning of gastrulation the bilaminar disk is oval and consists of the hypoblast layer and the epiblast layer. Gastrulation begins with formation of the **primitive streak** (Figure 1-6). This structure is a narrow trough with slightly bulging sides that develops in the midline of the epiblast toward the

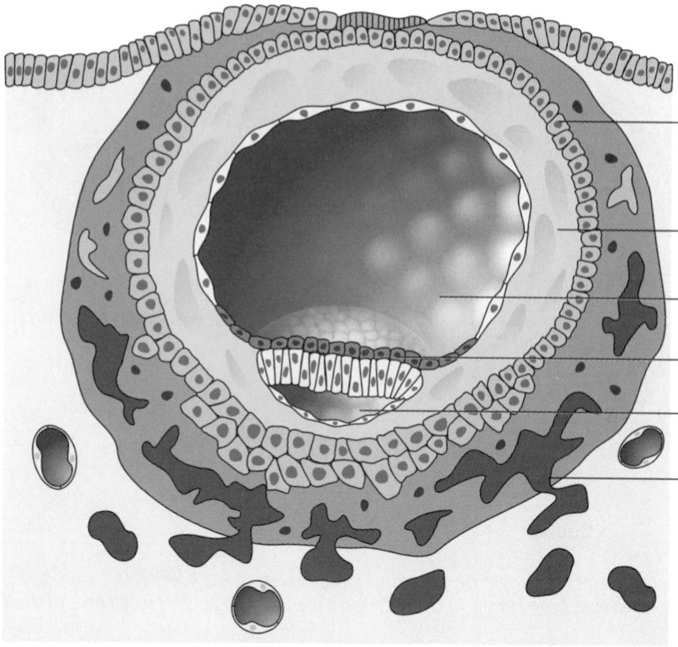

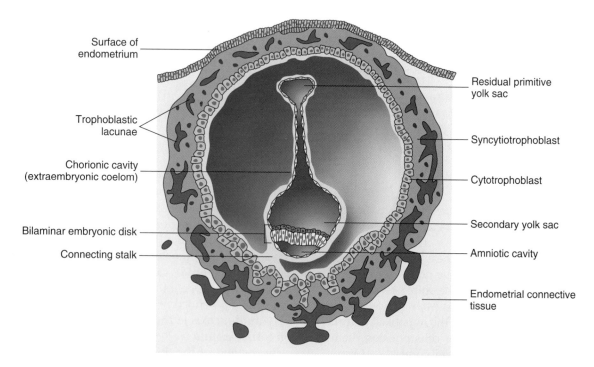

Figure 1-4 The blastocyst at approximately 12 days after fertilization. The extraembryonic mesoderm comprised of loose connective tissue has developed between the cytotrophoblast and the primitive yolk sac. The syncytiotrophoblast erodes maternal blood vessels in the endometrium, causing trophoblastic lacunae to fill with blood.

Cytotrophoblast

Extraembryonic mesoderm

Primitive yolk sac (exocoelomic cavity)

Hypoblast

Amniotic cavity

Syncytiotrophoblast with lacunae

Surface of endometrium

Trophoblastic lacunae

Chorionic cavity (extraembryonic coelom)

Bilaminar embryonic disk

Connecting stalk

Residual primitive yolk sac

Syncytiotrophoblast

Cytotrophoblast

Secondary yolk sac

Amniotic cavity

Endometrial connective tissue

Figure 1-5 The blastocyst at approximately 13 days after fertilization. Fluid-filled lacunae in the extraembryonic mesoderm have fused to create a new space called the *chorionic cavity (extraembryonic coelom)*. The chorionic cavity surrounds the primitive yolk sac and amniotic cavity except in the region of the connecting stalk. Cells from the hypoblast migrate along the inside of the primitive yolk sac, displace the primitive yolk sac, and form the secondary (definitive) yolk sac. The figure shows a residual portion of the primitive yolk sac.

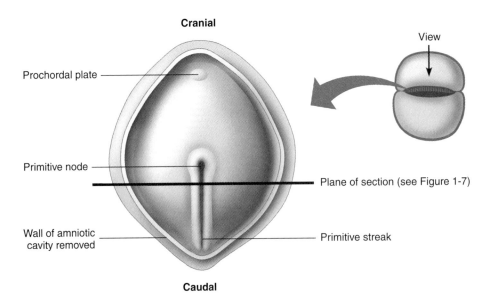

Figure 1-6 Dorsal view of bilaminar embryo at the beginning of gastrulation (third week). The primitive streak develops in the midline of the epiblast layer. The primitive pit and node are located at the cranial end of the primitive streak.

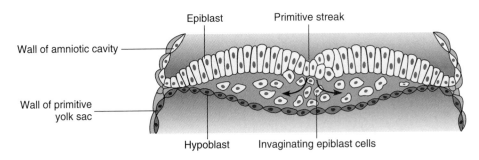

Figure 1-7 Invagination during gastrulation, transverse section through embryo along plane shown in Figure 1-6. Invagination involves epiblast cells migrating to the primitive streak and node, detaching from the epiblast, and growing beneath the epiblast. Some of the cells then displace the hypoblast to form the endoderm, whereas other cells migrate between endoderm and epiblast to form the embryonic mesoderm.

caudal end. The **primitive pit** surrounded by the elevated **primitive node** is located at the cranial end of the primitive streak.

During gastrulation, cells of the epiblast migrate to the primitive streak and primitive node, detach from the epiblast, and grow beneath the epiblast—a process called **invagination** (Figure 1-7). After the cells have invaginated, some cells displace the hypoblast to form the embryonic **endoderm.** Other cells position themselves between the endoderm and epiblast to form a third germ cell layer, the embryonic **mesoderm.** The remaining cells in the epiblast produce the **ectoderm.** The epiblast, therefore, forms all three embryonic germ layers: the ectoderm, the endoderm, and the mesoderm.[1]

Early in the third week, cells invaginating in the primitive pit and node region grow cranially until they reach the prochordal plate. They produce a cellular rod, the **notochordal process,** that runs longitudinally in the midline (Figure 1-8). The primitive pit extends into the notochordal process to form a small central **notochordal canal** (Figure 1-9). The canal eventually disappears, leaving a solid cylinder of cells, the **notochord.** The notochord represents the early midline axis of the embryo, and the axial skeleton forms around it.

By the end of the third week the mesoderm separates the ectoderm and endoderm everywhere in the embryonic disk, except for the cloacal membrane in the caudal region and the prochordal plate at the cranial midline area of the embryo (see Figure 1-8). In these two regions the endoderm and ectoderm are tightly adherent. The prochordal plate is the future region of the buccopharyngeal membrane.

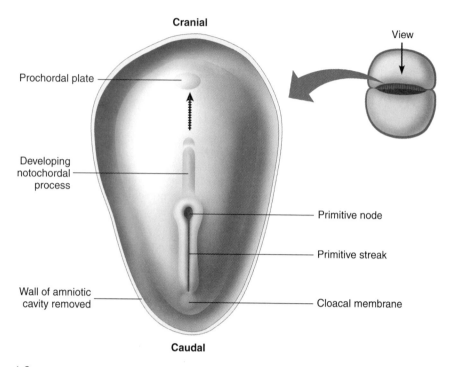

Figure 1-8 Developing notochordal process, dorsal view of epiblast. The notochordal process develops in the midline from cells in the primitive pit and grows in a cranial direction. The embryonic icon is for orientation purposes only and is not meant to be anatomically correct in its details.

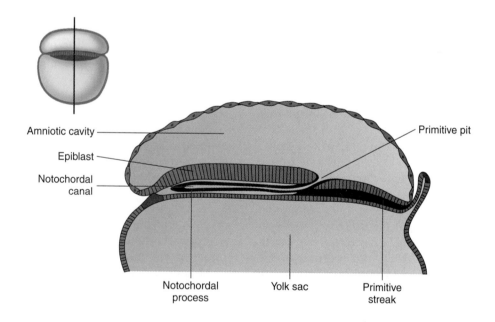

Figure 1-9 Developing notochordal process (midsagittal view). The primitive pit extends into the notochordal process to form the notochordal canal. The canal eventually disappears leaving the notochord as a solid structure.

Derivatives of Ectoderm The ectodermal germ layer generally forms structures that maintain contact with the outer environment. These include the central and peripheral nervous system; sensory epithelium of ear, nose, and eye; the epidermis and the skin appendages including the mammary gland; the pituitary gland; enamel; and other structures (Box 1-1).[2] Formation of the neuroectoderm and the neural crest are of particular importance and are described.

Neurulation is the process of development of the neural plate, neuroectoderm, and folding to produce the neural tube. During the third week of develop-

BOX 1-1	Derivatives of Three Germ Layers

Germ Layer	Derivative
Ectoderm	
Surface ectoderm	Epidermis, hair follicles, glands of skin, nails, mammary glands, adenohypophysis, lens of eye, inner ear, and tooth enamel
Neural crest ectoderm	Some connective tissue of head and neck (ectomesenchyme); pharyngeal arch cartilage, bone, and muscle; dentin and cementum; cells of spinal, cranial, and autonomic ganglia; meninges; adrenal medulla; melanocytes; and Schwann cells
Neural tube ectoderm	Central nervous system, retina, pineal gland, and neurohypophysis
Mesoderm	
Head	Skull and some connective tissue of head
Paraxial	Some muscles of head, muscles of trunk and limbs, skeleton (except skull), dermis, and connective tissue (except some in head and neck)
Intermediate	Kidneys, ovaries, testes, genital ducts, and accessory glands
Lateral	Connective tissue and muscle of viscera, serosa, primitive heart, blood and lymph cells, spleen, and adrenal cortex
Endoderm	Epithelial lining of digestive tract, respiratory tract, urinary bladder, and part of urethra; parenchymal cells of liver, pancreas, tonsils, thymus, thyroid gland, and parathyroid glands; epithelial lining of tympanic cavity and antrum, and auditory tube

ment the notochord induces the overlying ectoderm to thicken and differentiate into the **neural plate** (Figure 1-10). Viewed from above, the neural plate has an hourglass appearance along the cranial-caudal axis. Cells of the neural plate comprise the **neuroectoderm.** The neural plate grows caudally toward the primitive streak. The lateral edges of the neural plate become elevated to form the **neural folds.** A depressed groove called the **neural groove** forms between the neural folds (Figure 1-11). The neural folds approach each other and fuse in the midline to form the **neural tube.** The neural tube separates from the ectoderm with mesoderm in between. Fusion begins in the fourth week of development in the central portion of the embryo. The last parts of the neural tube to fuse are the cranial and caudal ends, known respectively as the **anterior neuropores** and the **posterior neuropores** (Figure 1-12).

The neural tube is the primordium of the central nervous system. The anterior region of the neural tube enlarges to form the forebrain, midbrain, and hindbrain. Eight bulges called **rhombomeres** develop in the hindbrain (Figure 1-13).

Neural crest cells arise from the neural folds and migrate throughout the body and differentiate into numerous varied structures (see Box 1-1). Neural crest cells from each rhombomere migrate to a specific location. Neural crest cells are important in providing mes-

enchyme (embryonic connective tissue) needed for craniofacial development. Neural crest cells needed for the development of the face and first pharyngeal arch structures originate in the midbrain and the first two rhombomeres.

Neural crest cells migrating from the rhombomeres express the **homeobox (HOX) genes** that were expressed in the rhombomeres of origin. HOX genes produce transcription factors that bind to the DNA of other genes and regulate gene expression. Homeobox genes are important in determining the identity and spatial arrangements of body regions, and they help determine the pattern and position of structures developing within the pharyngeal arches.[2,3]

Mutations of homeobox genes have been associated with congenital craniofacial anomalies such as Waardenburg's syndrome and one form of holoprosencephaly. Research in the molecular genetics of craniofacial development and the human genome project has yielded information about the location of mutations associated with these and other craniofacial anomalies. Research in this area is expected to continue to expand.

Differentiation of Embryonic Mesoderm and its Derivatives The mesoderm on either side of the notochord thickens to form longitudinal columns of tissue called the **paraxial mesoderm.** The paraxial mesoderm

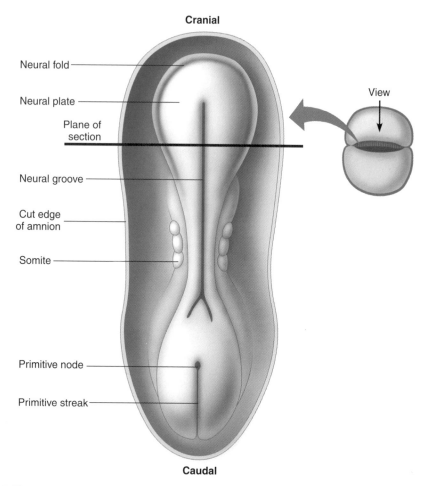

Figure 1-10 Neurulation (dorsal view) at approximately 20 days after fertilization. During neurulation the notochord induces the overlying ectoderm to form the neural plate. Note that from a dorsal perspective the neural plate has an hourglass appearance along the cranial-caudal axis. The lateral edges of the neural plate become elevated to form the neural folds. The neural groove is a depressed trough between the neural folds.

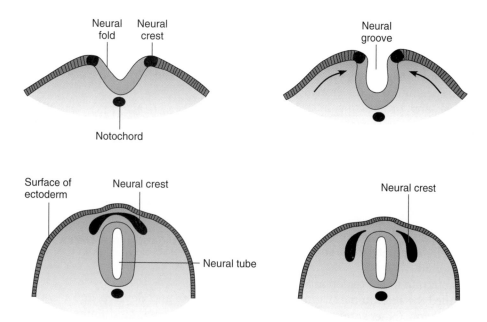

Figure 1-11 Neurulation, transverse view along plane shown in Figure 1-10. The neural folds approach each other and fuse to form the neural tube. The neural tube separates from the surface ectoderm. Note the origin of neural crest cells from the neural folds.

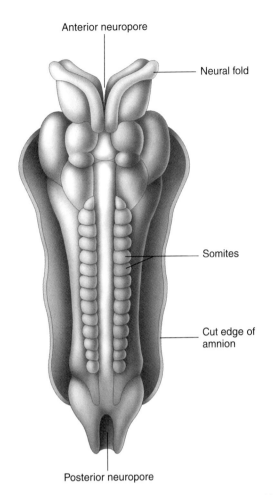

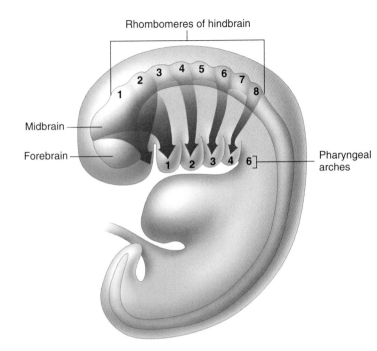

Figure 1-13 Paths of neural crest migration to the developing face and pharyngeal arches (sagittal view). Neural crest cells from the midbrain and the eight rhombomeres of the hindbrain migrate along the arrows in the figure to the face and pharyngeal arches where they provide embryonic connective tissue. Neural crest from the midbrain and first two rhombomeres contribute specifically to the face and first pharyngeal arch structures. (From Ten Cate AR [ed]: *Oral histology: development, structure, and function,* St Louis, 1998, Mosby.)

Figure 1-12 Somites and anterior and posterior neuropores (dorsal view). The anterior and posterior neuropores represent the last parts of the neural tube to fuse. The mesoderm on both sides of the notochord forms 48 paired blocks of tissue called *somites.* (From Sandra A, Coons WJ: *Core concepts in embryology,* Philadelphia, 1997, Lippincott-Raven.)

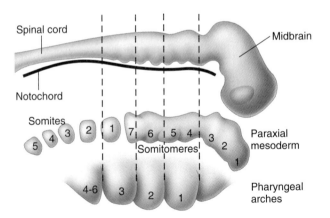

Figure 1-14 Somites and somitomeres (sagittal view). Somites are paired blocks of mesoderm. The most cranial somites are called *somitomeres,* and they are only partially segmented rather than being completely divided structures. Somites are numbered sequentially beginning with the most cranial somite. The same numbering system applies to somitomeres. The dotted lines illustrate that somitomeres are aligned with specific pharyngeal arches. (From Sandra A, Coons WJ: *Core concepts in embryology,* Philadelphia, 1997, Lippincott-Raven.)

segments into paired blocks of tissue called **somites** (see Figure 1-12). Of somites, 48 pairs develop in a regular repetitive pattern beginning in the cranial region during the third week and progressing in a caudal direction. A cavity called a **somitocoele** forms in the center of each somite.

The most cranial somites, called **somitomeres,** are only partially segmented structures (Figure 1-14). There are seven somitomeres approximately in register with the pharyngeal arches. The skeletal muscles of the head and neck develop from cells that migrate into the head and neck region and then differentiate into skeletal muscle cells. These cells originate from somitomeres and the most cranial somites.

Some somite cells migrate to the region around the notochord and are called the **sclerotome** (Figure 1-15). They form the axial skeleton. Other somite cells do not migrate and, instead, develop two other components. Superficial somite cells become the **dermatome** and form the dermis. Deeper somite cells become the

myotome and develop into most of the skeletal muscles of the trunk and limbs. Each somite, then, forms cartilage and bone components from sclerotome, muscle components from myotome, and skin components from dermatome.

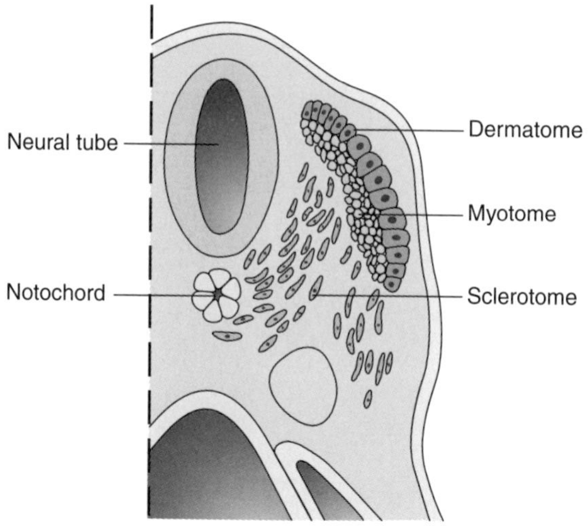

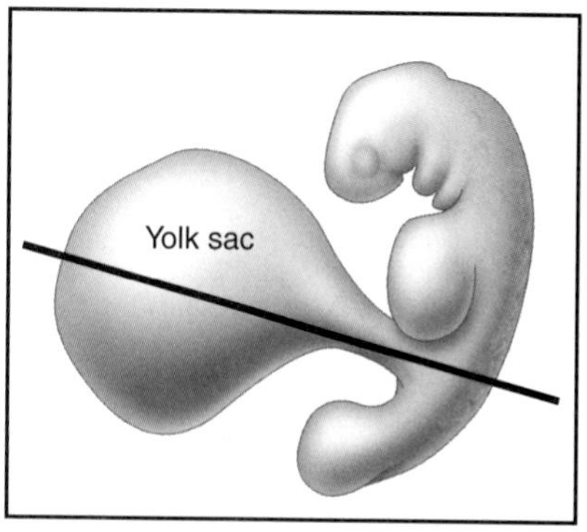

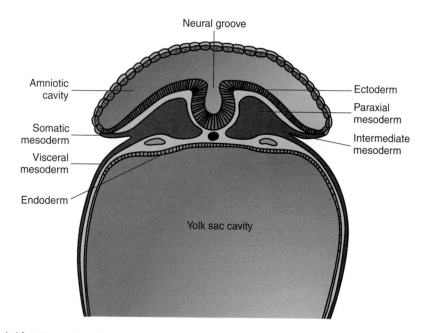

Figure 1-15 Differentiation of somites (transverse view showing half of embryo). The sclerotome forms the axial skeleton, the dermatome develops into the dermis, and the myotome differentiates into most of the skeletal muscle of the trunk and limbs. (From Sandra A, Coons WJ: *Core concepts in embryology*, Philadelphia, 1997, Lippincott-Raven.)

Figure 1-16 Differentiation of mesoderm (transverse view) at approximately 20 days after fertilization. The mesoderm at this stage consists of paraxial, intermediate, and lateral plate mesoderm. The lateral plate mesoderm is formed by two layers—the parietal (somatic) mesoderm and the visceral (splanchnic) mesoderm.

The **intermediate mesoderm** forms continuously with and lateral to the somites (Figure 1-16). It develops into the excretory units of the urinary system. More laterally the lateral plate mesoderm divides into two layers, the **visceral (splanchnic) mesoderm** and the **parietal (somatic) mesoderm.** The intraembryonic coelomic cavity forms between the visceral and parietal mesoderms. The visceral and parietal mesoderm contribute to the formation of the lateral and ventral body wall, the wall of the gut, and the serosa.[1]

Derivatives of Endoderm Derivatives of endoderm include components of the gastrointestinal, respiratory, urinary, and endocrine systems and the ear (see Box 1-1). Formation of the gastrointestinal system depends on folding of the embryo in the median and horizontal planes.

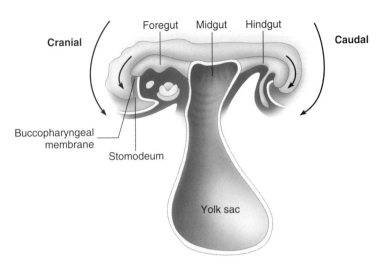

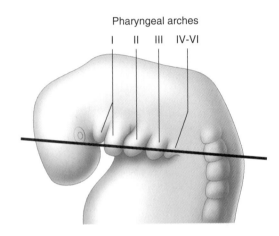

Figure 1-17 Folding of the embryo in the cranial-caudal plane, which creates the primordial gut. The head region folds ventrally, which brings part of the endoderm into the embryo as the foregut. The buccopharyngeal membrane separates the foregut and the stomodeum, the primitive oral cavity. The buccopharyngeal membrane degenerates by the end of the third week, and the foregut and stomodeum become continuous. (From Sandra A, Coons WJ: *Core concepts in embryology,* Philadelphia, 1997, Lippincott-Raven.)

Folding of the Embryo: Week 4 Beginning in the fourth week of development the flat trilaminar embryonic disk folds in two planes to form a more typical-appearing, cylindric, C-shaped embryo. Folding in the cranial-caudal plane is mainly a result of rapid longitudinal growth of the central nervous system. Growth of somites accounts for much of the lateral-medial folding.

Folding brings the endodermal-lined yolk sac into the embryo and creates the primordial gut: the foregut, midgut, and hindgut (Figure 1-17). Folding of the head region ventrally incorporates part of the endodermal lining into the embryo as the foregut. The **buccopharyngeal membrane** separates the foregut and the primitive oral cavity, which is called the **stomodeum.** The stomodeum is lined by ectoderm, and thus the buccopharyngeal membrane is lined by ectoderm on one side and endoderm on the other. The buccopharyngeal membrane breaks down at the end of the third week, allowing continuity between the foregut and stomodeum.[2]

DEVELOPMENT OF THE HEAD AND NECK

Pharyngeal (Branchial) Apparatus

The pharyngeal (branchial) arches begin to develop during the fourth week *in utero.* The pharyngeal apparatus gives rise to a significant number of structures of the head and neck. Understanding the development and derivations of the pharyngeal apparatus is important not only for understanding normal head and neck development but also for understanding the basis of many congenital abnormalities that involve these structures. Most congenital head and neck abnormalities occur when pharyngeal apparatus structures that should disappear during development persist.[4]

The pharyngeal apparatus consists of a series of bilaterally paired arches, pouches (clefts), grooves, and membranes. The structures of the pharyngeal apparatus are

Figure 1-18 The pharyngeal arch apparatus (lateral view of the external surface of the embryo) during the fourth week. Four pairs of pharyngeal arches are evident. The fourth arch is the result of fusion of arches IV and VI. Arch V regresses and does not give rise to structures in adults. (From Sandra A, Coons WJ: *Core concepts in embryology,* Philadelphia, 1997, Lippincott-Raven.)

numbered sequentially. For example, the four pairs of arches are numbered I, II, III, and IV beginning at the cranial end. The paired pharyngeal arches make up the lateral walls of the primordial pharynx, which develops from the foregut. As mentioned earlier, the stomodeum or primitive oral cavity is separated from the primordial pharynx by the buccopharyngeal membrane.

The buccopharyngeal membrane has an external surface comprised of ectoderm and an internal surface lined by endoderm. This membrane breaks down at approximately day 26, allowing the pharynx and foregut to communicate with the amniotic cavity.

The pharyngeal **arches** begin their development during the fourth week as a result of migration of neural crest cells into the head and neck region. Examination of the external surface of an embryo at the end of the fourth week of development reveals four distinct pairs of pharyngeal arches (Figure 1-18). Arches V and VI form in animals, but in humans they are poorly devel-

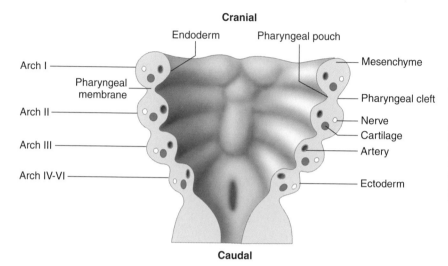

Cranial

Arch I

Pharyngeal membrane

Arch II

Arch III

Arch IV-VI

Endoderm

Pharyngeal pouch

Mesenchyme

Pharyngeal cleft

Nerve

Cartilage

Artery

Ectoderm

Caudal

Figure 1-19 The pharyngeal arch apparatus, as viewed along the plane of section shown in Figure 1-18. The pharyngeal arch apparatus gives rise to important head and neck structures. The pharyngeal arches are partially separated on the external surface by fissures called *grooves*, or *clefts*, and on the internal surface by pouches. The arches have a core of mesenchyme, an external surface of ectoderm, and an internal surface of endoderm. The arches have specific nerves, cartilages, muscles, and arteries associated with them.

oped and not visible on the external surface of the embryo. The fifth arch completely regresses and does not give rise to structures in the adult. Arch IV is the result of fusion of arches IV and VI.

The pharyngeal arches are partially separated on the external surface of the embryo by fissures called pharyngeal **grooves** or clefts (Figure 1-19). Pharyngeal **pouches** partially separate the arches on the internal aspect. The pharyngeal **membranes** represent the tissue interposed between pouches and clefts and connect adjacent arches. Pharyngeal arches, grooves, pouches, and membranes are important because they give rise to head and neck structures in the adult.[4,5]

Components of Pharyngeal Arches

Cellular Origins Ectoderm covers the external surface of each arch, and endoderm lines its internal surface (see Figure 1-19). Both are formed by epithelial cells. Each pharyngeal arch has a core of embryonic connective tissue called **mesenchyme.** The arch mesenchyme has two sources. During the third week mesenchyme originally develops from the mesoderm, and during the fourth week neural crest cells migrate from the brain into the arches and differentiate into mesenchyme. Neural crest cells have the potential to develop into different types of cells and tissues, including cartilage, bone, dentin, and cementum. Development of the head and neck, including tooth development, is unique in that neural crest cells make up a substantial portion of the mesenchyme. Some authorities acknowledge this contribution of neural crest cells by referring to head and neck mesenchyme as **ectomesenchyme.**[2]

Each pharyngeal arch has a specific cartilage that forms the skeleton of the arch (see Figure 1-19). It also has muscles, a nerve that supplies the muscles and mucosa derived from that arch, and arteries, called an

aortic arch.[4] All these components are well developed in the first and second arches except for the arteries.[3] The pharyngeal arches play the major role in the formation of the face, oral cavity and teeth, nasal cavities, pharynx, larynx, and neck. Knowledge of the specific nerve, cartilage, muscles, and arteries associated with each arch helps explain the development of head and neck structures. The following describes the derivatives of each component of the pharyngeal arches. This information is summarized in Table 1-1.

Nerve Components A specific cranial nerve grows from the brain and invades each arch (Figure 1-20). All structures, including muscles, dermis, and mucosa, arising from that arch are innervated by the associated cranial nerve.

Arch I: The trigeminal nerve (cranial nerve V) is the nerve for the first arch. The trigeminal nerve is the main sensory nerve of the head and neck, and it innervates the face, teeth, and mucosa of the oral cavity and anterior two thirds of the tongue. It also innervates the muscles of mastication. The mandibular division (V1) grows into the main portion of arch I, which is the mandibular process. The maxillary division (V2) supplies the maxillary process of arch I.

Arch II: The facial nerve (cranial nerve VII) is the second arch nerve.

Arch III: The glossopharyngeal nerve (cranial nerve IX) is the nerve for arch III.

Arches IV and VI: The vagus nerve (cranial nerve X) is the nerve for the fused fourth and sixth arches. The superior laryngeal branch of the vagus nerve innervates arch IV structures, and the recurrent laryngeal branch of the vagus supplies arch VI.

Cranial nerves VII, IX, and X supply muscles and part of the mucosa of the tongue, pharynx, and larynx.

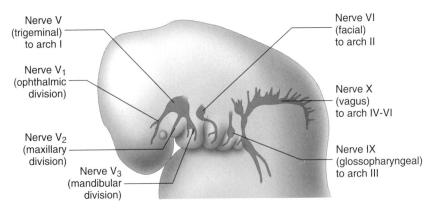

Figure 1-20 Lateral view of the embryo illustrating the cranial nerves to the pharyngeal arches. A specific cranial nerve is associated with each arch and innervates structures such as cartilages and muscles arising from that arch.

Nerve V (trigeminal) to arch I

Nerve V₁ (ophthalmic division)

Nerve V₂ (maxillary division)

Nerve V₃ (mandibular division)

Nerve VI (facial) to arch II

Nerve X (vagus) to arch IV-VI

Nerve IX (glossopharyngeal) to arch III

TABLE 1-1	Derivatives of the Pharyngeal Arches		
Arch	Cranial Nerve	Skeletal: Bone, Cartilage, Ligaments	Muscles
I	V: Trigeminal	Maxillary process: Maxilla, zygoma, zygomatic process of temporal bone Mandibular process: *Meckel's cartilage*, mandible, malleus, incus, sphenomandibular ligament	Muscles of mastication (masseter, temporalis, medial pterygoid, lateral pterygoid), anterior digastric muscle, mylohyoid, tensor veli palatini, tensor tympani
II	VII: Facial	*Reichert's cartilage*, stapes, styloid process of temporal bone, lesser horn and superior body of hyoid bone, stylohyoid ligament	Muscles of facial expression (frontalis, orbicularis oris, orbicularis oculi, zygomaticus, buccinator, platysma), stapedius, stylohyoid, and posterior belly of digastric muscle
III	IX: Glossopharyngeal	Greater horn and inferior body of hyoid bone	Stylopharyngeus muscle
IV and VI	X: Vagus	Laryngeal cartilages: thyroid, cricoid, arytenoid, and others	Cricothyroid, intrinsic muscles of larynx, constrictors of pharynx

NOTE: Structures in *italics* regress during development.

Cartilage Components Arch I, called the *mandibular arch*, is a major contributor to development of the face. This pair of arches has distinct maxillary and mandibular processes, or prominences (Figure 1-21). The processes form mainly from the migration of neural crest cells into the arches during the fourth week. Neural crest mesenchyme in the maxillary process undergoes intramembranous ossification to give rise to the zygomatic bone, the maxilla, and the squamous portion of the temporal bone.

The cartilage of the first arch is Meckel's cartilage (see Figure 1-21 and Figure 1-22). The dorsal end of Meckel's cartilage becomes ossified to form two of the middle ear ossicles—the malleus and incus. The middle portion of Meckel's cartilage regresses, but its perichondrium forms the sphenomandibular ligament. The ventral part of Meckel's cartilage forms a

horseshoe-shaped structure in the shape of the future mandible. The mesenchymal tissue lateral to the cartilage undergoes intramembranous ossification to produce the mandible as the original Meckel's cartilage disappears.

The cartilage of arch II is known as *Reichert's cartilage* (see Figure 1-21). Its dorsal end becomes ossified to produce the other middle ear ossicle, the stapes, and the styloid process of the temporal bone (see Figure 1-22). A portion of the perichondrium of Reichert's cartilage forms the stylohyoid ligament. Pharyngeal arch II is called the *hyoid arch* because of its contribution to development of the hyoid bone, specifically, the lesser horn and the superior portion of the body.

The cartilage of the third arch gives rise to the greater horn and the inferior part of the body of the hyoid bone (see Figure 1-22).

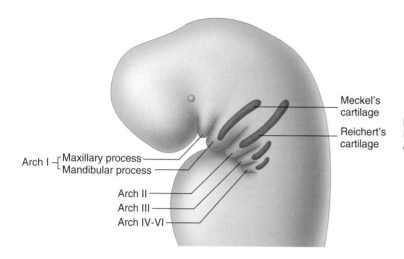

Arch I ⌈Maxillary process
       ⌊Mandibular process
Arch II
Arch III
Arch IV-VI

Meckel's cartilage

Reichert's cartilage

Figure 1-21 Lateral view of the embryo illustrating the cartilage components of the pharyngeal arches. Meckel's cartilage is associated with arch I and Reichert's cartilage with arch II.

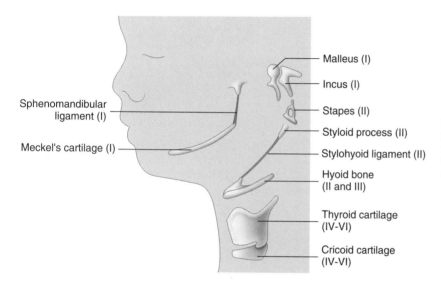

Sphenomandibular ligament (I)

Meckel's cartilage (I)

Malleus (I)
Incus (I)
Stapes (II)
Styloid process (II)
Stylohyoid ligament (II)
Hyoid bone (II and III)
Thyroid cartilage (IV-VI)
Cricoid cartilage (IV-VI)

Figure 1-22 Cartilaginous and skeletal derivatives of the pharyngeal arches. This schematic drawing summarizes the arch of origin of some head and neck structures. (From Sandra A, Coons WJ: *Core concepts in embryology,* Philadelphia, 1997, Lippincott-Raven.)

The cartilages of the fourth and sixth arches fuse to form the laryngeal cartilages, including the thyroid, cricoid, and arytenoid cartilages, but not the epiglottis (see Figure 1-22).

Muscle Components Skeletal muscles of the head and neck are derived from cells that migrate into this region from somitomeres and the most cranial somites (see Figure 1-14).

Arch I: These muscles include the important muscles of mastication: masseter, temporalis, medial pterygoid, and lateral pterygoid (Figure 1-23). Other muscular derivatives are the anterior belly of the digastric, mylohyoid, tensor veli palatini, and tensor tympani.

Arch II: The muscles of facial expression arise from the second arch. The facial muscles are characteristically thin, have their origin and insertion in the skin, and are found throughout the face and neck. Examples include the frontalis, orbicularis oris, orbicularis oculi, zygomaticus, and platysma (see Figure 1-23). Nonfacial muscles from the second arch include the stapedius, stylohyoid muscle, and posterior belly of the digastric muscle.

Arch III: These muscles gives rise to the stylopharyngeus muscle.

Arches IV and VI: These muscles form the muscles of the pharynx and larynx. Arch IV gives rise to the cricothyroid muscle, and arch VI produces the rest of the intrinsic muscles of the larynx.

Arterial Components The pharyngeal arch arteries are called the aortic arches. The arteries from arches I and II are significantly smaller than those from the remaining arches. Arch I contributes to part of the maxillary artery. Arch II gives rise to the hyoid and stapedial arteries. Arch III contributes to part of the carotid system. The left side of arch IV contributes to the arch of the aorta and the right side to the right subclavian artery. Arch VI is associated with the pulmonary arteries.

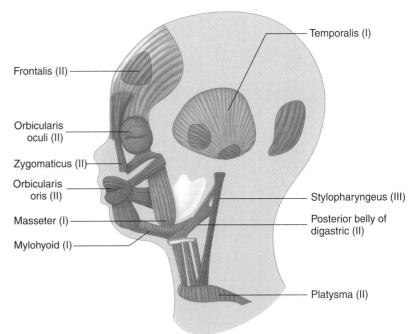

Figure 1-23 Skeletal muscle derivatives of the pharyngeal arches. This drawing summarizes some of the head and neck muscles and their pharyngeal arch of origin. (From Sandra A, Coons WJ: *Core concepts in embryology,* Philadelphia, 1997, Lippincott-Raven.)

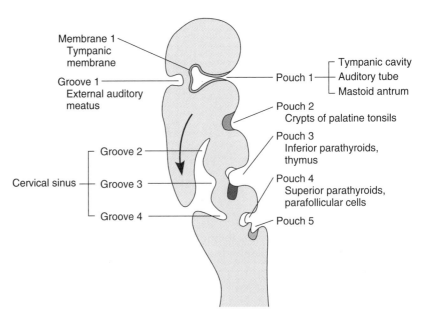

Figure 1-24 Derivatives of pharyngeal pouches, grooves, and membranes shown in anteroposterior longitudinal section. Note that pouch 5 and all grooves and membranes except the first regress.

Derivatives of Pharyngeal Pouches

Pharyngeal pouches represent extensions of the developing pharynx interposed between the inner surface of adjacent pairs of arches. The first pair of pouches is located between arches I and II (Figure 1-24).

Pouch 1 gives rise to the tympanic cavity, the pharyngotympanic tube (auditory or eustachian tube), and the mastoid antrum.

Pouch 2 endoderm forms the lining of the crypts of the palatine tonsils. The lymphoid tissue of the tonsils forms from mesenchyme surrounding the crypts rather than from pouch endoderm.

Pouch 3 has a dorsal part that gives rise to the inferior parathyroid glands and a ventral part that becomes the thymus. The early parathyroid glands and thymus lose their connection with the pharynx and migrate into the neck.

Pouch 4 also has dorsal and ventral portions. The dorsal part gives rise to the superior parathyroid glands, whereas the ventral part produces an ultimobranchial body. The ultimobranchial body fuses with the thyroid gland, and its cells become diffusely scattered throughout the thyroid and differentiate into parafollicular cells (C cells), which produce calcitonin.

Pouch 5 typically regresses.

BOX 1-2	Derivatives of Pharyngeal Pouches, Grooves, and Membranes

Pouch, Groove, Membrane Derivatives

Pouch 1	Tympanic cavity, auditory tube, mastoid antrum
Pouch 2	Crypt lining of palatine tonsils
Pouch 3	Inferior parathyroid glands, thymus
Pouch 4	Superior parathyroid glands, *ultimobranchial body* → parafollicular cells
Groove 1	External auditory meatus
Grooves 2 to 4	*Cervical sinus*
Membrane 1	Tympanic membrane

NOTE: Structures in *italics* regress during development.

Derivatives of Pharyngeal Grooves (Clefts)

The external surface of the head and neck region of an embryo displays four pairs of pharyngeal grooves, or clefts, located between the arches (see Figure 1-24). Groove 1 is located between arches I and II, and it is the only groove to give rise to structures in the adult, namely the external auditory meatus. Mesenchymal tissue of arches II and III proliferates and covers the remaining grooves, forming a temporary, fluid-filled cavity called the *cervical sinus.* Normally the cervical sinus and grooves 2 to 4 are obliterated during development of the neck. The cervical sinus rarely persists after birth. It may have a pathologic connection with the pharynx, called a *pharyngeal sinus,* or to both the pharynx and the outside of the neck, called a *pharyngeal fistula.*

Derivatives of Pharyngeal Membranes A

pharyngeal membrane consists of endoderm lining a pharyngeal pouch, ectoderm lining a pharyngeal groove, and a layer of mesenchyme in between. The first pharyngeal membrane forms the tympanic membrane, whereas the remaining membranes regress. Derivatives of pharyngeal pouches, grooves, and membranes are summarized in Box 1-2.

Development of the Face

Development of the face occurs primarily between weeks 4 and 8, so that by the end of the eighth week the face has taken on a human appearance. Facial development after week 8 occurs slowly and involves changes in facial proportions and relative positions of facial components. The discussion of facial and palatal development in this chapter concentrates on weeks 4 through 12.

Facial development results mainly from enlargement and movement of the **frontonasal prominence** and four prominences from pharyngeal arch I, the

paired **maxillary prominences,** and **mandibular prominences.** These structures surround the stomodeum. The maxillary and mandibular prominences develop as a result of neural crest cells migrating and proliferating into pharyngeal arch I.

One of the first events in formation of facial structures is fusion of the medial ends of the mandibular prominences in the midline to form the chin and lower lip. In the inferior and lateral portion of the frontonasal prominence, bilateral localized areas of surface ectoderm thicken to form **nasal placodes** (Figure 1-25, *A*). The mesenchyme along the periphery of the nasal placodes proliferates and forms horseshoe-shaped ridges called the **medial nasal prominences** and **lateral nasal prominences** (Figure 1-25, *B*). The center of the placode becomes thinner, eventually leading to loss of ectoderm and formation of **nasal pits.** The nasal pits are the precursors of the nostrils and nasal cavities.

Mesenchymal connective tissue in the maxillary prominences proliferates. The result is that the maxillary prominences become larger and move medially toward each other and toward the medial nasal prominences (Figure 1-25, *C*). The medial nasal prominences move toward each other, fuse in the midline, and form the **intermaxillary segment** (Figure 1-25, *D*). The intermaxillary segment is of special importance because it gives rise to the philtrum (middle portion) of the upper lip (Figure 1-25, *E*), four incisor teeth, alveolar bone and gingiva surrounding them, and primary palate.

A number of facial prominences fuse between weeks 7 and 10. The maxillary prominences fuse laterally with the mandibular prominences. The medial nasal prominences fuse with the maxillary prominences and lateral nasal prominences (see Figure 1-25, *C*).

The **nasolacrimal ducts** (originally called the *nasolacrimal grooves*) are bilateral epithelial structures that form at the line of fusion between lateral nasal

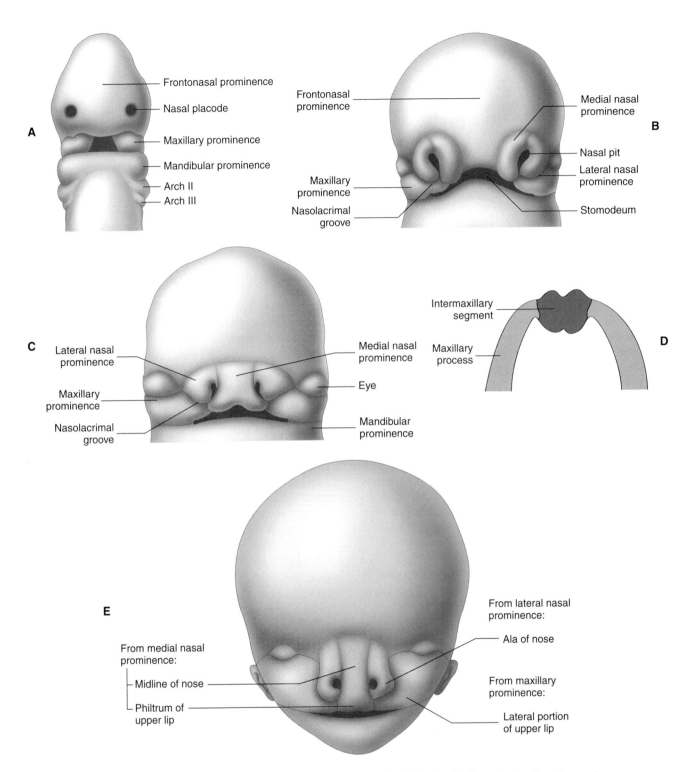

Figure 1-25 Development of the face. **A,** Approximately 4½ weeks. Thickening of surface ectoderm forms the nasal placodes. **B,** Approximately 6 weeks. Proliferation of mesenchyme forms the medial and lateral nasal prominences. The nasal pits develop in the center of the nasal placodes. **C,** Approximately 7 weeks. The maxillary prominences enlarge and push the medial nasal prominences toward each other. Fusion between the maxillary prominences and the medial nasal prominences occurs. The nasolacrimal groove develops at the line of fusion between the lateral nasal prominences and the maxillary prominences. **D,** Intermaxillary segment (occlusal view). The medial nasal prominences move toward each other, fuse in the midline, and form the intermaxillary segment. The intermaxillary segment is the origin of the philtrum of the upper lip, the four maxillary incisor teeth with their surrounding alveolar process, and the primary palate. **E,** Approximately 10 weeks. The entire upper lip is derived from the fused medial nasal prominences and maxillary prominences. The midline of the nose comes from the medial nasal prominence, whereas the ala of the nose is derived from the lateral nasal prominence.

Derivation of Facial Structures—A Summary

1. The maxillary prominences form the lateral portion of the upper lip and most of the maxilla (upper cheek region), including the secondary palate.
2. The frontonasal prominence forms the forehead and the dorsum and bridge of the nose.
3. The medial nasal prominences form the intermaxillary segment (see derivatives above), midline of the nose, and the nasal septum.
4. The lateral nasal prominences give rise to the alae of the nose.
5. The entire upper lip comes from the medial nasal prominences and the maxillary prominences.
6. The external nose comes from the frontonasal prominence, medial nasal prominences, and lateral nasal prominences.
7. The mandibular prominences form the lower lip, chin, and lower cheek region.
8. Mesenchymal connective tissue in the facial prominences give rise to various bones and ligaments in the facial region (discussed elsewhere).
9. As stated earlier, the muscles of mastication and the facial muscles are derived from the first and second pharyngeal arches.

prominences and maxillary prominences. Each nasolacrimal duct eventually connects the lacrimal sac to the nasal cavity.

It should be noted that fusion, or merging, of prominences involves first a breakdown of the surface epithelium at the area of contact. This allows the underlying mesenchymal cells in the two prominences to mingle with one another.[2]

Development of the Palate

The palate begins to develop early in week 6, but the process is not completed until week 12. The most critical period during palatal development is the end of the sixth week to the beginning of the ninth week.[4]

The entire palate develops from two structures—the primary palate (premaxilla) and the secondary palate (Figure 1-26, *A*). The **primary palate** is the triangular-shaped part of the palate anterior to the incisive foramen. The origin of the primary palate is the deep portion of the intermaxillary segment, which arises from the fusion of the two medial nasal prominences (Figure 1-26, *B*). The **secondary palate** gives rise to the hard and soft palate posterior to the incisive foramen. The secondary palate arises from paired **lateral palatine shelves** of the maxilla (see Figure 1-26, *B*). These shelves are comprised initially of mesenchymal connective tissue and are oriented in a superior-inferior plane with the tongue interposed (Figure 1-26, *C*). Later, the lateral palatine shelves become elongated and the tongue becomes relatively smaller and moves inferiorly. This allows the shelves to become oriented horizontally, to

approach one another, and to fuse in the midline (Figure 1-26, *D* and *E*). The median palatine raphe is a clinical remnant of fusion between the palatine shelves, and the incisive foramen is present at the junction of the primary palate and the lateral palatine shelves. The lateral palatine shelves also fuse with the primary palate and the nasal septum. Fusion between the nasal septum and palatine processes proceeds in an anteroposterior direction beginning in the ninth week.[2]

Pathogenesis of Cleft Lip and Cleft Palate

Cleft lip and palate occur when mesenchymal connective tissues from different embryologic structures fail to meet and merge with each other. The common form of cleft lip is a result of failure of fusion of the medial nasal process with the maxillary process. Cleft lip may be unilateral or bilateral and may extend into the alveolar process (see Chapter 2).

Cleft palate is the result of failure of the lateral palatine shelves to fuse with each other, with the nasal septum, or with the primary palate. Cleft lip and cleft palate are distinct and separate congenital abnormalities, but they often occur concomitantly.

Development of the Tongue

The tongue develops from several different sources. The mucosa of the **body of the tongue** or anterior two thirds of the tongue develops from the first pharyngeal arch, whereas the mucosa of the **base of the tongue** or posterior third develops from arch III. The skeletal muscle of the tongue develops from myoblasts that migrate into the tongue from occipital somites.

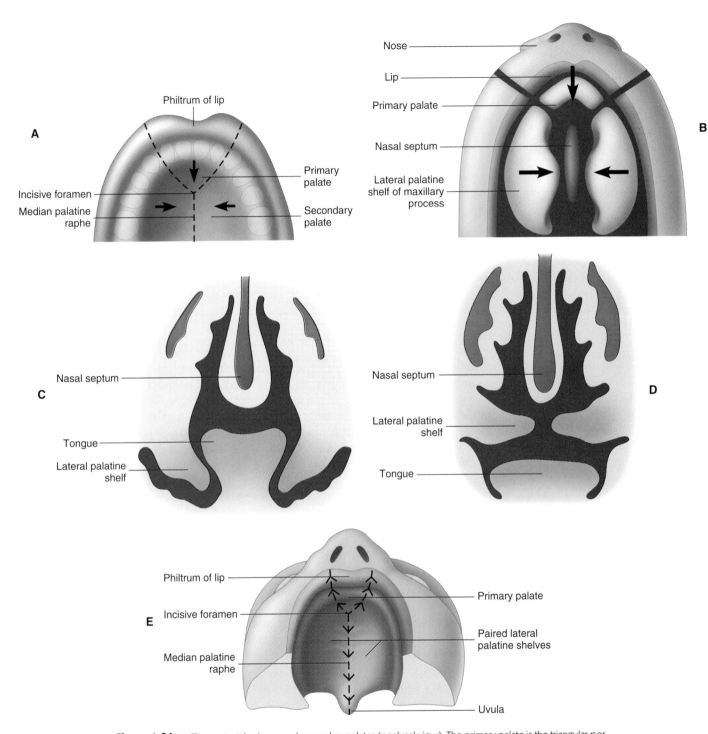

Figure 1-26 **A,** The postnatal primary and secondary palates (occlusal view). The primary palate is the triangular portion anterior to the incisive foramen. The secondary palate gives rise to the hard and soft palates posterior to the incisive foramen. **B,** Development of the palate (occlusal view). The primary palate develops from the deep portion of the intermaxillary segment. The secondary palate arises from paired lateral palatine shelves of the maxilla. **C,** Development of the palate (frontal view) at 6 to 7 weeks. The lateral palatine shelves are initially oriented in a superior-inferior plane with the tongue interposed. **D,** Development of the palate (frontal view) at 7 to 8 weeks. Later the tongue moves inferiorly and the lateral palatine shelves elongate, become oriented horizontally, and fuse in the midline. The lateral palatine shelves also fuse with the primary palate and the nasal septum. **E,** Occlusal view of the palate after fusion of the primary palate with lateral palatine processes. The incisive foramen is located at the junction of the primary and secondary palates. Fusion occurs progressively in the direction of the arrows.

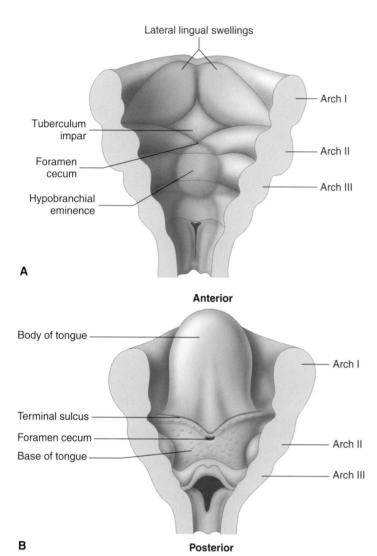

Anterior

B   **Posterior**

Figure 1-27 Development of the tongue. **A,** Anteroposterior longitudinal section at approximately 5 weeks. The mucosa of the anterior two thirds of the tongue (body) develops from the first pharyngeal arch. Two lateral lingual swellings overgrow a midline structure called the *tuberculum impar*. The mucosa of the posterior third (base) develops from the hypobranchial eminence, which is derived from the third pharyngeal arch. The hypobranchial eminence overgrows the second arch and fuses with the lateral lingual swellings and tuberculum impar. The skeletal muscles of the tongue arise from myoblasts that migrate into the tongue from the occipital somites. **B,** Dorsal view at approximately 5 months. The terminal sulcus is the line of demarcation between the body and base of the tongue. The foramen cecum is located in the midline of the terminal sulcus. The innervation of the mucosa of the tongue can be explained by its embryologic development. Cranial nerve V from the first arch innervates the body, and cranial nerve IX from the third arch innervates the base.

The tongue begins its development near the end of the fourth week as a midline enlargement in the floor of the primitive pharynx cranial to the foramen cecum. The enlargement is called the **tuberculum impar** (Figure 1-27, *A*). Two **lateral lingual swellings** form adjacent to the tuberculum impar. All three structures form as a result of proliferation of first arch mesenchyme. The lateral lingual swellings rapidly enlarge, fuse with one another, and overgrow the tuberculum impar. These three structures give rise to the body of the tongue (Figure 1-27, *B*).

The posterior third, or base, of the tongue develops from the **hypobranchial eminence,** which is a midline swelling caudal to the foramen cecum (see Figure 1-27, *A*). The hypobranchial eminence is comprised primarily of mesenchyme from arch III. The **copula** is a midline enlargement derived from arch II. The hypobranchial eminence overgrows the copula and fuses with the tuberculum impar and lateral lingual swellings. The copula disappears without contributing

to formation of the tongue. Thus the base of the tongue is derived from the third pharyngeal arch. The line of demarcation between the body and base is called the **terminal sulcus,** and the foramen cecum is found in the midline of this structure (see Figure 1-27, *B*).[1]

The innervation of the tongue can be explained by its embryologic origin. Sensory innervation to the mucosa of the body of the tongue is almost entirely from the nerve of the first arch, the trigeminal nerve (cranial nerve V). Sensory innervation to the mucosa of the base of the tongue comes mainly from the nerve of the third arch, the glossopharyngeal nerve (cranial nerve IX). The skeletal muscles of the tongue bring their nerve supply with them in the form of the hypoglossal nerve (cranial nerve XII).

Development of the Thyroid Gland

The thyroid gland begins its development as a thickening of endoderm in the midline of the floor of the

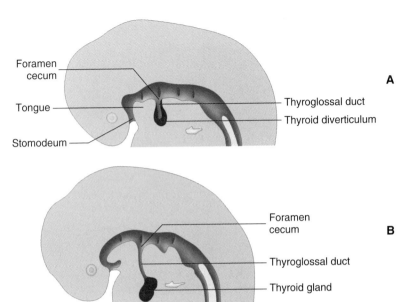

Figure 1-28 A, Development of the thyroid gland. A sagittal view at approximately 5 weeks. The thyroid gland develops close to the foramen cecum as an endodermal thickening and then as a pouch called the *thyroid diverticulum*. The diverticulum migrates ventrally but remains connected with the developing tongue by the thyroglossal duct. **B,** Development of the thyroid gland (sagittal view) at approximately 6 weeks. The thyroid gland reaches its final location in the neck by about the seventh week. The thyroglossal duct degenerates, but the foramen cecum persists on the dorsal surface of the tongue. (From Moore KL, Persaud TVN: *The developing human: clinically oriented embryology,* ed 6, Philadelphia, 1998, WB Saunders.)

primitive pharynx, close to where the tongue will soon develop (Figure 1-28, *A*). The endodermal thickening forms a pouch called the **thyroid diverticulum,** which migrates ventrally in the neck. The **thyroglossal duct** connects the developing and migrating thyroid gland with the developing tongue. By week 7 the thyroid gland has reached its final site in the neck (Figure 1-28, *B*). The thymus, parathyroid glands, and ultimobranchial bodies also migrate to this region. The ultimobranchial bodies become an intrinsic part of the thyroid gland and give rise to parafollicular cells, which produce calcitonin. The thyroglossal duct degenerates, but its proximal opening persists on the dorsum of the tongue as the **foramen cecum.**[1]

A number of pathologic conditions are associated with development of the thyroid gland. Remnants of the thyroglossal duct may persist after birth and give rise to thyroglossal duct cysts, most commonly in the neck. All or part of the developing thyroid may remain in the region of the foramen cecum, enlarge, differentiate, and produce a lingual thyroid.

Development of the Skull

The skull forms from mesenchymal connective tissue around the developing brain. The development of the skull is considered in two components. One is the development of the **neurocranium,** which is the calvaria and base of the skull. It is derived mainly from occipital somites and somitomeres. The other is the development of the **viscerocranium,** which includes the skeleton of the face and associated structures. The

viscerocranium is derived from neural crest ectoderm. Each component has some structures that form by endochondral ossification (cartilaginous component) and other structures that form by intramembranous ossification (membranous component) (Figure 1-29, *A* and *B*).[1]

Neurocranium The **cartilaginous neurocranium (chondrocranium)** consists of several cartilages that fuse and undergo endochondral ossification to give rise to the base of the skull. The cartilage junctions between two bones are called *synchondroses.* New cartilage cells continually form in the center of the synchondrosis, move peripherally, and then undergo endochondral ossification along the lateral margins. The occipital bone is formed first, followed by the body of the sphenoid bone and then the ethmoid bone. Other structures formed by the chondrocranium include the vomer bone of the nasal septum and the petrous and mastoid parts of the temporal bone.[6]

The **membranous neurocranium** gives rise to the flat bones of the calvaria, including the superior portion of the frontal, parietal, and occipital bones.[6] These bones arise by intramembranous ossification occurring in mesenchyme around the brain. Sutures and fontanelles are present during fetal and early neonatal life. **Sutures,** also called *syndesmoses,* are fibrous joints comprised of sheets of dense connective tissue that separate the bones of the calvaria. The sutures help the calvaria to change shape during birth, a process called *molding.* **Fontanelles** are regions of dense connective tissue where sutures come together. Sutures and fontanelles ossify at variable times after birth.

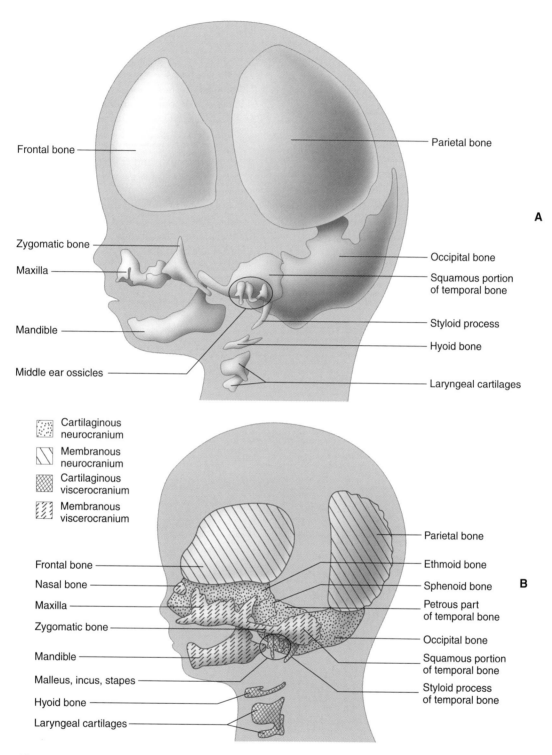

Figure 1-29 Development of the skull. **A,** A lateral view at approximately 12 weeks. The developing skull has two components. The neurocranium includes the calvaria and the base of the skull, and the viscerocranium includes the facial skeleton and associated structures. Each component has some structures that develop by endochondral ossification (cartilaginous) and others that develop by intramembranous ossification (membranous component). **B,** A lateral view at approximately 20 weeks. (**A** From Sandra A, Coons WJ: *Core concepts in embryology*, Philadelphia, 1997, Lippincott-Raven. **B** From Moore KL, Persaud TVN: *The developing human: clinically oriented embryology*, ed 6, Philadelphia, 1998, WB Saunders.)

Viscerocranium The viscerocranium, which includes the facial skeleton, arises from the pharyngeal arches. The earlier discussion in this chapter on cartilage components of the pharyngeal arches includes information about skeletal derivatives of the pharyngeal arches. The **cartilaginous viscerocranium** includes the middle ear ossicles, the styloid process of the temporal bone, the hyoid bone, and the laryngeal cartilages.

The **membranous viscerocranium** includes the maxilla, zygomatic bones, the squamous temporal bones, and the mandible. These bones form by intramembranous ossification except for the mandibular condyle and the midline of the chin. The squamous temporal bones later become part of the neurocranium.

REFERENCES

1. Sadler TW: *Langman's medical embryology,* ed 7, Baltimore, 1995, Williams & Wilkins.
2. Ten Cate AR (ed): *Oral histology: development, structure, and function,* St Louis, 1998, Mosby.
3. Thesleff I: Homeobox genes and growth factors in regulation of craniofacial and tooth morphogenesis, *Acta Odontol Scand* 53:129-134, 1995.
4. Moore KL, Persaud TVN: *The developing human: clinically oriented embryology,* ed 6, Philadelphia, 1998, WB Saunders.
5. Sandra A, Coons WJ: *Core concepts in embryology,* Philadelphia, 1997, Lippincott-Raven.
6. Avery JK: Development of cartilage and bones of the facial skeleton. In Avery JK (ed): *Oral development and histology,* ed 2, New York, 1994, Thieme Medical.

CHAPTER 2

Principles of Cleft Lip and Palate Formation

David C. Johnsen

KEY TERMS

clefting	peg-shaped	opacities	mineralization
supernumerary teeth	hypoplasia	apposition	

For the practicing dentist, lessons can be learned by linking developmental principles with clinical manifestations and treatment needs. The patient with developmental anomalies offers the dentist the chance to dramatically visualize the relationship between development and treatment needs. At times the dentist will be unable to determine the exact developmental infraction. However, the ongoing reference to embryologic development and anatomic systems will enhance recognition and eventually improve treatment. Genetic makeup is outside the scope of this chapter but is a constant consideration.

Common areas where the need for treatment is associated with developmental failure are the lip and the palate. A principle of development is presented followed by clinical examples of developmental failure. Also presented is a small sample of miscellaneous defects, each associated with a developmental failure.

CLEFT LIP AND PALATE

The most common major defect of the lip and palate is the occurrence of **clefting**. Although these two developmental defects are often associated, they are actually distinct. To begin with, the genetic aspects are different for the two processes. To picture various clinical outcomes, it is useful to orient oneself to the incisive foramen and think of a "zipper" effect when anticipating cleft formation. The secondary palate "zips" from the incisive canal posteriorly to complete the closure of the secondary palate. The process can be disturbed at any point from the time of rotation of the palatal shelves to the final closure of the uvula. In some cases the palatal soft tissues may successfully close but not the bony palate; the resulting submucous cleft can cause deficiencies in the palatal muscle attachments and a significant speech impediment. Similarly, the primary palate "zips" anteriorly from the incisive foramen bilaterally in a V configuration. As a result, defects of the primary palate are manifested either as a cleft lip only or as a cleft of the lip and alveolus.

Although schematic drawings of cleft classifications are a useful guide in learning, they are rarely useful in making final, individualized treatment decisions.[1,2] In addition, schematic drawings of clefts rarely represent the actual clinical manifestations. A major difference between clinical reality and the schematics is that the deviations are three dimensional in vivo.[3-5]

The clinical manifestations resulting from the presence of a cleft rarely fit into neat categories from a treatment planning perspective. Every treatment plan requires the skill of a coordinated team from different disciplines. In Figure 2-1 different clefts are illustrated, each needing individualized planning.[6]

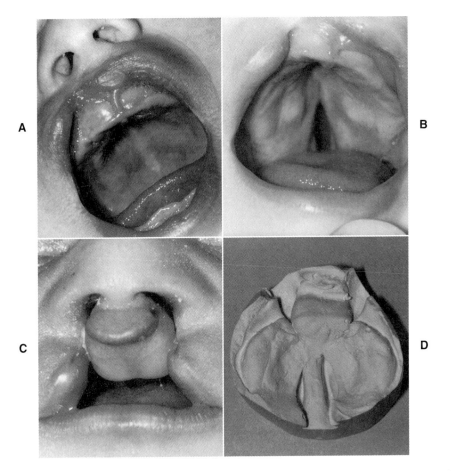

Figure 2-1 A series of infants and children showing variability of clefting along lines of expected embryologic fusion between the median nasal and maxillary processes and between the right and left palatal shelves. In addition to the cleft defect there is also a change in the orientation of the various arch segments. **A,** Infant with unilateral cleft of the lip and an intact dental alveolus and palate. The nose is symmetric compared with some of the subsequent examples. A small notch at the crest of the alveolar ridge is at the site of fusion of the right maxillary and median nasal processes. **B,** Infant with an isolated cleft of the lip and palate. The anterior portions of the palate and dental alveolus are intact. Some deviation of the arch is evident in three dimensions. **C** and **D,** Infant with bilateral cleft of the lip and palate but with portions of the anterior palate intact. The arch has a relatively normal configuration.

Dental Defects in the Lines of Clefting

Children with clefting of the dental alveolus frequently have various dental anomalies,[7-9] but it is important to realize that anomalies also occur along the lines of potential clefting (i.e., in the absence of an actual cleft). Thus the lessons from facial development can be used to better understand dental development. The suggested diagnostic approach adds perspective and awareness in anticipating patient needs.

Anomalies in Number of Teeth The developmental process of tooth initiation is affected by the embryologic defect of clefting.[10] Children with clefts frequently have either a missing or a supernumerary maxillary lateral incisor. The position of the lateral incisor is also unpredictable (i.e., the lateral incisor can be in the premaxillary segment, in the maxillary seg-

ment, in both segments, or completely missing).[11] This phenomenon can be explained by the migration of the initiating cells from near the neural crest to the site of tooth formation. Caution must be taken by the clinician in deciding on the fate of **supernumerary teeth,** particularly in cases with lateral incisors in both the premaxillary and maxillary segments. The decision may be to keep one or both teeth or to extract them.

Tooth shape is also affected in the area of an alveolar cleft. Thus the morphodifferentiation of the tooth could be affected by this embryologic failure. The most common example is the **peg-shaped,** or malformed, maxillary lateral incisor.

As stated previously, the area of the maxillary lateral incisor could also be a site for developmental anomalies in children without clefts. The notion has been advanced that anomalies in the lateral incisor

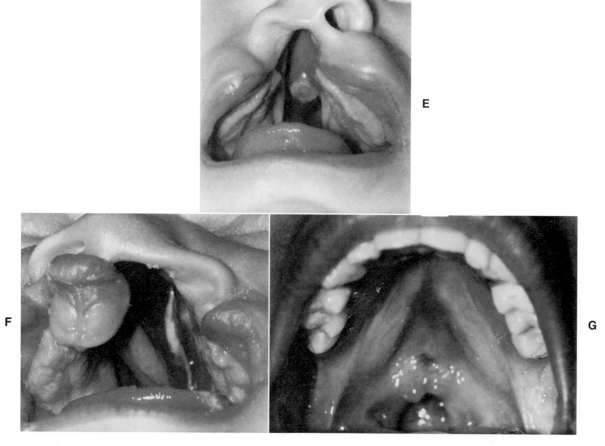

Figure 2-1, cont'd **E,** Infant with unilateral cleft of the lip and palate. In addition to the cleft, the arch is deviated in three dimensions, leaving the buccal segments in a rotated appearance. The nose is asymmetric as a result of the cleft. The nares—the site of fusion of the median nasal and maxillary processes—are affected by the cleft. **F,** Infant with complete bilateral cleft of the lip and palate. In addition to the marked clefting, the buccal segments appear rotated, the premaxilla is rotated upward, and the nasal septum is deviated. The nose is distorted by the presence of the cleft. The orbicularis oris muscle and its movements are limited to respective segments and cannot function coherently. **G,** Incomplete formation and fusion of the horizontal shelves of the hard palate result in a submucous cleft. The condition was detected only when speech difficulties were assessed. Deficiency in the hard palate apparently led to inadequate muscle movement for speech.

(missing supernumerary or malformed) could reflect lesser failures in the joining of the adjacent embryologic components. The frequency of the occurrence of peg-shaped lateral incisors and other anomalies must be viewed in the context of the major embryologic events in the area.[12,13]

Deviations in Tooth Eruption Teeth adjacent to alveolar clefts rarely erupt into good alignment.[14] One reason is related to the shape of the cleft defect. The cleft is larger beneath the mucosa than at the oral surface. This tear drop shape of the defect may not allow the tooth to erupt in its normal position and emerge with its roots upright. Therefore the embryologic defect has an effect on the eruptive phase of tooth development many years later. Moving the roots into

the cleft defect may compromise the viability of the tooth. Therefore it is important to coordinate the timing of alveolar bone grafting of the cleft defect with orthodontic tooth movement. Figure 2-2 illustrates radiographs of different clefts and root alignment without bone grafting and orthodontic treatment.

Emergence of the permanent canine is often at risk in children with alveolar clefting because of its mesial inclination. The canine crown is usually oriented mesially when the tooth begins its eruptive path (i.e., in the direction of the cleft defect), but the tooth cannot readily move into the submucosal cleft space. Therefore before orthodontic alignment of the canine is initiated, it is important to plan and perform the bone grafting of the alveolar defect to ensure proper tooth eruption.

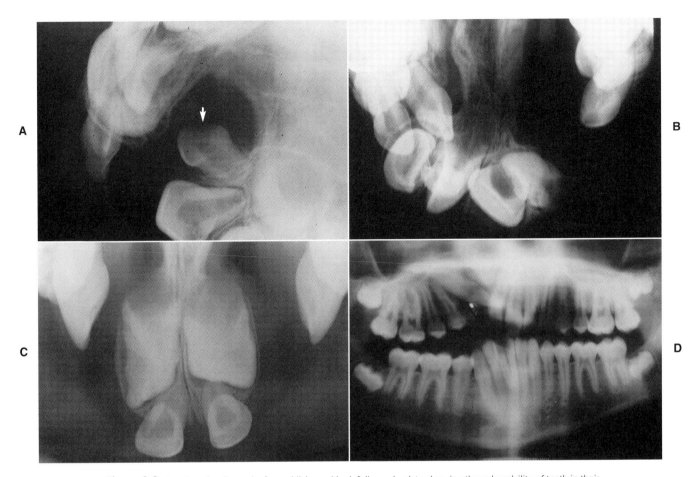

Figure 2-2 A series of radiographs from children with cleft lip and palate showing the vulnerability of teeth in their formation and eruption. The shape of the cleft influences the orientation of the teeth. Eruption and enamel integrity are often compromised. Bone grafting can facilitate the eruption of teeth adjacent to a cleft. Restoration by recontouring the tooth with dental composites can camouflage the tooth defects. **A,** Radiograph showing orientation of teeth to conform to the shape of the cleft. Such an orientation can divert the eruption path of the tooth in any of the three dimensions. Also note the defective enamel on the mesial surface of the lateral incisor adjacent to the cleft (*arrow*). It is also noteworthy that the lateral incisor is in the maxillary segment and not in the premaxillary segment. **B,** Radiograph showing a bilateral cleft of the dental alveolus and palate. Normal alignment of teeth would not be possible in this case without a bone graft. Attempts to align the teeth would result in the roots positioned into the cleft. **C,** Radiograph showing a bilateral cleft of the dental alveolus and palate. Lateral incisor teeth are missing and enamel is distorted. **D,** Radiograph from a child with a unilateral cleft of the lip, dental alveolus, and palate. The eruption path of the maxillary canine is medial to its normal course.

Defects of Enamel Defective enamel (**hypoplasia** and **opacities**) is common in the teeth adjacent to the cleft site.[15] This is an example of the influence of the embryologic defect (the cleft) at another stage of tooth development (**apposition** and **mineralization**) and further demonstrates the close connection between the two processes. Enamel defects occur in persons with untreated clefts of the lip and alveolus but increase in frequency following surgical intervention.

Because there is a higher occurrence of caries in teeth with enamel defects, the issue of prevention is of great importance in cleft children.

There are many lessons to be learned from nature's variability of expression. Some of these lessons help the dentist better understand common clinical problems. For example, the formation of lateral incisors on either side of the cleft supports the migratory idea for tooth-forming cells. Other lessons sharpen the dentist's observations such as the higher frequency of anomalies in the maxillary lateral incisor area.

Although the time for cleft occurrence is in the first few weeks of life, its impact on the subsequent stages of facial and dental development continues for the life of the individual. The child with a cleft often faces considerable social challenges and deserves the most empathetic care from the dentist.[16,17]

The correlation of developmental principles with clinical manifestations can be applied to other kinds of

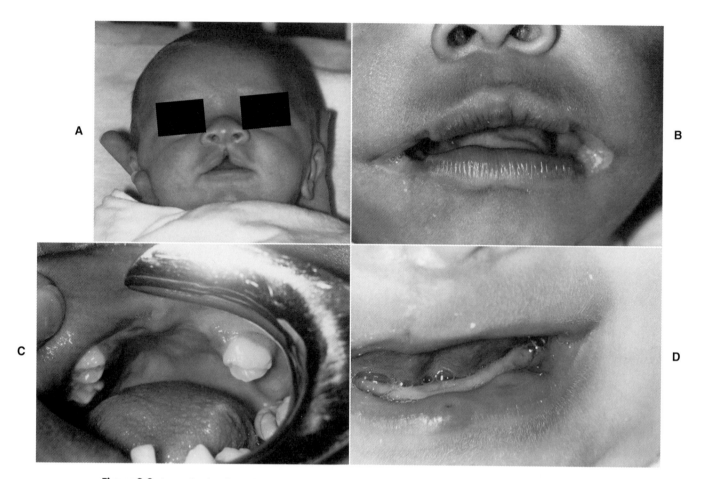

Figure 2-3 A sample of malformations resulting from failure of embryologic components to fuse or to form. **A,** Infant with midline cleft. The cleft is at the site of the midline groove. Midline clefts are less common than clefts from failed fusion of the maxillary and median nasal process. Midline clefts are commonly associated with neurologic deficits as was the case with this infant. **B,** Child with a bilateral horizontal facial cleft. The cleft is along the line of expected fusion between the first branchial (mandibular) arch and the maxilla. **C,** Child with agenesis of the premaxilla. **D,** Child with unilateral cleft of the lip, palate, and lip pits. The presence of lip pits increases the chance of clefting in offspring.

anomalies as illustrated in Figure 2-3.[18] These examples pose distinct problems for the clinician. In all the cases discussed, the clinician can learn much from these children and adults who happen to have a variation from the average physical presentation.

REFERENCES

1. Mortier PB et al: Evaluation of the results of cleft lip and palate surgical treatment: preliminary report, *Cleft Palate Craniofac J* 34(3): 247-253, 1997.
2. Enamark H et al: Lip and nose morphology in patients with unilateral cleft lip and palate from four Scandinavian centres, *Scand J Plast Reconstr Hand Surg* 27(1): 41-47, 1993.
3. Mazaheri M et al: Evaluation of maxillary dental arch form in unilateral clefts of lip, alveolus, and palate from one month to four years, *Cleft Palate Craniofac J* 30(1):90-93, 1993.
4. Mishima K et al: Three-dimensional comparison between the palatal forms in complete unilateral cleft lip and palate with and without Hotz plate from cheiloplasty to palatoplasty, *Cleft Palate Craniofac J* 33(4):312-317, 1996.
5. Honda Y et al: Longitudinal study of the changes of maxillary arch dimensions in Japanese children with cleft lip and/or palate: infancy to 4 years, *Cleft Palate Craniofac J* 32(2):149-155, 1995.
6. McComb HK, Coghlan BA: Primary repair of the unilateral cleft lip nose: completion of a longitudinal study, *Cleft Palate Craniofac J* 33(1):23-31, 1996.
7. Schroeder DC, Green LT: Frequency of dental trait anomalies in cleft, sibling, and noncleft groups, *J Dent Res* 54(4):802-807, 1975.
8. Ranta R: A review of tooth formation in children with cleft lip/palate, *Am J Orthod Dentofacial Orthop* 90(1):11-18, 1986.
9. Olin WH: Dental anomalies in cleft lip and palate patients, *Angle Orthod* 34:119-123, 1964.

10. Kraus BS, Jordan RE, Pruzansky S: Dental anomalies in the deciduous and permanent dentitions of individuals with cleft lip and palate, *J Dent Res* 45:1736-1746, 1966.

11. Tsai T-Z et al: Distribution patterns of primary and permanent dentition in children with unilateral complete cleft lip and palate, *Cleft Palate Craniofac J* 35(2):154-160, 1998.

12. Symons AL, Stritzel F, Stamation J: Anomalies associated with hypodontia of the permanent lateral incisor and second premolar, *J Clin Pediatr Dent* 17(2):109-111, 1993.

13. Neville BW et al: Abnormalities of the teeth. In Neville BW et al (eds): *Oral and maxillofacial pathology,* Philadelphia, 1995, WB Saunders.

14. Peterka M, Tvrdek M, Mullerova Z: Tooth eruption in patients with cleft lip and palate, *Acta Chir Plast* 34:154-158, 1993.

15. Johnsen DC, Dixon M: Dental caries of primary incisors in children with cleft lip and palate, *Cleft Palate Craniofac J* 21(2):104-109, 1984.

16. Pope AW: Points of risk and opportunity for parents of children with craniofacial conditions, *Cleft Palate Craniofac J* 36(1):36-39, 1999.

17. Thomas PT et al: Satisfaction with appearance among subjects affected by a cleft, *Cleft Palate Craniofac J* 34(3):226-231, 1997.

18. Onofre MA, Brosco HB, Taga R: Relationship between lower-lip fistulae and cleft lip and/or palate in Vander Woude syndrome, *Cleft Palate Craniofac J* 34(3):261-265, 1997.

CHAPTER 3

Summary of Human Postnatal Growth

Robert N. Staley

KEY TERMS

neotenous	maturity	general curve	genetically short
growth	old age	genital curve	morphologic age
size change	cross-sectional studies	adolescent spurt	dental age
positional change	longitudinal studies	(prepubertal acceleration	sexual age
proportional change	mixed longitudinal studies	or circumpubertal	skeletal age
functional change	distance curve (cumulative	acceleration)	hypothalamus
maturational change	curve)	average growers	growth hormone
compositional change	velocity curve (incremental	early maturing	(somatotropin)
timing and sequential change	curve)	genetically tall	malnutrition
prenatal growth	lymphoid curve	late maturing	secular trend
postnatal growth	neural curve		

Human growth encompasses physical, mental, psychologic, social, and moral development.[1] This summary focuses on physical growth. Human physical growth is a mind-boggling sequence of events that converts one cell into a vastly complex mature individual.

The growth of human children is studied for two basic reasons: (1) to assess the health and nutrition of children living in a nation and (2) to compare the growth of an individual child with the growth of a large sample of other children in the same population. The first reason is important for the epidemiology of the people of a nation; the second reason is important to health and education professionals and parents who care for growing children. Growth rate may be the best indicator of the physical and psychologic well being of children, a matter of great significance to a nation and its people.[2]

Humans are **neotenous,** or long growing, spending nearly 30% of their entire life span growing. This long

period of time provides for a large impact of environmental influence on the growing biologic system. **Growth** is the interplay between heredity and environment. Growth is increase and change. No simple definition can describe the complexity of growth.

Although most growth is completed at about 20 years of age, many tissues such as hair and nails continue to grow throughout life.

POSTNATAL GROWTH

Postnatal growth is defined as the first 20 years of growth after birth.[1] It is comprised of three periods: infancy, childhood, and adolescence. Infancy is the first postnatal year of life. Childhood is divided into an early phase (1 to 6 years), middle phase (6 to 10 years), and late phase (10 to 15 or 16 years). Puberty occurs in late childhood at about 13 to 14 years in males and 12 to 13 years in females. Adolescence is from 14 to 20 years in males

Different Kinds of Growth That Can Be Identified

1. **Size change:** Changes in size during growth are easily recognized and measured in many ways: weight (mass); height, length, and width (thickness); girth (circumference); area; and volume.
2. **Positional change:** Tissues and organs may migrate from one area to another during growth. Examples are neural crest cell migration, tooth eruption, and dropping of the diaphragm from the level of the fourth cervical vertebra to the level of the twelfth thoracic vertebra.
3. **Proportional change:** Parts of the body change in relationship with one another during growth. The head of an infant is, proportionally to the body, much larger than is the head of an adult.
4. **Functional change:** Tissues and organs undergo changes in functional capabilities during the growth process. The goal of growth is mature function in each tissue and organ.
5. **Maturational change:** Growth of the body as a whole is directed toward the achievement of the period of stability and adulthood.
6. **Compositional change:** Growth involves changes in composition of parts of the body. Eye pigmentation changes and body water content declines from 90% in the fetus to approximately 65% in the adult.
7. **Timing and sequential change:** Growth is continuous from conception to death, but for many reasons growth differs in rate and duration for various parts of the body. Certain phases of growth can be identified:
   a. **Prenatal growth** is characterized by a rapid increase in cell numbers and fast growth rates.
   b. **Postnatal growth** lasts for about the first 20 years of life and is characterized by declining growth rates and increasing maturation of tissues.
   c. **Maturity** is a period of stability during which the body achieves maximal function and growth processes are limited to the maintenance of an equilibrium state between cellular loss and gain.
   d. **Old age** is a period during which functional activity declines and growth processes slow.

and 13 to 20 years in females. These are general guidelines and do not include the extremes of variation, which may occur in postnatal growth.

Growth Study Types

Growth studies are of three basic types: cross-sectional, longitudinal, and mixed longitudinal.[2,3]

Cross-Sectional Studies In **cross-sectional studies** a large number of individuals of different ages are examined on one occasion to develop information on growth attained at a particular age. The method has the advantage of accumulating much information about growth at many ages in a short period of time. The majority of information about growth has been obtained using cross-sectional methods. Cross-sectional studies provide the best data for establishing national standards for growth and for comparing growth in different populations. A random or representative sample of 1000 boys and 1000 girls at each age is needed for construction of national standards. The number of children measured at each age should be proportional to the rate of growth. In the first year, samples should be taken at three intervals, the second year at two intervals, and during adolescence at two intervals each year. Although a mean rate of growth for a population can be estimated from cross-sectional data, nothing

can be learned from this data about the variability around that mean. Health professionals need to compare the rate or velocity of growth of a patient with standards for velocity at the patient's age. Standards for velocity can only be derived from a longitudinal study.

Longitudinal Studies **Longitudinal studies** involve the examination of a group of children repeatedly over a long period during active growth. This method produces the most valuable data for the study of growth rates and the variability of individual growth. However, the drawbacks of this kind of study include small sample size, difficulties in keeping subjects in the study, and long-term data collection. Analysis of the data must follow the period of data collection.

Mixed Longitudinal Studies **Mixed longitudinal studies** are a combination of the cross-sectional and longitudinal types. Subjects at different age levels are seen longitudinally for shorter periods (e.g., 6 years). In a 6-year span, growth can be studied between birth and 6 years for one group, between 5 and 11 years for another group, between 10 and 16 years for another group, and between 15 and 21 years in another group so that growth from birth to 21 years can be studied in 6 years.

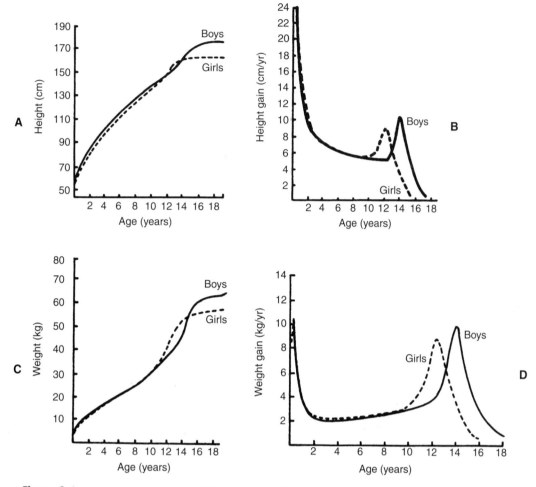

Figure 3-1 Height curves for distance, **(A)**, and velocity, **(B)**, and weight curves for distance, **(C)**, and velocity, **(D)**, for English boys and girls. (Modified from Tanner JM, Whitehouse RH, Takaishi M: *Arch Dis Child* 41:454-471, 1966.)

Graphic Interpretation of Growth Data

Growth data are presented in a graphic format, which reveals the substance of growth study findings in an easily grasped illustration. The two basic curves of growth are as follows:

1. The **distance curve,** or **cumulative curve,** indicates the distance a child has traversed along the growth path (Figure 3-1, *A* and *C*).[4] Data can be derived from cross-sectional and longitudinal studies.

2. The **velocity curve** or **incremental curve** indicates the rate of growth of a child over a period (see Figure 3-1, *B* and *D*). Data are derived from longitudinal studies.

Assessment of Normal Growth

Knowledge of normal human growth is essential to the recognition of abnormal or pathologic growth. Clinicians need norms or standards for height, weight, skeletal, and dental development to assess the normalcy of growth in patients. Growth studies of a representative sample of a population provide the data from which standards are developed. For example, the growth of North American white people should be assessed by standards derived from a representative sample from this population.

Normal height growth is commonly and arbitrarily referred to as the measurements that fall one standard deviation around the mean (Figure 3-2). One standard deviation above and below the mean contains measurements from approximately 68% of the subjects who participated in the growth study. The measurements from the remaining 32% of the subjects fall beyond the normal range. Patients who fall outside the normal range are unusual, but not necessarily abnormal. Standard deviations usefully describe data that fall into a normal distribution such as height and age at menarche. Data for body weight and skinfold thickness do not fall into a normal distribution.[5] Those

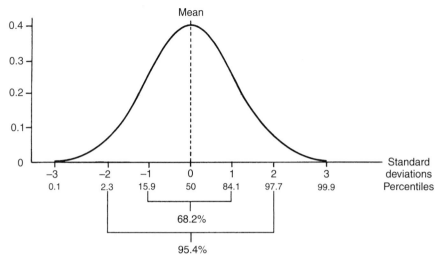

Figure 3-2 Normal distribution curve divided into percentiles and standard deviations. Clinically normal measurements are arbitrarily defined as those falling in the interval between one standard deviation above and below the mean (68.2% of all possible measurements).

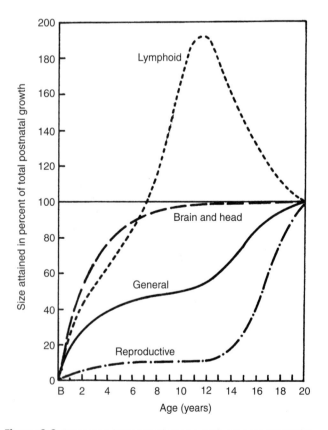

Figure 3-3 Scammon's basic growth curves. Each curve represents the tissue dimensions during postnatal growth as a percent of the adult dimension, which is 100%. (Redrawn from Scammon RE: The measurement of the body in childhood. In Harris JA et al [eds]: *The measurement of man*, Minneapolis, 1930, The University of Minnesota Press.)

kinds of data are best described in terms of percentiles. Height and weight data are usually represented in charts based on percentiles. The normal range of one standard deviation about the mean for a normal distribution falls between the 16th and 84th percentiles (see Figure 3-2).

Variation in Systemic Growth

Richard Scammon[6,7] reduced the growth curves of the tissues of the body to four basic curves. The curves cover the postnatal period of 20 years and assume that during that span of time adult dimensions have been achieved and have 100% of their value, starting at birth with 0%. For each year, each curve has a certain percentage of its adult value. He proposed four curves (from top to bottom): lymphoid, neural, general, and genital (Figure 3-3).

The **lymphoid curve** includes the thymus, pharyngeal and tonsillar adenoids, lymph nodes, and intestinal lymphatic masses. These tissues rise to a high point of nearly 200% between 10 and 15 years of age. The reduction from 200% to 100% is mainly achieved by involution of the thymus, which reverts to connective tissue.

The **neural curve** includes the brain, spinal cord, optic apparatus, and related bony parts of the skull, upper face, and vertebral column. The curve rises strongly during childhood. At the age of 8 years, the brain is nearly 95% of its adult size. Growth in size is accompanied by growth in internal structure, enabling the 8-year-old child to function mentally at nearly the same level as an adult.

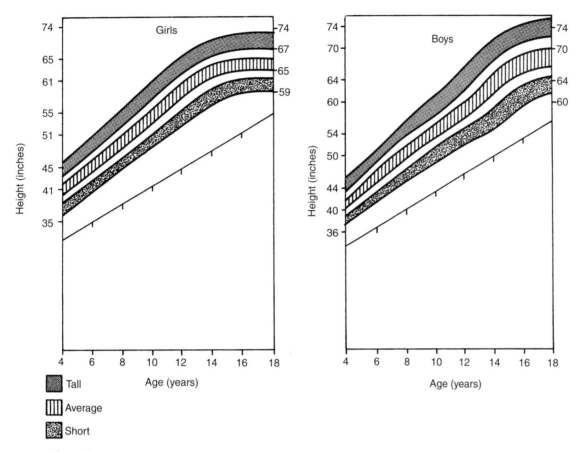

Figure 3-4 Growth curves for height of boys and girls. (Modified from Meredith HV, Knott VB: *Height-weight interpretation folder for boys and girls,* Chicago, 1967, Joint Committee on Health Problems in Education of the National Education Association and the American Medical Association.)

The **general curve** includes external dimensions of the body, respiratory and digestive organs, kidneys, aorta and pulmonary trunks, spleen, musculature, skeleton, and blood volume. This curve rises steadily from birth to 5 years of age and then reaches a plateau from 5 to 10 years, followed by another upsweep during adolescence and finally a slowdown in adulthood.

The **genital curve** includes the primary sex apparatus and all secondary sex traits. The curve has a small upturn in the first year of life and then is quiescent until after 10 years of age, at which time growth of these tissues increases during the time of puberty.

Growth in Height When a chart showing height for age is constructed from data taken from a large number of children, a wide spread of measurements is seen for each age.[8] Notice the increasing variability in height measurements with increasing age (Figure 3-4). The curve shown is a distance curve. Curves of males and females differ and are used separately in clinical applications. A child who falls beyond the average measurements for his or her age is not necessarily abnormal. Parental heights are important factors in determining the potential for height growth because

height is considered to be of polygenic inheritance. When the distance curves of boys and girls are compared, the girls' curve crosses the boys' curve at about 10 years of age, the beginning of the pubertal growth spurt, which occurs earlier in girls. From 10 to 13 years of age the girls are, on average, taller than the boys. At age 14 the boys overtake the girls in height (see Figure 3-1, *A*).[4]

When increments of growth are plotted on a chart to form a velocity curve the rate of growth is seen to decrease from birth to adolescence at which time a marked spurt in height growth is seen in both sexes at puberty. This is known as the **adolescent spurt,** the **prepubertal acceleration,** or the **circumpubertal acceleration.** The earlier onset of the spurt in females is illustrated in Figure 3-1, *B*.[4] The spurt begins at about age 10½ to 11 years in girls and at age 12½ to 13 years in boys. The spurt lasts for about 2 to 2½ years in both sexes. During the spurt boys grow about 8 inches in height, whereas girls grow about 6 inches. In girls, menarche always follows the peak velocity of the adolescent spurt in height.[9] The conclusion of the spurt is followed by rapid slowing of growth, girls reaching 98% of their final height by 16½ years and boys reach the same stage at 17¾ years. One reason the females are shorter on average than males is that they grow for a shorter period of time than males during postnatal growth.

When longitudinal measurements taken from several children are combined on the same velocity graph and averaged, the adolescent spurt is smoothed out and less dramatic. This happens because the spurt occurs at different ages in the children. When the peak velocity for each child is superimposed on the peak velocities of other children, the spectacular nature of the spurt and the variability in spurt onset, magnitude, duration, and cessation can be usefully described.[10]

Some children show a mild growth spurt in height at 6 or 7 years of age. Although growth in height stops at about 18 years in females and 20 years in males, there is evidence that height may slightly increase up to 30 years of age because of growth of the vertebral column. Loss of height begins at middle age and is caused by degeneration of intervertebral disks and to thinning of joint cartilages in the lower limbs.

On the basis of longitudinal data, it is possible to obtain a reasonably accurate prediction of adult height

Six Types of Height Growth in Children[11]

1. **Average growers** follow the middle range of the distance curve and comprise about ⅔ of all children.
2. **Early maturing** children are taller in childhood because they have matured faster than average. They are usually not particularly tall as adults.
3. **Genetically tall** children are taller than average children and will be tall as adults.
4. **Late maturing** children are shorter than average in childhood because of their late maturing and will eventually be adults of average stature.
5. **Genetically short** children are short as children and will be short adults.
6. The sixth group of children is made up of the children who start puberty either early or late and, subsequently, have either much less or much more growth in height than expected. Those children who enter puberty early finish growing much earlier than those entering puberty at a late age.

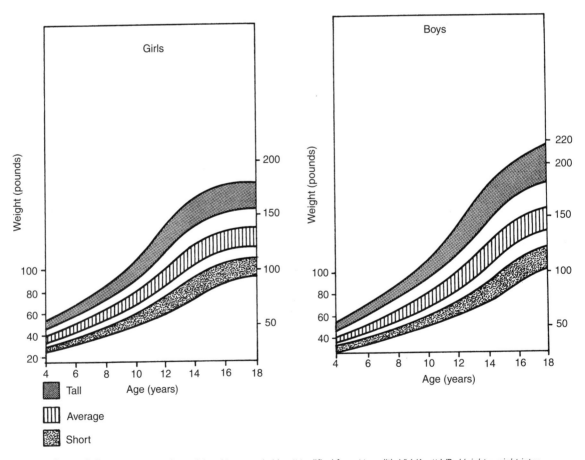

Figure 3-5 Growth curves for weight of boys and girls. (Modified from Meredith HV, Knott VB: *Height-weight interpretation folder for boys and girls,* Chicago, 1967, Joint Committee on Health Problems in Education of the National Education Association and the American Medical Association.)

beginning at 1 year of age for average growing children.[12] The prediction methods vary for males and females. From age 3 years to the adolescent spurt, the predictions are most reliable.

Growth in Weight

In comparison to height, there is much more variation in weight measurements (Figure 3-5).[8] With height, only three components are measured: the bones, cartilage, and skin. However, with weight, every tissue in the body is involved. The distance curves for height and weight illustrate this difference (see Figures 3-4 and 3-5).

Weight at birth is more variable than length. At birth, full-term females are on the average about 5 oz lighter than full-term males. Small mothers have small babies. Later children in a family are usually heavier than the first born. Weight gain is rapid during the first 2 years of postnatal growth. This is followed by a period of steady increase until the adolescent spurt. At ages 11 to 13 years of age, girls are, on average, heavier than boys. Following their adolescent spurt, boys become heavier (see Figure 3-1, C).[4] The velocity of weight growth decreases from birth to about 2 years of age after which it slowly accelerates until the onset of the adolescent spurt (see Figure 3-1, D).[4] During the spurt, boys may add 45 pounds and girls 35 pounds to their weight. The average age for the adolescent weight spurt in girls is 12 years and in boys is 14 years. The spurt is of less magnitude in girls compared with boys (see Figure 3-1, D).[4] The peak velocity for the weight spurt lags behind the peak velocity for height on an average of 3 months. The adolescent first becomes taller and then begins to fill out in weight. Similarly, body weight does not reach its adult value until after adult height has been attained.

Indices of Maturity

Several methods are used to assess the level of maturity attained by a child during postnatal growth.[2,10] Children of the same age vary in their maturity status a great deal, therefore, several biologic maturity indicators have been developed to assess the progress toward full maturation of an individual at various times during growth (Box 3-1). The dental age maturity indicator based on tooth crown and root calcification has an advantage over the maturity indicator based on eruption age because it is useful throughout the development of the teeth, not just during the narrow period covered by eruption.[13]

Maturity indicators differ for the sexes, females maturing earlier than males throughout postnatal growth.

Body Build and Proportions

A continual change in body proportions is seen during postnatal growth. Figure 3-7 shows some of the major changes that include shrinking proportions for the head and increasing proportions for the lower limbs.[7] Volume changes for the head and neck go from 30% of the total body at birth to 10% in the adult. The lower limb volume is 15% of the total body volume at birth compared with 30% of the total body volume in the adult. The trunk increases from 45% to 50%, and the upper limbs show no change in volume as a proportion of total body volume. These changes in proportions are related to the varying rates and duration of growth of the component parts of the body.

The center of gravity is higher in children than in adults, which makes children top heavy. At all ages the head is in advance of the trunk and the trunk is in advance of the limbs regarding maturity. The more peripheral parts of the limbs are in advance of the more

---

BOX 3-1 | **Biologic Maturity Indicators**

1. **Morphologic age** is based on height. A child's height can be compared with those of his same age group and other age groups to determine where he stands in relation to others. Height, or morphologic age, is useful as a maturity indicator from late infancy to early adulthood.
2. **Dental age** has been based on two different methods of assessment. The most commonly used method is the observation of age at eruption of the primary and permanent teeth. This might be called *tooth eruption age.* The second method involves rating of tooth development from crown calcification to root completion using x-rays of the unerupted and developing teeth.[13] Dental age maturity indicators are useful from birth to early adolescence (Figure 3-6).
3. **Sexual age** refers to the development of secondary sex characteristics, breast development, and menarche in females; penis and testis growth in males; and axillary and pubic hair development in both sexes. This type of indicator is useful only for adolescent growth.
4. **Skeletal age** is determined by assessing the development of bones in the hand and wrist. The development of bones from the appearance of calcification centers to epiphyseal plate closure occurs in the hand and wrist throughout the entire postnatal growth period and therefore provides a useful means for assessing biologic maturity. A total of 51 separate centers of bone growth are located in the hand and wrist. An atlas of hand-wrist development has been developed, which is useful in rating the maturity status of an individual child.[14]

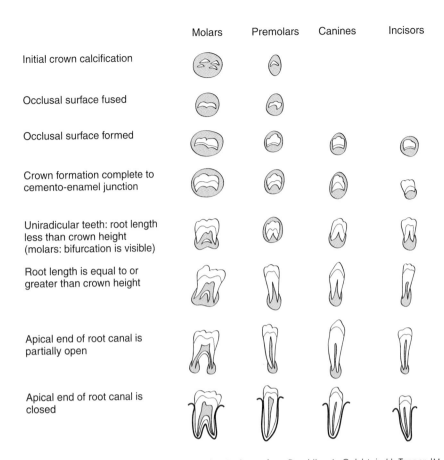

	Molars	Premolars	Canines	Incisors
Initial crown calcification				
Occlusal surface fused				
Occlusal surface formed				
Crown formation complete to cemento-enamel junction				
Uniradicular teeth: root length less than crown height (molars: bifurcation is visible)				
Root length is equal to or greater than crown height				
Apical end of root canal is partially open				
Apical end of root canal is closed				

Figure 3-6 Developmental stages of permanent teeth. (Redrawn from Demirjian A, Goldstein H, Tanner JM: *Human Biol* 45:211-227, 1973.)

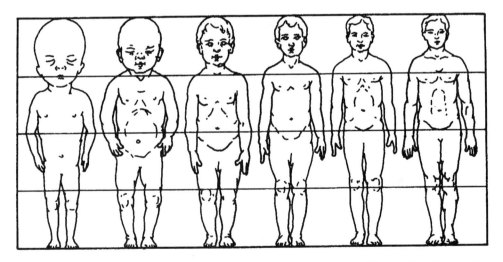

Figure 3-7 Changes in body proportions during growth (Redrawn from Robbins WJ et al: *Growth*, New Haven, Conn, 1928, Yale University Press.)

central parts. There is a transient stage during adolescence when the hands and feet are large and ungainly relative to the rest of the body. The foot stops growing early, before most other parts of the skeleton. In the later stages of adolescence, laterality overtakes linearity in growth.

In adolescence, male shoulders grow more than the pelvis, and the reverse occurs in females. Deposition of fat in the female body produces considerable alterations in body shape. In general, male and female differences are exaggerated in adolescence.[10]

TABLE 3-1	Body Composition Changes with Age (Percent of Total)		
Structure	Fetus	Newborn	Adult
Skin and fat	16%	26%	25%
Viscera	16%	16%	11%
Nervous system	21%	15%	3%
Muscle	25%	25%	43%
Skeleton	22%	18%	18%

From Krogman WM: *Child growth,* Ann Arbor, Mich, 1972, The University of Michigan Press.

Body Composition

In a breakdown that may be overly simple, it is possible to say that there are five major structural components of the human body: (1) skin and superficial fat, (2) viscera, heart included, (3) the central and peripheral nervous system, (4) muscle, and (5) bone. Changes in the proportional amounts of these five components occur during postnatal growth (Table 3-1).[1] Skin and fat, as a percent of total body composition, change little from birth to adulthood (26% to 25%). Viscera decreases slightly from 16% at birth to 11% in adulthood. The nervous tissues decrease markedly from 15% at birth to 3% in adulthood. Muscle tissue almost doubles from 25% at birth to 43% in adulthood. The skeleton does not change as a percent of total body composition from birth to adulthood (18%).

In regard to more elemental components, during postnatal growth there is a 17% decrease in total body water; protein and fat both increase by about 40%, and minerals increase by nearly 250%. The decrease in total body water is more marked in females who experience a decrease from 77% at birth to 54% at 18 years of age. Total body water in males decreases from 77% at birth to 65% at age 18.

Physiologic Changes

Many physiologic changes occur during postnatal growth, many of which show male-female differences.[10] The resting heart rate slows down from about 100 beats per minute at age 2 years to the adult value of 65 to 70 beats per minute. This agrees with the general biologic rule that the heart rate is inversely related to body size. Resting mouth temperature falls in females a degree or more from infancy to maturity, whereas in males the drop continues another half degree.

Some physiologic functions mature much earlier than others. The filtration rate of the glomeruli of the kidney reaches its adult value by age 2 to 3 years, but blood pressure rises throughout postnatal growth and the whole of life. Systolic pressure is about 80 mm Hg at age 5 and rises to the adult value of 120 mm Hg. Girls show a pubertal spurt in systolic blood pressure, which occurs earlier than the corresponding spurt in the male.

Heat production decreases during postnatal growth, with females experiencing a greater decrease in heat production than males. Differences are seen between the sexes in the increase in muscle strength during adolescence.

Sexual Development

At adolescence, a number of changes occur in the development of the primary and secondary sex apparatus. The earliest sign of male puberty is the growth of the testicles. In response to hormone production of the testes, the other parts of the sex apparatus begin their adolescent development. In the females, growth of the ovaries precedes growth of the rest of the sex apparatus. Menarche occurs after the peak velocity in height growth.

FACTORS INFLUENCING GROWTH AND MATURATION

Genetic Factors

The basic control of growth, both in magnitude and timing, is located in the genes.[1,2] The potential for growth is genetic. The actual outcome of growth depends on the interaction between the genetic potential and environmental influences.

Studies of twins have shown that body size, body shape, deposition of fat, and patterns of growth are all more under genetic control than under environmental control. Heredity controls both the end result and rate of progress toward the end result. The hand-wrist, dental, sexual, and other biologic ages of identical twins are similar, whereas the maturity indicators for nonidentical twins may differ considerably. Genetic factors most likely play a leading role in male-female growth differences. The marked advancement of girls over boys in the rate of maturation is attributed to the delaying action of the Y chromosome in males. By delaying growth, the Y chromosome allows males to grow over a longer period of time than females, therefore making possible greater overall growth. Individuals with the chromosome pattern XXY (Klinefelter's syndrome) are long legged and have a growth pattern similar to males even with the presence of two X chromosomes. Individuals with Turner's syndrome, having only one X chromosome, develop with a female pattern of growth becoming more like a female at adulthood. Individuals with an XYY chromosome constitution are very tall (6 feet or more), which lends support to the hypothesis that the Y chromosome has a delaying effect on growth.

Neural Control

It is thought that a growth center exists in the region of the **hypothalamus,** which keeps children on their genetically determined growth curves. Although the correlation between birth size and adult size is low, by the age of 2 the correlation becomes reasonably high. The interpretation of this fact is that during the first 2 years of postnatal growth, the neural control system has got the child on its predetermined genetic curve. At birth, body size is limited to accommodate the birth process. After birth, those children destined to become large experience a burst of growth activity, which levels off during the first 2 years. Not all children experience this burst of early growth, thus some mechanism is obviously operating to make these early changes. The hypothalamus is located above the pituitary gland, and it is thought that the hypothalamus sends messages to the pituitary gland through an elaborate feedback system.

There is also evidence that the peripheral nervous system plays a part in growth control. If a somatic muscle is denervated, it atrophies. It is suggested that peripheral nerve fibers exert a nutritive or trophic effect on the structures they innervate.

Hormonal Control

Probably all of the endocrine glands influence growth.[1,10] The anterior lobe of the pituitary gland produces a protein called **growth hormone,** or **somatotropin.** This can be detected at the end of the second fetal month, soon after the pituitary has formed. It is thought that the growth hormone, although not essential for fetal growth, is essential to growth from birth onward. Growth hormone maintains the normal rate of protein synthesis and appears to inhibit the synthesis of fat and the oxidation of carbohydrate. It is necessary for the proliferation of cartilage cells thus it has a great effect on bone growth and, consequently, height growth. Its growth functions become ineffective when the epiphyses close, but it probably maintains its effects on protein synthesis throughout life. Production of growth hormone is thought to be controlled by the hypothalamus. An excess of growth hormone produces a pituitary giant, and a deficiency of the hormone produces a pituitary dwarf. Human growth hormone is used in the treatment of pituitary dwarfism.

A complicated interaction exists between growth hormone and insulin. Insulin is important in protein synthesis, and growth hormone is incapable of causing the formation of normal amounts of ribonucleic acid without the help of insulin. Other evidence suggests that, in diabetes, excess production of growth hormone may depress insulin production. There may be an antagonism between the production of growth hormone and production of cortisone by the cortex of the suprarenal glands. Growth hormone is produced in a daily rhythmic secretion, the amount varying inversely with cortisone secretion. The peak of daily secretion of growth hormone is in the early stages of sleep.

The anterior lobe of the pituitary gland also secretes thyrotrophic hormone, which affects growth by stimulating the thyroid gland to secrete. The hormones of the thyroid gland, thyroxine and triiodothyronine, both stimulate general metabolism and are important in growth of the bones, teeth, and brain. Iodine deficiency reduces the production of these hormones. Deficiency in childhood of the thyroid hormones produces a mentally retarded dwarf. Thyroid secretion decreases from birth to adolescence and then increases for the duration of the adolescent spurt.

It is agreed that the pituitary and thyroid hormones play little direct role in growth during the adolescent spurt. The changes seen at adolescence are caused by the secretion of androgens and gonadal hormones. Androgens are produced by the suprarenal cortex, which is controlled by the adrenocorticotrophic hormone (ACTH) produced by the pituitary gland. No change in the amount of the ACTH occurs during adolescence, thus it is thought that perhaps an inhibiting mechanism to androgen production is removed at adolescence to permit secretion of the androgens. The androgens play a major role during adolescent growth in both sexes.

The gonadotrophic hormone of the pituitary gland stimulates production of testosterone in males and estrogen and progesterone in females. Testosterone and the adrenal androgens both stimulate growth of muscle, bone, blood red cells, and secondary sex characteristics in males. Ovarian secretions have less general affects on growth, and in females the androgen production from the adrenal gland is primarily responsible for growth at adolescence. The ovarian secretions do control secondary sex changes, including alterations in body shape.

The parathyroid secretions, parathormone and calcitonin, control the amount of calcium in the blood and its interchange with calcium in the bone. The two hormones are mutually antagonistic. They affect bone growth.

The timing sequence of maturation is undoubtedly under hormonal control. Bone and dental growth from birth to the adolescent spurt are under thyroid control. At adolescence, bones fall under increasing influence of the gonadal hormones.

Nutrition

Sufficient intake of nutritious food is essential for normal growth.[1,2] **Malnutrition** involves deficiency in calories and required food elements. Rats fed on a calorie-deficient diet, otherwise satisfactory, ceased to grow. When adequate calories are added to the diet, they begin to grow again. This kind of adjustment of the body to varying dietary sufficiency also occurs in humans. Undernutrition tends to accentuate the normal differential growth of the body tissues. Growth of teeth takes precedence over bone growth, and bones grow better than soft tissues such as muscle and fat. Starvation alters the composition of the body. In starvation, protein in the body is not accumulated but becomes consumed so that the cell mass of the body is reduced. Fat is consumed and depleted. Extracellular body fluid is increased. Loss of weight is thereby masked by famine edema.

A sufficient diet includes an adequate supply of protein. Nine amino acids are essential for growth. Absence of any one results in disordered growth. Calcium, phosphorus, magnesium, manganese, and fluorides are essential for proper bone and tooth growth. Iron is needed for hemoglobin production. Vitamins are also essential for normal growth. Vitamin A controls activities of both osteoblasts and osteoclasts. Defects in bone growth occur with vitamin A deficiency. Vitamin B2 has considerable influence on growth. Vitamin C is necessary for proper bone and connective tissue growth. Vitamin D is required for normal bone growth. Oxygen is also a necessary component of normal growth. Children born with congenital cardiac defects may show stunting and retardation of growth, which is often reversed by surgical repair.

Secular Trend

There is considerable evidence that children today are growing faster than they grew in the past.[1,2] Figures from England indicate that the height of 16-year-old boys increased by more than ½ inch every 10 years from 1873 to 1943. Secular change in the height of North American boys between 1880 and 1960 is shown in Figure 3-8. Boys at 15 years of age were 5 inches taller in 1960 than their counterparts in 1880. A similar trend has been seen in younger children. Between 1880 and 1950 the average height of American and West European children increased

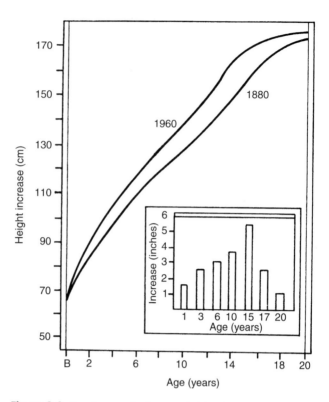

Figure 3-8 Growth curves for the mean height of North American white boys in 1880 and 1960. (Redrawn from Meredith HV: Changes in the stature and body weight of North American boys during the last 80 years. In Lipsitt LP, Spiker CC [eds]: *Advances in child development and behavior*, New York, 1963, Academic Press.)

by more than ½ inch each ten years for a total of 4 inches. The trend is probably the result of both more food and better balanced diets. Other benefits such as decreased illness and improved health care have also contributed to **secular trend.**

Although children are growing at a faster rate, they are also stopping growth sooner. The adolescent height spurt is earlier now, but not more accentuated today than in the past. Early in the 20th century men reached their final height at 25 years of age. Now final height is reached at about 20 years of age. Secular change has been more marked in children than in total adult height. Adults are getting larger but less dramatically than children. An interesting feature of the secular trend is the progressive advancement in the timing of menarche. This change may be related to better nutrition. Finally, there is evidence that the secular trend in height and weight has hit a plateau in the United States during the past 30 years.[2]

Season and Circadian Rhythm

Growth in height is faster in the spring than in the autumn.[15] On the contrary, weight growth proceeds faster in the autumn than in the spring. There is evidence that growth in height and eruption of teeth is greater at night than in the daytime. The reason for these differences is probably related to fluctuations in hormone release.

Disease

The effects of disease are similar to those of malnutrition.[15] After an illness, a catch up growth period usually brings the child back to the predetermined growth curve. Females compensate better than males, following illness. Diseases that slow growth probably have the effect of reducing growth hormone production as a result of increased production of cortisone during the disease. Cartilage cell growth is stopped temporarily and the result is seen on x-rays as a line of arrested growth. Similar lines can be found in the teeth.

Cultural Factors

Cultural factors have various effects on growth. For example, a secular trend increase in height occurred in Japan between males born in 1900 and those born near the middle of the 20th century. However, males of Japanese heritage born near the middle of the century in the United States grew taller on average than both groups born in Japan because of different cultural influences.[16] Evidence that psychologic abuse can adversely affect growth was discovered accidentally in 1948 by a physician who studied height and weight gain for 1 year in children at two German orphanages. The children in an orphanage governed by a harsh headmistress grew less in height and weight than the children in another orphanage, even after they were given additional food equal to 20% more calories than the other orphanage.[17]

Orthodontic treatment represents a cultural influence on the growth and development of the dentition and face. The most effective time for orthodontic treatment is during the period of postnatal growth, when alteration of the developing dentition and surrounding facial structures can be accomplished in conjunction with growth.

REFERENCES

1. Krogman WM: *Child growth,* Ann Arbor, Mich, 1972, The University of Michigan Press.
2. Eveleth PB, Tanner JM: *World wide variation in human growth,* ed 2, Cambridge, Mass, 1990, Cambridge University Press.
3. Malina RM: *Growth and development: the first twenty years,* Minneapolis, 1975, Burgess Publishing.
4. Tanner JM, Whitehouse RH, Takaishi M: Standards from birth to maturity for height, weight, height velocity and weight velocity in British children, *Arch Dis Child* 41:454-471, 1966.
5. Cederquist R: General body growth and development. In Enlow DH (ed): *Facial growth,* ed 3, Philadelphia, 1990, WB Saunders.
6. Scammon RE: The measurement of the body in childhood. In Harris JA et al (eds): *The measurement of man,* Minneapolis, 1930, The University of Minnesota Press.
7. Scammon RE: Developmental anatomy. In Schaeffer JP (ed): *Morris' human anatomy,* ed 11, New York, 1953, Blakiston.
8. Meredith HV, Knott VB: *Height-weight interpretation folder for boys and girls,* Chicago, 1967, Joint Committee on Health Problems in Education of the National Education Association and the American Medical Association.
9. Simmons K, Greulich WW: Menarcheal age and the height, weight, and skeletal age of girls age 7 to 17 years, *J Pediatr* 22:518-548, 1943.
10. Tanner JM: Growth at adolescence, ed 2, Oxford, 1962, Blackwell Scientific.
11. Roche AF: Predictions. In Johnston FE, Roche AF, Susanne C (eds): *Human physical growth and maturation: methodologies and factors,* New York, 1980, Plenum Press.
12. Bayley N: Growth curves of height and weight for boys and girls, scaled according to physical maturity, *J Pediatr* 48:187-194, 1956.
13. Demirjian A, Goldstein H, Tanner JM: A new system of dental age assessment, *Hum Biol* 45:211-227, 1973.
14. Greulich WW, Pyle LI: *Radiographic atlas of skeletal development of the hand and wrist,* Stanford, Calif, 1959, Stanford University Press.
15. Sinclair D: *Human growth after birth,* London, 1969, Oxford University Press.
16. Greulich WW: A comparison of the physical growth and development of American-born and native Japanese children, *Am J Phys Anthropol* 15:489-515, 1957.
17. Widdowson EM: Mental contentment and physical growth, *Lancet* 260(1):1316-1318, 1951.

CHAPTER 4

Introduction to the Growth of the Face

Samir E. Bishara and Donald Ferguson

KEY TERMS

growth	intramembranous bone	secondary translation	spheno-occipital
development	formation	synchondrosis	synchondrosis
maturation	endochondral ossification	craniofacial sutures	mandibular condyles
chondrogenesis	remodeling	cranial base synchondrosis	nasal septum
endochondral bone formation	primary translation		

Studying the normal changes that occur in the facial complex helps the clinician identify and diagnose any existing abnormalities with the purpose of providing optimal treatment to the patient. It is, therefore, essential for clinicians to be aware of how the face changes, where these changes occur, and when these changes usually take place. Such knowledge enables the practitioner to modify the growth processes to meet the needs of those patients who seek treatment for various malocclusions.

Astute clinicians are interested in both the immediate outcome of treatment as well as the long-term stability and benefits of the treatment rendered because the changes in the face and dentition continue throughout life. At certain stages of development these changes are drastic and easily observable,[1] whereas at other times the changes are more subtle but equally significant.[2] For example, when normal individuals were followed between 25 and 45 years of age, significant changes in the dentofacial complex were found. These changes included a greater prominence of the nose and an increase in maxillary and mandibular tooth size–arch length discrepancies expressed as crowding and averaging 2.0 mm in both males and females.[2]

The terms *growth, development,* and *maturation* are often used interchangeably to describe the changes

that occur throughout life. According to *Webster's Dictionary,* **growth** is defined as size development, progressive development (i.e., evolution, emergence, increase, or expansion). **Development** is defined as going through natural growth, differentiation, or evolution by successive changes. **Maturation** is defined as the emergence of personal characteristics and behavioral phenomena through growth processes.

Obviously these three words form a continuum of the same concept and are often used interchangeably.

BONE FORMATION

Embryogenesis of Craniofacial Skeletal Tissues

The craniofacial skeleton is derived from three unique processes: **chondrogenesis,** which is the formation of cartilage; **endochondral bone formation,** which is the process of converting cartilage into bone; and **intramembranous bone formation,** which is the process of bone formation from undifferentiated mesenchymal tissue.[3,4] Bone can either form directly from osteoblasts, a process called *intramembranous ossification,* or have a cartilaginous precursor called **endochondral ossifica-**

The Five Steps of Chondrogenesis

1. Chondroblasts produce matrix: The intercellular matrix produced by cartilage cells is hard but flexible and capable of providing rigid support.
2. Cells become encased in matrix: When the chondroblasts become fully encased within their own secretory matrix material, the cartilage cells become chondrocytes. New chondroblasts are differentiated from the surface membrane (perichondrium), and this results in increased cartilage size (i.e., cartilage can increase in size by appositional growth).
3. Chondrocytes enlarge, divide, and produce matrix: Cells continue to grow and secrete matrix, thereby increasing the cartilage mass from within. Growth resulting from internal expansion is called *interstitial growth*.

4. Matrix remains uncalcified: Cartilage matrix is rich in chondroitin sulfate associated with noncollagenous protein. This combination has the special property of marked hydrophilia. Nutrients and metabolic wastes diffuse directly through the soft matrix to and from cells. Hence, blood vessels are not required in cartilage.
5. Membrane covers the surface but is not essential: Cartilage has an enclosing, vascular membrane called the *perichondrium,* but cartilage can also exist without one. This property enables cartilage to grow and adapt in sites involving pressure (e.g., joints). Cartilage is pressure tolerant.

The Five Steps of Intramembranous Bone Formation

1. Osteoblasts produce osteoid tissue: Osteoblasts differentiate from the ectomesenchymal condensation centers and produce a fibrous bone matrix (osteoid).
2. Cells and blood vessels are encased: As osteoid deposition by osteoblasts continues, cells are encased and become osteocytes. Blood vessels are retained within the spaces and eventually become surrounded by bone, and a haversian system starts to form to nourish the bone.
3. Osteoid tissue is produced by membrane cells: Osteocytes lose their capacity to contribute directly to an increase in bone size, but the osteoblasts in the surface periosteum produce more osteoid tissue thereby

adding layers to the surface of the existing bone (i.e., appositional bone growth).
4. Osteoid calcifies: Bone matrix eventually becomes mineralized and makes bone relatively impermeable to nutrients and metabolic wastes. Entrapped blood vessels serve to supply nutrients to osteocytes and bone tissue as well as to remove waste products.
5. Essential membrane covers bone: An outside bone membrane called the *periosteum* and an internal membrane called the *endosteum* are essential for bone survival. Disruption of the membrane or its vascular supply may directly result in bone cell death and eventual bone loss. Bone is pressure sensitive. Calcified bone is hard and relatively inflexible.

tion. In the latter case chondroblasts initially form cartilage, which, in turn, is calcified and invaded by osteogenic tissue to form bone. A comparison between bone and cartilage properties is presented in Table 4-1.

Intramembranous Bone Formation
As with craniofacial cartilage, intramembranous bone is derived from neural crest cells. The earliest evidence of intramembranous bone formation in the skull occurs in the mandible during the latter portion of the sixth prenatal week. By the eighth week, centers of ossification appear in the calvarial and facial regions in areas where mild tension forces are present. By fol-

lowing the same five steps used with chondrogenesis, one is able to compare and contrast chondrogenesis with intramembranous bone formation.

Endochondral Bone Formation
The first evidence that cartilage is converted into bone in the craniofacial skeleton occurs during the eighth prenatal week. In the craniofacial skeleton, only the bones of the cranial base and portions of the calvarium are derived by way of endochondral bone formation. For the sake of comparing and contrasting endochondral bone formation with chondrogenesis and intramembranous bone formation, a five-step sequence is used.

The Five Steps of Endochondral Bone Formation

1. Hypertrophy of chondrocytes and matrix calcifies: Within the cartilage primordium matrix a center of calcification appears. Chondrocytes show hypertrophic changes, and calcification of the cartilage matrix continues.
2. Invasion of blood vessels and connective tissue cells: Blood vessels invade from the perichondrium into the calcifying matrix, bringing undifferentiated connective tissue cells.
3. Osteoblasts differentiate and produce osteoid tissue: From the connective tissue precursor cells, osteoblasts

differentiate and deposit osteoid on the remnants of the calcified cartilage matrix.
4. Osteoid tissue calcifies: The fibrous bone matrix mineralizes.
5. Membrane covers bone and is essential: Bone, whether it be of intramembranous or of endochondral origin, requires a membrane if it is going to survive. It is not possible to detect qualitatively any differences between bone of either origin in the mature craniofacial skeleton. In Table 4-1, cartilage and bone are compared in relation to their properties during growth and development.

TABLE 4-1	Comparison of Selected Physiologic Properties of Bone and Primary Cartilage Important During Growth	
Characteristics	Cartilage	Bone
Calcification	Noncalcified	Calcified
Vascularity	Nonvascular	Vascular
Surface membrane	Nonessential	Essential
Rigidity	Flexible	Inflexible
Pressure resistance	Tolerant of pressure	Sensitive to pressure

Changes in the Shape and Position of Bone

Any change in bone morphology or spatial relationship can be accomplished by one of two processes: remodeling and translation.[3,5]

Remodeling **Remodeling** is the selective bone apposition by osteoblasts and resorption by osteoclasts (see Chapter 28). Although these changes may occur simultaneously in the same bone, they are not necessarily equal in amount or opposite in direction. This results in differential changes and alterations in the size as well as the morphology (shape) of a given bone.

Translation or Displacement As a result of bone remodeling and changes in its shape and size, the bone itself will change its position in space. This phenomenon is called **primary translation** (Figure 4-1, *A*). **Secondary translation,** on the other hand, occurs when the growth of one bone results in a change in the spatial position of an adjacent bone (see Figure 4-1, *B*). For example, the

growth changes in a long bone like the humerus displaces the radius.[3] Primary and secondary translations can occur simultaneously.

GROWTH OF THE CRANIUM AND FACE[3,6,7]

Growth of the Cranial Vault

To accommodate the rapidly expanding brain, adaptive growth occurs at the coronal, sagittal, parietal, temporal, and occipital sutures. This intramembranous sutural growth system replaces the fontanels, which are present at birth. One of the last functions of the fontanels is to allow the cranium sufficient flexibility during parturition.

The cranial cavity achieves 87% of its adult size by age 2 years, 90% by 5 years and 98% by 15 years of age.[8] Between 15 years and adulthood the growth changes are mostly secondary to the pneumatization of the frontal sinuses and thickening of the anterior part of the frontal bone. Therefore it is reasonable to assume that the growth of the cranial vault follows the

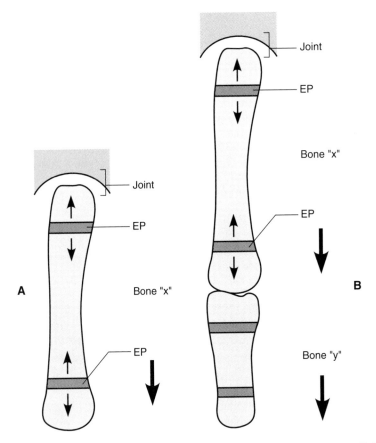

Figure 4-1 A, Changes occurring within bone "x" cause the bone to change its position in space. **B,** Changes occurring in bone "x" result in the translation or displacement of bone "y." Changes may also occur independently in bone "y." *EP,* Epiphyseal plate.

TABLE 4-2	Percentage of Craniofacial Growth Completed at Different Stages		
		Stages	
	1 to 5 Years	5 to 10 Years	10 to 20 Years
Cranium	85%	11%	4%
Maxilla	45%	20%	35%
Mandible	40%	25%	35%

Modified from Graber TM: *Orthodontics,* ed 3, Philadelphia, 1972, WB Saunders.

neural curve. In other words, rapid development during the first few years of life is followed by a decelerated growth rate (Table 4-2).

Growth of the Cranial Base

The changes in the cranial base occur primarily as a result of endochondral growth through a system of synchondroses. A **synchondrosis** is a cartilaginous joint where the hyaline cartilage divides and subsequently is converted into bone. Prenatally, the cranial base has a series of synchondroses within and between the ethmoid, sphenoid, and occipital bones. This arrangement allows for a rapid increase in the length of the cranial base early in life to accommodate the growing brain. The intraethmoidal and intrasphe-

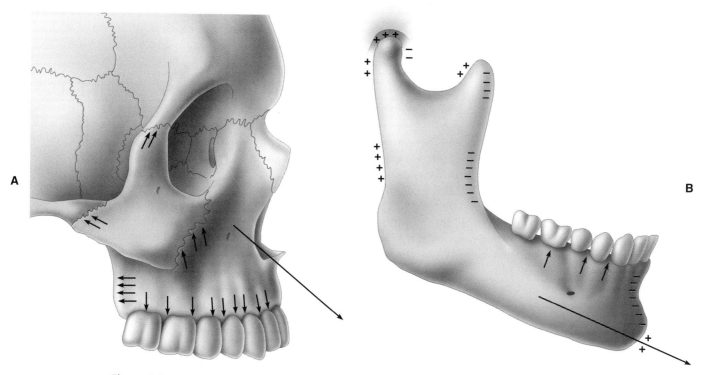

Figure 4-2 A, Different aspects of the growth of the nasomaxillary complex. **B,** Different aspects of the growth of the mandible.

noidal synchondroses close before birth, whereas the intraoccipital synchondrosis closes before 5 years of age. The sphenoethmoidal synchondrosis closes around 6 years of age, and the segment of the anterior cranial base designated as the planum sphenoidale becomes relatively stable early in life.[9] As a result, this segment is used for cephalometric superimpositions to evaluate the changes in the face that occur as a result of growth or treatment.

The spheno-occipital synchondrosis, on the other hand, is closed by 13 to 15 years of age. Therefore any subsequent changes that occur in either the length or the flexure of the cranial base are the result of surface deposition or resorption.[10]

Growth of the Nasomaxillary Complex (Figure 4-2, A)

The growth of the cartilaginous nasal septum, particularly the vomer and the perpendicular plate of the ethmoid, carries the nasomaxillary complex downward and forward.[9] This displacement allows for growth at the posterior aspect of the maxilla as well as at the maxillary tuberosities to accommodate for the eruption of the permanent molars. The forward movement of the maxilla also allows for the enlargement of the nasal and oral pharynx to accommodate

for the increased respiratory functional demands of the growing child.

The maxillary complex is surrounded by a system of sutures that allows for the growth and the displacement of the various bones both anteroposteriorly and laterally. The circummaxillary suture system includes the zygomaticomaxillary, frontozygomatic, sphenopalatine, and palatomaxillary sutures.

To allow for the increased functional demands in the nasal cavities, the nasal floor is lowered by being translated bodily downward and simultaneously undergoing surface resorption. This is accompanied by bone deposition on the oral side of the palatal shelves of the maxillary bone. It is of interest to note that in spite of the significant bone deposition on the oral side of the palatal vault, the depth of the vault actually continues to increase with age. This increase is the result of the significant growth of the alveolar processes that accompanies the eruption of the primary and permanent dentitions.

Changes in Maxillary Width Growth in width at the palatal suture occurs during the first 5 years of life, mostly at the intermaxillary and interpalatine suture (midpalatal). At later stages of development, any additional increase in the width of the anterior maxilla occurs as a result of bone deposition on the outer surfaces of the maxilla and by the buccal eruption of the permanent teeth.

Growth of the Mandible (see Figure 4-2, B)

In the neonate the mandible is made of two halves (i.e., it is not completely united at the midline). By the end of the first year the two halves of the mandible are essentially united as one parabolic bone. The various parts of the mandible include a body and two rami that support the condyles and coronoid processes.

The mandible is formed from intramembranous tissues. It needs to be remembered that the original (embryonic) primary cartilage of the mandible (Meckel's cartilage) disappears early during intrauterine life with only few remnants, namely the malleus and incus ossicles in the middle ear and the sphenomandibular ligament (see Chapter 1). Therefore the condylar cartilage is solely derived from secondary cartilage.

In general, the growth at the head of the condyle occurs in an upward and backward direction. Mandibular growth is expressed as a downward and forward displacement, which is an example of primary translation. This displacement and that of the nasomaxillary complex allow for the growth of the pharynx, tongue, and other related structures.

The growth at the condyles compensates for the vertical displacement of the mandible and accommodates for the eruption of the teeth vertically. On the other hand, bone resorption at the anterior border and deposition at the posterior border of the two rami account for the anteroposterior growth of the mandibular rami and body. These changes increase the posterior length of the body of the mandible to accommodate for the erupting permanent molars.

Growth of the Alveolar Processes

The growth of the alveolar bone is completely dependent on the presence and eruption of teeth. Following tooth extraction, the alveolar processes start to resorb; the rate of resorption can be slowed by restoring function through the placement of well-fitting dentures. The increase in the vertical height of the face is the result of the growth of the maxillary and mandibular alveolar processes, which is associated with the eruption of teeth.

Surface Remodeling

In addition to the specific sites of bone formation that have been discussed, all bony surfaces undergo selective remodeling through deposition and resorption. As an example, the bony chin becomes more prominent with age mostly as a result of bone resorption above the chin (rather than bone deposition on the chin) accompanied with forward mandibular growth.[11]

DIFFERENTIAL GROWTH OF THE FACE[12]

Although the growth of the various areas of the dentofacial complex has been discussed separately, it must be emphasized that most of these changes occur simultaneously and are interdependent (Box 4-1). For example, the forward growth of the cranial base may carry the maxilla forward, whereas a decrease in the cranial base flexure (more obtuse cranial base angle) may carry the mandible backward. Similarly, the downward descent of the maxilla causes the mandible to rotate backward.

As a result, growth of the mandibular body and condylar heads does not proceed in a proportional manner throughout life. For example, in the fetus the size of the head is almost ⅓ the size of the total body. On the other hand, at birth, the head is ¼ the size of the total body length, whereas at adulthood it becomes only ⅛ the size of the total body length. Similar differential growth occurs in the various parts of the craniofacial complex as illustrated in Table 4-2. The table indicates that almost ⅔ of the total growth of the maxilla and mandible would have been expressed by the time most patients seek orthodontic treatment around 10 to 12 years of age. Still the clinician may be able to influence the remaining growth potential of the patient when attempting to correct any existing skeletal discrepancies between the maxilla and mandible.

Differences in size, as well as growth direction, velocity or timing, are observed among individuals. Therefore any measured attribute, whether linear, angular, or volume, demonstrates a range of expression about a central tendency. Incremental growth curves for healthy males and females demonstrate the same general trends and show marked differences in maturation timing. Generally, females mature 2 years earlier than males, but variations are so great that an early-maturing boy may mature earlier than a late-maturing girl. In general, males tend to grow larger than females (see Chapter 3).

THE HISTORY OF CRANIOFACIAL GROWTH THEORIES[6]

Growth Centers vs. Growth Sites

Before the 1950s it was commonly believed that the head and face grew from growth centers that were under strict genetic control. The concept of a "growth center" evolved from the observation of

BOX 4-1 — Directional Changes in the Growth of Various Parts of the Craniofacial Complex

Students of craniofacial growth need to be familiar with the directional changes of the various parts of the craniofacial complex to be able to design an appropriate plan to optimally treat various skeletal discrepancies.

The changes in the cranial base, nasomaxillary complex, and mandible are described separately, although these changes often occur simultaneously. In addition to presenting the average changes, the range of variation is illustrated. Although the average trends are useful in simplifying the description of these changes, it must be emphasized that there is a significant amount of individual variation that occurs, which is the reason why it is difficult to predict the overall changes in any one individual.

Changes in the Cranial Base Relationships (Figure 4-3)

According to Knott,[13] the cranial base flexure increased (i.e., the angle decreased by an average of -3.8 ± 0.6 degree in males and -1.5 ± 0.4 degree in females between 6 and 25 years of age). Of great interest is the variation in the change in the angle, which ranged between -12.0 to 3.0 degrees in males and -6.0 to 3.0 degrees in females.

In an individual case the extreme changes can significantly influence either positively or adversely the other parts of the craniofacial complex that are directly and indirectly related to the cranial base.

Changes in the Nasomaxillary Complex (Figure 4-4)

Bjork,[14] using metallic implants, evaluated the changes in the growth direction of the nasomaxillary complex between 7 and 19 years of age. When related to the anterior cranial base (SN plane), the change was in a downward and forward direction at an average angle of 51.0 degrees with a range between 0 degrees (pure vertical growth) and 82.0 degrees (almost horizontal growth). Such a large individual variation partly explains why the same orthopedic appliance can have differing results when applied to two individuals with significantly different maxillary growth potentials.

Changes in Condylar Growth (Figure 4-5)

Bjork,[11] using metallic implants, determined the direction of condylar growth between 5 and 19 years of age in a male Scandinavian sample. On the average the condyle grew upward and backward, the angle between the direction of condylar growth and the posterior border of the ramus was, on average, 6.0 degrees with a range between -25.0 and 16.0 degrees. As a result, condylar growth can vary between a sagittal (backward and upward) and a vertical (upward and forward) direction in any one individual. Such variation significantly influences the mandibular growth direction at pogonion. Furthermore, the expression of mandibular growth is also influenced by the location of the center of rotation of the mandible.[15] In other words, similar condylar growth direction and amounts can be expressed differently at pogonion depending on whether the center of rotation is at the condyle, premolar, or incisor area.[15]

In summary, the difficulty that the clinician is facing when predicting the growth of the facial structures is influenced not only by the individual variation within that structure (cranial base, maxilla or mandible), but also by the compounding and cumulative effects of the variation of each of the parts on the overall growth of the face.

---

long bone growth. The epiphyseal plates of long bones were noted for their ability to grow under conditions of mechanical loading. Eventually, among craniofacial theorists, a growth center came to mean a center with the ability to generate tissue-separating forces.[14]

It was also believed that **craniofacial sutures** generated tissue-separating forces during growth, thereby pushing apart the various bones of the craniofacial complex. At this point in time, there is an overwhelming and convincing body of research evidence to support the view that sutures are adaptive, compensatory growth mechanisms (i.e., they are "growth sites"). Therefore craniofacial sutures are important growth sites that serve to facilitate calvarial and midface growth.[6,16] Most calvarial sutures close by 5 years of age, but some facial sutures remain patent throughout puberty. Sutures respond to mild tension forces by surface deposition of bone, thereby enabling bones of the face and skull to adapt.

Primary cartilage initially forms the **cranial base synchondrosis,** which grows by way of endochondral bone formation. The anterior cranial base becomes completely ossified by age 6 years. However, cartilage separating the sphenoid and occipital bones remains patent and viable through puberty. Early in life this cartilaginous junction, called the **spheno-occipital synchondrosis,** has a growth-directing capacity.

The **mandibular condyles,** once considered a growth center with directive capacity, are now

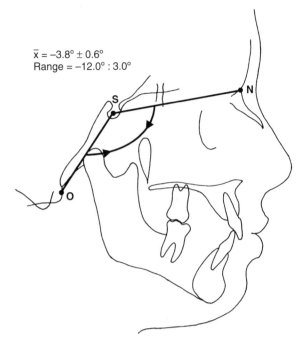

$\bar{x} = -3.8° \pm 0.6°$
Range = $-12.0° : 3.0°$

Figure 4-3 Changes in the cranial base angle of males between 6 and 25 years of age. (From Bishara SE, Peterson L, Bishara EC: *Am J Orthod* 85:238-252, 1984.)

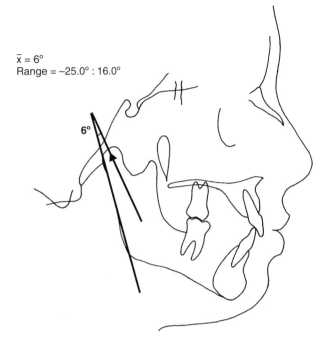

$\bar{x} = 6°$
Range = $-25.0° : 16.0°$

Figure 4-5 Directional changes in the growth of the condyles from 7 to 19 years of age. (From Enlow DH: *Facial growth,* ed 3, Philadelphia, 1990, WB Saunders.)

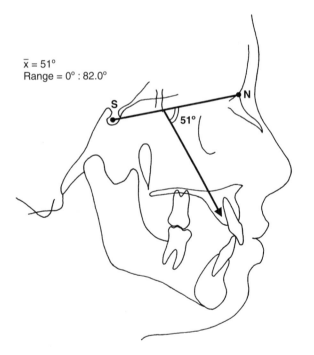

$\bar{x} = 51°$
Range = $0° : 82.0°$

Figure 4-4 Directional changes in the growth of the nasomaxillary complex from 7 to 19 years of age. (From Bishara SE, Treder JE, Jakobsen JR: *Am J Orthod Dentofacial Orthop* 106[2]:175-186, 1994.)

regarded as having primarily an adaptive growth mechanism.[16] Cartilage found at the head of the condyle is a secondary, fibrous-type cartilage and differs substantially from the primary, growth-plate type cartilage considered to be under strong genetic

control. Condylar cartilage does not originate from a primary cartilage precursor. It grows peripherally (appositionally) and is highly responsive to mechanical stimulation. During craniofacial growth, the mandible is repositioned continuously to its best possible functional advantage. This reposturing alters the anatomic position of the condyle in the glenoid fossa through remodeling of the fossa and compensatory growth of the condylar cartilage. Both mechanisms facilitate maintenance of mandibular posture. Mandibular condylar cartilage also has some intrinsic growth of its own but does not generate tissue-separating forces similar to epiphyseal plates. To a large extent the mandibular condyles behave the same way as the sutures (i.e., in an adaptive and compensatory fashion).

Scott[7] suggested that the primary cartilage present in the **nasal septum** is the primary mechanism responsible for the growth of the nasomaxillary complex. Latham[17] proposed a mechanism that could explain how the nasal septum exerts its downward and forward influence on the maxillary complex. He described a ligament extending from the nasal septal cartilage to the anterior premaxillary region, which he termed the *septopremaxillary ligament.* He proposed that this distinct connection is an important relationship, particularly before birth, between midfacial and nasal septal growth. This theory is called the *nasal septum theory of craniofacial growth.* In general, the nasal septum cartilage is regarded as a growth center.[7,17]

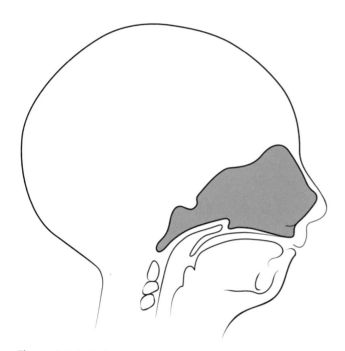

Figure 4-6 Sagittal section of the head of a human fetus to show the relationship of septal cartilage to cranial base.

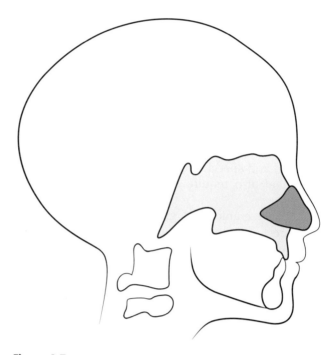

Figure 4-7 Midsagittal section of the nasal cavity illustrating the relative size of the nasal cartilage at about 6 years of age.

The Role of Primary Cartilage during Growth

Primary cartilage is singular in form, has the capacity to grow from within (interstitial growth), is pressure tolerant, noncalcified, flexible, nonvascular, and does not require a nutrient membrane covering for survival.[5] Primary cartilage found in the head and face is identical to the growth-plate cartilage of long bones. It is regarded as genetically predisposed, acts during growth as an autonomous tissue, and has the capacity to directly influence craniofacial pattern.[7]

Primary cartilage first appears in the head during the fifth week prenatally.[18] By the eighth prenatal week, independent sites of craniofacial cartilage have coalesced into a cartilaginous mass called the chondrocranium, which is the precursor to the adult cranial base and nasal and otic structures (Figure 4-6). By mid-childhood, most primary cartilage is replaced by bone through endochondral bone formation (Figure 4-7).

The overall influence of primary cartilage on craniofacial growth is most profound in early life. By birth, cartilage comprises a substantial portion of the nasal septum and cranial base. Interstitial expansion of primary cartilage probably has a direct influence on the position of the maxilla.[7,17,19] The maxilla is most likely thrust downward and forward during prenatal life, infancy, and early childhood. After mid-childhood the contributions to midface growth by primary cartilage is greatly diminished. Likewise, the spheno-occipital

synchondrosis significantly contributes to craniofacial growth, but after 6 years of age its relative contribution is small.

The Role of the Functional Matrix

In the 1960s Moss and Salentijn[20] reintroduced a concept regarding the controlling influence of functional space development on craniofacial growth. This concept came to be known as the *functional matrix theory.* Moss and Salentijn[21] suggested that the head carries out several vital functions and that the craniofacial structures respond to the changing requirements for those functions. According to this theory, craniofacial growth is the result of both changes in the "capsular matrices," causing spatial changes in the position of bones (translation), and by "periosteal matrices," causing more local changes in the size and shape of the skeleton (remodeling).

Moss and Salentijn[21] contend that there are several capsular matrices in the head such as the neurocranial capsule, which is controlled by the growing brain, thrusting the bony calvarial plates outward. On the other hand, alteration of the size and shape of the individual bones of the calvaria are under the influence of the periosteal matrices.[20] A periosteal matrix such as muscles and tendons act directly upon a skeletal unit via the periosteum, resulting in bone apposition and resorption.

As stated, there are a number of functions carried out by the head. Some functions are more essential than others, but all require the development and maintenance of spaces. Neural growth and integration is a critical function, and space is required for the brain as well as the central and peripheral nervous system expansion. Respiration and deglutition are also essential to life and require development of nasal, pharyngeal, and oral spaces. Sight, olfaction, hearing, and speech are important craniofacial functions that also require development of functioning spaces.

A likely craniofacial growth scenario describing the direct influence of functioning space development on head and face pattern includes rapid size increase of the brain during prenatal and early postnatal life that thrusts the calvarial bony plates outward and the midface forward and downward.[21] Birth invokes a set of functional processes that were previously not essential for the life of the embryo (e.g., breathing and swallowing). Repositioning of the mandible and tongue takes place to ensure patency of the nasooropharyngeal spaces. The mandible is depressed and thrusts forward for these functions to be supported and maintained.

REFERENCES

1. Bishara SE, Peterson L, Bishara EC: Changes in facial dimensions and relationships between the ages of 5 and 25 years, *Am J Orthod* 85:238-252, 1984.
2. Bishara SE, Treder JE, Jakobsen JR: Facial and dental changes in adulthood, *Am J Orthod Dentofacial Orthop* 106(2):175-186, 1994.
3. Enlow DH: *Facial growth,* ed 3, Philadelphia, 1990, WB Saunders.
4. Scott JH: The growth of the human face, *Proc Roy Soc Med* 47:5, 1954.
5. Enlow DH: *Handbook of facial growth,* ed 2, Philadelphia, 1982, WB Saunders.
6. Sarnat BG: Craniofacial change and non-change after experimental surgery in young and adult animals, *Angle Orthod* 58:321-342, 1988.
7. Scott JH: The nasal septum, *Br Dent J* 95:37, 1953.
8. Graber TM: *Orthodontics,* ed 3, Philadelphia, 1972, WB Saunders.
9. Knott VB: Changes in cranial base measures of human males and females from age 6 years to early adulthood, *Growth* 35:145-158, 1971.
10. Hight JR: The correlation of spheno-occipital synchondrosis fusion to hand-wrist maturation, *Am J Orthod* 79:464-465, 1981.
11. Bjork A: Variations in the growth pattern of the human mandible: a longitudinal radiographic study by the implant method, *J Dent Res* 42:400-411, 1963.
12. Moyers RE: *Handbook of orthodontics,* Chicago, 1988, Year Book Medical.
13. Knott VB: Changes in cranial base measures of human males and females from age 6 years to early adulthood, *Growth* 35:145-158, 1971.
14. Bjork A: Sutural growth of the upper face studied by the implant method, *Acta Odont Scand* 24:109-127, 1996.
15. Bjork A: Prediction of mandibular growth rotation, *Am J Orthod* 55(6):585-599, 1969.
16. Koski KL: Cranial growth centers: facts or fallacies? *Am J Orthod* 54:566-583, 1968.
17. Latham RA: Maxillary development and growth: the septopremaxillary ligament, *J Anat* 107:471, 1974.
18. Sperber GH: *Craniofacial embryology,* ed 3, Boston, 1981, John Wright-PSG.
19. Gange RJ, Johnston LE: The septopremaxillary attachment and midfacial growth, *Am J Orthod* 66:71-81, 1979.
20. Moss ML, Salentijn L: The primary role of functional matrices in facial growth, *Am J Orthod* 55:566-577, 1969.
21. Moss ML, Salentijn L: The capsular matrix, *Am J Orthod* 56:474-490, 1969.

CHAPTER 5

Development of the Dental Occlusion

Samir E. Bishara

KEY TERMS

occlusion
overbite
open bite
overjet
underjet
generalized spacings

primate spaces
crowding
terminal planes
flush terminal plane
mesial step
distal step

eruption of the first
  permanent tooth
temporary open bite
diastema
Blanche test

Class I molar relationship
Class II molar relationship
Class III molar relationship
leeway space
  deficiency

WHAT IS OCCLUSION?

In its simplest definition **occlusion** is the way the maxillary and mandibular teeth articulate. In reality dental occlusion is a much more complex relationship because it involves the study of the teeth, their morphology and angulations, the muscles of mastication, the skeletal structures, the temporomandibular joint, and the functional jaw movements. In addition, it involves the relationship of the teeth in centric occlusion, in centric relation, and during function. Because all this requires neuromuscular coordination, occlusion also involves an understanding of the neuromuscular systems.

CHANGES IN THE DENTAL OCCLUSION WITH AGE

From birth until adulthood and beyond, dental occlusion undergoes significant changes. At times these changes are drastic, as in the mixed dentition stage, and at other times they are more subtle (e.g., after the complete eruption of the permanent teeth between early and late adulthood). It is important for the clinician to understand and recognize the scope of the

changes that are normally occurring in the dentition to be able to diagnose any abnormal developments. Such an understanding also prevents an eager, well-intentioned but not adequately informed clinician from treating "normal" conditions in the mixed dentition stage that are often part of the normal clinical manifestation of the early stages of dental development.

STAGES OF DENTAL DEVELOPMENT

To simplify the description of the continuum of changes in the dental relationships during the various stages of the dentition, this continuum is arbitrarily divided into four stages: gum pads, primary dentition, mixed dentition, and permanent dentition.

Gum Pads Stage

The gum pads stage of dental development extends from birth until the eruption of the first primary tooth, usually a lower central incisor, around 6 to 7 months of age. The gum pads in the maxillary and mandibular arches show elevations and grooves that outline the position of the various primary teeth that are still developing in the alveolar ridges. A few babies are born with one or more primary incisors already erupted, which can cause a painful situation for a breastfeeding mother.

The maxillary and mandibular gum pads have been frequently illustrated to describe an anterior open bite relationship while the posterior segments are touching. More often, the maxillary gum pad slightly overlaps the mandibular gum pad both horizontally and vertically. In this manner the opposing surfaces of the pads provide for a more efficient way of squeezing milk during breastfeeding.

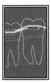

CLINICAL CONSIDERATIONS

The timing of the eruption of the first primary tooth varies between babies; therefore it is prudent for the clinician to provide the parents with an age range for the expected eruption time of the various teeth. Such variations are present in both the primary and permanent dentition stages. For example, the average timing of eruption of the lower permanent central incisor is around 6 years of age (±6 months) in 68% of the population. In 95% of the population the timing of eruption might vary by 1 year around the mean age (i.e., it can occur anytime between 5 and 7 years of age).

Primary Dentition Stage

The primary dentition stage extends from the time of eruption of the primary teeth until the eruption of the first permanent tooth around 6 years of age. Four characteristics of the primary dentition stage are discussed in some detail, namely, overbite, overjet, spacing, and the relationship of the second primary molars.[1-6]

Overbite **Overbite** is the amount of vertical overlap between the maxillary and mandibular central incisors. This relationship can be described either in millimeters or more often as a percentage of how much the upper central incisors overlap the crowns of the lower incisors. The overbite in the primary dentition normally varies between 10% and 40%.

When the incisal edges of the incisors are at the same level, the condition is described as "edge to edge or zero overbite." When there is a lack of overlap, the condition is described as **open bite** and quantified in millimeters.

Foster[2] in a study of 100 British children between 2 and 3 years of age described the overbite relationship as ideal (19%), reduced (37%), open bite (24%), and excessive overbite (20%). The fact that more than 60%

of the children in this population have a reduced overbite or an open bite is attributed to the effects of the various oral habits (finger or pacifier sucking) that are common in this age group.

Overjet **Overjet** is the horizontal relationship or the distance between the most protruded maxillary central incisor and the opposing mandibular central incisor. This relationship is expressed in millimeters. If the maxillary incisors are lingual to the mandibular incisors, the relationship is described as an **underjet.** The normal range of overjet in the primary dentition varies between 0 and 4.0 mm.

In the same study by Foster,[2] the overjet was ideal in 28% of the cases and excessive in 72% of the children. Again, the presence of excessive overjet was attributed to the effects of the oral habits.

Spacings In the primary dentition stage a child may have generalized spaces between the teeth, localized spaces, no spaces, or a crowded dentition. The presence of spacing in the primary dentition stage is a common occurrence. According to Foster,[2] **generalized spacings** occur in almost ⅔ of the individuals in the primary dentition stage.

In addition to the generalized spacings, localized spacings are often present and are referred to as **primate spaces.** Such spaces are present in 87% of the maxillary arches usually between the lateral incisors and canines. The primate spaces are also present in 78% of the mandibular arches, usually between the canines and first primary molars.

A tooth size-arch length discrepancy (TSALD) in the form of **crowding** is less common and occurs in approximately 3% of the children in the primary dentition stage.

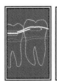

CLINICAL CONSIDERATIONS

Clinicians need to realize that the presence of spacings in the primary dentition stage does not mean that there will be adequate space for the erupting permanent teeth.[4] On the other hand, the presence of crowding in the primary dentition stage increases the probability of crowding occurring in the permanent dentition stage. This is because the arch length available anterior to the mandibular second primary molars does not increase after their eruption. Actually, the anterior dental arch length decreases with age.[4,6] As a result, the presence of a tooth size-arch length discrepancy in the form of crowding in the primary dentition stage should not be expected to resolve itself by spontaneous growth in the anterior part of the dental arches.

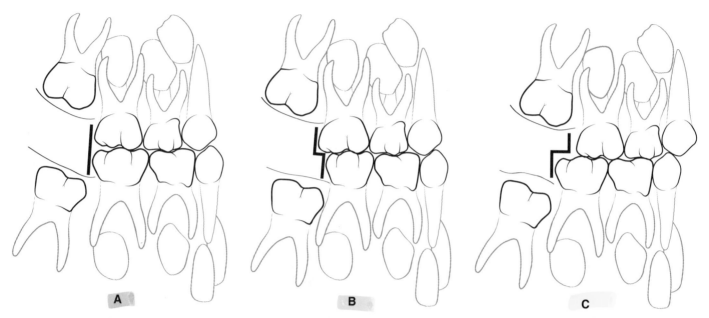

Figure 5-1 Terminal plane relationship between the distal surfaces of the maxillary and mandibular second primary molars. **A,** Flush terminal planes. **B,** Mesial step with the mandibular plane mesial to the maxillary plane. **C,** Distal step with the mandibular plane distal to the maxillary plane.

Molar Relationship In the primary dentition stage the anteroposterior molar relationship is described in terms of the relationship between terminal planes. The **terminal planes** are the distal surfaces of the maxillary and mandibular second primary molars. Essentially the two terminal planes can be related to each other in one of three ways (Figure 5-1).

In the **flush terminal plane** relationship, both the maxillary and mandibular planes are at the same level anteroposteriorly (see Figure 5-1, *A*). In the **mesial step** relationship, the maxillary terminal plane is relatively more posterior than the mandibular terminal plane (see Figure 5-1, *B*). Lastly, in the **distal step** relationship, the maxillary terminal plane is relatively more anterior than the mandibular terminal plane (see Figure 5-1, *C*).

The word *relative* needs to be emphasized; the description of a mesial or distal step does not identify which of the two arches is ahead or behind the other. In a study on 121 Iowa children at age 5 years, the distribution of the terminal plane relationships of the primary second molars were found to be as follows[1]:

Distal step	10%
Flush terminal plane	29%
Mesial step of 1.0 mm	42%
Mesial step >1.0 mm	19%

Therefore almost 90% of the cases had a terminal plane relationship, which was either flush or with a 1.0-mm or greater mesial step.

Determining the terminal plane relationships in the primary dentition stage is of great importance to the clinician because the erupting first permanent molars are guided by the distal surfaces of the second primary molars as they erupt into occlusion (see Figure 5-1).

During the primary dentition stage the overbite, overjet, and anteroposterior relationship of the dentition do not undergo significant changes unless they are influenced by environmental factors such as trauma, habits, or caries.

At the late primary dentition stage of development, the maxilla and mandible are housing the greatest number of teeth ever, including 20 erupted primary teeth and at least 28 unerupted but partially forming permanent teeth.

Mixed Dentition Stage

The mixed dentition stage starts with the **eruption of the first permanent tooth,** usually the mandibular central incisor, and is normally completed at the time the last primary tooth is shed. The mixed dentition period is characterized by significant changes in the dentition as a result of the loss of 20 primary teeth and the eruption of their succedaneous permanent teeth.

In the early stages of the mixed dentition period there may be a **temporary open bite,** usually either a result of the still incomplete eruption of the incisors or because of mechanical interference from a persistent finger habit. During normal development this open bite is often transitory in nature; the open bite is present until the incisors complete their eruption process, unless the abnormal habit persists.

As each tooth erupts the clinician should expect that its antimere (the same tooth on the opposite side [e.g., the right and left central incisors]) would erupt within 6 months of each other. The sequence of eruption of the primary and permanent teeth are detailed in Chapter 6.

Spacing A **diastema** is a space between any two neighboring teeth. During the mixed dentition stage the presence of a midline diastema between the maxillary central incisors is a normal occurrence. In most cases the size of the diastema may vary between 1.0 and 3.0 mm. These diastemas usually close by the time the maxillary canines fully erupt and do not require any orthodontic intervention. If the diastema persists in the permanent dentition stage and if the patient is concerned, the clinician may consider closing it orthodontically or with composite buildups to the teeth.

Molar Relationship As stated previously, the terminal planes of the second primary molars influence the path of eruption of the permanent first molars (see Figure 5-1). For example, when the terminal plane relationship in the primary dentition stage is flush, the permanent molars erupt in a "cusp-to-cusp" or "end-to-end" first permanent molar relationship in the mixed dentition stage.

Before we elaborate further on the molar relationship, a number of definitions are in order. These definitions are based on Angle's classification (see Chapter 9).[7]

In a **Class I molar relationship** the mesiobuccal cusp of the maxillary first permanent molar occludes with the buccal groove of the mandibular first molar. This is considered the normal relationship of these teeth (Figure 5-2, *A*).

In a **Class II molar relationship** the mesiobuccal cusp of the maxillary first permanent molar occludes mesial to the buccal groove of the mandibular first molar (see Figure 5-2, *B*).

In a **Class III molar relationship** the mesiobuccal cusp of the maxillary first permanent molar occludes distal to the buccal groove of the mandibular first molar (see Figure 5-2, *C*).

Bishara et al[1] evaluated the changes in the molar relationship from the primary dentition stage to the permanent dentition stage on 121 Iowa subjects (242 sides) followed for an average period of 8 years between 5 and 13 years of age. The findings from this study indicated all cases that started with a distal step in the primary dentition stage developed into a Class II molar relationship in the permanent dentition stage. Because none of these cases self-correct, treatment could be initiated by the clinician as early as it is advisable.

Of the cases with a flush terminal plane relationship in the primary dentition stage, 56% developed into a Class I molar relationship and 44% developed into a

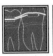

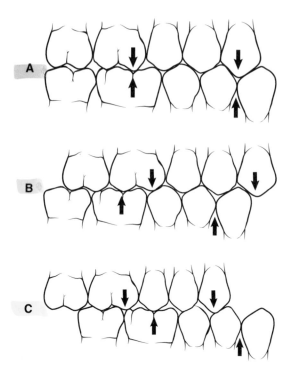

Figure 5-2 Molar classification according to Angle. **A,** Class I with the mesiobuccal cusp of the maxillary first permanent molar in the buccal groove of the mandibular first molar. **B,** Class II with the mesiobuccal cusp of the maxillary first molar mesial to the buccal groove of the mandibular first molar. **C,** Class III with the mesiobuccal cusp of the maxillary first molar distal to the buccal groove of the mandibular first molar.

Class II molar relationship in the permanent dentition stage. Because a flush terminal plane in the primary and mixed dentition stages could develop into an unfavorable relationship (i.e., a Class II molar relationship in the permanent dentition stage), these cases should be closely observed to initiate orthodontic treatment when indicated.

In cases with a mesial step in the primary dentition stage, the findings indicated that the greater the mesial step, the greater the probability for the molar relationship to develop into a Class I or Class III. Furthermore, the development of a Class II molar relationship, although still possible, was less probable. Conversely, the incidence of a Class III molar relationship increased. More specifically, of the cases with a 1-mm mesial step, 76% became Class I molar relationships, 23% became Class II molar relationships, and 1% became Class III molar relationships. In cases with a mesial step of 2 mm or more in the primary dentition stage, 68% became Class I molar relationships, 13% became Class II molar relationships, and 19% became Class III molar relationships. Of the total group, 61.6% of the cases ended up as Class I molar relationships, 34.3% were Class II molar relationships, and 4.1% were Class III molar relationship in the permanent dentition stage (see Chapter 7 for more details).

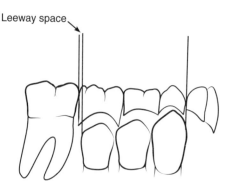

Figure 5-3 Leeway space is the difference in space between the combined mesial-distal crown dimensions of the unerupted permanent canine, first and second premolars, and the primary canine and the primary first and second molars.

Causes of Change in the Molar Relationship

A number of factors are involved in the changes of the molar relationship from the flush terminal plane relationship, which is considered "normal" in the early mixed dentition stage, to a Class I molar relationship, which is "normal" in the permanent dentition stage.

The Leeway Spaces In general, the sum of the mesiodistal width of the primary canine and the primary first and second molars is larger than the sum of their succedaneous teeth, namely, the permanent canine and first and second premolars. This difference is called the *leeway space* and is present in both the maxillary and mandibular arches (Figure 5-3). The most favorable dental arch pattern is when leeway space is excessive (i.e., the combined size of unerupted canine and premolars is smaller than the available arch space).

The leeway space is larger in the mandibular arch than in the maxillary arch. On the average, the unerupted canine and premolars are 1.8 mm smaller, per side, in the lower arch. In the upper arch, the leeway space averages only 0.9 mm per side.[1] Sometimes the combined sizes of the unerupted teeth are larger than the space available. This condition is called a **leeway space deficiency,** and dental arch crowding often results. It is important to note that, for most individuals, the growth changes in other dental arch dimensions will not typically be great enough to compensate for leeway deficiencies. The leeway space differential between the two arches allows the first permanent molars to move mesially relatively more in the mandibular arch than in the maxillary arch.

Mandibular Growth In general, both the maxilla and mandible grow downward and forward, but during this developmental stage the mandible grows relatively more forward than the maxilla. It was thought that these relative growth changes may contribute to

CLINICAL CONSIDERATIONS

The observations on the changes in the molar relationship are of importance to clinicians involved in the management and treatment of young patients in the primary and mixed dentition stages. The findings imply that cases with distal steps in the primary dentition stage should be observed on a regular basis and treatment started as soon as the clinician and the patient are ready to initiate it because the condition will not self-correct with time.

Patients with a flush terminal plane relationship present a more challenging diagnostic question. This is because the findings suggest that slightly more than half of these cases progress to a normal Class I molar relationship, whereas 44% of the cases progress to a Class II, or end-to-end, occlusion. These findings imply that what is considered "normal" occlusion in the primary or mixed dentition stage does not necessarily lead to a "normal" occlusion in the permanent dentition stage. Therefore it is important for the clinician to closely observe these cases and, when needed, initiate orthodontic treatment at the appropriate time.

The findings also indicate that the presence of a favorable difference in the leeway spaces between the maxillary and mandibular arches is not a good predictor of whether a Class I molar relationship will be estab-

lished in the permanent dentition stage. In addition, the final molar occlusion is dependent on a number of dental and skeletal facial changes, both genetic and environmental, that interact to achieve or not achieve a normal occlusion.

These findings indicate that the change in the molar relationship might be more complex than was previously assumed and is associated with changes in a number of variables in both of the dental arches and the rest of the dentofacial structures. This complexity may explain why none of the cases with a distal step and many of the cases with a flush terminal plane or a mesial step in the primary dentition stage did not change to a Class I permanent molar relationship. Maintaining the Class II occlusion occurred in spite of the fact that these cases also exhibited positive leeway spaces and significant mandibular growth.

In conclusion, clinicians need to realize that some of the dental relationships such as midline diastema or an end-to-end molar relationship are considered normal occurrences in the mixed dentition stage but not in the permanent dentition stage. Such an understanding should prevent the clinician from treating these conditions too early.

the transition from an end-to-end to a Class I molar relationship. The findings from the Iowa study indicated that a weak correlation was present between the changes in the molar relationship and the changes in the anteroposterior jaw relationship.[1] Furthermore, there were no significant correlations between these two variables and the difference in the leeway space between the maxillary and mandibular arches.

The Iowa results further indicated that changes in other variables such as intercanine widths, arch lengths, and maxillary and mandibular relationships were associated with, and indirectly contributed to, the changes in the molar relationship. In other words the factors involved in the changes in the molar relationship are more complex than previously thought and are not solely dependent on one or two variables such as leeway spaces or mandibular growth.

Characteristics of a "Normal" Dental Arch Pattern in the Mixed Dentition Stage The status of the dental arch at mid-adolescence is contingent upon clinical features that can be easily recognized during the mixed dentition stage. The simplest method of evaluating the status of the dental arches for either the presence or predisposition to a malocclusion, is to conceptually compare the patient's arches in the mixed dentition stage to what is considered to be an ideal dental arch pattern.

The ideal dental arch pattern in the mixed dentition stage after the eruption of the central and lateral incisors has the following characteristics:

Class I molar and canine relationship
Positive leeway space (i.e., no TSALD)
Minor or no rotations or incisor crowding
Normal buccolingual axial inclinations
Normal mesiodistal axial inclinations
Tight proximal contacts
Even marginal ridges vertically
Flat occlusal plane or a mild curve of Spee

Environmental Factors That May Influence the Dental Arch Pattern The primary determinant of a malocclusion is the genetic predisposition. On the other hand, there are secondary environmental factors that can dramatically influence the disposition of the dental arches including early loss of primary teeth, interproximal caries, a pathologic condition, ankylosis of primary teeth, oral habits, and trauma.

The environmental factors most commonly affecting dental arch status are probably caries and premature loss of the primary teeth. According to Northway, Wainright, and Demirjian,[8] early caries as well as early loss of the primary first or second molars result in a decrease in dental arch length. For example, the loss of the primary second molars had the most deleterious effect on dental arch length and resulted in 2 to 4 mm

CLINICAL CONSIDERATIONS

In an earlier study on the same population, tooth size–arch length discrepancies (TSALD) significantly increased from early adolescence (13 years of age) until early adulthood (25 years of age).[11] When the changes in the anterior TSALD between 13 and 45 years were calculated, the total mandibular arch and maxillary arch change amounted to 2.7 mm and 1.9 mm, respectively, in male subjects and 3.5 and 2.0 mm, respectively, in female subjects. As a result, one may speculate that without long-term retention, adolescents who were orthodontically treated to a perfectly aligned dentition should expect some crowding to occur in the anterior part of the dental arches. This should be considered part of the normal maturation process. Clearly, these findings have important clinical implications regarding the long-term stability and retention of the treatment results. The patient should be made aware of the probability of these changes occurring after the retention appliances are discontinued.

of space closure per quadrant in both arches. In addition, the loss of the upper primary first molar typically resulted in blocked out canines, whereas upper primary second molar loss usually resulted in an impacted second premolar. The greatest space loss was the result of the mesial movement of the permanent molars (see Chapter 17).

In general, more space was lost in the first year after the premature tooth loss of a primary tooth than in successive years. It needs to be emphasized that no reattainment of space was demonstrated during growth in either the upper or lower arches without treatment.

Permanent Dentition Stage

The permanent dentition stage of dental development starts after the shedding of the last primary tooth and the eruption of all the permanent teeth excluding third molars. Some of the characteristics of the "normal" occlusion in the permanent dentition stage include the following:

Overlap: In a normally occluding dentition, the maxillary teeth are labial/buccal to the mandibular teeth.

Angulations: In the primary dentition stage the teeth are, in general, vertically positioned in the alveolar bone. On the other hand, in the permanent dentition stage the teeth have buccolingual and mesiodistal angulations.

Occlusion: With the exception of the mandibular central incisors and the maxillary second molars, each permanent tooth occludes with two teeth from the opposite arch.

Arch curvatures: The anteroposterior curvature in the mandibular arch is called the *curve of Spee*. The corresponding curve in the maxillary arch is called the *compensating curve*. The buccolingual curvature from the one side to the other is called the *Monson curve* or the *Wilson curve*.

Overbite and overjet: The overbite often ranges between 10% and 50%, and the overjet ranges between 1.0 and 3.0 mm.

Posterior relationships: The maxillary and mandibular molars are in a Class I occlusion (i.e., the mesiobuccal cusp of the maxillary first molar is in the buccal groove of the mandibular first molar). In addition, the whole posterior segment needs to be well interdigitated. More specifically, the maxillary canines should also be occluding in the embrasure between the mandibular canines and first premolars (see Figure 5-2, *A*).

Late Changes in the Permanent Dentition Stage

Because of the increasing number of adults seeking orthodontic care, an understanding of the changes that normally take place in the adult craniofacial structures becomes critical. In general, after the eruption of the permanent teeth, the dentition is relatively stable when compared with the cascade of changes observed in the mixed dentition stage. But change is the rule when it comes to the dentofacial complex.

The changes in the various craniofacial skeletal profile and dental arch parameters between 25 and 45 years of age were investigated.[9] The average time span between young and mid-adulthood observations for female subjects was 20.0 ± 0.8 years and for male subjects was 20.3 ± 1.2 years. The findings suggested that age-related changes in the craniofacial complex do not cease with the onset of adulthood but continue, albeit at a significantly slower rate, throughout adult life. With a few important exceptions, these changes tend to be of small magnitude so that their clinical relevance is somewhat limited and generally would not significantly influence orthodontic treatment planning.[9]

Two findings are considered to be of clinical importance and need elaboration. In both male and female subjects the lips became more retruded relative to the nose and chin between 25 and 45 years of age. The implication is that orthodontic treatment at earlier ages should not result in an overly straight soft tissue profile and overly retrusive lips because the expected changes in the relative positions of the nose, lips, and chin may exaggerate these characteristics. In both male and female subjects, interincisor and intercanine arch widths decreased. Also total arch lengths decreased and, as a result, anterior crowding increased.[9,10]

REFERENCES

1. Bishara SE et al: Changes in the molar relationship between the primary and permanent dentitions: a longitudinal study, *Am J Orthod Dentofacial Orthop* 93(1):19-28, 1988.
2. Foster TD: *A textbook of orthodontics*, ed 2, St Louis, 1982, Blackwell Scientific Publications.
3. Knott VB: Longitudinal study of dental arch width at four stages of dentition, *Angle Orthod* 42:387-394, 1972.
4. Moorrees CFA: *The dentition of the growing child*, Cambridge, 1959, Harvard University Press.
5. Moorrees CFA: Growth studies of the dentition: a review, *Am J Orthod* 55:600-616, 1969.
6. Sillman JH: Dimensional changes of the dental arches: longitudinal study from birth to 25 years, *Am J Orthod* 50:824-842, 1964.
7. Angle EH: *Treatment of malocclusion of the teeth*, ed 7, Philadelphia, 1907, SS White Dental Manufacturing.
8. Northway WM, Wainright RL, Demirjian A: Effects of premature loss of deciduous molars, *Angle Orthod* 54:295-329, 1984.
9. Bishara SE, Treder JE, Jakobsen JR: Facial and dental changes in adulthood, *Am J Orthod Dentofacial Orthop* 106(2):175-186, 1994.
10. Bishara SE et al: Arch width changes from 6 weeks to 45 years of age, *Am J Orthod Dentofacial Orthop* 111:401-409, 1997.
11. Bishara SE et al: Changes in the maxillary and mandibular tooth size-arch length relationship from early adolescence to early adulthood, *Am J Orthod Dentofacial Orthop* 95(1):46-59, 1989.

CHAPTER 6

Dental Arch Development

Donald Ferguson and Samir E. Bishara

KEY TERMS

dental arches　　　　　calcification　　　　　maxillary arch　　　　　mandibular arch

OVERALL SEQUENCE OF DENTAL ARCH DEVELOPMENT

In Chapter 5 the development of dental occlusion from the primary to the mixed and permanent dentition stages was described. These changes are associated with the eruption of the primary and permanent teeth and with changes in arch length and width as well as relationships. Furthermore, there is a significant difference between the primary and permanent tooth size, particularly in the anterior part of the arch (i.e., incisors and canines).

The purpose of this chapter is to explain and describe the changes in the dimensions of the dental arches and the changes in their relationships. Furthermore, the sequence of eruption of the primary and permanent teeth, the timing of their calcification, and the difference in tooth size between groups of teeth are described.

DIMENSIONAL CHANGES IN THE DENTAL ARCHES

The transition from the primary dentition stage to the permanent dentition stage has an impact on dental arch length, circumference, and intermolar and intercanine widths.[1-4] The following narrative summarizes and Figure 6-1 illustrates the average dimensional changes for the maxillary and mandibular arches.

Changes in the Maxillary Arch
(see Figure 6-1, *A*)

The intercanine width increases by an average of 6.0 mm in a child between 3 and 13 years of age. It continues to increase between 13 and 45 years of age by approximately 1.7 mm. In the primary dentition stage there is an increase of intermolar width of 2.0 mm between 3 and 5 years of age. The first permanent intermolar width increases by 2.2 mm between 8 and 13 years of age and decreases by 1.0 mm by 45 years of age. There is a slight decrease in arch length with age because of the uprighting of the incisors.

Changes in the Mandibular Arch
(see Figure 6-1, *B*)

Between 3 and 13 years of age the intercanine width increases by an average of 3.7 mm. Then between 13 and 45 years of age the intercanine width decreases by 1.2 mm.[2] It should be noted that after the eruption of the mandibular incisors there is little change to be expected in the intercanine width.

In the primary dentition stage there is an increase of intermolar width of 1.5 mm between 3 and 5 years of age. The first permanent intermolar width increases by

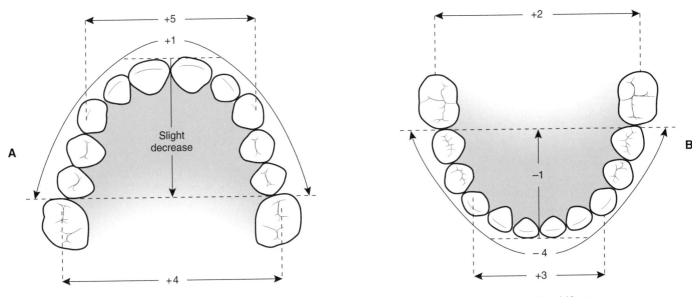

Figure 6-1 Diagram representing average dental arch dimensional changes (in millimeters) between 6 and 18 years of age for **A,** maxillary arch, and **B,** mandibular arch. (Redrawn from Moorrees CFA: *Am J Orthod* 55:600-616, 1969.)

1.0 mm between 8 and 13 years of age and then decreases by 1.0 mm by age 45.

The arch length decreases in the mixed and permanent dentition stages as a result of the uprighting of the incisors and the loss of the leeway space by the mesial movement of the first permanent molars.

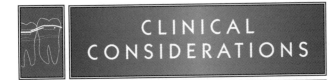

CLINICAL CONSIDERATIONS

Following the eruption of the mandibular central and lateral incisors, the arch width measurements in the lower arch are essentially established. Lower arch length after the eruption of the first permanent molars does not increase. Actually, the arch length may decrease with the loss of the primary molars and the mesial movement of the first permanent molars in the leeway space. Because of these limitations, most clinicians consider the lower arch as the key to orthodontic diagnosis (see Chapters 9 and 12).

CHANGES IN THE RELATIONSHIP OF THE DENTAL ARCHES

The clinician must realize that there are differences between the preeruptive and posteruptive shapes and relationships of the upper and lower **dental arches.** Early in development the maxilla is anterior to the mandible, but in the adult the upper anterior apical alveolar area is typically more posterior than the lower anterior apical area. The upper incisors are usually more labially inclined than the lower incisors. The shape of the mandibular posterior area is wider, transversely, than the upper posterior area during the prenatal period. This relationship carries on into adulthood. Hence, the apices of the teeth are more lateral in the lower posterior segment than in the upper posterior segment. In addition, the buccolingual inclination of the lower posterior teeth is usually more pronounced.

Two aspects of dental development are briefly discussed, including the timing of initial calcification of the teeth and their sequence of eruption for both the primary and permanent dentitions.

Primary Dentition

Calcification The primary teeth begin **calcification** between the third and fourth prenatal months. Mandibular primary teeth usually begin calcification before the maxillary primary teeth. The central incisors typically are first, and the second molars are last to begin calcification. Males usually begin calcification before females.

Sequence of Tooth Eruption Usually no teeth are present at birth. The first primary tooth to erupt is the central incisor at about 6 or 7 months of age, and the last to erupt is the second primary molar at about 2 to 3 years of age. The usual sequence for eruption is the central incisor (designated by the letter *A* when using

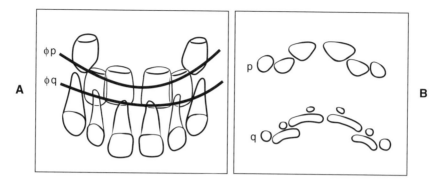

Figure 6-2 Maxillary anterior region from mesial of canine to mesial of canine. **A,** Facial view. **B,** Cross-sectional view. (Redrawn from Van der Linden FPGM: *Transition of the human dentition,* Monograph no 13, Ann Arbor, Mich, 1982, Craniofacial Growth Series, University of Michigan.)

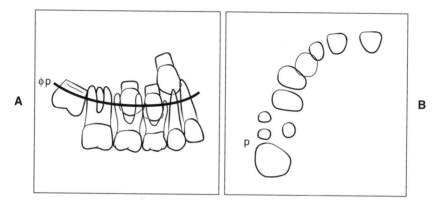

Figure 6-3 Maxillary posterior region from the distal of the lateral incisors to the mesial of the first permanent molars. **A,** Facial view. **B,** Cross-sectional view. (Redrawn from Van der Linden FPGM: *Transition of the human dentition,* Monograph no 13, Ann Arbor, Mich, 1982, Craniofacial Growth Series, University of Michigan.)

Palmer notation), the lateral incisor *(B)*, the first primary molar *(D)*, the canine *(C)*, and the second primary molar *(E)*. Thus the typical eruption sequence is *A-B-D-C-E*.[1]

Permanent Dentition

Calcification The permanent teeth usually do not begin to calcify until shortly after birth. The first permanent molar is the first tooth to show evidence of calcification during the second postnatal month. The third molar is the last tooth to begin calcification at about 8 to 9 years of age.

Sequence of Tooth Eruption In the **mandibular arch** the sequence is as follows: the first molar (designated by the number *6* using Palmer notation), central incisor *(1)*, the lateral incisor *(2)*, the canine *(3)*, the first premolar *(4)*, the second premolar *(5)*, the second molar *(7)*, and the third molar *(8)*, or *6-1-2-3-4-5-7-8*. For the **maxillary arch** the usual sequence of eruption is *6-1-2-4-5-3-7-8*. Females generally precede males in the eruption timing by an average of 5 months.[5]

Replacement of the primary teeth by the permanent teeth often takes place between the ages of 6 and 12 years. However, eruption times for the permanent teeth can vary considerably, depending on the specific tooth. The lower incisor has the least amount of variation in eruption timing. In other words, 90% of lower permanent incisors erupt within a span of 3.1 years. On the other hand, excluding third molars, which have the largest variation in eruption timing, the lower second premolar shows the greatest variation in eruption timing with a 6.6-year span.

TOOTH SIZE DIFFERENCES DURING THE MIXED DENTITION STAGE

For the sake of clarity, tooth size differences during the mixed dentition stage will be described on a regional basis: upper anterior, upper posterior, lower anterior, and lower posterior.[5] Figures 6-2 through 6-5 represent each region with a narrative that outlines various developmental features (primary to permanent tooth

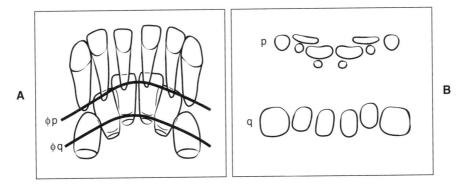

Figure 6-4 Mandibular anterior region from the mesial of canine to the mesial of canine. **A,** Facial view. **B,** Cross-sectional view. (Redrawn from Van der Linden FPGM: *Transition of the human dentition,* Monograph no 13, Ann Arbor, Mich, 1982, Craniofacial Growth Series, University of Michigan.)

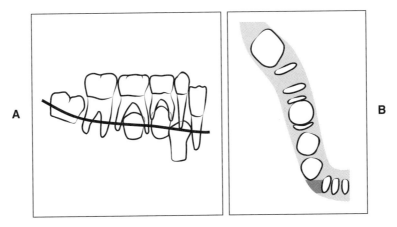

Figure 6-5 Mandibular posterior segment from the distal of lateral incisors to the mesial of the first permanent molars. **A,** Facial view. **B,** Cross-sectional view. (Redrawn from Van der Linden FPGM: *Transition of the human dentition,* Monograph no 13, Ann Arbor, Mich, 1982, Craniofacial Growth Series, University of Michigan.)

size comparisons, preeruption positions of the permanent teeth, and features in permanent eruption dynamics).

Maxillary Anterior Region

The size of the primary incisor mesiodistal crown dimensions are, on the average, 75% the size of their permanent successors. As a result, the average total combined permanent incisor tooth width is 8 mm larger than the primary teeth. Before eruption, the central incisor is lingual to its predecessor. The lateral incisor is lingual to the central incisor and canine (see Figure 6-2).

After eruption the position of the permanent incisors is slightly different. The incisors erupt in a more labial position than the primary incisors. Although the eruption is frequently not symmetric, it tends to occur within a 6-month interval. Eruption of the permanent canines causes mesial movement of the lateral incisors and closure of midline diastemas.

Maxillary Posterior Region

The average size of the primary teeth relative to their permanent successors differs greatly. The primary canines are 85% of the size of the permanent canines. The primary first molars may equal the size of the first premolars whereas the primary second molars are larger than the second premolars. On the other hand, there is significant variation between the size of the primary and permanent teeth. As a result the correlation coefficient (*r*) between the mesiodistal width of individual primary teeth to their permanent successors ranges between 0.2 and 0.5 mm. For example, the sum of the mesiodistal width of *C-D-E* to the sum of the mesiodistal width of *3-4-5* has a correlation coefficient of 0.5.

In the alveolar processes during the preeruptive phase, relatively speaking, the first premolars are typically more occlusal (i.e., the second premolars and canines are relatively more apical) (see Figure 6-3). The average leeway space is 0.9 mm per side with a range from +6.0 mm to −5.8 mm. An excess leeway space of 2 mm or more is optimal. When the leeway space is less than optimal, a *4-5-3* eruption sequence is more advantageous because it allows for the extraction of first premolars as part of a serial extraction procedure when indicated (see Chapter 18).

Mandibular Anterior Region

The average total permanent lower incisor mesiodistal crown widths are 6 mm more than the total primary incisor widths. Similar to the maxillary dentition, the individual tooth correlation coefficients between the primary and permanent teeth range between 0.2 and 0.6. The primary incisor crown dimensions average 75% of the size of their successors, but the correlation coefficient for the combined incisor width is only 0.4.

Preeruptively, the central incisors are usually lingual to their predecessors and the lateral incisors are lingual to the permanent central incisors. The central incisor crypts overlap the lateral incisor crypts (see Figure 6-4). The permanent central incisors and lateral incisors erupt lingual to their predecessors and then move labially following their eruption. Often the incisors emerge rotated and then realign if sufficient space is available.

Mandibular Posterior Segment

As with the maxillary teeth, the average primary tooth size relative to their permanent successors differs significantly. The primary canines are 85% of the size of the permanent canines, the primary first molars are 115% of the size of the first premolars, and the primary second molars are 138% of the size of the second premolars. On the other hand, the correlation coefficients between individual teeth range between 0.2 and 0.5, whereas the correlation coefficient of the sum of the mesiodistal widths of *C-D-E* to that of *3-4-5* is 0.5.

The first premolars are typically positioned in the alveolar processes, more occlusal than the canines and second premolars before their emergence. The canine is relatively more apically positioned (see Figure 6-5). When these teeth erupt the average leeway space is 1.7

mm per side with a range from +3.8 mm to −5.6 mm. An excess leeway space of 1 mm or more is preferable. The optimal eruption sequence is *3-4-5*. The eruption sequence in the posterior region is frequently asymmetric and may vary by 6 months between the two sides of the arch.

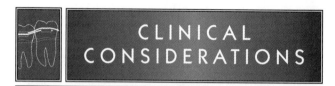

CLINICAL CONSIDERATIONS

The sequence of eruption of the permanent teeth can play an important role when considering a guidance of eruption/serial extraction procedures (see Chapter 18). Therefore the clinician needs to obtain appropriate radiographic records to make such an evaluation. Because of the relatively low correlation coefficients between the size of the primary teeth and their permanent predecessors, it is difficult to predict the future size of the permanent teeth by measuring the primary teeth. As a result, other methods of prediction were developed that provide a more accurate assessment that would be helpful to the clinician in estimating the size of the unerupted permanent teeth in the mixed dentition (see Chapter 12).

REFERENCES

1. Moorrees CFA: *The dentition of the growing child,* Cambridge, 1959, Harvard University Press.
2. Bishara SE et al: Arch width changes from 6 weeks to 45 years of age, *Am J Orthod Dentofacial Orthop* 111:401-409, 1997.
3. Foster TD: *A textbook of orthodontics,* ed 2, St Louis, 1982, Blackwell Scientific Publications.
4. Moorrees CFA: Growth studies of the dentition: a review, *Am J Orthod* 55:600-616, 1969.
5. Van der Linden FPGM: *Transition of the human dentition,* Monograph no 13, Ann Arbor, Mich, 1982, Craniofacial Growth Series, University of Michigan.

CHAPTER 7

Facial and Dental Changes in Adolescence

Samir E. Bishara

KEY TERMS

growth changes
standing height
maxillary length
maxillary relationship

maxillary-mandibular
   relationship
face types
condylar growth

growth prediction
growth spurt
distal step

flush terminal plane
   relationship
mesial step

Assessment and prediction of dentofacial growth is perhaps the most essential yet, to a great extent, the most subjective area, in the field of clinical orthodontics. Although the percentage of adult orthodontic patients has increased in recent years, the majority of treatment is directed toward preadolescent and adolescent patients. These individuals are still undergoing significant growth changes in their occlusion, facial skeleton, and profile.

Such changes are fairly complex because each person has a unique growth pattern that is influenced by their particular genetic makeup (i.e., the biologic or internal environment, as well as external environmental factors such as function, disease, habits, and orthodontic treatment).[1]

Cephalometric superimpositions often demonstrate dramatic dental, skeletal, and soft tissue changes during orthodontic treatment. Many orthodontists give themselves full credit when they take advantage of the patient's favorable growth combined with a reasonable orthodontic treatment plan. These same clinicians, however, blame unfavorable growth and lack of patient cooperation when the treatment results are anything short of their expectations.

Because growth can be either a friend or a foe, it becomes important to determine the timing, magnitude, and direction of facial growth. Such an understanding should enable orthodontists to better plan the treatment of skeletal discrepancies in their attempt to achieve a more stable and pleasing result. To accomplish such an objective in a consistent manner is a complex and difficult task. Therefore it behooves all clinicians to discern between the science and the fiction in facial growth or, as Professor Koski[2] once said, "the facts and fallacies" in facial growth.

The purpose of this chapter is to review pertinent longitudinal facial growth data as well as some of the methods used to predict facial growth. The clinical implications of the available information are discussed. When appropriate, the subject matter is arranged in a question-and-answer format (Box 7-1).

IOWA GROWTH STUDIES

To avoid repetition during various parts of this chapter, it may be expeditious to first describe the Iowa Growth Study material. Collection of the data started at The University of Iowa in 1946 by Drs. Meredith and Higley. Cephalograms, study casts and other records were obtained on the participants from ages 4 through 18 years. Another set of records was taken at adulthood around 25 years of age and a final set was taken at 45 years of age.[3] All subjects were Caucasian, and 97% were of northern European ancestry. This population provided the material for the series of Iowa

Facial Growth Studies published during the last 50 years.

The subjects chosen for the current series of studies had clinically acceptable occlusion with no apparent facial disharmony. In other words, they exhibited a Class I molar and canine relationship, less than 3 mm crowding at the time of the eruption of the permanent dentition, and no gross asymmetries in the dental arches. None of the subjects had orthodontic treatment.

These criteria for the selection of the sample had the disadvantage of limiting the number of persons to be included in the study to only 35 subjects—20 males and 15 females. On the other hand, these selection criteria had the advantage of providing a purely longitudinal set of data rather than a mixed longitudinal set of data. With mixed longitudinal data the absolute and incremental values may vary between consecutive ages. This variation, whether it is an increase or decrease, is partly related to the changes in the composition of the sample as well as the actual growth changes that occurred.

For example, in the Michigan standards, fluctuation in the size of parameter in successive years may not be solely the result of changes in the spatial position of the parts, but it could also be the result of the increase and decrease in the number of individuals included in the sample at different ages.[4] Such variation in sample size could cause the fluctuation in both the mean value as well as its standard deviation. Similar trends can also be observed in the Bolton standards.[5] Therefore the variability related to the composition of the sample can be eliminated by examining only those subjects for whom complete sets of data are available.

The author would like to emphasize that both the Bolton and Michigan data are unique treasures, and the profession is grateful to the people who have been involved in the acquisition and analysis of this important data. The previously mentioned facts merely point to some of the limitations that investigators face in working with longitudinal data, specifically the difficult choice between sample size and the homogeneity of the data.

OVERALL CHANGES BETWEEN 5 AND 25 YEARS OF AGE

The **growth changes** between 5 and 25 years of age in standing height and various craniofacial parameters were divided arbitrarily into three stages, specifically 5 to 10, 10 to 15, and 15 to 25 years of age.[6] This was an attempt to better understand what happens in the face in broad terms at various stages of development that are of particular interest to the orthodontist.

Standing height is usually used as a standard or indicator of skeletal body maturation and, as a result, it was included in these evaluations. Approximately 40% of the total change in standing height occurs between 5 and 10 years of age, another 40% occurs between 10 and 15 years of age, and the balance occurs after 15 years of age (Table 7-1). Females, when compared with males, have relatively greater growth increments between 5 and 10 years than between 10 and 15 years. These relative differences, in the magnitude of the changes in standing height between males and females, are also found in most linear facial dimensions such as face heights and depths but were not as readily observed when the facial relationships were evaluated (see Tables 7-1 and 7-2).

The relative changes in **maxillary length** were approximately 40%, 40%, and 20% in males and 50%, 30%, and 20% in females (see Table 7-1). The changes in **maxillary relationship** were 11%, 78%, and 11% in males and −25%, 50%, and 75% in females. Two observations worth emphasizing are that the percentages are different in males and females and that the timing of the linear and positional changes of the maxillary complex do not closely correspond in the three periods. For example, maxillary length expressed 50% of its total increase between 5 and 10 years of age in females. On the other hand, SNA angle actually decreased (i.e., point A moved relatively further back in relation to the cranial base). This change could be the result of a relatively

TABLE 7-1	Changes in Different Parameters Between 5 and 25 Years of Age			

Parameters	Total Change 5-25 Years	Percentage Change 5-10 Years	10-15 Years	15-25 Years
Standing Height				
Males	59.6 cm	41%	44%	15%
Females	55.5 cm	54%	41%	5%
Ans-Pns				
Males	10.6 mm	37%	42%	21%
Females	7.2 mm	49%	33%	18%
SNA				
Males	1.8 degrees	11%	78%	11%
Females	0.4 degrees	−25%	50%	75%
Ar-Pog				
Males	31.0 mm	34%	39%	27%
Females	21.0 mm	48%	41%	11%
SN-Pog				
Males	5.0 degrees	37%	33%	30%
Females	3.0 degrees	41%	50%	9%
ANB				
Males	−1.6 degrees	−31%	−6%	−63%
Females	−1.4 degrees	−57%	−71%	−28%

TABLE 7-2	Changes in Face Heights and Soft Tissue Convexity Between 5 and 25 Years of Age			

Parameters	Total Change 5-25	Percentage Change 5-10	10-15	15-25
Anterior Face Height (N-Me)				
Males	29.8 mm	42%	39%	19%
Females	21.9 mm	48%	37%	15%
Posterior Face Height (S-Go)				
Males	29.1 mm	35%	36%	28%
Females	18.5 mm	45%	40%	15%
Soft Tissue Convexity with Nose (Gl'-Pr -Pog')				
Males	−7.3 degrees	−44%	−70%	−14%
Females	−9.2 degrees	−53%	−37%	−10%
Soft Tissue Convexity without Nose (Gl' SLs - Pog')				
Males	3.3 degrees	−48%	−36%	185%
Females	1.0 degrees	−280%	−280%	170%

greater forward movement at nasion or a clockwise rotation of the maxillary complex.

The changes in mandibular length in males were 34%, 39%, and 27% in the three growth periods (see Table 7-1). The corresponding changes in relationship (SNPog) were more or less similar (i.e., 37%, 33%, and 30%). In females the changes in mandibular length were 48%, 41%, and 11% with similar percent changes in mandibular relationship, namely 41%, 50%, and 9%.

If one looks at the **maxillary-mandibular relationship** as described by the ANB angle, some interesting differences can be seen (see Table 7-1). In males the relative decrease in the angle was 31%, 6%, and 63% in the three periods of growth, whereas in females there was an increase in the angle in the last period.

After evaluating other parameters in the dentofacial complex (see Tables 7-1 and 7-2), the following conclusions can be reached:

1. There are significant changes that occur in the periods between 5 and 10 and 10 and 15 years of age and they are, in general, significantly more than the changes between 15 and 25 years.
2. The changes occur earlier in females than in males.
3. The changes in the different parts of the face are not necessarily similar in either their timing or their magnitude.
4. The timing of change between the linear and angular changes in a structure do not often occur at the same time or in the same direction.
5. There are significant changes in the last period of growth (i.e., between 15 and 25 years of age) in certain facial parameters, specifically face height, soft tissue facial convexity, and the ANB angle.

Actually, most of the effective changes in the soft tissue profile occurred between 15 and 25 years of age. This is an interesting observation because it indicated that most of the decrease in the convexity of the profile occurred in late adolescence.

CHANGES IN VARIOUS FACE TYPES WITH AGE

In a study that characterized **face types** as being either long, average or short as determined from an evaluation of both the cant of the mandibular plane (MP:SN angle) and the ratio of posterior/anterior face heights (S-Go:NMe), several questions were addressed.[7]

How Often Do People Change Their Facial Types Between 5 and 25 Years of Age?

The findings from the study indicated that most persons (77%) were categorized as having the same facial type both at 5 and at 25 years of age. This means that as facial growth progressed with age, there was a

strong tendency to maintain the overall facial pattern in most individuals. It was also observed that the differences between the three facial types, particularly in the vertical relationships, were more pronounced at adulthood than in childhood. This indicated that the facial pattern became more expressed with age.[7]

This concept of genetic predisposition has been illustrated previously in other parameters. For example, resemblance between the size of children and parents is small in infancy as compared to later in life. This is thought to be because of the ability of some genes to be more strongly expressed sometime after birth. In other words, children with a genetic predisposition to be large but who were born small actually increased to a higher percentile of height and weight within the first 6 months of life. Similarly, children born large but who had a genetic predisposition to be small took approximately 18 months to move downward in the height and weight percentiles. It seems that size at birth reflects uterine conditions much more than the baby's genetic makeup.[8]

On the other hand, the case for the environment is illustrated in a study on a set of monozygotic twins. The twins were compared as adults after having been separated at birth. They were raised separately until adulthood under extremely different conditions.[9] One was raised in a "normal" home environment, while the other was raised in a physically and mentally adverse environment. The difference in height between the twins was significant, with the "normal" infant being 8.3 cm taller than the other. Skeletal shape of the twins, however, was similar.

It seems that the facial growth data is supportive of this genetic predisposition in the majority of cases because 77% of the faces in the study maintained their face type.[7] But it should still be remembered that in 23% of the subjects there was a change in the categorization of facial type between 5 and 25 years of age. This "shifting" from one face type to another mostly occurred in cases with borderline characteristics between two facial types (i.e., from average to long or from short to average). Whether these changes were a late genetic expression or whether they resulted from environmental influences or both is difficult to determine, but they provide the basis for the dilemma that the clinician faces in planning the treatment of these cases.

How Does the Growth of Long, Average, and Short Facial Types Differ from Each Other?

When the growth curves of the three facial types in people between 5 and 25 years of age were evaluated, there was a lack of significant differences in the profile of the curves (i.e., the shape or slope of the absolute growth curves). This finding indicated that the curves

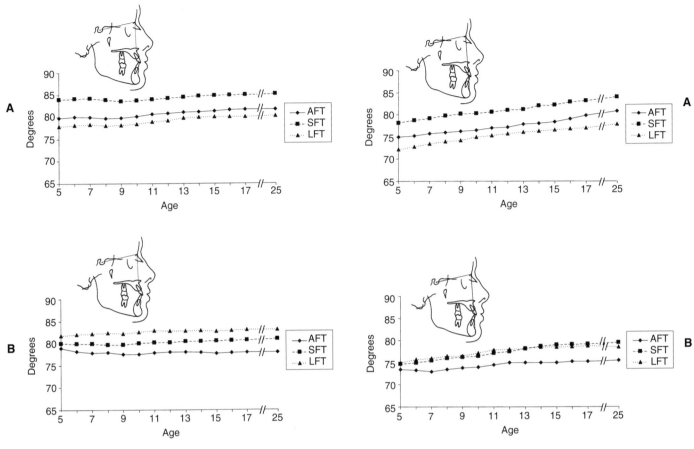

Figure 7-1 Graphs illustrating the absolute changes in SNA between 5 and 25 years of age for males (**A**) and females (**B**) for three different facial types; average (AFT), short (SFT), and long (LFT).

Figure 7-2 Graphs illustrating the absolute changes in SNPog between 5 and 25 years of age for males (**A**) and females (**B**) for three different facial types; average (AFT), short (SFT), and long (LFT).

were fairly parallel for the three face types. For example, the mean curves for SNA and SNPog that are illustrated in Figures 7-1 and 7-2 essentially describe similar trends.[7]

This overall pattern of parallelism was observed in most of the curves for the 48 dentofacial parameters evaluated and indicated that, regardless of facial type, the curves demonstrate a parallel relationship (i.e., similar growth behavior and similar growth direction). As interesting as this finding might seem in the context of facial growth, such a phenomenon parallels the findings in the well-publicized standards for standing height for tall, average, and short persons.[10]

This consistency in curve parallelism observed was matched by a consistent presence of significant differences among the three facial types in the curve magnitude (i.e., in the amount of growth expressed).[7] For example, the short face type expressed relatively larger curves for most of the anteroposterior dentofacial parameters evaluated such as SNA and SNPog. On the other hand, the magnitude of the curves for the vertical facial dimensions was larger in the long face type.

What Causes the Differences Between the Various Facial Types?

It seems that the outcome of facial growth in the various facial types is influenced at least in part by the original size and original relationships of the different parts of the face superimposed on the differences in the magnitude of change between the successive ages (i.e., the rate of change). For example, the comparisons of the curves for SNPog indicate that the three facial types have parallel growth curves. Yet the overall magnitudes of both the absolute and incremental curves for the three facial types were different, being smaller for the long face and larger for the short face.

How Much Variation Is There in the Dentofacial Characteristics Within Each Facial Type?

Even within a relatively homogenous and small sample, each face type expressed a considerable amount of variation.[7] Individuals *within* each facial type were neither of similar size, nor did they have similar dentofacial relationships. In other words, there is obviously more than one combination in both the size and relationship of the different parts of the dentofacial complex, but they all end up with the same face type. Therefore subtle changes in various parameters can influence the overall direction of facial growth as well as the ultimate facial relationships. As a result, during treatment planning, the clinician should evaluate both the overall general face type as well as the individual facial characteristics of each patient. These characteristics make the patient a unique individual who needs a unique treatment plan.

METHODS OF PREDICTING FACIAL GROWTH CHANGES

All the variations that have just been described represent the range of normal relationships within a normal population. On the other hand, persons with more severe skeletal discrepancies (i.e., with an abnormally long or short face) have more accentuated characteristics and relatively more predictable facial changes. So how clinically applicable is the ability to predict the growth of the face?

According to Bjork,[11] **growth prediction** can be accomplished by three general methods: longitudinal, metric, and structural.

Longitudinal Approach

With the longitudinal approach, an individual may be evaluated over a specified period to determine the pattern of growth. This concept was clinically applied by Tweed[12] on his growing patients. He advocated taking two lateral cephalograms 12 to 18 months apart to evaluate the skeletal facial changes. Consequently, the patient was placed into one of three categories that are used to predict future growth trends. In type A the growth of the middle and lower face proceeds in unison with changes in the vertical and horizontal dimensions being approximately equal. In type B the middle face grows downward and forward more rapidly than the lower face. This type of growth is predominantly in a vertical direction. In type C the lower face develops at a faster rate than the middle face. Tweed's basic assumption was that the growth pattern would remain constant.

Subscribing to the concept of constancy of the growth pattern was presented in the early 1950s by Brodie.[13] Soon after, Moore[14] and other investigators and clinicians concluded that this constancy can only be observed with population averages but that it is not useful in predicting the changes occurring in any one individual.

The obvious limitation of the longitudinal approach is that it is accurate only when it is performed retrospectively but not prospectively. Often the pattern and rate of growth in one period is not similar to that occurring in a subsequent period in any given individual. Therefore it can be concluded that the longitudinal approach is not an accurate method of predicting future dentofacial changes.

Metric Approach

The metric method of predicting growth consists of measuring different structures on a single x-ray film then relating these measurements to future growth changes. From a clinical perspective, this should be an ideal method of prediction because of its simplicity. But how successful is this method of prediction (i.e., how strong is the interrelationship of the changes) within a facial structure, between the various facial structures, and between the facial structures and other body dimensions? At this juncture it might be helpful to explain the scientific determination and clinical application of the strength of the relationships between any two variables.

A correlation coefficient symbolized by a small r describes the association or the strength of the relationship between two variables. A correlation coefficient also gives the direction, positive or negative, of this relationship. Its use in prediction is derived from squaring the value of r, which is called the *coefficient of determination,* or r^2. This coefficient describes the amount of variation of the second variable that can be eliminated if the first variable is known.[15]

According to Horowitz and Hixon,[15] a correlation coefficient may be statistically significant at the 0.001 level of confidence but is still of no clinical significance for prediction. As a rule they suggested an r value of 0.8 to be the dividing line for use in clinical prediction because the coefficient of determination, or r^2, is 0.64 (i.e., 64% of the variation can be accounted for in the variable that is being predicted).[15] It is with these facts in mind that the available data are interpreted.

In independent studies by Bjork and Palling,[16] Bjork,[17] Harvold,[18] Lande,[19] Solow and Siersbaek-Nielsen,[20] and others,[21,22] correlation coefficients for facial dimensions, be it linear or angular, when related to future growth of that same dimension did not exceed an r of 0.4 or 0.5 (i.e., they only explain 16% to 25% of the variation). Meredith[23,24] earlier examined this concept in considerable detail on the Iowa growth data. He related the growth changes for a series of head, face, and other body dimensions and calculated correlations between (1) the size at one age to the size of the same parameter at another age, (2) the size of the parameter at one age to the amount of change at a subsequent age, and (3) the amount of change at one period to the changes at subsequent periods. These correlations were performed both within a variable as well as between different variables. Of hundreds of correlation coefficients calculated, 60% had an r value of less than 0.4.[23-25] The highest correlation found was between the growth in face width and the growth in shoulder width with an r of 0.65. This is still a fairly low correlation for clinical use.

From a clinical perspective the metric method of prediction has its own limitation in predicting facial changes.

Structural Approach

The structural method for predicting mandibular growth direction was developed by Bjork[26] from superimpositions on metallic implants. The method consists of recognizing specific structural (i.e., morphologic) features in the mandible that indicate future growth trends.

When evaluating mandibular morphology, Bjork[11,26] listed seven areas on the cephalogram that should be evaluated to help predict future mandibular growth direction:

1. The inclination of the condyle as an indication of its growth direction, whether vertically or sagittally. For example, with vertical condylar growth, the mandible rotates forward.
2. The curvature of the mandibular canal (i.e., the more curved the canal is the more forward mandibular rotation will be).
3. Inclination of the symphysis. If it is inclined lingually, the mandible rotates forward.
4. Shape of the lower border of the mandible.
5. The interincisal angle, which is more acute in forward rotators.
6. The interpremolar or molar angles are also more acute in forward rotators.
7. The anterior lower face height.

Bjork's comprehensive work[11,17,26,27] on both maxillary and mandibular changes also demonstrated the wide range of variation in the growth of the nasomaxillary complex, condyles, and mandibular position within a given population. Such variation is to be expected because the future direction of mandibular growth is influenced by the changes in other parts of the craniofacial complex (i.e., the changes in the cranial base, the position of the glenoid fossa, the nasomaxillary complex, growth of the alveolar processes, and what should be considered as "the great unknown" [see Chapter 4]). More specifically, one of the unknowns is the effect of future changes in the environment and function on the growth of the face. These variables are difficult to quantify by any prediction method because they are essentially unknown to both the clinician and to the patient.

In a later study, Skieller, Bjork, and Linde-Hansen[28] attempted to refine this prediction approach by quantifying it. They found that the combination of four variables gives the best prognostic estimate of future mandibular growth direction. The variables were (1) mandibular inclination measured as MP:SN angle or as the ratio of posterior/anterior face heights, (2) the intermolar angle, (3) the shape of the lower border of the mandible measured as the angle between Go-Me and a tangent to the lower border of the mandible, and (4) the inclination of the symphysis measured as the angle between the tangent of the anterior surface of the symphysis and the SN.

When the measurements of these variables were included in the multiple regression analysis, the R^2 was calculated to be 0.8612. This is a fairly high R^2, as it explains more than 86% of the variation in the direction of mandibular growth. But, unfortunately, there was a catch. According to Skieller, Bjork, and Linde-Hansen,[28] the high R^2 value obtained may be related to the fact that the sample they evaluated contained a number of extremes whose growth usually proceeds in a more consistent and predictable direction. They suggested that if the extremes were eliminated, prediction of the direction of growth would be much less reliable.

From a clinical perspective, one can conclude that if a patient has a very steep mandibular plane with an obtuse gonial angle and an open bite tendency with a Class II or Class III malocclusion, it becomes fairly obvious that there is a high probability that the future direction of mandibular growth will be unfavorable regardless of the best efforts of the clinician.

Because the prediction of how the extreme facial types grow does not seem to be a great challenge to the average clinician, the discussion will focus on the various methods of predicting the changes that occur in the average adolescent population. This group comprises most of the patients that the clinician manages on a day-to-day basis. The longitudinal, metric, and structural methods of prediction are of a limited clinical value. Recent computer technology has provided more sophisticated approaches to this ongoing problem.

Computerized Prediction Methods

At this point it needs to be emphasized that computerization is essentially a tool of analysis and not a method of analysis. This is because computers are programmed to use equations based on either the longitudinal, metric, structural, or other methods of prediction. The biggest advantage of computer technology is that it facilitates testing and applying more complex formulas to growth prediction.

In the 1970s Ricketts et al[29-32] were among the first to realize that the clinician could be provided with a much more complete analysis of a cephalogram, including diagnosis, treatment planning, and a short- and long-term growth forecast of the dentofacial changes, with and without treatment. So Ricketts[29] introduced his method of computer analysis based on the concept of the cubic root combined with a vast clinical experience.

Greenberg and Johnston[33] tested these computer predictions. They selected cephalograms on 100 orthodontically untreated subjects from the Bolton-Brush Growth Study at both 10 and 15 years of age. From this sample, 20 subjects were selected at random as experimental subjects and their lateral cephalograms at 10 years of age were submitted for a 5-year computer forecast. Upon receipt of the forecasts, the cephalograms of children at 15 years of age were also sent for tracing. From the remaining 80 subjects they calculated the average changes in various parameters between 10 and 15 years of age. Comparisons were made between three types of calculations: (1) the computer forecast of the changes between 10 and 15 years on the 20 cases, (2) the actual changes that occurred in the same 20 cases, and (3) adding the average changes that occurred in the other 80 subjects to the dimensions at 10 years in the 20 experimental subjects. Greenberg and Johnston[33] found that the computer forecasts were essentially no better than the assumption of "average growth." In other words, there were no significant differences in accuracy between the predictions generated by the computer and those based on the simple addition of the average changes. Furthermore, both methods (i.e., the computer predictions and adding average changes) were not accurate representations of the actual changes for most of the facial parameters evaluated.

Cangialosi et al[34] evaluated the reliability of another commercially available computer program using pretreatment and posttreatment cephalograms of 30 patients treated during an active period of growth. The computer predictions were compared with the actual treatment results. In addition, the growth forecast from the computer program was compared with the growth forecast using a manual method. Of the 10 variables predicted, five were found to be statistically reliable. The computer forecast came close to the actual measurements in four variables, and the manual method came closer for three variables. Two of the four parameters predicted by the computer were related to the dentition. On the other hand, predicting the skeletal and soft tissue changes was much less accurate. However, one should remember that the dental changes as a result of treatment are more predictable because, to a great extent, these changes are dictated by the clinician.

The different methodologies presented by the computerized techniques may appear complex, yet they have inherently the same limitations described previously.[30,34-36] According to Hixon[37] and Hixon and Klein,[38] "To err is human; to really foul things up requires a poorly programmed computer." This is not intended to mean that clinicians should not use the various computer programs available, but they need to realize that such programs are useful for general patient education as well as average growth or treatment simulations and not for individualized predictions.

In conclusion, the overall changes in the size and relationship of the human face in the 20-year period from childhood to adulthood are, in general, difficult to accurately predict for an individual at this time. This is because the changes are under the influence of the combined and complex effects of the hard-to-predict, genetic, and environmental factors. The situation is rendered even more complex because we are using a two-dimensional image—the cephalogram—to predict a three-dimensional multifunctional object—the face.

FACIAL CHANGES IN ADOLESCENCE AND THE GROWTH SPURT

The adolescent **growth spurt** in the dentofacial structures, specifically in the mandible, is one of the most frequently mentioned concepts in facial growth. Clinicians have been told to gear their treatment timing so that it coincides with the adolescent growth spurt. This subject is best addressed by answering three commonly asked questions.

Is There a Mandibular Growth Spurt and How Often Does It Occur?

The most accurate and reliable data on the subject of mandibular growth spurts can be obtained from studies using metallic implants. In a 1963 study, Bjork[11] evaluated the growth of the condyles on 45 boys between 7 and 21 years of age. Of the 45 boys evaluated, only 11 individuals (less than 25%) had what was able to be described as a *discernible puberal growth variation.*

What is the Magnitude of the Spurt?

For the 11 subjects in Bjork's 1963 study,[11] he described a slower **condylar growth** rate around 12 years of age, amounting to a mean of 1.5 mm and a spurt 2.0 years later that averaged 5.5 mm and ranged between 4.0 and 8.0 mm (Table 7-3). For the rest of the 34 subjects in the study, there was a more steady annual

TABLE 7-3	Changes in Condylar Growth in the 11 Cases (Out of 45) that Exhibited Puberal Growth Changes	
Condylar Growth	Age (Years)	Change (mm)
Prepuberal minimum	11.8 (9.3 - 13.5)	1.5 (0.5 - 2.0)
Puberal maximum	14.5 (12.9 - 15.5)	5.5 (4.0 - 8.0)

condylar growth that averaged 3.0 mm during the same period. As for the timing of the spurt, the mean age for its occurrence was 14.0 years with a range between 12 and 15 years.[11]

Bjork's findings and conclusions point to the following:

1. There was a discernible, but not necessarily significant, spurt in condylar growth in less than 25% of the sample.
2. The magnitude, duration, and timing of the spurt varied widely even in this selected subsample of 11 subjects.
3. There was no relationship between the intensity of the growth and its direction.

These are the facts that need to be kept in mind particularly when planning the orthodontic treatment of patients with skeletal discrepancies.

How Do Other Nonimplant Longitudinal Studies Describe the Adolescent Changes in Mandibular Growth?

A slightly different picture is presented when the studies by Riolo et al[4] and Broadbent, Broadbent, and Bolton[5] are examined.

In Riolo's et al data,[4] the mean change in the mandibular linear dimension (Ar-Gn) was fairly gradual. Similarly, the change in the anteroposterior relationship of the mandible (SNPog) also described a gradual increase with age. The data from Broadbent, Broadbent, and Bolton[5] on the same parameters also showed a small consistent increase in their magnitude in both males and females with no significant spurts evident.

So how did many orthodontists believe in the universal existence of a mandibular growth spurt? Probably it has to do with the fact that, in some studies, the sample was divided into persons who actually demonstrated a pubertal acceleration in mandibular dimensions and those who did not demonstrate such a change. Only the findings on the first group (i.e., the exceptions) were highlighted.[11] Another possible explanation is that if the scale of any curve is sufficiently enlarged, a small and clinically insignificant acceleration may be made to look fairly impressive.[39-41]

What Do These Findings Mean to the Clinician?

The presence of a significant pubertal acceleration in mandibular parameters may occur in less than 25% of the cases but not in all or even most persons. To expect anything else is wishful thinking. As a result, to routinely postpone or delay treatment in cases with skeletal anteroposterior discrepancies in anticipation of a spurt is not scientifically justifiable. This should not be interpreted to mean that such accelerations do not occur in any one person; it only indicates that changes, which could be described as clinically significant spurts, do not occur in a consistent pattern in the majority of patients.

In reality the clinician is facing two problems: (1) the formidable task of determining which of the subjects within a given population will experience an adolescent growth spurt and (2) for those few who will experience a spurt, the need to predict the timing and magnitude of its occurrence as well as its direction.

In the absence of a consistent and significant growth spurt in adolescence, how can we explain the fact that we are successfully treating most of our growing and cooperating patients who have mild to moderate skeletal discrepancies?

OVERALL GROWTH CHANGES DURING EARLY ADOLESCENCE

In a series of studies on the Iowa Growth sample, the subjects were grouped according to the timing of the greatest change in the rate of growth in any 2 consecutive years between 8 and 17 years of age.[20,21] Such an arrangement accentuates the amount of change in the 2 years that were labeled the *maximum growth period*, and compared with the 2 years before (premaximum) and the 2 years following (postmaximum) this period.

TABLE 7-4	Mean Changes During the 2 Years of Maximum Growth Velocity (Maximum Period), the 2 Years Prior (Premaximum Period), and the 2 Years Following (Postmaximum Period)						
		Maximum Period		Premaximum Period		Postmaximum Period	
Parameter	Sex	$\bar{x}$	SD	$\bar{x}$	SD	$\bar{x}$	SD
Height (cm)	Male	14.1	2.4	12.2	1.2	7.4	2.3
	Female	13.8	1.9	11.8	1.5	5.7	1.9
Ar-Pog (mm)	Male	6.3	1.3	5.4	1.5	3.7	1.6
	Female	4.8	1.0	3.8	0.9	2.8	1.0
SNPog (degrees)	Male	1.2	0.9	1.0	0.5	0.7	0.4
	Female	1.2	0.6	0.8	0.6	0.2	0.2

$\bar{x}$, Mean; *SD*, standard deviation.

Mandibular Growth Changes in the Maximum, Premaximum, and Postmaximum Periods

As stated previously, the comparisons between maximum, premaximum, and postmaximum growth were made with the subjects grouped according to the amount of growth and not according to either their chronologic or skeletal age.

Comparisons between the changes in standing height in the maximum, premaximum, and postmaximum periods indicated that significant differences were present between the three periods of growth for both boys and girls.[21] Similar results were obtained for mandibular length (Ar-Pog). In general, the changes in girls occurred earlier and were of smaller magnitude, but the trends were similar.[21]

Table 7-4 indicates that, for males, the average changes in standing height in the three periods were 14.1, 12.2, and 7.4 cm. The average changes in mandibular length were 6.3, 5.4, and 3.7 mm. The changes in mandibular relationship were 1.2, 1.0, and 0.7 degrees. The results further indicated that no significant differences were present between the premaximum and maximum periods in the changes in mandibular relationships.

The logical conclusion from these findings is that significant growth occurs during adolescence for a relatively long period in most individuals. This is not meant to advocate a particular age for treatment (i.e., early vs. late) because the timing of treatment is dependent on a number of factors including the following:

1. The nature of the malocclusion and its cause
2. The severity of the skeletal discrepancy
3. The presence of a functional shift
4. The stage of dental development, including the relationship of the erupting permanent second molars to the roots of the first molars

5. Growth expectations
6. The ability of the patient to cooperate
7. The need for tooth extractions

PREDICTION OF FACIAL CHANGES FROM SKELETAL BODY CHANGES

Is There a Relationship Between the Timing of Changes in the Facial Parameters and in Standing Height?

In the same series of studies a special type of analysis referred to as *autocorrelation analysis* was used to determine the relationship between the timing of various growth events in the face and standing height.[21,22] In other words, the analysis compares, on a longitudinal basis, the growth profile of the various facial parameters to that of standing height between 8 and 15 years of age.

The findings indicated that, with one exception, all the correlations between the timing of the changes in height and those for the changes in mandibular, maxillary, and cranial base length and relationships were below 0.5. Only mandibular length in girls had a clinically significant correlation with the timing of changes in standing height ($r = 0.83$).

What About the Correlations Between the Timing of Facial Growth Events and the General Skeletal Maturation, as Determined from Wrist X-rays?

In 1990 Moore, Moyer, and DuBois[42] assessed the relevance of hand-wrist radiographs to craniofacial growth and clinical orthodontics. They evaluated serial cephalometric and hand-wrist radiographs on 86 children between 11 and 16 years of age. They used

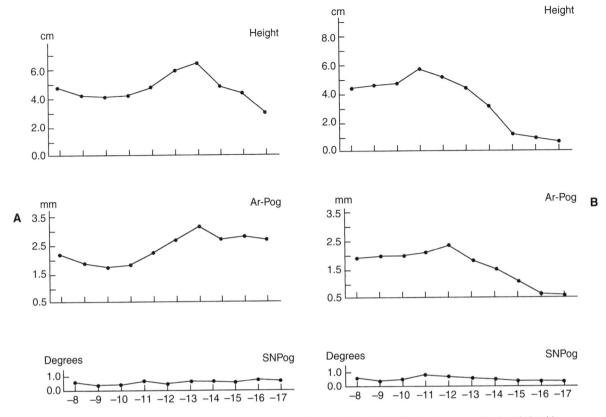

Figure 7-3 Mean incremental changes in standing height, mandibular length (Ar-Pog), and mandibular relationship (SNPog) for 20 male (**A**) and 15 female (**B**) subjects illustrating the yearly changes between 8 and 17 years of age.

four skeletal linear measurements that are known to have statistically significant increases during that period. Their results indicated that growth spurts could not be consistently observed on an individual basis and that the correlations between adolescent growth acceleration and deceleration in the facial dimensions, with both standing height and skeletal maturity as determined from wrist x-rays, were not clinically significant for prediction.

Therefore this brief review strongly suggests that, in general, there is a lack of clinically useful correlations between the timing of change in either standing height or wrist x-rays as indicators of skeletal maturation and the changes in the various dentofacial parameters that clinicians are interested in predicting.

Is the Change in Mandibular Length Accompanied by a Corresponding Forward Positioning of the Mandible?

Clinicians are interested in finding out whether the increase in mandibular length is going to be translated as a forward positioning of pogonion. It can be readily illustrated from the graphs of the mean curves that as mandibular length increases, we do not observe a corresponding forward position at the chin point (Figure 7-3).

Individual curves further indicated that the changes in mandibular relationship are expressed as a relatively constant change between 8 and 17 years of age. Even in those cases that expressed a spurt in mandibular length, the change in mandibular relationship did not express a corresponding significant spurt in the forward positioning of the chin point (Figure 7-4). Therefore the forward positioning of the chin is more dependent on forward mandibular rotation/translation than on the simple increase in mandibular length! This has been previously illustrated by Bjork,[27] who found that similar amounts and directions of growth at the condyles can be expressed differently at pogonion depending on whether the center of rotation of the mandible is at the condyles, the premolars, or the incisors.

Is There a Difference in the Treatment Results If Orthopedic/Orthodontic Changes Are Initiated at Different Stages of Development?

Tulloch, Philips, and Proffit[43] prospectively evaluated 166 children in the mixed dentition stage between 7 and 12 years of age. The children had an increased overjet ranging from 7 to 12 mm. Tulloch and her colleagues[43] randomly assigned these patients to one of

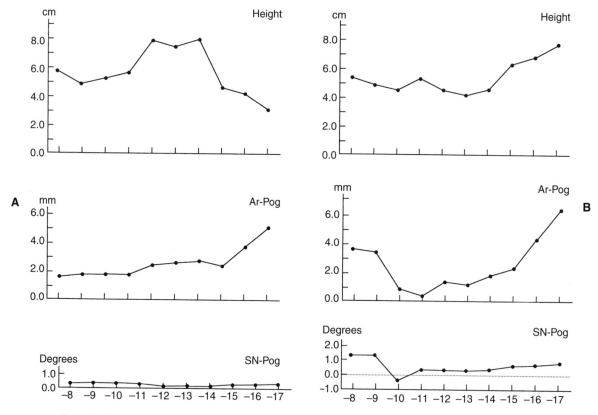

Figure 7-4 Individual incremental curves for two male subjects illustrating the variation in the yearly changes of various parameters between 8 and 17 years of age.

three groups: observation only with no treatment (N = 61), bionator treatment (N = 53), and headgear only treatment (N = 52).

In one part of the study the effects of treatment on the dentofacial structures were related to the time treatment was initiated as it relates to chronologic age, dental age, and skeletal age as determined from wrist x-rays. The overall changes in the dentofacial structures over 15 months of treatment were correlated to each of the three maturity indicators. Their findings indicated that these correlations were close to 0 (i.e., a low association between the magnitude of treatment changes and treatment timing). Data from Keeling et al[44] and Ghafari et al,[45] in similar prospective studies in Florida and Pennsylvania, respectively, confirmed the results obtained by Tulloch, Philips, and Proffit[43] in North Carolina.

CLINICAL IMPLICATIONS

The conclusions from these studies strongly suggest that there is little to be gained from timing growth modification treatment to a particular stage of maturation, whether it is chronologic, dental, or skeletal. Therefore similar treatment results can be obtained over a wider age range in the child's development.[43]

That fact explains why treating most patients, in spite of scientific and clinical biases, is successful.

In treatment planning cases with anteroposterior discrepancies in growing individuals, the clinician should consider four important points:

1. The timing of mandibular changes in both size and relationship are not closely correlated to each other as well as to the changes in standing height or wrist x-rays; hence it is not accurately predictable from these parameters.

2. There are significant mandibular changes in size and relationship between the ages of 8 and 17 years. The changes in mandibular relationship were not significantly different in the maximum and premaximum periods in either boys or girls. The magnitude of change in the postmaximum period tended to be smaller than in the other two periods.

3. The treatment of anteroposterior discrepancies should be initiated as soon as the orthodontist believes that treatment is indicated instead of waiting for the pubertal spurt. This is because the occurrence, magnitude, and timing of the spurt in a particular patient is highly unpredictable, at least to the degree that renders them clinically useful to the orthodontist and profitable to the patient.

CLINICAL CONSIDERATIONS

Instead of the clinician attempting a hit-and-miss approach to prediction, it may be wiser to use more straightforward concepts that can be applied in the treatment planning of growing patients with antero-posterior skeletal discrepancies.

Cases with Severe Skeletal Discrepancies
In general, it can be assumed that the existing growth pattern prevails in most of these cases. For example, if a patient has a steep mandibular plane, open bite tendency, long anterior face, and a Class II malocclusion at age 10 years, the probability is high that in most of these cases a vertical growth pattern will continue. As a result the orthopedic correction should include the use of an extraoral high pull force to the molars or any other appropriate appliance that the clinician prefers to use.

Average Skeletal Discrepancy
For the majority of cases, future growth is less predictable. When dealing with these cases, one should assume what can be referred to as the *worst case scenario*. In other words, for the milder version of the case described earlier, the assumption will be that growth is going to proceed in an unfavorable direction relative to the needed correction. The treatment mechanics should avoid extrusive forces whether extraoral or intraoral. As treatment progresses, two possible outcomes may occur. If the case significantly improves as a result of favorable growth and treatment changes, the clinician can easily modify or adjust the mechanics accordingly. On the other hand, if the growth proceeds in an unfavorable direction, the mechanics are already designed with this eventuality in mind.

4. Patient cooperation in wearing extraoral or functional appliances does not seem to improve at the later stages of adolescence. If anything, most of these patients are involved in various activities that would often distract them from wearing such appliances. Actually, Tung and Kiyak[46] performed a study in which they found that younger children, in general, are more cooperative than adolescents.

THE EFFECTS OF ALVEOLAR GROWTH ON THE PLACEMENT OF IMPLANTS

In patients with either a missing central incisor as a result of trauma or a congenitally missing lateral incisor, the treatment options for replacing the lost tooth following orthodontic treatment may include adding a tooth to the Hawley retainer as a temporary solution, acid etched or conventional prosthetic replacement, or placing a single tooth implant.

In the context of this chapter the effects of alveolar growth on the timing of implant placement are briefly discussed. In a 1996 study, Iseri and Solow[47] evaluated cephalograms on patients from the original Bjork material with metallic implants placed in the maxilla and mandible. They found significant anterior alveolar growth that continued into late adolescence and early adulthood. As a result, clinicians should postpone placing an implant in younger patients until alveolar growth is completed. Such growth could result in the implant being progressively in infraocclusion.

CHANGES IN THE MOLAR RELATIONSHIP BETWEEN THE PRIMARY AND PERMANENT DENTITIONS

The changes in the molar relationship were evaluated on 121 individuals (60 males and 61 females) from the Iowa Growth Study.[48] None of these subjects had congenitally missing teeth and none had early loss of primary first or second molars or had undergone orthodontic therapy.

At each developmental stage and for each individual, the molar relationship was measured as the distance (in millimeters) between perpendicular projections on the occlusal plane from the distal surfaces of the upper and lower primary second molar crowns. Similar measurements were obtained from the mesial surfaces of the permanent first molar crowns in the mixed and permanent dentitions. The findings on the 121 subjects were presented for the right and left sides separately for a total of 242 sides.

Terminal Plane Relationship in the Primary Dentition

The terminal plane relationship of the second primary molars can be described as flush, occurring in 29.4% of the individuals; mesial step, occurring in 61.1% of the individuals; or distal step, occurring in 9.5% of the individuals.[48]

Changes from the Primary to the Permanent Dentitions

At the time of eruption of the permanent first molars, their initial occlusion is dependent on the terminal plane relationship of the primary second molars. Therefore in about 30% of the population, the first molars erupt into a cusp-to-cusp relationship (i.e.,

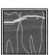

CLINICAL CONSIDERATIONS

It is crucial for the clinician who is involved in early orthodontic treatment to have a good understanding of the anteroposterior occlusal changes that occur from the primary to the permanent dentitions.

Distal Step
If the initial occlusion in the permanent dentition has a **distal step,** the molar relationship in the permanent dentition develops into a Class II. This provides credence to a frequently repeated axiom: "Once a Class II, always a Class II."[48]

Because the distoocclusion in the primary or mixed dentitions does not self-correct with growth, it needs to be emphasized that cases with distal steps in the primary dentition should be observed on a regular basis and treatment started as soon as the clinician and the patient are ready to initiate it.

Flush Terminal Plane Relationship
Individuals with a **flush terminal plane relationship** present a more challenging diagnostic question. Of these cases, 56% became Class I and 44% became Class II in the permanent dentition. In other words, slightly less than half of these cases progress to a Class II or end-to-end occlusion.[48] These findings imply that what was previously considered as "normal" occlusion in the primary or mixed dentition in reality does not often result in a "normal" occlusion in the permanent dentition. Therefore it is important for the clinician to closely observe these cases and to initiate treatment when needed.

It needs to be emphasized that, in the 56.4% of the individuals with flush terminal plane, placing a lower lingual holding arch to maintain space may have an adverse effect on the developing dentition (i.e., it may prevent more cases with a flush terminal plane from becoming Class I). This is important to remember because orthodontists, pediatric dentists, and general dentists often consider placing a lower lingual arch as a preventive or interceptive but noninvasive procedure.

One can readily imagine how maintaining arch length and preventing the mesial drift of the mandibular permanent molars can adversely affect the changes in the molar relationship from the mixed dentition to the permanent dentition. As a result, in cases with an end-to-end molar relationship in which a lingual arch is placed, the clinician should consider the possibility of placing a headgear or other appliances to obtain a Class I occlusion. The parents should be made aware of such a possibility beforehand.

1-mm Mesial Step
Of the cases with a 1-mm **mesial step,** 76% became Class I, 23% changed to a Class II, and 1% became a Class III relationship. In cases with a mesial step of 2 mm or more in the primary dentition, 68% became a Class I, 13% became a Class II, and 19% became a Class III relationship. These findings indicated that the greater the mesial step, the greater the probability for the molar relationship to develop into a Class I or Class III occlusion. The findings also indicated that a more favorable molar relationship in the primary dentition lessens the chance for a Class II occlusion developing in the permanent dentition but does not prevent it! Thus some cases with a mesial step may still develop into Class II molars in the permanent dentition, but such changes occur in a smaller percentage of cases.[48]

Class III Molar Relationship
Finally, the incidence of a Class III molar relationship in the permanent dentition increased as the magnitude of the mesial step increased in the primary dentition. The incidence was 1% with a 1-mm mesial step and increased to 19% with a mesial step of 2 mm or more.[48]

In summary, it is necessary to periodically evaluate the changes in the occlusal relationship in young patients to inform the parents of any developing adverse relationships that may require future treatment.

---

with the mesiobuccal cusp of the maxillary first permanent molar anterior to the buccal groove of the mandibular first permanent molar).

The 23 sides with distal steps in the initial occlusion (9.5% of the total) all progressed to either have a Class II tendency or a full Class II molar relationship in the permanent dentition. In general, there was a tendency for the distal occlusion to improve slightly with age but not to the extent of becoming a Class I relationship.

A change to a Class I molar relationship occurred in two cases as a result of the premature loss of the mandibular second primary molars caused by dental caries. These two cases were not included in the study.

In the 71 sides with flush terminal planes (29.4% of the total), 56.3% became Class I and 43.7% became Class II in the permanent dentition. These findings indicated that the presence of a flush terminal plane in the primary dentition would result in an end-to-end relationship at the time of eruption of the first permanent molars. Unfortunately, 44% of these cases will end up with a Class II occlusion.

Of the 101 sides with a 1.0-mm mesial step in the primary dentition (41.7% of the total), 76.2% became

---

BOX 7-2

Summary of Facial Changes

1. The growth changes in the face are both complex and highly variable, as has been demonstrated from the low correlations between the changes in the various facial parameters.
2. The same can be said about the relationship between the changes in the facial parameters to the various indices of skeletal maturation such as standing height and wrist x-rays. Contemporary methods are generally incapable of providing an efficient estimate of individual changes attributable to growth.
3. The adolescent growth spurt in the mandible occurs in less than 25% of the cases, but the presence, onset, duration, and magnitude of the pubertal growth spurt in facial dimensions cannot be accurately predicted for any one individual.
4. Substantial mandibular growth occurs during adolescence over a number of years. Therefore in the presence of significant skeletal discrepancies, treatment should not be postponed in anticipation of the elusive spurt, particularly if treatment is indicated at an earlier age.

5. At the present time the simplest method of predicting changes in facial dimensions is to start with the facial type presented by the patient and add the average growth changes expected for that face type. Obviously this method has its limitations regarding the prediction of individual changes, but it is as good, or as bad, as any other more complex method.
6. In regards to the future changes in facial relationships, treatment planning should be based on a worst case scenario. In other words, for individuals with unfavorable skeletal relationships, it is wiser to design a treatment plan with the assumption that the same facial growth pattern will be maintained during the treatment period. Favorable growth changes, if they occur, make the treatment objectives easier to accomplish.
7. Orthodontists should be familiar with the effects of the mechanics used on the facial and dental structures. Therefore growth projections require careful attention to the mechanics used.

Class I, 22.8% became Class II, and only one side became Class III in the permanent dentition. Of the 47 sides with a mesial step of 2.0 mm or more in the primary dentition (19.4% of the total), 68.1% became Class I, 12.8% became Class II, and 19.1% became Class III in the permanent dentition.

SUMMARY

The ability to forecast or predict growth lies at the very heart of contemporary clinical orthodontics. The orthodontist, in formulating a treatment plan, relies largely on subjective criteria in conceiving the outcome of treatment. This intuitive perception is necessary, but the overall approach should be based on the available scientific information.

There are at least five components to be dealt with in the prediction of craniofacial changes: the direction, the magnitude, the timing, the rate of change, and the effects of treatment.[32]

In general, orthodontists are well informed regarding the effects of orthodontic treatment on the patient but are not yet able to accurately predict the direction, timing, and magnitude of the facial changes that occur with growth in any one individual (Box 7-2).

REFERENCES

1. Kraus BS, Wise WJ, Frei RH: Heredity and the craniofacial complex, *Am J Orthod* 45:172-217, 1959.
2. Koski K: Cranial growth centers: facts or fallacies, *Am J Orthod* 54:566-583, 1968.
3. Bishara SE et al: Arch width changes from 6 weeks to 45 years of age, *Am J Orthod Dentofacial Orthop* 111:401-409, 1997.
4. Riolo ML et al: *An atlas of craniofacial growth,* Monograph no 2, Craniofacial Growth Series, Ann Arbor, Mich, 1974, Center for Human Growth and Development.
5. Broadbent BH Sr, Broadbent BH Jr, Golden WH: *Bolton standards of dentofacial developmental growth,* St Louis, 1975, Mosby.
6. Bishara SE, Peterson L, Bishara EC: Changes in facial dimensions and relationships between the ages of 5 and 25 years, *Am J Orthod* 85:238-252, 1984.
7. Bishara SE, Jakobsen JR: Longitudinal changes in three facial types, *Am J Orthod* 88:466-502, 1985.
8. Smith DW et al: Shifting linear growth during infancy: illustration of genetic factors in growth from fetal life through infancy, *J Pediatr* 89:225-230, 1976.
9. Shields J: *Monozygotic twins brought up apart and brought up together,* London, 1962, O.U.P.
10. Meredith HV, Knott VB: *Height weight interpretation folder for boys and girls,* Washington, D.C., 1963, Joint Committee on Health Problems in Education of the National Education Association and the American Medical Association.

11. Bjork A: Variation in the growth pattern of the human mandible: longitudinal radiographic study by the implant method, *J Dent Res* 42:400-411, 1963.

12. Tweed C: *Clinical orthodontics,* St Louis, 1966, Mosby.

13. Brodie AG: Research in the department of orthodontics graduate college: University of Illinois from 1951 to 1956, *Angle Orthod* 27:196-216, 1957.

14. Moore HW: Observations of facial growth and its clinical significance, *Am J Orthod* 45:399-423, 1959.

15. Horowitz SL, Hixon EH: *The nature of orthodontic diagnosis,* St Louis, 1996, Mosby.

16. Bjork A, Palling M: Adolescent age changes in sagittal jaw relation, alveolar prognathy and incisal inclination, *Acta Odont Scand* 12:201, 1955.

17. Bjork A: The significance of growth changes in facial pattern and their relationship to changes in occlusion, *Dental Rec* 71:197, 1951.

18. Harvold E: Some biologic aspects of orthodontic treatment in the transitional dentition, *Am J Orthod* 49:1, 1962.

19. Lande MJ: Growth behavior of the human bony facial profile as revealed by serial cephalometric roentgenology, *Angle Orthod* 22:78-90, 1952.

20. Solow B, Siersbaek-Nielsen S: Growth changes in head posture related to craniofacial development, *Am J Orthod* 89:132-140, 1986.

21. Bishara SE et al: Longitudinal changes in standing height and mandibular parameters between the ages of 8 and 17 years, *Am J Orthod* 80:115-135, 1981.

22. Jamison J et al: Longitudinal changes in the maxilla and the maxillary-mandibular relationship between 8 and 17 years of age, *Am J Orthod* 82:217-220, 1982.

23. Meredith HV: Changes in form of the head and face during childhood, *Growth* 24:215-264, 1960.

24. Meredith HV: Childhood interrelations of anatomic growth rates, *Growth* 26:23, 1962.

25. Meredith HV: Interage relations of anatomic measures, *Adv Child Dev Behav* 2:222-253, 1963.

26. Bjork A: The face in profile, *Sven Tandlak Tidskr* 40, 1947.

27. Bjork A: Prediction of mandibular growth rotation, *Am J Orthod* 55:585-599, 1966.

28. Skieller V, Bjork A, Linde-Hansen T: Prediction of mandibular growth rotation evaluated from a longitudinal implant sample, *Am J Orthod* 86:359-370, 1984.

29. Ricketts RM: The value of cephalometrics and computerized technology, *Angle Orthod* 42:179-199, 1972.

30. Ricketts R et al: An overview of computerized cephalometrics, *Am J Orthod* 61:1-28, 1972.

31. Ricketts RJ et al: An overview of computerized prediction: the accuracy of a contemporary long-range forecast, *Am J Orthod* 67:243-252, 1975.

32. Ricketts RM: The influence of orthodontic treatment on facial growth and development, *Angle Orthod* 30:103-133, 1960.

33. Greenberg L, Johnston L: Computerized prediction: the accuracy of a contemporary long-range forecast, *Am J Orthod* 67:243-251, 1975.

34. Cangialosi TJ et al: Reliability of computer generated prediction tracing, *Angle Orthod* 65:277-284, 1995.

35. Hirschfield W: Time series and exponential smoothing methods applied to the analysis and prediction of growth, *Growth* 35:129-143, 1970.

36. Hirschfield W, Moyers R: Prediction of craniofacial growth: the state of the art, *Am J Orthod* 60:435-443, 1971.

37. Hixon EH: Cephalometrics: a perspective, *Angle Orthod* 42:200-211, 1972.

38. Hixon EH, Klein P: Simplified mechanics: a means of treatment based on available scientific information, *Am J Orthod* 62:113-141, 1972.

39. Bambha JK: Longitudinal cephalometric roentgenographic study of face and cranium in relation to body height, *J Am Dent Assoc* 63:776-799, 1961.

40. Bambha JK, Von Natta P: Longitudinal study of facial growth in relation to skeletal maturation during adolescence, *Am J Orthod* 49:481-492, 1963.

41. Bergersen E: The male adolescent facial growth spurt: its prediction and relation to skeletal maturation, *Angle Orthod* 42:319-338, 1972.

42. Moore RN, Moyer BA, DuBois LM: Skeletal maturation and craniofacial growth, *Am J Orthod Dentofacial Orthop* 98:33-40, 1990.

43. Tulloch JFC, Philips C, Proffit WR: Benefit of early Class II treatment: progress report of a two-phase randomized clinical trial, *Am J Orthod Dentofacial Orthop* 113:62-72, 1998.

44. Keeling SD et al: Anteroposterior skeletal and dental changes after early Class II treatment with bionators and headgear, *Am J Orthod Dentofacial Orthop* 113:40-50, 1998.

45. Ghafari J et al: Headgear versus function regulator in the early treatment of Class II, division 1 malocclusion: a randomized clinical trial, *Am J Orthod Dentofacial Orthop* 113:51-61, 1998.

46. Tung AW, Kiyak HA: Psychological influences on the timing of orthodontic treatment, *Am J Orthod Dentofacial Orthop* 113:29-39, 1998.

47. Iseri H, Solow B: Continued eruption of maxillary incisors and first molars in girls from 9 to 25 years: studied by the implant method, *Eur J Orthod* 18:245-256, 1996.

48. Bishara SE et al: Changes in the molar relationship between the deciduous and permanent dentitions: a longitudinal study, *Am J Orthod Dentofacial Orthop* 93:19-28, 1988.

SUGGESTED READINGS

1. Balbach DR: The cephalometric relationship between the morphology of the mandible and its future occlusal position, *Angle Orthod* 39:29-41, 1969.

2. Bennett GG, Kronman JH: A cephalometric study of mandibular development and its relationship to the mandibular and occlusal planes, *Angle Orthod* 40:119-128, 1970.

3. Bergersen E: The male adolescent facial growth spurt: its prediction and relation to skeletal maturation, *Angle Orthod* 42:319-338, 1972.

4. Bjork A: The significance of growth changes in facial pattern and their relationship to changes in occlusion, *Dental Rec* 71:197, 1951.

5. Bjork A: Prediction of mandibular growth rotation, *Am J Orthod* 55:585-599, 1966.

6. Bjork A, Helm S: Prediction of the age of maximum puberal growth in body height, *Angle Orthod* 37:134-143, 1967.

7. Bookstein F: On the cephalometrics of skeletal change, *Am J Orthod* 82:177-198, 1982.

8. Brown T, Barrett MJ, Grave KC: Facial growth and skeletal maturation at adolescence, *Tandlaegebladet* 75:1211-1222, 1971.

9. Burstone C: Process of maturation and growth prediction, *Am J Orthod* 49:907-919, 1963.

10. Chapman SM: Ossification of the adductor sesamoid and the adolescent growth spurt, *Angle Orthod* 42:236-244, 1972.

11. Creekmore TD: Inhibition or stimulation of the vertical growth of the facial complex: its significance to treatment, *Angle Orthod* 37:285-297, 1967.

12. DeMisch A, Waterman P: Calcification of the mandibular third molar and its relation to skeletal and chronologic age in children, *Child Dev* 27:459, 1956.

13. Frisancho R, Garn S, Rohmann C: Age at menarche: a new method of prediction and retrospective assessment based on hand x-rays, *Hum Biol* 41:42-50, 1969.

14. Gilda JE: Analysis of linear facial growth, *Angle Orthod* 44:1-14, 1974.

15. Graber TM: *Orthodontics: current principles and techniques*, ed 3, St Louis, 2000, Mosby.

16. Greulich WW, Pyle SI: *Radiographic atlas of skeletal development of the hand and wrist*, ed 2, Stanford, Calif, 1959, Standford University Press.

17. Hagg U, Taranger J: Maturation indicators and the pubertal growth spurt, *Am J Orthod* 82:299-309, 1982.

18. Harvold E: Some biologic aspects of orthodontic treatment in the transitional dentition, *Am J Orthod* 49:1, 1962.

19. Hirschfield W: Time series and exponential smoothing methods applied to the analysis and prediction of growth, *Growth* 35:129-143, 1970.

20. Hirschfield W, Moyers R: Prediction of craniofacial growth: the state of the art, *Am J Orthod* 60:435-443, 1971.

21. Hunter WS, Balbach R, Lamphier E: The heritability of attained growth in the human face, *Am J Orthod* 58:128-134, 1970.

22. Jamison J et al: Longitudinal changes in the maxilla and the maxillary-mandibular relationship between 8 and 17 years of age, *Am J Orthod* 82:217-230, 1982.

23. Johnston LE: A statistical evaluation of cephalometric prediction, *Angle Orthod* 38:284-304, 1968.

24. King EW: Variations in profile change and their significance in timing treatment, *Angle Orthod* 30:141-153, 1960.

25. Knott VB: Changes in cranial base measures of human males and females from age 6 years to early adulthood, *Growth* 35:145-158, 1971.

26. Kraus S, Wise J, Frei H: Heredity and the craniofacial complex, *Am J Orthod* 45:172-217, 1959.

27. Lauterstein AM: A cross-sectional study in dental development and skeletal age, *J Am Dent Assoc* 62:161-167, 1961.

28. Maj G, Luzi C: The role of cephalometrics in the diagnosis and prognosis of malocclusions, *Am J Orthod* 48:911-923, 1962.

29. Meredith HV: Changes in form of the head and face during childhood, *Growth* 24:215-264, 1960.

30. Meredith HV: Childhood interrelations of anatomic growth rates, *Growth* 24:23, 1962.

31. Moore HW: Observations of facial growth and its clinical significance, *Am J Orthod* 45:399-423, 1959.

32. Nanda RS: The rates of growth of several facial components measured from serial cephalometric roentgenograms, *Am J Orthod* 41:658-673, 1955.

33. Poulton DR: Changes in Class II malocclusions with and without occipital headgear therapy, *Angle Orthod* 29:234-250, 1959.

34. Ricketts RM: Planning treatment on the basis of the facial pattern and an estimate of its growth, *Angle Orthod* 27:14, 1957.

35. Ricketts RM: Cephalometric synthesis, *Am J Orthod* 46:647-672, 1960.

36. Ricketts RM: Cephalometric analysis and synthesis, *Angle Orthod* 31:141-156, 1961.

37. Ricketts RM: The value of cephalometrics and computerized technology, *Angle Orthod* 42:179-199, 1972.

38. Schudy FF: The rotation of the mandible resulting from growth: its implications in orthodontic treatment, *Angle Orthod* 35:36-50, 1965.

39. Silverstein A: Changes in the bony facial profile with treatment of Class II, Division I (Angle) malocclusion, *Angle Orthod* 24:214-237, 1954.

40. Sutow WW, Terasalei T, Onwada K: Comparison of skeletal maturation with dental status in Japanese children, *Pediatrics* 14:327-333, 1954.

41. Tofani MI: Mandibular growth at puberty, *Am J Orthod* 61:176-195, 1972.

CHAPTER 8

Etiology and Prevalence of Malocclusion

Robert N. Staley

KEY TERMS

etiology	arch form	overjet	maxillary diastema
hereditary	near-ideal occlusion	posterior crossbites	overbite
genetic	crowding	incisor alignment	open bite
environmental factors	malalignment		

ETIOLOGY OF MALOCCLUSION

Clinicians who treat malocclusions need information about their **etiology** to prevent, intercept, and treat occlusal problems. The etiology of a malocclusion is the study of its cause or causes. Malocclusions have two basic causes: (1) **hereditary,** or **genetic,** factors and (2) **environmental factors.** Knowledge of hereditary factors helps a clinician plan and execute treatment that effectively addresses genetic causes. Knowledge of environmental factors also directs treatment decisions and involves strategies to prevent the continued influence of environmental factors on the occlusion of the teeth. For example, malocclusions resulting from an environmental factor such as thumbsucking can be prevented if the habit is stopped before the age of 5 or 6 years in a child who is experiencing normal craniofacial and occlusal development. Thumbsucking intercepted in older children with mixed dentitions may, if stopped, require no additional treatment; however, many older children and adolescents may need orthodontic treatment to correct the effects of the habit. On the other hand, when thumbsucking occurs in a child who has a developing Class II Division 1 malocclusion, the habit is one etiologic factor superimposed on perhaps several other factors including heredity. Stopping the habit in the child with a Class II maloc-

clusion addresses only one, albeit important, etiologic factor. Therefore knowledge about the cause of a patient's malocclusion is important for the appropriate diagnosis and treatment of that patient.

Influence of Heredity on Skeletal and Dental Variables

Harris and Johnson[1] studied the heritability of skeletal and tooth-based variables in a longitudinal study of 30 sibships at 4, 14, and 20 years of age. Estimates of heritability for each phenotypic or morphologic variable studied were derived from intraclass correlation (between siblings) computed by analysis of variance. *Heritability* for measured variables in siblings was defined as twice the intraclass correlation. The theoretic upper limit of the genetic contribution for a first-degree relative (a sibling) is a heritability estimate of 50%, but, because of sampling fluctuation and environmental covariation (enhanced acquired similarity), heritability estimates can exceed 50% with an upper boundary greater than 100%. A heritability estimate of 50% implies that a measured variable is under considerable genetic control, whereas a heritability estimate near 0% implies that a variable is influenced primarily by environmental factors. Twenty-nine skeletal craniometric variables showed significant heritability that increased from an average of 62% at 4 years of age to an average correlation of 80% at 20 years of age. Craniofacial parameters that showed significant heritability at all three ages included the following distances: sella-gnathion, sella-A point, sella-gonion, nasion-anterior nasal spine, articulare-pogonion, bimaxillofrontale breadth, bizygomatic breadth, bialare breadth, and anterior face height index (nasion-anterior nasal spine distance divided by nasion-menton distance). The average heritability estimates for these particular distances increased from 80% at 4 years of age to 120% at 20 years of age. These parameters are important in craniofacial growth and can have an important impact on the development of malocclusions. In contrast, Harris and Johnson[1] found much lower heritability estimates for arch and occlusal parameters, and the trend was a decrease in heritability from 4 to 20 years of age. The average heritability estimate of seven arch dimensions and indices was 80% at 4 years of age and −5% at 20 years of age. The average heritability estimate for 11 occlusal parameters including interincisal angle, overbite, arch crowding, incisor irregularity, posterior crossbites, and tooth rotations was 43% at 4 years of age and 24% at 20 years of age. In other words, the occlusal and arch parameters were affected minimally by genetic influences and experienced increasing influence from environmental factors throughout postnatal growth.

Heredity and Arch Form

Cassidy et al[2] studied the genetic influence on dental **arch form** in 320 adolescent orthodontic patients in 155 sibships. Heritability estimates were computed as described previously for Harris and Johnson.[1] Forty-eight parameters grouped as tooth rotations, arch widths, arch depths, arch chords, and arch interrelationships were measured on plaster casts. Tooth rotations had heritability estimates essentially equal to 0%. Twelve different arch width variables had a mean heritability of 57%, indicating that arch widths are under considerable genetic influence. The mean heritability estimates for 9 different arch depth variables was 45%, for 12 different arch chord variables was 40%, and for 6 different arch shape variables was 39%, all significantly lower than the estimate for arch widths. Arch interrelationships were defined as (1) the distance along the occlusal plane between the mesiobuccal cusp tip of the maxillary permanent first molar and buccal groove of the mandibular permanent first molar—basically, a quantitative measure of Angle's classification, and (2) incisor overjet. The heritability estimate for anteroposterior relationship of the first molars (Angle classification) was 56%, showing appreciable genetic influence. The heritability estimate for incisor

overjet was 23%, indicating that overjet is primarily influenced by environmental factors.

These findings support the view that an important aspect of the etiology of malocclusions is environmental in origin. A number of primarily environmental causes are known such as habits, trauma, caries, periodontal disease, chronic nasal obstruction with mouth breathing,[3] and reduced masticatory stress resulting from the soft consistency of foods in urbanized societies. The association between soft dietary consistency and the development of malocclusion has been supported by several studies conducted by Corruccini and fellow investigators.[4-7] This factor probably plays a major role in the large frequency of crowded and rotated teeth observed in people living in urban societies. Future investigations need to further explore the environmental etiologic factors that lead to malocclusion so that malocclusions can be more easily prevented and treated more successfully.

Other known causes of malocclusion include clefts of the alveolus and palate that occur during fetal growth, genetic syndromes that affect the development of craniofacial structures, and supernumerary and congenitally absent teeth that predominantly result from heritable factors.

PREVALENCE OF MALOCCLUSION

A modern country knows the frequencies of different malocclusion problems among its citizens so that it can inform its dental profession about the scope of these problems and better serve the needs of those who suffer from malocclusion. Epidemiologists who collect information about malocclusion frequency gather data about the prevalence and severity of malocclusions in the sex and race subgroups. Epidemiologists cooperate with dental professionals, especially orthodontists, so that the information obtained about malocclusions is relevant to those who treat patients.

Several methods have been used to collect data on the prevalence of malocclusion in populations. Many surveys have included the classification system of Angle[17] in the collection of data related to the incidence of malocclusion. Before Angle introduced his system for classifying malocclusions, an array of complicated and confusing classification methods were used by clinicians. Malocclusion occurs in all three planes of space and affects each tooth in all three planes. Angle brilliantly perceived that malocclusions could be meaningfully grouped into three major classes based on the anteroposterior relationship of the maxillary and mandibular permanent first molars (see Chapters 5 and 9). Angle's classes include most of the problems that motivate patients to seek treatment.

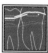

CLINICAL CONSIDERATIONS

Knowledge of the contribution of genetic and environmental causes of malocclusion obligates clinicians to differentiate between patients whose malocclusions are primarily of genetic origin from patients whose malocclusions are primarily of environmental origin. Abnormal morphologic structures in the face and dentition that have a high degree of heritability require different treatment approaches from those structures that are influenced primarily by environmental factors. For example, a young patient with a Class II malocclusion who has a maxilla in normal position but a mandible that is retrusive is a good candidate for orthopedic headgear treatment aimed at redirecting maxillary growth and allowing the mandible to catch up with the maxilla. Orthopedic treatments with headgears, activators, and chin cups address heritable etiologic factors. The widening of an abnormally narrow palate and dental arch with a rapid maxillary expander is another example of orthopedic treatment of a predominantly heritable etiologic factor. In adults, abnormal craniofacial structures that probably have a high degree of heritability, such as retrusive and prognathic mandibles, can be treated with orthognathic surgery.

In contrast, growing and adult patients with more normal anteroposterior, vertical, and transverse relationships for the maxilla and mandible who also happen to have a Class I, Class II, or a Class III malocclusion are candidates for treatments that focus on moving teeth as opposed to influencing facial structures. For most patients the differentiation between genetic and local

environmental factors is of great importance when choosing the appropriate treatment and retention plans.

Retention of a treated malocclusion is a challenge because the genetic and environmental etiologic factors responsible for the malocclusion may continue to draw the treated teeth back into malocclusion.[8-12] Stability of treated malocclusions appears to be similar in growing and adult patients.[13] Addressing known etiologic factors during treatment can produce more stable occlusions after treatment. For example, rotated teeth have strong tendencies to return to their pretreatment irregularity.[14] Gingival fibers are one of the factors that cause relapse of teeth that were rotated during treatment. Gingival fibrotomies help stabilize rotated teeth.[15] Placement of teeth in appropriate positions, angulations, inclinations, and occlusal relations during treatment is important for stability following active tooth movement. The wearing of well-designed retainers is another important factor in stabilizing treated malocclusions.

Prevention of genetic causes for malocclusion is not possible at this time. In contrast, the prevention of environmental causes holds much promise. The control of habits, the prevention of caries[16] and periodontal disease, and the wearing of devices that protect the teeth during athletic events are examples of effective preventative measures. Corruccini and others[4-7] have provided convincing evidence that a diet of soft food causes malocclusion; however, the prevention of malocclusion by avoiding a soft food diet is difficult for a patient whose entire culture is deeply immersed in a cooked, soft, and cariogenic diet.

Limitations of Angle's Classification in Assessing the Prevalence of Malocclusion

Angle's classes do not differentiate malocclusions having dental arch anteroposterior discrepancies from those associated with anteroposterior imbalances in facial structures. Also, the Angle classification system does not include any assessment of vertical and transverse problems. Overbite is a commonly used measure of vertical occlusal relations in the dentition but is not a measure of vertical relationships of the skeletal facial structures. Crossbites in the transverse plane can be simple two-teeth problems or complex discrepancies involving most of the maxillary and mandibular posterior teeth. The Angle classification system does not assess tooth malalignment problems such as rotation, crowding, and spacing of teeth that occur frequently in residents of the United States. Other factors such as congenital absence and impaction of teeth that require

orthodontic treatment are not accounted for in the Angle classification system. Therefore an epidemiologic survey cannot rely solely on the Angle classification system because important factors such as tooth alignment, overbite, overjet, and crossbites are not assessed.

Knowledge of the association between the Angle classes and tooth alignment, transverse, and vertical problems is useful to health care providers. These associations help differentiate simpler malocclusion problems such as an alignment problem in a Class I malocclusion from more complex problems such as a Class II Division 1 malocclusion with a posterior crossbite and anterior open bite.

Some claim the Angle classification system is too subjective for use in epidemiology.[18,19] This criticism is valid when investigators do not set objective limits on continuous variables such as tooth crowding and first molar anteroposterior position. For instance, persons with Class I molar relations can have ideal occlusion, normal occlusion, and Class I malocclusion. For example, these three groups can be differentiated by obtaining an objective measure of incisor irregularity[20] and assigning ideal occlusion to a score of 0 (perfect alignment), normal occlusion to a score of 1, and a Class I malocclusion to a score above 1. Similarly some first molar relations fall between Classes I and II and between Classes I and III. Class I, II, and III molar relations can be differentiated by establishing an objective range of, say, 2 mm mesial and distal to the buccal groove of the lower first molar in which the mesiobuccal cusp tip of the upper first molar is considered to be Class I. These methodologic problems probably account for much of the variability observed in studies that used the Angle classification system to assess the prevalence of malocclusion.

Indices of Malocclusion

Grainger[21] developed the orthodontic Treatment Priority Index (TPI), which summed six occlusal features into a score that differentiated persons with normal occlusion from those with varying degrees of malocclusion. The six occlusal features were (1) first molar relationship, (2) overjet (horizontal incisor relation), (3) overbite and open bite (vertical incisor relation), (4) tooth displacement (crowding, rotations), (5) congenitally missing teeth, and (6) posterior crossbite. Scores were assigned as follows: 0 = normal; 1 to 3 = minor deviations; 4 to 6 = definite deviations, treatment elective; 7 to 9 = handicapping malocclusion, treatment desirable; and 10+ = severe handicapping malocclusion, treatment necessary. The TPI was used by the United States Public Health Service when it surveyed occlusion in children and adolescents between 1963 and 1970.[22,23]

Several additional methods for assessing malocclusion in populations, such as the epidemiologic registration method of Bjork, Krebs, and Solow,[24] the method developed by the Federation Dentaire Internationale,[25] the Dental Aesthetic Index,[26] and the Malocclusion Severity Index,[27] have been developed and used. Other indices that have been developed but not widely used include Salzmann's Handicapping Malocclusion Assessment Record,[28] Summer's Occplusal Index,[29] and Uniform Methods for the Epidemiologic Assessment of Malocclusion developed by the World Health Organization.[30]

STUDIES OF THE PREVALENCE OF MALOCCLUSION USING ANGLE CLASSIFICATION

Because the Angle classification method is relevant to clinicians, and encompasses the majority of malocclusions observed in patients, a review of some of the studies that have used this method seems appropriate.

The variability among studies is evident in a summary of earlier publications.[31]

The United States

Several studies conducted among white American adolescents are summarized in Table 8-1.[32-37] Total malocclusion frequencies varied from 46% to 87% with a mean of 66.7%. The frequency of Class I malocclusion varied from 28% to 72% with a mean of 45.8%. The frequency of Class II malocclusion varied from 6.6% to 29% with a mean of 18%. The frequency of Class III malocclusion varied from 1% to 9.4% with a mean of 3%. It is probable that white American adolescents do not actually have such a wide range of malocclusion frequencies and that the variability in Table 8-1 is most likely related to a lack of agreement among observers in their definitions of the Angle classes.

A study of Angle's classes in a sample of African-American adolescents in the United States is summarized in Table 8-2.[38] Total malocclusion frequency in the sample was high, the frequency of Class I malocclusion was high, the frequency of Class II malocclusion was lower when compared to most of the studies of white American adolescents in Table 8-1, and the frequency of Class III malocclusion was somewhat higher than most of the studies of white American adolescents (see Table 8-1).

A survey of Angle's classes in a sample of Native American Chippewa Indian children and adolescents (6 to 18 years of age) living in Minnesota is summarized in Table 8-3.[39] The frequencies of total malocclusion and Class I malocclusion in Chippewa Indian children were high, whereas the frequencies of Class II and Class III malocclusion were lower or similar to that of white or black American adolescents (see Tables 8-1 and 8-2).

Other Societies

Helm[40] studied malocclusion in 1700 Danish children and adolescents 9 to 18 years of age and found that about 14% had normal occlusion, 58% had Class I malocclusion, 24% had Class II malocclusion, and about 4% had Class III malocclusion. The Danish white youth had a malocclusion distribution according to Angle's classification that differed from the averages reported in Table 8-1 for white American adolescents. The Danish children had fewer normal occlusions and more Class I, Class II, and Class III malocclusions than the averages for white Americans. A study of 2349 Norwegian children ages 7 to 8 years yielded the following results: normal occlusion (41.3%), Class I (30.1%), Class II (21.3%), and Class III

TABLE 8-1	Frequency of Malocclusion in American White Children and Adolescents According to Angle's Classification						
					Percent		
Author	N	Ages	Normal Occlusion	Total Malocclusion	Class I	Class II	Class III
Brehm, Jackson (1961)[32]	6328	6-18	16.6	83.4	60.1	22.8	0.5
Emrich, Brodie, Blayney (1965)[33]	13,475	12-14	54.0	46.0	30.0	15.0	1.0
Krogman (1951)[34]	586	6.5-12.5	45.9	54.1	28.0	24.4	1.7
Mills (1966)[35]	1337	13-14	17.5	82.5	72.2	6.6	3.7
Newman (1956)[36]	3355	6-14	48.1	51.9	38.2	13.2	0.5
Savara (1955)[37]	2774	14-17	21.1	78.9	50.1	19.4	9.4
Mean %			33.9	66.1	46.4	16.9	2.8

N, Sample size.

TABLE 8-2	Frequency of Malocclusion in American Black Adolescents 12 to 14 Years Old According to Angle's Classification[38]					
				Percent		
Sex	N	Normal Occlusion	Total Malocclusion	Class I	Class II	Class III
Males	1470	16.5	83.5	67.8	11.4	4.3
Females	1819	16.5	83.5	65.3	12.7	5.5
Both	3289	16.5	83.5	66.4	12.1	5.0

N, Sample size.

TABLE 8-3	Frequency of Malocclusion in American Chippewa Indian Children and Adolescents 6 to 18 Years Old According to Angle's Classification[39]					
				Percent		
Sex	N	Normal Occlusion	Total Malocclusion	Class I	Class II	Class III
Males	329	35.9	64.1	53.8	7.3	3.0
Females	322	33.2	66.8	52.2	11.8	2.8
Both	651	34.6	65.4	53.0	9.5	2.9

N, Sample size.

(7.3%).[41] The Norwegian white children had fewer Class I malocclusions and more normal occlusions and more Class II and Class III malocclusions than the averages for white American children. A survey of 3087 Hungarian youths ages 15 to 20 years yielded fewer malocclusions than the averages for white Americans: normal occlusion (52%), Class I (35.9%), Class II (13%), and Class III (1.1%).[42] A study of 592 Greek young adults produced overall percentages of Angle classes similar to the averaged data for American adolescents in Table 8-1: normal occlusion (38.2%), Class I (36.3%), Class II (23%), Class III (2.5%).[43]

A survey of 335 Polynesians from 12 to 70 years of age of which 150 were male and 185 were female yielded findings significantly different from those reported for white Americans in Table 8-1.[44] The percentages of occlusions were as follows: normal occlusion (57.6%), Class I (24.4%), Class II (3.5%), and Class III (14.4%). No significant sex differences were observed for the incidence of malocclusion. A dental survey of 715 children ages 4 to 18 years was conducted in Ghana, a country on the west coast of Africa.[45] Those with normal occlusion numbered 61.4%, and the malocclusion group had the following frequencies: all abnormal occlusions (38.6%), Class I (36.1%), Class II (1.2%), and Class III (1.3%). A comparison with Canadian children showed that the children of Ghana had fewer overall abnormal occlusions (38.6% compared to 54.9% for Canadians), fewer Class II malocclusions (1.2% compared to 10.4% for Canadians), and fewer Class III malocclusions (1.3% compared to 8.4% in Canadians). A study of 1050 ethnically Chinese children 12 to 14 years of age in Australia[46] showed that 7.1% of the Chinese children had normal occlusion, 58.8% had Class I malocclusion, 21.5% had Class II malocclusion, and 12.6% had Class III malocclusion.

The preceding studies are only a few of the many that have been conducted. They give some insight into the variations found in different ethnic and racial groups. Because the incidence of malocclusions may well change or fluctuate in populations with time, follow-up studies are needed.

STUDIES OF THE PREVALENCE OF MALOCCLUSION USING SPECIFIC CHARACTERISTICS

U.S. Public Health Service Survey, 1963-1970

Information about the dental occlusions of white and black ethnic groups in the United States was gathered in an examination of approximately 8000 children 6 to 11 years of age and adolescents 12 to 17 years of age.[22,23] Specific characteristics of malocclusion such as tooth displacement scores (qualitative measures) and quantitative measures for overjet, overbite, open bite, and numbers of teeth in posterior crossbite were evaluated. The TPI discussed previously was scored to provide and indicate the overall severity of a malocclusion.[21] The results of this survey are summarized in Tables 8-4 and 8-5. **Near-ideal occlusion** was found in about 23% of the whites 6 to 11 years old and in only 10.5% of the whites 12 to 17 years old. Near-ideal occlusion was found in about 33% of blacks 6 to 11 years old and in about 15% of blacks 12 to 17 years old (see Table 8-4). The decrease in the frequency of near-ideal occlusion from childhood to adolescence was also reflected in the data from Illinois children.[33] Moderate and severe malocclusions increased in frequency from childhood to adolescence (see Table 8-4).

Crowding and **malalignment** of the teeth increased in whites and blacks from childhood to adolescence, especially in the severe category in which whites had an increase of about 39% and blacks had an increase of about 32%. In contrast, the percentages of individuals with ideal alignment of the teeth decreased from 57%

TABLE 8-4	Treatment Priority Index Scores for United States Children and Youths, 1963-1970[22,23]			
	Percent Distribution			
	Ages 6-11 Years		Ages 12-17 Years	
Treatment Priority Index Score	White	Black	White	Black
0 (near ideal occlusion)	22.9	33.1	10.5	14.7
1 to 3 (mild malocclusion)	39.7	35.0	34.6	36.9
4 to 6 (moderate malocclusion)	23.7	15.0	25.7	21.0
>6 (severe or very severe malocclusion)	13.7	16.9	29.2	27.4

to 13% in whites and 65% to 16% in blacks (see Table 8-5). Large **overjets** were seen in about 16% of whites and in about 12.5% of black children and adolescents (see Table 8-5). **Posterior crossbites** were observed in 5.4% of the white sample and in 6.6% of the black sample with small increases in both samples from childhood to adolescence (see Table 8-5).

U.S. Public Health Service Survey, 1988-1991

Brunelle, Bhat, and Lipton[47] reported the incidence of certain occlusal traits in noninstitutionalized people in the United States. The data were collected in the Third National Health and Nutrition Examination Survey, Phase I, conducted by the National Center for Health Statistics from 1988-1991. Three racial groups (whites, blacks, and Mexican-Americans) were examined from age 8 years through 50 years.

Incisor Alignment   Incisor alignment was measured in millimeters of irregularity that were summed to form an index.[21] A total score of zero means that the incisors were perfectly aligned mesial to the canine crowns. The distribution of incisor alignment scores is shown in Table 8-6. About one fourth of the persons surveyed had perfect alignment of their maxillary incisors and somewhat fewer persons (21.9%) had perfectly aligned mandibular incisors. Severe irregularity (sum of scores 5 and 6+) was observed in 17.4% of the

maxillary arches and in 20.6% of the mandibular arches—a rather large group, all of whom would be potential orthodontic patients.

The average incisor irregularity score was 2.4 mm in the maxillary arch and 2.7 mm in the mandibular arch (Table 8-7). Blacks had significantly lower maxillary and mandibular incisor alignment scores than the whites and Mexican-Americans, who had statistically similar alignment scores in both arches. Mean incisor alignment scores increased from 8 through 11 years of age to 18 through 50 years of age in both dental arches of all race-ethnicity groups (see Table 8-7). The trend for an increase in incisor irregularity with age is an important factor in the diagnosis, treatment planning, and retention of orthodontic patients who have this problem.

Maxillary Diastema   The prevalence of a diastema between the maxillary central incisors **(maxillary diastema)** of 2 mm or more in width is shown in Table 8-8. When all race-ethnicity groups are pooled, males had a diastema significantly more frequently than females. The prevalence of diastemas in blacks (16.2%) was significantly higher than the prevalences in whites (4.9%) and Mexican-Americans (6.6%) who had statistically similar frequencies of occurrence. The 8- to 11-year-old children in all groups had a higher prevalence of maxillary diastemas than the 12- to 17-year-old adolescents and 18- to 50-year-old adults, primarily because the younger subjects did not have a full complement of erupted permanent teeth.

TABLE 8-5	Percent of United States Children and Youths with Different Malocclusion Characteristics, 1963-1970[22,23]			
	Ages 6-11 Years		Ages 12-17 Years	
Malocclusion Categories	White	Black	White	Black
Crowding/Malalignment				
Tooth displacement score 0 (ideal)	56.8	64.6	13.0	16.0
Tooth displacement score 1 to 5 (moderate)	38.9	32.6	43.6	49.5
Tooth displacement score >5 (severe)	4.3	2.6	43.4	34.5
Anteroposterior				
Overjet 6 mm or more	17.3	13.5	15.3	11.8
Underjet 1 mm or more	0.8	0.6	0.8	1.2
Vertical				
Open bite 2 mm or more	1.4	9.6	1.2	10.1
Overbite 6 mm or more	7.6	0.8	11.7	1.4
Transverse				
Lingual crossbite two or more teeth	4.9	5.3	5.9	8.0
Buccal crossbite two or more teeth	1.0	0.4	1.6	1.0

TABLE 8-6	Distribution of Maxillary and Mandibular Incisor Alignment Scores Among Americans Ages 8 to 50 Years, 1988-1991[47]

	Maxillary			Mandibular	
mm	N	Percent	mm	N	Percent
0	1699	24.6	0	1718	21.9
1	1609	23.2	1	1451	20.5
2	1095	16.7	2	1190	16.9
3	702	9.6	3	742	10.9
4	535	8.4	4	586	9.2
5	321	6.0	5	368	5.9
6+	750	11.4	6+	983	14.7

N, Sample size.

TABLE 8-7	Average Maxillary and Mandibular Incisor Alignment Scores by Age Group, Gender, and Race-Ethnicity of Americans Ages 8 to 50 Years, 1988-1991[47]

	Age Groups (Mean [SE] in mm)			
	All Ages	8-11 Years	12-17 Years	18-50 Years
Maxillary Alignment				
All persons*	2.4 (0.08)	1.7 (0.10)	2.4 (0.15)	2.6 (0.10)
Males	2.6 (0.10)	1.5 (0.17)	2.6 (0.18)	2.7 (0.12)
Females	2.3 (0.10)	1.9 (0.15)	2.1 (0.18)	2.4 (0.11)
Race-Ethnicity				
Whites	2.5 (0.09)	1.7 (0.12)	2.2 (0.20)	2.6 (0.11)
Blacks	2.1 (0.13)†	1.6 (0.14)	2.2 (0.15)	2.2 (0.14)
Mexican-Americans	2.6 (0.10)	1.9 (0.12)	3.0 (0.28)	2.7 (0.12)
Mandibular Alignment				
All persons*	2.7 (0.07)	1.6 (0.14)	2.5 (0.15)	2.9 (0.09)
Males	2.9 (0.09)‡	1.5 (0.14)	2.8 (0.16)	3.1 (0.12)
Females	2.6 (0.09)	1.8 (0.19)	2.1 (0.21)	2.8 (0.10)
Race-Ethnicity				
Whites	2.8 (0.07)	1.6 (0.17)	2.5 (0.20)	3.0 (0.09)
Blacks	2.2 (0.16)†	1.6 (0.15)	1.8 (0.20)	2.3 (0.17)
Mexican-Americans	3.0 (0.11)	1.7 (0.13)	3.1 (0.17)	3.2 (0.13)

*Includes persons of "other" race-ethnicity designations.
†Blacks are different from whites and Mexican-Americans, $p \leq 0.01$.
‡Males are different from females, $p < 0.01$.
SE, Standard error.

TABLE 8-8	Prevalence of Maxillary Diastema ≥2 mm by Age Group, Gender, and Race-Ethnicity of Americans Ages 8 to 50 Years, 1988-1991[47]			
	Age Groups (Percent of Persons [SE])			
	All Ages	8-11 Years	12-17 Years	18-50 Years
All persons	6.5 (0.6)	19.3 (2.4)	6.0 (0.7)	4.8 (0.6)
Males	7.7 (0.9)*	20.0 (3.7)	7.2 (1.5)	6.2 (0.9)
Females	5.3 (0.5)	18.7 (2.2)	4.8 (1.1)	3.5 (0.5)
Race-Ethnicity				
Whites	4.9 (0.6)	17.7 (2.7)	5.5 (0.9)	3.2 (0.6)
Males	6.2 (1.0)	18.5 (4.7)	7.1 (2.2)	4.6 (1.0)
Females	3.8 (0.5)	17.0 (2.6)	3.9 (1.4)	1.9 (0.4)
Blacks	16.2 (0.9)†	29.4 (3.0)	12.5 (2.5)	14.7 (0.8)
Males	16.8 (1.3)	27.4 (3.0)	12.4 (4.0)	16.0 (1.4)
Females	15.6 (1.4)	31.5 (4.2)	12.6 (2.0)	13.7 (1.3)
Mexican-Americans	6.6 (0.8)	18.2 (3.4)	4.1 (1.8)	5.0 (0.6)
Males	7.6 (1.1)	19.3 (4.0)	5.0 (2.2)	6.1 (0.9)
Females	5.4 (0.8)	17.0 (3.2)	3.2 (1.5)	3.6 (0.5)

*Males are different from females, p <0.01.
†Blacks are different from whites and Mexican-Americans, p <0.001.
SE, Standard error.

TABLE 8-9	Prevalence of Posterior Crossbite by Age Group, Gender, and Race-Ethnicity of Americans Ages 8 to 50 Years, 1988-1991[47]			
	Age Groups (Percent of Persons [SE])			
	All Ages	8-11 Years	12-17 Years	18-50 Years
All persons	9.4 (0.8)	8.5 (1.2)	7.9 (1.5)	9.9 (1.0)
Males	9.1 (1.2)	7.2 (2.6)	6.0 (1.5)	10.2 (1.3)
Females	9.6 (0.8)	9.9 (2.0)	9.7 (2.1)	9.5 (1.0)
Race-Ethnicity				
Whites	9.6 (1.0)	8.8 (1.4)	7.6 (2.1)	10.2 (1.3)
Blacks	9.2 (1.1)	6.6 (1.1)	7.7 (2.2)	10.4 (1.2)
Mexican-Americans	8.5 (0.9)	6.9 (1.7)	8.4 (1.2)	8.9 (0.9)

SE, Standard error.

Posterior Crossbite The prevalence of posterior crossbites in all groups combined was 9.4% with little change from 8 to 50 years of age (Table 8-9). No significant differences in prevalence of posterior crossbite were observed between the race-ethnicity groups and sexes. All persons were assigned to four groups according to their maxillary alignment scores, and the prevalence of posterior crossbite was estimated for the four alignment groups (Table 8-10). The trend was for an increased prevalence of posterior crossbite in those groups with more poorly aligned incisors. No sex differences were observed. Blacks with poor incisor alignment had a significantly higher prevalence of posterior crossbite (23.2%) than did whites (10.0%) and

TABLE 8-10	Distribution of Persons with Posterior Crossbite by Maxillary Alignment Category, Age Group, Gender, and Race-Ethnicity of Americans Ages 8 to 50 Years, 1988-1991[47]

	Maxillary Alignment Group (Percent of Persons [SE])			
	Excellent (0)	Good (1-2 mm)	Fair (3-5 mm)	Poor (6+ mm)
All ages	7.8 (1.4)	8.0 (0.9)	11.6 (1.6)	11.8 (2.2)
8-11 years	5.4 (1.7)	9.5 (2.2)	10.3 (3.3)	17.9 (7.2)
12-17 years	8.1 (2.7)	5.4 (1.5)	8.1 (3.0)	17.1 (4.7)
18-50 years	8.5 (2.2)	8.6 (1.2)	12.5 (1.9)	10.1 (2.2)
Gender				
Males	7.8 (2.4)	7.7 (1.2)	11.6 (2.1)	10.9 (2.7)
Females	7.7 (1.3)	8.4 (1.3)	11.7 (2.0)	13.1 (2.4)
Race-Ethnicity				
Whites	8.3 (1.8)	8.0 (1.0)	13.0 (1.9)	10.0 (2.6)
Blacks	5.2 (1.2)	9.0 (1.4)	7.9 (1.3)	23.2 (4.8)*
Mexican-Americans	6.1 (1.3)	7.9 (0.9)	8.6 (1.5)	15.3 (6.7)

*Blacks with poor alignment are different from whites and Mexican-Americans, p <0.01.
SE, Standard error.

TABLE 8-11	Distribution of Overjet Among Americans Ages 8 to 50 Years, 1988-1991[47]

	Overjet (mm)	Percent of Persons	Cumulative Percent
Mandibular incisors	−4	0.3	0.3
	−3	0.1	0.4
	−2	0.1	0.5
	−1	0.3	0.8
Maxillary incisors	0	4.4	5.2
	1	14.0	19.2
	2	25.9	45.1
	3	23.7	68.8
	4	15.2	84.0
	5	7.7	91.7
	6+	8.3	100.0

*Blacks with poor alignment are different from whites and Mexican-Americans, p <0.01.
SE, Standard error.

TABLE 8-12	Average Overjet Score by Age, Gender, and Race-Ethnicity for Americans Ages 8 to 50 Years with Zero or Positive Scores, 1988-1991[47]			
		Age Groups (Mean [SE] in mm)		
	All Ages	8-11 Years	12-17 Years	18-50 Years
All persons*	2.9 (0.06)	3.4 (0.05)	3.0 (0.08)	2.9 (0.06)
Males	2.9 (0.08)	3.4 (0.05)	3.3 (0.13)	2.7 (0.09)
Females	3.0 (0.05)	3.3 (0.10)	2.8 (0.09)	3.0 (0.05)
Race-Ethnicity				
Whites	2.9 (0.07)	3.3 (0.07)	3.0 (0.11)	2.9 (0.07)
Blacks	3.1 (0.07)	3.7 (0.15)	3.3 (0.13)	2.9 (0.06)
Mexican-Americans†	2.8 (0.06)	3.3 (0.11)	3.0 (0.09)	2.6 (0.05)

*Includes persons of "other" race-ethnicity designations.
†Mexican-Americans are different from non-Hispanic blacks, p ≤0.03.
SE, Standard error.

TABLE 8-13	Distribution of Overbite for Americans Ages 8 to 50 Years, 1988-1991[47]	
mm	Number	Percent of Persons
0	743	8.8
1	1163	14.5
2	1478	22.9
3	1243	20.5
4	908	16.5
5	438	9.1
6+	360	7.8

Mexican-Americans (15.3%), who had statistically similar prevalences of posterior crossbite.

Overjet Overjet is the horizontal distance parallel to the occlusal plane from the midpoint of the labial surface on the most anterior lower central incisor to the midpoint of the labial surface on the most anterior upper central incisor. Overjet is positive when the upper incisor is anterior to the lower incisor, zero when the upper incisor is directly above the lower incisor, and negative when the lower incisor is anterior to the upper incisor. The distribution of overjet among persons between 8 and 50 years of age is shown in Table 8-11.

Less than 1% of this sample had negative overjet. Approximately 8% of the sample had severe overjet of 6 mm or more. Overjet by age, gender, and race-ethnicity for persons with zero and positive overjet measurements are listed in Table 8-12. Average overjet in this sample was 2.9 mm. A trend for overjet to decrease from younger to older persons was observed in both genders and all race-ethnicity groups. Blacks had significantly greater average overjet than the Mexican-Americans (see Table 8-12).

Overbite and Open Bite Overbite is the vertical overlap of the incisor teeth when the posterior teeth are in contact. Overbite is positive when incisors overlap, zero when the incisal edges of the upper and lower incisors are in contact, and negative when the incisal edges are vertically separated. Negative overbite is equivalent to open bite.

The distribution of persons 8 to 50 years of age who had zero or positive overbite is shown in Table 8-13. About 8% of the sample had severe overbite of 6 mm or more. About 9% of this sample had zero overbite. Average overbite in the sample having positive and zero overbites was about 3 mm (Table 8-14). No differences were observed between the genders and age groups. Whites had a significantly greater average overbite (3.1 mm) than blacks (2.3 mm) and Mexican-Americans (2.2 mm) (see Table 8-14).

Less than 5% of the sample had an anterior open bite when the posterior teeth were in occlusion. Average open bite for all persons having this condi-

TABLE 8-14	Average Overbite by Age Group, Gender, and Race-Ethnicity of Americans Ages 8 to 50 Years, 1988-1991[47]

	Age Groups (Mean [SE] in mm)			
	All Ages	8-11 Years	12-17 Years	18-50 Years
All persons	2.9 (0.06)	3.0 (0.06)	3.0 (0.09)	2.8 (0.06)
Males	3.0 (0.07)	3.2 (0.11)	3.1 (0.14)	2.9 (0.08)
Females	2.8 (0.06)	2.9 (0.11)	2.8 (0.12)	2.7 (0.06)
Race-Ethnicity				
Whites*	3.1 (0.05)	3.2 (0.09)	3.1 (0.12)	3.0 (0.06)
Blacks	2.3 (0.08)	2.6 (0.12)	2.3 (0.11)	2.2 (0.07)
Mexican-Americans	2.2 (0.08)	2.7 (0.10)	2.6 (0.18)	2.1 (0.07)

*Whites are different from Blacks and Mexican-Americans, p <0.001.
SE, Standard error.

TABLE 8-15	Average Open Bite for Americans Ages 8 to 50 Years with Open Bite by Age Group, Gender, and Race-Ethnicity, 1988-1991[47]

	Age Groups (Mean [SE] in mm)			
	All Ages	8-11 Years	12-17 Years	18-50 Years
All persons	1.1 (0.13)	1.9 (0.34)	1.0 (0.25)	1.0 (0.13)
Males	1.0 (0.17)	1.5 (0.42)	0.9 (0.42)	1.0 (0.19)
Females	1.2 (0.14)	2.1 (0.40)	1.2 (0.33)	1.0 (0.13)
Race-Ethnicity				
Whites	0.8 (0.12)	2.1 (0.51)	0.6 (0.33)	0.6 (0.09)
Blacks*	1.6 (0.16)	1.8 (0.42)	1.6 (0.36)	1.6 (0.19)
Mexican-Americans	1.1 (0.09)	1.2 (0.19)	1.3 (0.26)	1.1 (0.13)

*Blacks are different from whites and Mexican-Americans, p<0.001.
SE, Standard error.

tion was 1.1 mm (Table 8-15). Average open bite was similar in males and females. In all persons with open bite, the younger ages 8 to 11 had numerically greater average open bite (1.9 mm) than the 12 to 17 age group (1.0 mm) and the 18 to 50 age group (1.0 mm). This decrease may be related to growth and environmental influences such as oral habits. Blacks had significantly greater average anterior open bite (1.6 mm) than whites (0.8 mm) and Mexican-Americans (1.1 mm).

SUMMARY

Although the Angle classification system is useful to clinicians, its use in epidemiologic surveys has been questioned because past investigators did not agree on definitions of the classes. Furthermore, many aspects of malocclusion are not included in the Angle system.[48] More recent surveys in the United States have measured specific variables such as incisor irregularity, overbite, and overjet. From these data it has been discovered that the frequency of near-ideal occlusion decreases from childhood to adolescence, whereas the frequency of severe malocclusion increases during this same growth transition in white and black Americans. More specifically, incisor malalignment increased from childhood to adulthood in white and black Americans and Mexican-Americans, whereas maxillary diastemas and overjet decreased during growth in these same groups.

The prevalence of malocclusion is high in the United States—a reason to continue training professionals to care for those patients in need of treatment. The functional, esthetic, and psychologic benefits of orthodontic treatment ensure a continued seeking out of these services by those afflicted with malocclusion.

REFERENCES

1. Harris EF, Johnson MG: Heritability of craniometric and occlusal variables: a longitudinal sib analysis, *Am J Orthod Dentofacial Orthop* 99:258-268, 1991.
2. Cassidy KM et al: Genetic influence on dental arch form in orthodontic patients, *Angle Orthod* 68:445-454, 1998.
3. Woodside DG et al: Mandibular and maxillary growth after changed mode of breathing, *Am J Orthod Dentofacial Orthop* 100:1-18, 1991.
4. Corruccini RS, Whitley LD: Occlusal variation in a rural Kentucky community, *Am J Orthod* 79:250-262, 1981.
5. Beecher RM, Corruccini RS, Freeman M: Craniofacial correlates of dietary consistency in a nonhuman primate, *J Craniofac Genet Dev Biol* 3:193-202, 1983.
6. Corruccini RS, Beecher RM: Occlusal variation related to soft diet in a nonhuman primate, *Science* 21:74-76, 1982.
7. Corruccini RS, Beecher RM: Occlusal morphological integration lowered in baboons raised on a soft diet, *J Craniofac Genet Dev Biol* 4:135-142, 1984.
8. Little RM, Wallen TR, Riedel RA: Stability and relapse of mandibular anterior alignment: first premolar extraction cases treated by traditional edgewise orthodontics, *Am J Orthod* 80(4):349-365, 1981.
9. Sadowsky C, Sakols EI: Long-term assessment of orthodontic relapse, *Am J Orthod* 82:456-463, 1982.
10. Uhde MD, Sadowsky C, BeGole EA: Long-term stability of dental relationships after orthodontic treatment, *Angle Orthod* 53(3):240-252, 1983.
11. Puneky PJ, Sadowsky C, BeGole EA: Tooth morphology and lower incisor alignment many years after orthodontic therapy, *Am J Orthod* 86(4):299-305, 1984.
12. Shields TE, Little RM, Chapko MK: Stability and relapse of mandibular anterior alignment: a cephalometric appraisal of first premolar extraction cases treated by traditional edgewise orthodontics, *Am J Orthod* 87(1):27-38, 1985.
13. Harris EF et al: Effects of patient age on postorthodontic stability in Class II, division 1 malocclusions, *Am J Orthod Dentofacial Orthop* 105:25-34, 1994.
14. Swanson WD, Riedel RA, D'Anna JA: Postretention study: incidence and stability of rotated teeth in humans, *Angle Orthod* 45(3):198-203, 1975.
15. Edwards JG: A long-term prospective evaluation of the circumferential supracrestal fiberotomy in alleviating orthodontic relapse, *Am J Orthod Dentofacial Orthop* 93:380-387, 1988.
16. Ast DB, Alaway M, Draker HL: The prevalence of malocclusion, related to dental caries and lost first permanent molars, in a fluoridated city and a fluoride deficient city, *Am J Orthod* 48:106-113, 1962.
17. Angle EH: Classification of malocclusion, *Dental Cosmos* 41:248-264; 350-357, 1899.
18. Massler M, Frankel JM: Prevalence of malocclusion in children aged 14 to 18 years, *Am J Orthod* 37:751-758, 1951.
19. Savara BS: Incidence of dental caries, gingivitis, and malocclusion in Chicago children (14 to 17 years of age), *J Dent Res* 34:546-552, 1955.
20. Little RM: The irregularity index: a quantitative score of mandibular anterior alignment, *Am J Orthod* 75:554-563, 1975.
21. Grainger RM: Orthodontic treatment priority index, *Vital Heath Stat* 2:1-49, 1967.
22. Kelly JE, Sanchez M, Van Kirk LE: *An assessment of the occlusion of the teeth of children aged 6-11 years,* United States PHS Pub No 74-1612, Washington, DC, 1973, US Government Printing Office.
23. Kelly JE, Harvey CR: *An assessment of the occlusion of the teeth of youths 12-17 years,* United States PHS Pub No 77-1644, Washington, DC, 1977, US Government Printing Office.
24. Bjork A, Krebs A, Solow B: A method for epidemiological registration of malocclusion, *Acta Odont Scand* 22:27-41, 1964.
25. Federation Dentaire Internationale: Commission on classification and statistics for oral conditions: a method for measuring occlusal traits, *Int Dent J* 23:530-537, 1973.
26. Cons NC et al: Perceptions of occlusal conditions in Australia, the German Democratic Republic, and the United States, *Int Dent J* 33:200-206, 1983.
27. Hill PA: The prevalence and severity of malocclusion and the need for orthodontic treatment in 9-, 12-, and 15-year-old Glasgow schoolchildren, *Br J Orthod* 19:87-96, 1992.
28. Salzmann JD: Handicapping malocclusion assessment to establish treatment priority, *Am J Orthod* 54:766-768, 1968.
29. Summers CJ: A system for identifying and scoring occlusal disorders, *Am J Orthod* 59:552-567, 1971.
30. Baume LJ: Uniform methods for the epidemiologic assessment of malocclusion, *Am J Orthod* 66:251-272, 1974.
31. Dockrell RB: Co-report: population differences in prevalence of malocclusion, *Int Dent J* 8:278-282, 1958.
32. Brehm HL, Jackson DL: An investigation of the extent of the need for orthodontic services, *Am J Orthod* 47:148-149, 1961.
33. Emrich RE, Brodie AG, Blayney JR: Prevalence of Class I, Class II, and Class III malocclusions (Angle) in an urban population: an epidemiological study, *J Dent Res* 44:947-953, 1965.

34. Krogman WM: The problem of timing in facial growth, with special reference to the period of the changing dentition, *Am J Orthod* 37:253, 1951.

35. Mills LF: Epidemiologic studies of occlusion IV: the prevalence of malocclusion in a population of 1455 school children, *J Dent Res* 45:332-336, 1966.

36. Newman GV: Prevalence of malocclusion in children six to fourteen years of age and treatment in preventable cases, *J Am Dent Assoc* 52:566-575, 1956.

37. Savara BS: Incidence of dental caries, gingivitis, and malocclusion in Chicago children (14 to 17 years of age), *J Dent Res* 34:546-552, 1955.

38. Altemus LA: Frequency of the incidence of malocclusion in American Negro children aged twelve to sixteen, *Angle Orthod* 29:189-200, 1959.

39. Grewe JM et al: Prevalence of malocclusion in Chippewa Indian children, *J Dent Res* 47:302-305, 1968.

40. Helm S: Malocclusion in Danish children with adolescent dentition: an epidemiologic study, *Am J Orthod* 54:352-366, 1968.

41. Telle ES: Study of the frequency of malocclusion in the county of Hedmark, Norway: a preliminary report, *Trans Eur Orthod Soc* 192-198, 1951.

42. Gergely (1958) as reported by Graber TM: *Orthodontics: principles and practice,* ed 3, Philadelphia, 1972, WB Saunders.

43. Haralabakis H: Incidence of malocclusion among dental students at Athens University, *Trans Europ Orthod Soc* 310-311, 1957.

44. Davies GN: Dental conditions among the Polynesians of Pukapuka (Danger Island). I. General background and the prevalence of malocclusion, *J Dent Res* 35:115-131, 1956.

45. Houpt MI, Adu-Aryee S, Grainger RM: Dental survey in the Brong Ahafo region of Ghana, *Arch Oral Biol* 12:1337-1341, 1967.

46. Lew KK, Foong WC, Loh E: Malocclusion prevalence in an ethnic Chinese population, *Aust Dent J* 38:442-449, 1993.

47. Brunelle JA, Bhat M, Lipton JA: Prevalence and distribution of selected occlusal characteristics in the US population, 1988-1991, *J Dent Res* 75(Spec Iss):706-713, 1996.

48. Ackerman JL, Proffit WR: The characteristics of malocclusion: a modern approach to classification and diagnosis, *Am J Orthod* 56:443-454, 1969.

SECTION II

DIAGNOSIS

CHAPTER 9

Orthodontic Diagnosis and Treatment Planning

Robert N. Staley

KEY TERMS

normal occlusion	Class II	malocclusion	posterior crossbites
facial morphology	Division 1	chief concern	lateral functional shift
diagnostic norm	Subdivision	pertinent health issues	scissors bite
objective norm	Division 2	dental history	Brodie syndrome
biometric norm	Subdivision	temporomandibular joint	panoramic radiograph
subjective norm	Class III	facial form	periapical mouth survey
therapeutic norm	Subdivision	interlabial gaps	congenitally missing teeth
mean value	Venn diagram	gummy smile	impacted teeth
range of values	alignment	anteroposterior relationship	root dilaceration
molar relationship	profile	of the first molars and	alveolar bone height
crown angulation	transverse deviation	canines	periodontal status
crown inclination	sagittal deviation	overjet	supernumerary teeth
rotations	vertical deviation	anterior crossbite	root resorption
spaces	transsagittal deviation	anterior functional shift	pathologic conditions
occlusal plane	sagittovertical deviation	overbite	lateral cephalometric
Angle classification	verticotransverse deviation	open bite	radiograph
Class I	transsagittovertical deviation		

Dentists must acquire a number of skills to provide a patient with an orthodontic diagnosis. Clinicians must recognize **normal occlusion** and normal **facial morphology,** differentiate normal from abnormal, and be able to do this in the primary, mixed, and adult dentitions. Additionally, dentists must know when to treat and when to refer patients with malocclusions to an appropriately trained caregiver.

The recognition and reporting of a malocclusion or a condition that could lead to a malocclusion is the most important orthodontic service that a dentist can provide to his patients. Malocclusion occurs all too frequently in patients (see Chapter 8) and has an important impact on the function and esthetics of the entire dentition. In fact, malocclusion has a detrimental impact on the self-esteem of many children, adolescents, and adults.[1] If a malocclusion is not recognized by either the dentist or the patient, it cannot be assessed and treated. An orthodontic assessment should also provide the patient with treatment options that need to be considered.

The following sequence of steps is taken with a patient who has a malocclusion:

1. Recognize the malocclusion in an initial examination or screening, and report the discovery to a patient or parent.
2. Gather records or refer the patient to a fully trained colleague.

3. Develop a diagnosis from the records.
4. Develop a treatment plan.
5. Consult with the patient and parent about the diagnosis and treatment plan.

Treatment begins after an agreement has been made by all parties at the consultation appointment.

Concept of Normal Occlusion and Facial Morphology

To adequately describe abnormal occlusion, what is meant by normal occlusion and normal facial form must be agreed upon. Koski[2] defined various norms that need to be used by orthodontists.

A **diagnostic norm** is a standard that helps to determine the extent to which a patient deviates from normal. An **objective norm** is a norm based on a measurement technique that is repeatable, reliable, and based on scientific method. A **biometric norm** is an objective norm derived from the measurement of a biologic variable in a random sample of persons who are considered normal. Cephalometric and arch width norms are examples of quantitative biometric norms. Angle's classes of malocclusion are examples of qualitative biometric norms.[3] A **subjective norm** is a norm based solely on personal judgment and prejudice. A **therapeutic norm** is essentially a treatment goal for a particular patient. Diagnostic norms and treatment goals are usually not synonymous because of the great variation seen in the morphology, physiology, and growth status of patients.

The Mean versus the Range of Normal Relationships

The mean derived from quantitative measurements of a biologic variable such as those used in orthodontic diagnosis is considered the norm by some. However, usually no single individual in a random sample of normal persons is likely to have the **mean value** for one particular variable, let alone several variables. "Normal," with respect to orthodontic biologic variables, consists of a **range of values,** rather than just the mean value. Most investigators and clinicians have arbitrarily defined the range of normal to include all measurement values of a normally distributed biologic variable that lie one standard deviation above and below the mean value for a representative sample of normal subjects (see Chapter 3). Normal values for a particular variable, therefore, comprise about 68% of all measurement values obtained from a sample of normal individuals, assuming that the measurements of the variable fall into a normal statistical distribution. This spread of values describes the normal variability inherent in humans.

The concept of a therapeutic norm or treatment goal is valuable in orthodontics because it gives the clinician a reasonable goal for treatment that recognizes the limitations imposed by a particular patient's morphology, growth status, and function. As a result, in some instances treatment goals can include abnormal values. For example, all patients should not be treated to the mean value of a biometric norm such as a lower incisor to mandibular plane angle of 90 degrees. Some patients can be beneficially treated to this angular relation. However, patients with a high (i.e., steep mandibular plane angle) are often best treated to a lower incisor to mandibular plane angle of less than 90 degrees. Similarly, patients with low (i.e., flat mandibular plane angles) are usually best treated to a lower incisor to mandibular plane angle higher than 90 degrees.

Most people probably agree that objective norms are preferable to subjective norms, but that mean values of diagnostic norms are best not used as absolute treatment goals.

Normal and Ideal Occlusion

Normal occlusion occurs frequently in a population, whereas ideal occlusion is a rarity. Normal occlusion includes variations in tooth positions and relationships that diverge in minor ways from the ideal (Figure 9-1).

Angle Angle[3] described normal occlusion as an evenly placed row of teeth arranged in a graceful curve with harmony between the upper and lower arches. According to Angle, the key to normal occlusion in adults is the anteroposterior relationship between the upper and lower first molars. Angle's concept of normal occlusion is essentially the description of an ideal occlusion. He stated that knowledge of normal occlusion should include knowledge of the normal relations of the occlusal surfaces of permanent and primary teeth, their forms and structures, and the growth and development of the teeth, jaws, and muscles. Angle thought that the first molars and canines were the most reliable teeth. His description of first molar and canine relationships in normal occlusion was and remains a fundamental observation on which dental and orthodontic diagnoses are based. Angle stated the following:

In normal occlusion, the mesiobuccal cusp of the upper first molar is received in the sulcus between the mesial and distal buccal cusps of the lower [first molar]. The mesial and distal inclines of the mesiobuccal cusp of the upper first molar are received between the mesial and distal buccal cusps of the lower first molar. The inclines of the distobuccal cusp [of the upper first molar] are received between the distobuccal cusp of the first lower [molar] and the mesiobuccal cusp of the second lower [molar]. The mesial incline of the upper [canine oc-

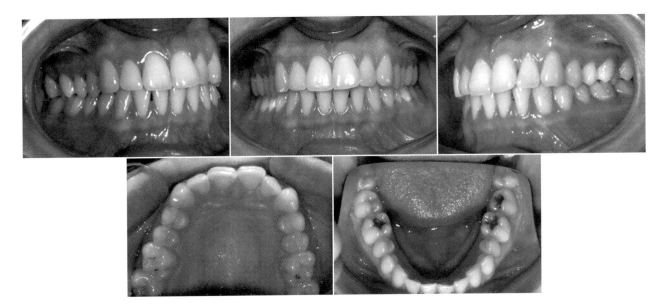

Figure 9-1 Normal occlusion in an adult female.

cludes] with the distal incline of the lower [canine]; the distal incline of the upper [canine] occludes with the mesial incline of the buccal cusp of the lower first [premolar]. Each of the teeth in both jaws has two antagonists or supports in the opposite jaw, except the lower centrals and the upper third molars.

Angle stressed the importance of cuspal interdigitation to the establishment of normal occlusion during eruption of the teeth and to the maintenance of good occlusion. He stated that normal occlusion of the teeth is maintained first by the occlusal inclined planes of the cusps, second by the support given by the harmony in size of the upper and lower arches, and third by the influence of the muscles labially, buccally, and lingually. He concluded that these same three factors are also powerful in maintaining a malocclusion.

Begg Begg's concept of normal occlusion[4] differs greatly from that of Angle. Begg concluded that the normal occlusion of tribal peoples is the true normal occlusion of humans. The dentitions of the rural Australian Aborigines that he studied were characterized by a great deal of attrition that produced in the majority of adults an end-to-end incisor relation, mesial placement of the mandibular arch, and occlusal and interproximal wear that reduced the size of the teeth and reduced the incidence of crowding. He referred to the relatively unworn canine teeth of urban Europeans as abnormal and the root of periodontal, caries, and occlusal problems so prevalent in these people. The interproximal tooth wear that Begg saw in the skeletal remains of Australian Aborigines provided him with a rationale for the extraction of teeth in urban Europeans who had malocclusions. Begg's tendency to extract permanent teeth in the course of orthodontic treatment contrasted greatly with Angle's determination to avoid the extraction of teeth during treatment.

KEYS TO NORMAL OCCLUSION

It is apparent that Andrews[5] described an ideal occlusion rather than a normal occlusion (Box 9-1). The ideal occlusion described by Angle and Andrews serves as a paragon of occlusal excellence that gives clinicians a treatment goal to which they can aspire. Figure 9-2 illustrates an ideal occlusion in skeletal remains in which all 32 adult teeth are present. Figure 9-3 illustrates ideal occlusion in the primary dentition (see Chapter 5). Morphologic variation in the dentition and supporting structures dictate that treated occlusions are not always ideal but sometimes contain one or more abnormal features. One of the challenges of diagnosis is to decide whether the goal for orthodontic treatment in a patient is normal occlusion or an acceptable occlusion that incorporates some abnormal features.

CLASSIFICATION OF MALOCCLUSION

Etiologic classification is commonly used in medicine. However, malocclusion has a complex or unknown etiology in most instances (see Chapter 8). Because malocclusion is a morphologic abnormality, most classifications are based primarily on morphology. There is a misleading nature of morphologic classifications, namely the assumption that all individuals in a given class or type of malocclusion share

BOX 9-1   Andrews' Six Keys to Normal Occlusion in the Adult Dentition

1. **Molar relationship:** The mesiobuccal cusp of the upper first molar occludes with the groove between the mesiobuccal and middle buccal cusp of the lower first molar. The distobuccal cusp of the upper first molar contacts the mesiobuccal cusp of the lower second molar.
2. **Crown angulation:** All tooth crowns are angulated mesially (mesiodistal tip).
3. **Crown inclination:** Inclination refers to the labiolingual or buccolingual inclination of the crowns of the teeth.
   a. Incisors are inclined toward the buccal or labial surface.
   b. Upper posterior teeth are inclined lingually, similarly from the canine to the premolars. Upper molar crowns are inclined slightly more than the canines and premolars.
   c. Lower posterior teeth are inclined lingually, progressively more from canine to molars.
4. **Rotations:** Rotations are not present.
5. **Spaces:** Spaces are not present between teeth.
6. **Occlusal plane:** The plane is either flat or slightly curved.

From Andrews LF: *Am J Orthod* 62:296-309, 1972.

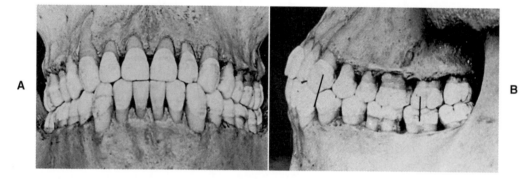

Figure 9-2 A, Frontal view of an ideal occlusion in the skeletal remains of an adult. **(B)** Lateral view of the same skull. The vertical axial line passing through the mesiobuccal cusp tip of the maxillary first molar meets the vertical axial line passing through the buccal groove of the mandibular first molar. The vertical axial line passing through the cusp tip of the maxillary canine meets the vertical line bisecting the embrasure between the mandibular canine and first premolar.

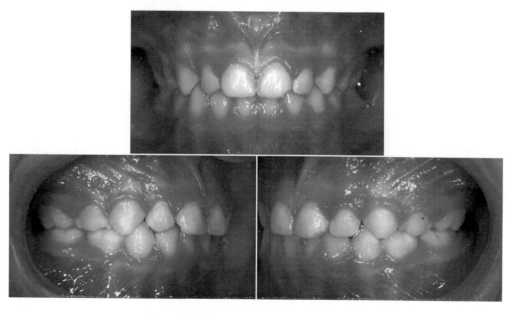

Figure 9-3 Ideal occlusion in a primary dentition.

a common cause. Orthodontists have often referred to Class I or Class II treatment as if the causes of all Class I and Class II malocclusions were the same. This is an inappropriate use of the morphologic classification of malocclusions.

Angle Classification

Angle[3] described seven malpositions of individual teeth: (1) buccal or labial, (2) lingual, (3) mesial, (4) distal, (5) torso (rotated), (6) infra (not erupted sufficiently to reach the occlusal plane), and (7) supra (erupted through and beyond the occlusal plane). These individual tooth malpositions can be used to describe a malocclusion more fully.

The **Angle classification** system for malocclusions proposed by Angle[3] is widely used and serves as an excellent means of general description that has facilitated the communication about different malocclusions within the profession (Figure 9-4). The system basically describes anteroposterior relationships of the permanent first molars and canines.

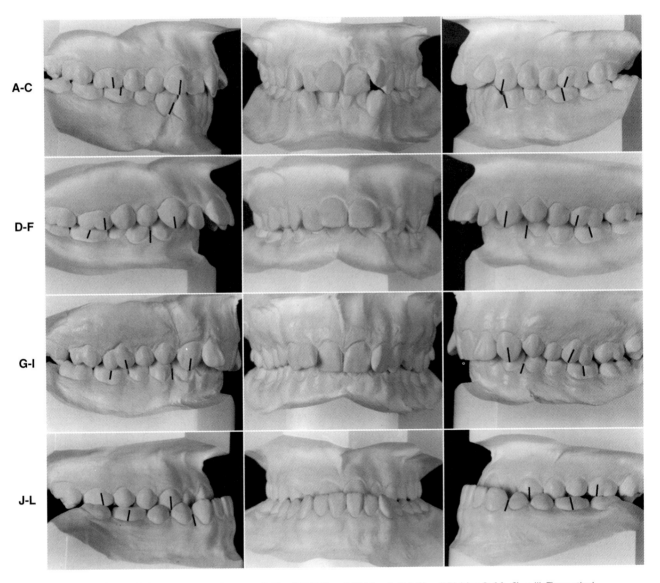

Figure 9-4 Malocclusion classes. **A-C,** Class I. **D-F,** Class II Division 1. **G-I,** Class II Division 2. **J-L,** Class III. The vertical axial lines passing through the mesiobuccal cusp tips of the maxillary first molars have different relationships with the vertical axial lines passing through the buccal grooves of the mandibular first molars in different malocclusion classes. A similar variation among malocclusion classes is observed in the relationships between the vertical axial lines passing through the cusp tips of the maxillary canines and the vertical lines bisecting the embrasures between the mandibular canines and first premolars.

As can be noted from the information in Box 9-2, Angle[3] included in his description of malocclusions not only the positions and relations of the teeth, but also information about arch width, the retrusion or protrusion of the mandible, the effects of the malocclusion on the face, abnormal lip function, and the association of nasal obstruction and mouth breathing with malocclusion. Angle wrote his descriptions of malocclusions more than 30 years before the advent of cephalometric radiographs. Cephalometric measurements help clinicians differentiate Class II and Class III malocclusions more accurately in patients who have normal skeletal relations between the maxilla and mandible from those who have abnormal relations between the maxilla and mandible. Furthermore, the determination of whether the discrepancy is in one or both jaws is made easier with cephalometric radiographs (see Chapter 10).

Clinical Notation of the Malocclusion

The occlusion of the first molars and canines on both sides of the arch is recorded at the screening visit. For a Class I occlusion the occlusal notation should be I, I, I, I from right molars to left molars. This notation quickly alerts the clinician to the presence or absence of anteroposterior problems in an occlusion.

Molar and canine positions are often not fully Class I, II, or III, but rather in an intermediate relationship. As a result molars and canines that fall between Class I and Class II are called *end-to-end malocclusions* (notation E) and those between Class I and Class III are called *super I malocclusions* (notation SI). These refinements in Angle's qualitative classes help clinicians better describe an occlusion. The occlusal notation reveals bilateral asymmetries, and the severity of a malocclusion, for example, a mild Class II occlusion (E-E-E-E) can be differentiated from one that is fully Class II (II, II, II, II).

The broad principles of the Angle classification system can be applied to the primary and mixed dentitions (see Chapters 5).

Severity of Malocclusion and Problem List

J.L. Ackerman and W.R. Proffit[6] developed a **Venn diagram** to assist in describing more fully the severity of a malocclusion. This was an attempt to differentiate the many different kinds of problems seen in each of the malocclusion cases defined by Angle. They added

---

BOX 9-2   Angle's Classification System

Class I: The relative mesiodistal position of the dental arches is normal with the permanent first molars usually in normal occlusion, although one or more teeth may be in lingual or buccal malposition with malocclusions usually confined to the anterior teeth.

Class II: The relative mesiodistal relations of the dental arches is abnormal with all the lower teeth occluding distal to normal, producing a marked disharmony in the incisor region and in the facial lines. In full Class II the distobuccal cusp of the permanent upper first molar fits into the sulcus between the mesial and middle buccal cusps of the lower first molar. The mandible is retrusive (in a more posterior or dorsal position than normal).

Division 1: A Class II Division 1 malocclusion is characterized by a narrowing of the upper arch, lengthened and protruding upper incisors, abnormal function of the lips, and some form of nasal obstruction and mouth breathing.

Subdivision: A Class II Division 1 Subdivision malocclusion has a normal occlusal relation on one side of the arches and a Class II occlusion on the other side. These patients are also mouth breathers.

Division 2: Class II Division 2 malocclusions are characterized by a slight narrowing of the upper arch, bunching (crowding) of the upper incisors with overlapping and lingual inclination, and normal nasal and lip function.

Subdivision: Class II Division 2 Subdivision malocclusions have a normal occlusal relation on one side of the arches and a Class II occlusion on the other side.

Class III: The relative mesiodistal relations of the arches are abnormal with all the lower teeth occluding mesial to normal, producing a marked disharmony in the incisor region and in the facial lines. In full Class III the buccal cusp of the upper second premolar fits into the sulcus between the mesiobuccal and middle buccal cusps of the lower first molar. The arrangement of teeth varies from even alignment to crowding and overlapping, especially in the upper arch. The lower incisors and canines are inclined lingually because of the pressure of the lower lip in its effort to close the mouth. The mandible is protrusive (in a more anterior or ventral position than normal). Marring of the facial lines is noticeable, in some instances becoming a pronounced deformity.

Subdivision: The disharmony is of a lesser degree with a normal occlusion one side of the arches and a Class III occlusion on the other side.

From Angle EH: *Dental Cosmos* 41:248-264; 350-357, 1899.

to Angle's mesiodistal (sagittal) classes of malocclusion four other factors, namely, an assessment of tooth alignment, facial profile, transverse problems, and vertical problems. Patients with combinations of problems in two or all three planes of space had more severe malocclusions than did those patients having fewer problems.

Nine Categories of the Ackerman and Proffit Diagram

1. **Alignment** (spacing, crowding)
2. **Profile** (convex, straight, concave)
3. **Transverse deviation** (crossbites)
4. **Sagittal deviation** (Angle class)
5. **Vertical deviation** (deep bite, open bite)
6. **Transsagittal deviation** (combination of crossbite and Angle class)
7. **Sagittovertical deviation** (combination of Angle class and deep bite or open bite)
8. **Verticotransverse deviation** (combination of deep bite or open bite with crossbite)
9. **Transsagittovertical deviation** (combination of problems in three planes of space)

It is obvious that an alignment problem alone in a patient is more easily treated than a problem involving all three planes of space. This system can help an orthodontist organize a list of problems for a patient and, in turn, give the patient a better understanding of the length and difficulty of the proposed treatment. After making a problem list, a treatment plan is created that addresses each of the problems.[7] Some occlusal and associated facial problems cannot be corrected to a fully normal form and function by orthodontic treatment or even by combined orthodontic surgical treatment. Nevertheless, the orthodontic treatment plan should attempt to correct as many of the patient's problems as possible.

FACIAL MORPHOLOGY, OCCLUSION, AND MALOCCLUSION

Facial profiles can sometimes reveal underlying **malocclusion** problems. Anteroposterior relations between the maxilla and mandible are observed in the three basic types of profiles. Patients with a straight profile usually have normal occlusions or Class I malocclusions. Those having convex profiles have an increased probability of having a Class II malocclusion associated with a retrusive mandible or perhaps a protrusive maxilla (Figure 9-5). Patients with a concave profile have an increased probability of having a Class III malocclusion associated with a retruded maxilla, a protrusive mandible, or both.

Facial profiles can also reveal growth problems in the vertical dimension. Excessive vertical growth of the face can lead to an anterior open bite malocclusion, lips apart at rest, a gummy smile, and an increased angle between the ramus and body of the mandible. Long vertical face heights may be associated with Class I, II, and III malocclusions (Figure 9-6). Insufficient vertical growth of the face can produce a deep overbite (overclosed) malocclusion, with redundant, overlapped lips and decreased angle between the ramus and body of the mandible. Short vertical face heights may be associated with Class I, II, and III malocclusions (Figure 9-7). As a result of these observations, the clinician should realize that the presence of a particular type of facial profile is not always indicative of the Angle malocclusion class.

Therefore an examination of the patient's face is an important part of an orthodontic chairside evaluation. Patients who have convex or concave profiles or obvious vertical abnormalities in facial form associated with a malocclusion have severe problems that require comprehensive treatment and sometimes orthognathic surgery. On the other hand, patients who have malocclusions associated with normal facial proportions have a better prognosis for treatment than those who have malocclusions associated with abnormal facial proportions.

ORTHODONTIC EXAMINATION AND RECORDS

The collection of data from direct observations of a patient, from questioning the patient, and from x-rays, plaster models, and photographs constitutes a body of information essential to the formulation of a diagnosis and treatment plan. The care taken in record collection is reflected in the diagnosis and treatment of the patient.

Records commonly taken before treating a patient needing orthodontic treatment include a clinical examination with a recording of the general health and oral history of the patient, impressions for plaster casts of the teeth, intraoral and facial photographs (frontal and lateral views), a full-mouth survey of periapical x-rays and/or a panoramic x-ray, and a lateral cephalometric radiograph. From the evaluation of these records, impressions are formed concerning the growth status of the patient, the severity of the malocclusion, the appropriate appliance plan, and the prognosis of treatment. Patients with complex Class I malocclusions or facial growth imbalances associated with Class II and Class III malocclusions should be treated by an orthodontist.

When treatment begins, record taking continues in the form of treatment progress notes taken at each visit. Periodically during treatment, x-rays and other records

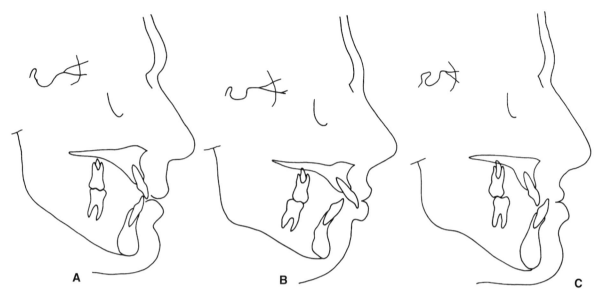

Figure 9-5 **A,** Straight profile, Class I. **B,** Convex profile, Class II Division 1. **C,** Concave profile, Class III.

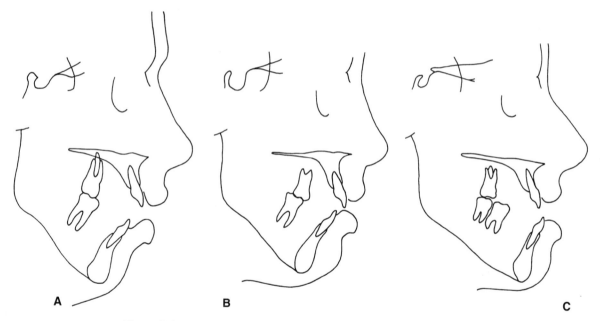

Figure 9-6 Long vertical growth profiles. **A,** Class I. **B,** Class II Division 1. **C,** Class III.

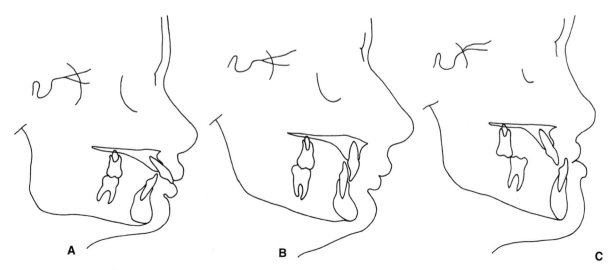

Figure 9-7 Short vertical growth profiles. **A,** Class II Division 1. **B,** Class II Division 2. **C,** Class III.

may be taken to assess treatment progress. When active treatment is completed, new records are taken. The patient is then followed during the retention phase of treatment. Retention records allow evaluation of any changes in the occlusion occurring after treatment.

Patient History and Facial Assessment

The patient examination and the analysis of records are summarized on clinical forms (Figures 9-8 and 9-9). The **chief concern** of the patient should first be recorded. Why did the patient seek treatment? In some cases or-

---

ORTHODONTIC EXAMINATION AND DIAGNOSIS

Date of Examination _____

Patient's Name _____ Birthdate _____ Sex _____
                          (last)   (first)   (initial)

1. **Chief Concern** _____
2. **Medical History and Airway Exam**
    a. General health_____
    b. Significant conditions (e.g., requiring antibiotic premedication)_____
    c. Prescribed drugs _____
    d. Tonsils and adenoids   normal _____ enlarged _____
    e. Nasal airway: open _____ obstructed _____mouth breathing_____
3. **Dental History**
    a. Habits: finger _____tongue _____lip _____
        Bruxism _____ musical instruments_____
    b. Trauma to face and teeth: _____
    c. Previous orthodontic treatment _____
4. **TEMPEROMANDIBULAR JOINT EXAM:** symptoms _____
        pain _____ history _____
5. **Facial Form**
    a. <u>Frontal:</u>
        1) Bilateral: symmetry _____asymmetry _____
    b. <u>Profile:</u> straight _____convex _____concave_____
    c. <u>Anteroposterior jaw positions:</u>
        1) Maxilla: normal _____ protrusive _____ retrusive _____
        2) Mandible: normal _____ protrusive _____ retrusive _____
    d. <u>Vertical:</u>
        a. Face: normal _____ long _____ short _____
    e. <u>Lips:</u>
        1) Together in Centric occlusion when relaxed _____
        2) Apart in Centric occlusion when relaxed _____
        3) Gummy Smile_____
6. **Dentition**
    A. <u>Stage of Dentition:</u> Primary _____Mixed (Early) _____ (Late)_____ Permanent _____
    B. Number of erupted adult teeth: Inc U____L____, Can U____L____, P1 U____L____, P2 U____L____
                                M1 U____L____, M2 U____L____.
    C. <u>Periodontal status:</u> (All adults **must have** recent periodontal probings). _____
        Gingival Recession _____Abnormal Frenum _____
    D. <u>Restorative Status:</u> Caries_____ Endodontics _____
            Prosthetic restorations_____

Figure 9-8 Orthodontic examination and diagnosis form.

Anteroposterior

E. Angle Classification: Class I _____Class II-1 _____Class II-2 _____ Class III _____

  Right Molar _____ Right Canine _____Left Canine _____Left Molar_____

  (Choices: III, SI [Super I], I, E, II)

F. Incisor Overjet: (mm) _____   Edge to Edge_____   Anterior Crossbite_____

Vertical

G. Overbite (%) _____Anterior Openbite (mm) _____Posterior Openbite (mm) _____

Transverse

H. Dental midlines to face (mm):   Upper _____   Lower _____

I. Posterior Crossbite: Unilateral _____   Bilateral _____

  Scissors Bite _____Intermolar width difference (mm) _____

J. Asymmetry in dental arches _____

Functional Shifts on Closure: Anteroposterior _____Transverse _____

Premature loss of deciduous teeth: _____

Toothsize/Arch Size: Excess Space   Adequate   Crowding

  Maxilla   _____   _____   _____

  Mandible   _____   _____   _____

Radiographic Analysis:

  Missing Teeth _____   Supernumerary Teeth _____

  Impacted Teeth _____   Root Resorption _____

  Root Dilaceration _____   Periapical Pathology _____

  Alveolar Bone Height _____   Other _____

Summary of Diagnostic Findings and Problem List

1. **Chief Concern** _____

2. **Medical History** _____

3. **Dental History** _____

4. **Facial Form** _____

5. **Dentition:**

  a. **Periodontal status** _____

  b. **Restorative status** _____

  c. **Angle Class:** _____; RM_____ RC_____ LC_____ LM_____

  d. **Overbite (%)**_____ **Overjet (mm)** _____

  e. **Crossbites (anterior)**_____ **(posterior)** _____

  f. **Functional Shifts**_____

  g. **Crowding/Spacing (mm)** U_____ L _____ **Molar Width Difference (mm)**_____

  h. **Radiographic Findings**_____

6. **Orthodontic Problem List:**

  1.

  2.

  3.

  4.

Figure 9-8, cont'd For legend see opposite page.

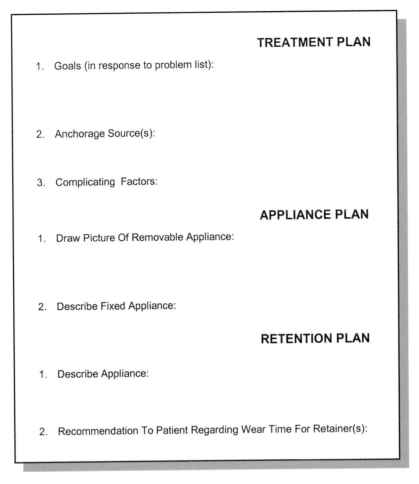

TREATMENT PLAN

1. Goals (in response to problem list):

2. Anchorage Source(s):

3. Complicating Factors:

APPLIANCE PLAN

1. Draw Picture Of Removable Appliance:

2. Describe Fixed Appliance:

RETENTION PLAN

1. Describe Appliance:

2. Recommendation To Patient Regarding Wear Time For Retainer(s):

Figure 9-9 Treatment planning form.

thodontic treatment is not required or advisable. For example, a maxillary anterior diastema with an otherwise normal occlusion may be best closed with composite restorative material. If the clinical examination reveals occlusal problems in need of treatment, additional record collection is initiated with the patient's consent.

Pertinent health issues that could influence treatment are listed, including prescribed medications. Consultation with the patient's physician may be necessary to determine if premedication is needed. Also, if a patient has significant difficulty in breathing through the nose, a referral should be made to an otolaryngologist. With older adults, information on bone density is important (see Chapter 28).

The patient's **dental history** is then recorded, including notations about any trauma to the face and teeth.

A **temporomandibular joint** (TMJ) examination is imperative. Studies indicate that TMJ disease is neither improved nor worsened as a result of orthodontic treatment, thus a record of TMJ symptoms before treatment

is needed for all concerned. Some TMJ disorders that are detected at the pretreatment examination may benefit from orthodontic treatment, whereas other disorders may either complicate treatment or be a contraindication for orthodontic treatment. Referral to a specialist in the diagnosis and treatment of TMJ disorders is a wise decision when symptoms, radiographic evidence, and history suggest the presence of a complicated disorder. Informed consent before orthodontic treatment should be obtained from patients who have positive findings.

Facial form can be assessed from direct observation and from facial photographs. Patients with normal occlusion have a wide variety of facial forms. However, as facial form deviates further from normal, the probability that an associated malocclusion is present increases. Precise description of facial form requires anthropometric measurements or analysis of cephalograms. In people with normal facial features, the lips are together at rest or only slightly apart.

Patients with large **interlabial gaps** have either short lips or excessive anterior vertical growth.

A **gummy smile,** that is a smile that reveals a great deal of gingiva above the maxillary incisors, is another sign of a short upper lip or excessive maxillary anterior vertical growth.

DENTAL EXAMINATION

An examination of the dentition includes counting the erupted primary and permanent teeth and recording the periodontal and restorative status of the patient. Any periodontal disease, caries, or endodontic problems must be treated before the start of orthodontic treatment.

Anteroposterior Dental Relations

Dental relationships are recorded from a chairside examination and then confirmed and supplemented by an evaluation of the dental casts. The Angle classification is an important observation for an orthodontic assessment. Limited treatment is best confined to Class I malocclusions with minor deviations from normal occlusion. The **anteroposterior relationship** of the first molars and canines with the teeth in centric occlusion (CO) is recorded. After recording the molar and canine relationships, the occlusion is classified according to Angle's classification system.[3] Some patients have a Class I molar relation and a Class II canine relation. These patients' occlusions are classified as Class I, and it should be noted that it has Class II characteristics. When molars in the permanent dentition are end to end or cusp tip to cusp tip, the occlusion is classified as a Class II malocclusion. An end-to-end molar relationship is considered normal in the early mixed dentition (see Chapter 5) but not in the permanent dentition.

Overjet is the distance between the labial surface of the most labial mandibular central incisor and the incisal edge of the most labial maxillary central incisor when the teeth are in CO. The distance is measured parallel to the occlusal plane with the use of calipers (Figure 9-10). Overjet is best measured on study casts that are positioned in CO. Mean overjet in white adults with normal occlusion is 2.2 mm ± 0.8 mm for males and 2.5 mm ± 1.1 mm for females.[8]

When the labial surfaces of the maxillary incisors occlude posterior to the lingual surfaces of the mandibular incisors, the resulting **anterior crossbite** is measured as illustrated in Figure 9-10. Anterior crossbites may involve two or all the anterior teeth. Those associated with Class III molar relations are much more difficult to treat than those associated with Class I molar relations.

Some anterior crossbites are associated with an **anterior functional shift** on closure from centric relation (CR) to CO. If the patient can touch his or her upper and lower incisors together in CR, the occlusion is referred to as psuedo-Class III. Anterior crossbites associated with a large anterior CR-CO functional shift are much easier to correct than those showing no evidence of a CR-CO shift. Anterior crossbites associated with average to deeper overbite are more easily treated and successfully retained than are those associated with little or no overbite.

Vertical Dental Relations

Overbite is expressed as the percentage of the mandibular incisor crown that is overlapped vertically by the maxillary incisors when the teeth are in CO (see Figure 9-10). Overbite values range from 0% to more than 100%. The mean values of white adults with normal occlusion are 45% ± 20% for males and 36% ± 13% for females.[8] The vertical distance between the maxillary and mandibular incisor edges should be measured in **open bite** cases. A notation should be made when the mandibular incisors are impinging on the palatal tissues.

Habits, such as thumbsucking and abnormal tongue resting position, and abnormal facial growth (excessive vertical growth) may cause an open bite malocclusion. Anterior open bites occur more often than posterior open bites. Record the extent and location of the open bite. Successful treatment depends on a correct diagnosis of the cause, therefore the patient should be asked to establish a history of the open bite problem. In general, anterior open bites are among the most difficult problems to treat and in some patients may require a combined orthodontic-surgical treatment.

Transverse Dental Relations

The most common **posterior crossbites** involve only two teeth in which the upper tooth is placed, in relative terms, too far lingually in relation to the opposing lower tooth. Posterior crossbites that involve many teeth are classified as either unilateral or bilateral, depending on the position of the teeth in CO.

A true unilateral crossbite occurs when the patient exhibits no lateral functional shift of the mandible during closure from CR into CO. Most patients with a unilateral posterior crossbite do exhibit some CR-CO **lateral functional shift** upon closure of the mandible and thus actually have a bilateral posterior crossbite associated with a lateral functional shift. In unilateral posterior crossbite, the lower dental midline is usually deviated away from the upper dental midline toward the side of the crossbite. The patient should be asked to open his mouth. If the lower dental midline is coincident with the upper dental midline when the mouth is open, a lateral shift is occurring as the teeth are brought into occlusion. Pa-

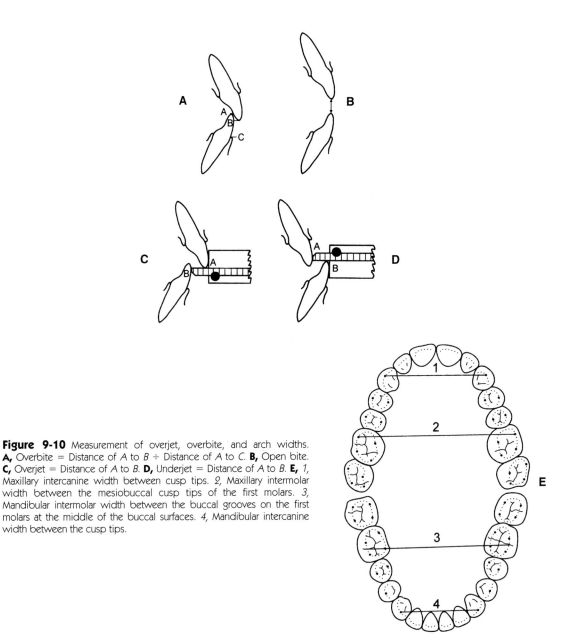

Figure 9-10 Measurement of overjet, overbite, and arch widths. **A,** Overbite = Distance of *A* to *B* ÷ Distance of *A* to *C*. **B,** Open bite. **C,** Overjet = Distance of *A* to *B*. **D,** Underjet = Distance of *A* to *B*. **E,** *1,* Maxillary intercanine width between cusp tips. *2,* Maxillary intermolar width between the mesiobuccal cusp tips of the first molars. *3,* Mandibular intermolar width between the buccal grooves on the first molars at the middle of the buccal surfaces. *4,* Mandibular intercanine width between the cusp tips.

tients having true or skeletal unilateral posterior cross-bites are difficult to treat and may require surgical orthodontic treatment to successfully resolve the malocclusion. Bilateral posterior crossbites and unilateral posterior crossbites with a significant lateral CR-CO shift can be treated with a variety of appliances that deliver bilateral forces (see Chapters 17, 19, and 23).

A **scissors bite** in the posterior teeth occurs when the upper teeth are positioned totally buccal to the lower teeth in CO. This is found most frequently in the premolar region of Class II Division I malocclusions. A rare buccal crossbite in which all of the lower teeth are positioned lingual to the upper teeth occurs in patients having a retrusive and small mandible or a large maxilla. This is referred to as the **Brodie syndrome.**

Arch Width Measurements

Patients with posterior crossbite problems should be carefully assessed to determine the best feasible treatment plan. To make this important clinical judgment, the intermolar measurements in all patients who have unilateral and bilateral posterior crossbites are taken (see Figure 9-10). The distance between the tips of the mesiobuccal cusps of the maxillary first molars is measured. The distance between the buccal grooves of the mandibular first molars, at a point in the middle of the buccal surface, is measured. Intercanine and intermolar widths for the maxillary and mandibular arches of white adults who have normal occlusion are listed in Table 9-1.[8] The mean differences between the wider upper and narrower lower intermolar widths

TABLE 9-1	Arch Widths in White Adults with Normal Occlusion							
	Males (N = 19)				*Females (N = 17)*			
Arch Width	Mean (mm)	SD	Minimum	Maximum	Mean (mm)	SD	Minimum	Maximum
Maxillary intercanine*	36.2	2.3	32.9	41.9	33.2	1.4	31.3	35.4
Mandibular intercanine	26.3	1.8	23.3	31.0	25.3	1.5	22.6	28.2
Maxillary intermolar*	54.7	2.1	51.4	58.0	50.2	2.0	46.6	54.1
Mandibular intermolar*	53.1	1.6	50.2	56.0	49.0	1.8	46.4	52.9
Intermolar width difference†	1.6	1.4	−0.5	4.4	1.2	1.2	−1.3	4.3

*Difference between sexes significant ($p < 0.05$).
†Molar difference = Maxillary intermolar distance − Mandibular intermolar distance.
N, Sample size; SD, standard deviation.

are small and positive: males 1.6 mm ± 1.4 mm and females 1.2 mm ± 1.2 mm. In patients with posterior crossbites, the upper intermolar width is smaller than the lower intermolar distance. This difference is used to determine how much expansion of the maxillary arch is required to correct the crossbite. If the crossbite is minimal, requiring that the distance between the upper molars be expanded less than 4 mm, treatment may be accomplished with either a removable appliance, such as an expansion plate, or a fixed appliance, such as a quad helix (see Chapters 17 and 19). If the distance between the upper molars must be expanded from 4 to 12 mm, the patient will need rapid maxillary expansion (see Chapter 23). Adult patients who need the distance between the upper molars expanded more than 4 mm may need a surgically assisted rapid maxillary expansion procedure performed on them.

Asymmetry in Dental Arches

Asymmetry in canine and molar relations should be noted. Premature loss of a primary tooth on only one side of the arch is a common cause of asymmetry in the adult occlusion. Early correction of the shift of the dental midline in the mixed dentition may either prevent future asymmetric occlusion and orthodontic treatment or simplify any required future treatment. Restoration of carious primary teeth and the prompt placement of space maintainer appliances can prevent the development of asymmetric occlusions that are difficult to treat

in adult patients. More pronounced asymmetries could be an expression of skeletal discrepancies and should be evaluated appropriately (see Chapter 29).

Functional Shifts on Closure

It is important to note the presence or absence of lateral and anteroposterior functional shifts of the mandible during closure in all patients with anterior and posterior crossbites, as explained previously.

Premature Loss of Primary Teeth

The premature unilateral loss of a primary canine is invariably associated with a deviation in the dental midline. Extraction of the contralateral primary canine, if done soon, may prevent deviation of the midline. Premature loss of a primary second molar invites undesirable mesial movement of the permanent first molar. When this happens, a space maintenance appliance, if promptly inserted, can prevent the need or improve the prognosis for future orthodontic treatment. Maintenance of a healthy primary dentition is an important means of preventing malocclusions (see Chapter 17).

Tooth Size-Arch Length Relation

The crowding that exists in the adult dentition or the crowding that is predicted in a mixed dentition is recorded on the clinical form. A detailed description of the procedure used to measure crowding is presented in Chapter 12.

RADIOGRAPHIC ANALYSIS

It is essential to have a **panoramic radiograph** or a complete **periapical mouth survey** in the diagnostic records of potential orthodontic patients.

Congenitally missing teeth, except for third molars, most often require orthodontic treatment to resolve resulting occlusion problems. **Impacted teeth** need to be assessed radiographically for position and relationship to other teeth. **Root dilaceration** can have an impact on the successful movement of a tooth. **Alveolar bone height** and **periodontal status** are important factors for orthodontic diagnosis. Unerupted **supernumerary teeth** should be removed before orthodontic treatment. Significant **root resorption** is a contraindication for orthodontic treatment and needs to be identified and assessed before placement of appliances. Periapical **pathologic conditions** should be addressed by appropriate endodontic procedures before a patient begins orthodontic treatment.

A **lateral cephalometric radiograph** of the head is taken routinely by specialists and is essential to the successful diagnosis and treatment planning of patients who have convex or concave facial profiles and either long or short anterior face heights (see Chapter 10).

DIAGNOSTIC SUMMARY AND PROBLEM LIST

A summary of findings should be made by the clinician that highlights the important information gleaned from an examination and work up of all the diagnostic records. From this summary, a list of problems is assembled.

TREATMENT PLAN

The treatment plan is created as a response to the problem list. Ideally, the treatment plan describes the procedures meant to correct each problem on the list. Sometimes a problem is listed for which no orthodontic treatment is planned. For example, a retrusive chin may be corrected with a genioplasty surgery, an option requiring a referral to an oral surgeon.

Anchorage sources such as headgear, transpalatal arches, interarch elastics, or specific appliances,

whether removable or fixed, are listed. Complicating factors such as periodontal bone loss or root resorption are noted.

APPLIANCE PLAN

A description of the appliances planned for use in the treatment is recorded. Changes in appliance type occurring during treatment should be entered as an update.

RETENTION PLAN

Before treatment begins, the patient and clinician must discuss the kinds of retainers recommended and their importance. The daily wear time and overall duration for wear should be discussed. For routine orthodontic treatment, removable retainers are worn full-time (except for while eating) for 6 to 12 months and nightly thereafter for an indefinite extended time by adolescents and adults. Fixed banded or bonded retainers in the mandibular arch do not depend on patient cooperation and are more reliable than removable retainers, but they interfere with flossing and entail monitoring over long periods. Children in the mixed dentition do not usually wear retainers for longer than a year so that tooth eruption is not restricted.

REFERENCES

1. Tung AW, Kiyak HA: Psychological influences on the timing of orthodontic treatment, *Am J Orthod Dentofacial Orthop* 113:29-39, 1998.
2. Koski K: The norm concept in dental orthopedics, *Angle Orthod* 25:113-117, 1955.
3. Angle EH: Classification of malocclusion, *Dental Cosmos* 41:248-264; 350-357, 1899.
4. Begg PR: *Begg orthodontic theory and technique,* Philadelphia, 1965, WB Saunders.
5. Andrews LF: The six keys to normal occlusion, *Am J Orthod* 62:296-309, 1972.
6. Ackerman JL, Proffit WR: The characteristics of malocclusion: a modern approach to classification and diagnosis, *Am J Orthod* 56:443-454, 1969.
7. Proffit WR, Ackerman JL: Rating the characteristics of malocclusion: a systematic approach for planning treatment, *Am J Orthod* 64(3):258-269, 1973.
8. Staley RN, Stuntz WR, Peterson LC: A comparison of arch widths in adults with normal occlusion and adults with class II Division 1 malocclusion, *Am J Orthod* 88:163-169, 1985.

CHAPTER 10

Cephalometric Analysis

Robert N. Staley

KEY TERMS

enlargement
focal spot
penumbra
rotating anode
collimator
grid
aluminum shield
lead shield

sella
nasion
orbitale
point A
point B
pogonion
gnathion

menton
articulare
gonion
porion
soft tissue glabella
pronasale
labrale superius

labrale inferius
soft tissue pogonion
Frankfort horizontal plane
sella-nasion plane
facial plane
mandibular plane
ramus plane

Using direct observation, clinicians can learn to recognize patients with significant mandibular retrusion, mandibular prognathism, long and short anterior face heights, and excessive vertical growth of the maxilla. These features are associated with the three facial profile types: straight, convex, and concave. Cephalometric radiographs enable clinicians to quantify facial and dental relationships and thereby assess more accurately the extent to which a patient deviates from normal facial and dental morphologies. By comparing anatomic relationships in an individual patient to the relationships found in a group of persons with normal occlusion, the normality of a patient can be determined.

Standardized cephalometric x-rays are taken by orthodontists as an aid in diagnosis to evaluate the pretreatment dental and facial relationships of a patient, to evaluate changes during treatment, and to assess tooth movement and facial growth at the end of treatment. On the cephalometric film, teeth can be related to other teeth, to the jaw in which they reside, and to cranial structures. The maxilla and mandible can be

related to one another and other structures in the cranium, and the soft tissue profile can be evaluated.

A cephalometric analysis is one of several diagnostic aids. An orthodontic diagnosis cannot be made solely on the basis of a cephalometric analysis. It is a valuable aid in orthodontic diagnosis only if its findings are correctly and wisely interpreted with the help of other diagnostic aids.

CEPHALOMETRIC RADIOGRAPHY (TECHNICAL CONSIDERATIONS)

A cephalometric x-ray apparatus consists of an x-ray–producing machine that is placed a fixed distance from a device that holds the x-ray film and positions the patient's head. The standard lateral and posteroanterior x-rays are usually taken with the patient in centric occlusion. Repeated standardized films can be taken of an individual in the same cephalometric x-ray apparatus. Standardization is necessary for the study of growth and treatment progress.

The x-ray source is placed as far as is practically possible (5 to 6 feet) away from the patient to reduce the **enlargement** of the head structures. The film is placed as close to the patient as possible, while still accommodating the largest head, to reduce enlargement. The patient is held firmly in a head holder, which orients the Frankfort horizontal plane (porion-orbitale) parallel with the floor. This is accomplished by placing the ear rods of the head holder into the external auditory orifices and relating orbitale to the head holder. The central x-ray beam passes through the right and left ear rods. For this reason, bilateral facial structures on the right and left sides of the mid-sagittal plane are not perfectly superimposed. Asymmetry between the two sides of the face compounds the differences.

The **focal spot** is the area from which the roentgen radiation is emitted. The **penumbra** is the secondary shadow cast by a radiated structure on the film that results in a blurring of the borders of an image. The penumbra increases as the focal spot and tube-subject-film distances increase. A **rotating anode** permits the use of higher energy levels with a small focal spot. A variable white light **collimator** allows precise limitation of the primary x-ray beam to the area of the face. A **grid,** a series of thin strips of lead, is placed between the patient and the film. The grid absorbs secondary radiation, and thereby reduces the image blurring caused by secondary radiation. Intensifying screens within the film cassette permit film exposure with lower radiation exposure. An adjustable **aluminum shield** is placed between the x-ray source and the patient's profile to reduce radiation exposure to the soft tissues. The soft tissue profile can then be observed and studied on the same x-ray film. To protect the patient from unnecessary radiation, a **lead shield** is worn by the patient and the variable collimator is adjusted so that the lower neck structures are not included in the primary radiation beam.

ANATOMIC LANDMARKS

A knowledge of craniofacial anatomy is required for the interpretation of a cephalometric film. Structures are overlapped and often difficult to observe on the two-dimensional x-ray film. Anatomic structures commonly observed in lateral cephalograms are il-

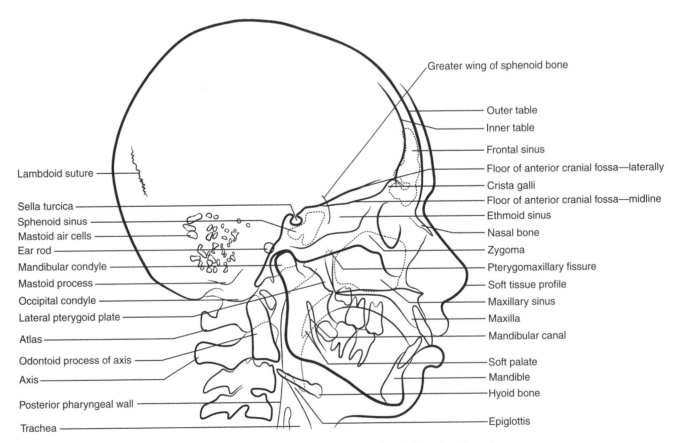

Figure 10-1 Anatomic landmarks on a lateral cephalometric radiograph.

lustrated in Figure 10-1. Skeletal structures are often more easily identified in children than in adults because bone density in adults obscures details. Soft tissue structures such as the pharyngeal walls, adenoidal tissues, and tongue should be recognized. For a more comprehensive description of cephalometric anatomy and interpretations, other texts should be consulted.[1-3]

CEPHALOMETRIC LANDMARKS

Radiographic cephalometry was first used in the fourth and fifth decades of the twentieth century as a research tool by anthropologists and orthodontists for the study of human variation and growth. In the fifth decade of this century, orthodontists began to use cephalograms to assist in clinical diagnosis and treatment. Subsequently, the cephalometric analyses in present use were developed.

Clinicians have chosen landmarks and relationships most relevant to diagnosis and treatment (Box 10-1). Many of the most frequently used landmarks are illustrated in Figure 10-2. Most landmark points are located on anatomic structures, but one important point, sella, is located in the middle of the bony outline of the pituitary fossa. Some points are more easily and reliably located than others. For example, nasion is relatively easy to locate when compared with the posterior nasal spine. Location of a point may be

---

BOX 10-1   Cephalometric Landmark Definitions and Locations (see Figure 10-2)

Hard Tissue Points [1-3]

1. **Sella** (S) is located in the center of the outline of the pituitary fossa (sella turcica). Locating the point before tracing the shadow of the anterior and posterior clinoid processes and floor of the fossa is probably more accurate than locating the point after tracing the structures.
2. **Nasion** (N) is located at the most inferior, anterior point on the frontal bone adjacent to the frontonasal suture. Again, point location should precede tracing of the bony outlines.
3. **Orbitale** (Or) is located on the lowermost point on the outline of the bony orbit. Usually, both right and left orbital outlines are visible. Orbitale is then located at the bisection of the two orbit outlines. Orbitale may be difficult to locate in some subjects.
4. **Point A** (A) is located at the most posterior part of the anterior shadow of the maxilla, usually near the apex of the central incisor root.
5. **Point B** (B) is located at the most posterior point on the shadow of the anterior border of the mandible, usually near the apex of the central incisor root.
6. **Pogonion** (Pog) is located at the most anterior point on the shadow of the chin.
7. **Gnathion** (Gn) is located at a point on the shadow of the chin midway between pogonion and menton.
8. **Menton** (Me) is located at the most inferior point on the shadow of the chin.
9. **Articulare** (Ar) is the point of intersection of the inferior border of the cranial base and the averaged posterior surfaces of the mandibular condyles.
10. **Gonion** (Go) is the midpoint of the angle of the mandible found by bisecting the angle formed by the mandibular and ramus planes.
11. **Porion** (Po) is located at the most superior point on the shadow of the ear rod at the superior border of the external auditory meatus. The correct location of porion is thus directly dependent on the placement of the ear rods at the time of x-ray film exposure. Porion is sometimes inaccurately positioned for this reason. The ear rods are difficult to locate in underexposed films in which the roentgen rays have not sufficiently penetrated the temporal bone.

Anatomic porion is used instead of porion by some clinicians. It is the superior point on the shadow of each external auditory meatus. Anatomic porion is at the bisection of bilateral radiolucent areas posterior and superior to the heads of the mandibular condyles. The ear rods must be translucent to allow these structures to be identified. Most published standards for cephalometric measurements involving porion are based on ear rod porion.

Soft Tissue Points[1-3] (Figure 10-3)

1. **Soft tissue glabella** (G′) is the most prominent point in the midsagittal plane of the forehead (see Figure 10-3).
2. **Pronasale** (Pr) is the most prominent point on the tip of the nose.
3. **Labrale superius** (Ls) is the median point in the upper margin of the upper membranous lip.
4. **Labrale inferius** (Li) is the median point in the lower margin of the lower membranous lip.
5. **Soft tissue pogonion** (Pog′) is the most prominent point on the soft tissue contour of the chin.

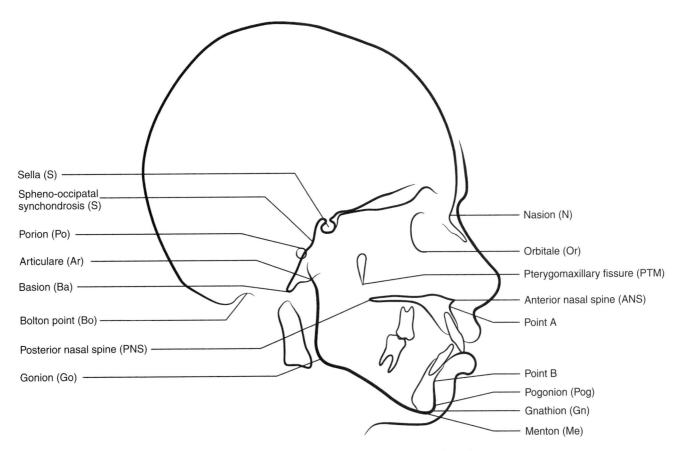

Figure 10-2 Major landmarks on a lateral cephalometric tracing.

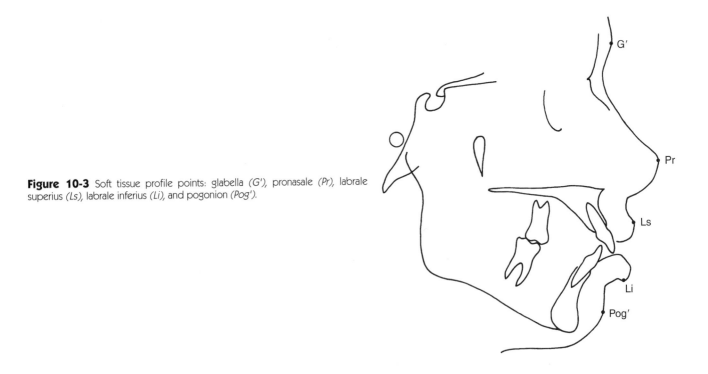

Figure 10-3 Soft tissue profile points: glabella *(G')*, pronasale *(Pr)*, labrale superius *(Ls)*, labrale inferius *(Li)*, and pogonion *(Pog')*.

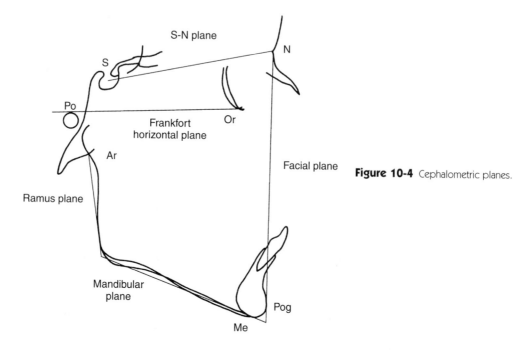

Figure 10-4 Cephalometric planes.

BOX
10-2

Cephalometric Planes

A plane requires three points for definition; however, the cephalometric planes illustrated in Figure 10-4 are only just lines connecting two points.

1. The **Frankfort horizontal plane** (Po-Or) is formed by a line passing through points porion and orbitale. Misplacement of the ear rods results in an incorrect location of porion, which should be located at the superior border of the external auditory meatus. Careful and firm placement of the ear rods is, therefore, essential for obtaining a correctly positioned Frankfort plane. To properly orient a cephalometric tracing, the Frankfort plane should be oriented parallel to the top and bottom borders of the tracing sheet.

2. The **sella-nasion plane** (S-N) is easily located and has been used for the superimposition of tracings from two or more sequentially exposed cephalograms.

3. The **facial plane** (N-Pog) is formed by passing a line through the nasion and pogonion points.

4. The **mandibular plane** (Go-Me) is drawn between menton and a point tangent to the posterior portion of the lower border of the mandible just as it turns upward to the posterior border of the ramus. The mandibular plane is incorrectly positioned if the x-ray is taken while the patient is not in centric occlusion.

5. The **ramus plane** is tangent to the averaged inferior, posterior surface of the ramus and passes through articulare.

---

easier in one plane of space than another. For example, the vertical position of the posterior nasal spine is usually more easily located than its anteroposterior position. Accuracy in point selection has an important impact on the reliability of a cephalometric analysis. From the various landmarks, various cephalometric planes are constructed (Box 10-2).

CEPHALOMETRIC ANGLES AND DISTANCES

A cephalometric analysis is divided into skeletal, dental, and soft tissue components (Boxes 10-3 and 10-4). The skeletal measurements are designed to evaluate the relationships of the jaws to the cranial base. The dental measurements relate the teeth to one another and to the

BOX 10-3

Angles Describing Skeletal Relationships (Figures 10-5 and 10-6)

1. The SN-Pog angle relates the anteroposterior position of the chin to a line passing through the anterior cranial base.
2. The SNA angle relates the anteroposterior position of the maxillary apical base to a line passing through the anterior cranial base.
3. The SNB angle relates the anteroposterior position of the mandibular apical base to a line passing through the anterior cranial base. NOTE: All measurements using the S-N plane are affected by the tilt or cant (steepness) of this plane as related to the Frankfort horizontal plane. When the S-N plane approaches a location horizontal to the Frankfort plane, the angles SN-Pog, SNA, and SNB are larger. When the S-N plane has a greater tilt in relation to the Frankfort horizontal plane, the angles are smaller. As a result, these changes in the cant of S-N plane should be taken into consideration when interpreting the measurements.
4. The ANB angle relates the anteroposterior position of the maxilla to the anteroposterior position of the mandible. Severe Class II malocclusions are often associated with large ANB values.
5. The facial angle (N-Pog:FH) relates the anteroposterior position of the chin to the Frankfort horizontal plane.
6. The mandibular plane-Frankfort horizontal plane angle (FMA or MP-FH) relates the cant of the mandibular plane to the Frankfort horizontal plane. NOTE: The accuracy of measurements involving the Frankfort horizontal plane is dependent on correct placement of the ear rods when the x-ray is taken.
7. The mandibular plane–S-N plane angle (MP-SN) relates the cant of the mandibular plane to a line passing through the anterior cranial base. NOTE: The MP-FH and MP-SN angles are accurate only if the teeth are in centric occlusion when the x-ray is taken.

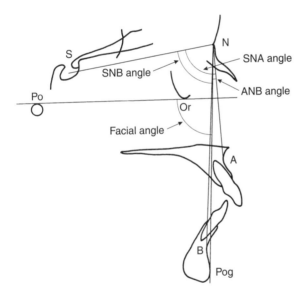

Figure 10-5 Angles relating the anterior cranial base to the maxilla and mandible.

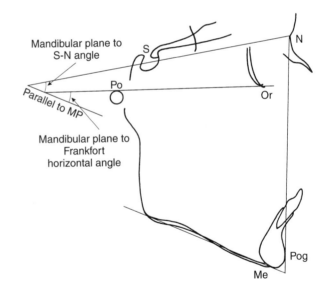

Figure 10-6 Mandibular plane angles.

BOX 10-4   Angles and Distances Describing Dental Relationships

1. The maxillary incisor to S-N plane angle (⊥:SN) relates the axial inclination of the most labial maxillary incisor to a line passing through the anterior cranial base (Figure 10-7).
2. The FH plane to mandibular incisor angle (FMIA or ⊤:FH) relates the axial inclination of the most labial mandibular incisor to the Frankfort horizontal plane (Figure 10-8).
3. The mandibular incisor to mandibular plane angle (IMPA or ⊤:MP) relates the axial inclination of the most labial mandibular incisor to the mandibular plane (see Figure 10-8). This relationship is affected by the morphology of the mandible. In general, as the lower border of the mandible becomes more horizontal, the IMPA increases, and as the lower border of the mandible becomes canted more vertically, the IMPA decreases.
4. The maxillary incisor to mandibular incisor angle (⊥:⊤) relates the axial inclination of the maxillary incisor to the axial inclination of the mandibular incisor (see Figure 10-7). As the incisors incline more labially, the angle becomes smaller; as the incisors incline more lingually, the angle becomes larger.
5. The maxillary incisor to line A-Pog (⊥:APog) distance, measured in millimeters, locates the anteroposterior position of the incisal tip of the most labial maxillary incisor crown in relation to a line connecting the maxillary base and chin (Figure 10-9).
6. The mandibular incisor to line NB (⊤:NB) distance measures the anteroposterior position of the incisal tip of the most labial mandibular incisor crown in relation to a line connecting the frontal bone and mandibular base (see Figure 10-9).

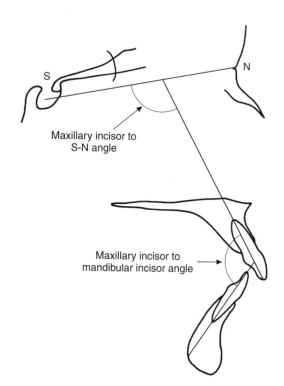

Figure 10-7 Upper incisor angle to the anterior cranial base and interincisal angle.

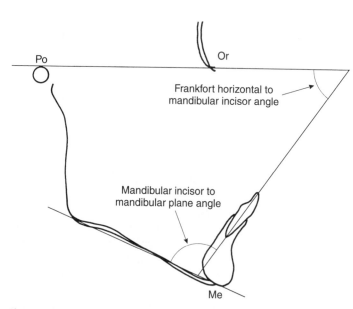

Figure 10-8 Mandibular incisor angles to the mandibular and Frankfort horizontal planes.

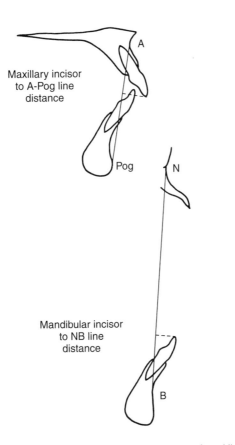

Maxillary incisor
to A-Pog line
distance

Pog

N

Mandibular incisor
to NB line
distance

B

Figure 10-9 The distances of upper and lower incisors to frontal lines.

jaw and cranial structures. The angular and linear measurements suggested in this chapter are taken from a number of cephalometric analyses.[4-9]

Soft tissue profile analyses have been developed for diagnostic purposes and mainly describe the overall profile as well as the relationships of the lips to the tip of the nose and soft tissue chin (see Chapter 11).

CEPHALOMETRIC NORMS

The normality of a patient is evaluated by relating the angular and distance measurements taken from the cephalogram to normative cephalometric values obtained from a sample of normal peers. The patient should belong to the same population from which the normative sample was taken.

The cephalometric normative values in Tables 10-1 and 10-2 are taken from the Iowa Facial Growth Study.[9] The Iowa longitudinal sample numbered 35 white subjects (20 males and 15 females) having normal occlusion. None of the subjects had received orthodontic treatment.

Table 10-1 gives cephalometric norms for males at 12 years of age that can be used in patients ranging from

10 to 17 years of age. Table 10-2 gives cephalometric norms for females at 14 years of age that are useful in patients ranging from 12 years of age to adulthood. The norms listed in Tables 10-1 and 10-2 use landmarks and planes that are defined and illustrated in this chapter. More comprehensive cephalometric norms for patients from 5 years of age to adulthood that are age- and gender-specific are listed in Chapter 11.

The distance measurements in Tables 10-1 and 10-2 and those in Chapter 11 were corrected to absolute values from their magnified values as measured on cephalograms. To compare the absolute distance values given in Tables 10-1 and 10-2 to those of a patient, the specific magnification factor associated with the cephalometric apparatus from which the radiographs are obtained should be used to correct the magnified measurements to absolute values comparable to those in Tables 10-1 and 10-2. The magnification factors from different cephalometric machines range from 8% to 14%. Therefore knowledge of the magnification factor of a particular machine is important when comparing distances measured on cephalograms.

For each angle or distance, the mean, standard deviation, and range (maximum and minimum values) have been recorded. The mean value is a mathematic central point derived from measurements taken from many individuals. None of the individuals of the norm group were likely to have a measurement identical to the mean. Because variability is basic to human physiognomy, the likelihood that any patient will have several of the mean values is remote. For our purposes, all measurements falling within 1 standard deviation above and below the mean are considered normal.

Although the normative values of a cephalometric analysis are useful as diagnostic tools, the mean values should not be used as treatment goals. Each patient has a unique set of cephalometric measurements and relationships. The objective of treatment must be the attainment of tooth relationships that are in harmony with the facial and dental morphology of the individual patient.

TRACING OF ANATOMIC STRUCTURES

In bilaterally symmetric faces, facial structures on the left side (including teeth) are usually superior and posterior to structures on the right side. Because of variations in anatomy and head position, the sides may be difficult to identify. Therefore a tracing of bilateral landmarks should bisect the images of the right and left sides. In the tracing of a bilaterally symmetric molar relationship, either side can be traced or the images of the two sides can be bisected. If the molar relationship is asymmetric, the side with the

TABLE 10-1	Cephalometric Standards for 12-Year-Old Males			
Measurement	Mean	SD	Minimum	Maximum
Skeletal Anteroposterior				
SNA°	82	3.7	76	89
SNB°	80	3.7	73	86
ANB°	2	2.4	−2	6
SN:Pog°	81	4.2	72	88
FH:N-Pog°	86	4.5	79	94
Skeletal Vertical				
N:Me mm	122	6.0	113	135
S:Go mm	90	6.8	80	102
S:Go/N:Me%	74	6.5	61	87
MP:SN°	28	7.2	13	43
MP:FH°	23	7.4	7	42
Dental Angular				
⊥:T°	134	9.8	115	152
⊥:SN°	102	6.3	89	115
T:FH°	62	10.9	48	85
T:MP°	96	9.2	78	108
Dental Linear				
⊥:A-Pog mm	4	1.9	0	7
T:NB mm	4	2.5	−1	9

From Bishara SE: *Am J Orthod* 79:35-44, 1981.
SD, Standard deviation.

TABLE 10-2	Cephalometric Standards for 14-Year-Old Females			
Measurement	Mean	SD	Minimum	Maximum
Skeletal Anteroposterior				
SNA°	80	3.8	74	90
SNB°	77	3.3	71	84
ANB°	3	2.1	0	7
SN:Pog°	77	3.3	72	84
FH:N-Pog°	84	2.5	79	89
Skeletal Vertical				
N:Me mm	107	5.0	96	116
S:Go mm	72	3.7	61	78
S:Go/N:Me%	68	3.5	63	75
MP:SN°	34	4.2	24	39
MP:FH°	28	4.9	19	35
Dental Angular				
⊥:T°	129	9.0	111	142
⊥:SN°	102	5.4	96	110
T:FH°	58	6.5	46	65
T:MP°	95	5.5	86	106
Dental Linear				
⊥:A-Pog mm	6	1.7	3	9
T:NB mm	4	2.0	2	8

From Bishara SE: *Am J Orthod* 79:35-44, 1981.
SD, Standard deviation.

greater discrepancy is traced. Being consistent in the tracing of sequential cephalograms of a patient is important for the meaningful interpretation of growth and treatment changes.

Structures in the middle of the head such as the sella turcica, nasal bones, and the central incisors are easily observed and traced. The most anterior upper and lower incisors are traced.

CEPHALOMETRIC X-RAY TRACING TECHNIQUE

The facial profile is customarily placed on the right side of the tracing sheet. Masking tape is used to attach the tracing acetate to the x-ray. The tracing is made on the frosted surface of the acetate sheet. An x-ray viewbox providing adequate illumination and a sharpened pencil are essential for tracing. A completed tracing is illustrated in Figure 10-10.

The tracing is begun by marking the points needed for the analysis on the tracing sheet. The soft tissue profile is traced and then the sella turcica going forward to the planum sphenoidale along the floor of the anterior cranial fossa and the shadows of the greater wings of the sphenoid bone are traced. The anterior surface of the frontal and nasal bones are then traced followed by tracing the outline of the maxilla from the anterior nasal spine along the floor of the nasal cavity back to the posterior nasal spine. The pointed end of the pterygomaxillary fissure is directed toward the posterior

nasal spine and is, therefore, a guide to the anteroposterior position of the posterior nasal spine. From the posterior nasal spine, trace forward along the palatal surface of the maxilla to the lingual alveolar bone around the incisors. The anterior surface of the maxilla is then traced. The most anterior central incisors are outlined, and after referring to the models or diagnostic record, the first molars are traced in their correct occlusal relationship. If the molar relationship is different on the right and left sides, the relationship for both sides should be written on the tracing. The symphysis and its inner cortical bone should be traced, and the lower and posterior borders of the mandible should be bisected until the borders intersect the posterior cranial base. The orbital rims are often difficult to trace. Both rims may be traced and bisected. The ear rod is traced, unless anatomic porion is used.

SUPERIMPOSITION OF SERIAL CEPHALOGRAMS

Clinicians and researchers are interested in studying the growth and treatment changes seen in patients. From the study of facial growth, techniques have been developed that allow accurate superimposition of lateral cephalograms taken from the same person at two or more different times. It is important that the serial cephalograms be made from the same cephalometric machine. Superimposition is more accurate in nongrowing adults than in growing persons.[10]

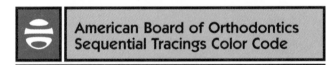

American Board of Orthodontics Sequential Tracings Color Code

1. Pretreatment (initial)—black
2. Progress—blue
3. End of treatment—red
4. Retention—green

OVERALL SUPERIMPOSITION OF THE FACE

The purpose of an overall superimposition is to assess growth and treatment changes of the maxilla, mandible, and soft tissue profile. In some nongrowing patients, movement of maxillary teeth can be assessed as well. Anatomic structures that experience the least amount of growth changes during the ages when orthodontic treatment is performed are superimposed in order to most accurately depict facial growth and treatment changes. After the age of 6 or 7

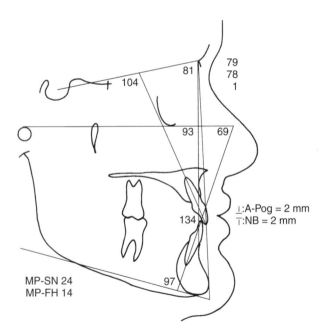

Figure 10-10 A cephalometric tracing with measurements placed on the tracing.

years, the planum sphenoidale and the ethmoidal part of the anterior cranial base change little in the antero-posterior direction.[10] The most accurate structure for the overall superimposition of the face is illustrated in Figure 10-11.

The overall superimposition method described has a high degree of validity and a medium to high degree of reproducibility.[10] An overall superimposition is illustrated in Figure 10-12.

SUPERIMPOSITION OF THE MAXILLA

Maxillary superimposition permits a clinician to assess the movement of maxillary teeth in relation to the maxilla. Two methods provide the most accurate superimposition, the structural and modified best-fit methods. If the details of the zygomatic process of the maxilla are clearly identifiable on the cephalogram, the structural method is recommended. The structural method has a medium

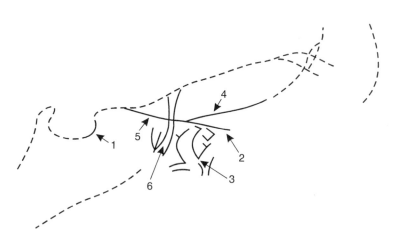

Figure 10-11 Anatomic structures used in an overall facial superimposition. *1,* The anterior wall of sella turcica. *2,* The contour of the cribriform plate of the ethmoid cells (lamina cribrosa), if identifiable. *3,* Details in the trabecular system of the ethmoid cells, if identifiable. *4,* Floor of the anterior cranial base lateral to the cribriform plate. *5,* The plane of the sphenoid bone (planum sphenoidale). *6,* Register on the midpoints between the right and left shadows of the anterior curvatures of the great wings of the sphenoid bone where they intersect the planum sphenoidale.

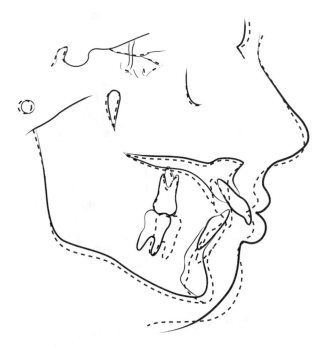

Figure 10-12 An overall superimposition of tracings from serial cephalograms of an orthodontic patient. *Solid line,* Pretreatment; *broken line,* end of treatment.

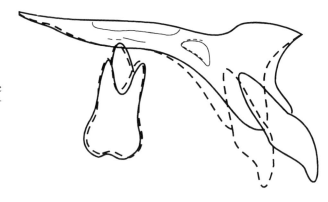

Figure 10-13 A superimposition of tracings from serial cephalograms of the maxilla of an orthodontic patient. *Solid line,* Pretreatment; *broken line,* end of treatment.

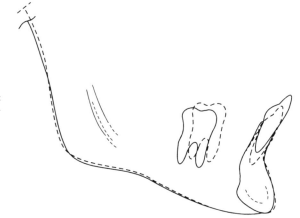

Figure 10-14 A superimposition of tracings from serial cephalograms of the mandible of an orthodontic patient. *Solid line,* Pretreatment; *broken line,* end of treatment.

to high validity and a low degree of reproducibility.[10] Because details of the zygomatic processes and orbital floors are not always identifiable, the structural method is not described here. Those interested in this method can find it described by Bishara and Athanasiou.[10]

The modified best-fit method for superimposing maxillary structures has a low degree of validity and a medium degree of reproducibility.[10] The method involves the following steps:

1. The outline of the palate, the permanent first molars, the most labially positioned incisor, and the incisal canal, when visible, are traced from the two cephalograms of the patient using different colors.
2. The two tracings are superimposed to a best fit of the contour of the nasal floor, oral part of the palate, and entrance of the incisal canal.

A maxillary superimposition is illustrated in Figure 10-13.

SUPERIMPOSITION OF THE MANDIBLE

Mandibular superimposition is used to assess the movement of mandibular teeth in relation to the

mandible. The method described is based on Bjork's implant studies and has a medium to high degree of both validity and reproducibility.[10]

Relatively Stable Structures of the Mandible

1. The anterior contour of the bony chin
2. The inner contour of the cortical plates at the inferior border of the symphysis, and any surrounding distinct trabecular structures
3. The contours of the mandibular nerve canals
4. The inferior contour of a mineralized third molar germ

The third molar tooth germ can only be used from the beginning of crown mineralization until the beginning of root formation.

Recommended Procedures for Mandibular Superimpositions

1. Trace the following structures on each cephalogram
   a. The symphysis and inner cortical bone
   b. The inferior and posterior borders of the mandible (bisect right and left sides)
   c. Articulare
   d. The anterior contour of the ramus
   e. The mandibular canals, if identifiable
   f. Third molar tooth buds before roots have formed
   g. The most labially positioned incisor
   h. The first molars

2. The four stable areas are used to superimpose the two tracings. In many patients, the third molar buds have developed roots, making them unusable for superimposition. The mandibular canals may be difficult to locate. However, the symphysis and its structures are routinely available for super-imposition.

A mandibular superimposition is illustrated in Figure 10-14.

REFERENCES

1. Athanasiou AE: *Orthodontic cephalometry,* London, 1995, Mosby-Wolfe.
2. Krogman W, Sassouni V: *A syllabus in roentgenographic cephalometry,* Philadelphia, 1957, Philadelphia Center for Research in Child Growth.
3. Riolo ML et al: *An atlas of craniofacial growth: cephalometric standards from the University School Growth Study,* Ann Arbor, Mich, 1974, The University of Michigan.
4. Downs WB: Variation in facial relationships: their significance in treatment and prognosis, *Am J Orthod* 34:812-840, 1948.
5. Reidel RA: A cephalometric roentgenographic study of the relation of the maxilla and associated parts to the cranial base in normal and malocclusion of the teeth, master's thesis, Evanston, Ill, 1948, Northwestern University.
6. Steiner CC: Cephalometrics for you and me, *Am J Orthod* 39:729-755, 1953.
7. Tweed CH: Was the development of the diagnostic facial triangle as an accurate analysis based on facts or fancy? *Am J Orthod* 48:823-840, 1962.
8. Wylie WL: Rapid evaluation of facial dysplasia in the vertical plane, *Angle Orthod* 22:165-182, 1952.
9. Bishara SE: Longitudinal cephalometric standards from 5 years of age to adulthood, *Am J Orthod* 79:35-44, 1981.
10. Bishara SE, Athanasiou AE: Cephalometric methods for assessment of dentofacial changes. In Athanasiou AE (ed): *Orthodontic cephalometry,* London, 1995, Mosby-Wolfe.

CHAPTER 11

Iowa Longitudinal Cephalometric Standards from 5 Years of Age to Adulthood

Samir E. Bishara

KEY TERMS

longitudinal studies
cephalometric standards
normative cephalometric
    standards

Iowa cephalometric
    standards
skeletal anteroposterior
    relationship

skeletal vertical relationship
dental linear relationship

dental angular relationship
soft tissue relationship

Numerous scientific reports in the orthodontic literature describe and classify the various components of the craniofacial complex in terms of the changes in their linear dimensions and angular relationships.[1-5] Many of these measurements have been subsequently used in the diagnosis and treatment planning of dentofacial malrelationships. Most of the studies were cross-sectional in nature and provided a large number of cephalometric standards for males and females at different ages and for various ethnic groups. In contrast, only a limited number of longitudinal or semi-longitudinal studies have been reported in which measurements were obtained on the same subjects from early childhood to adulthood.[6-8] Such a scarcity is not surprising because longitudinal studies are, by their nature, lengthy, costly, and dependent on the continuous cooperation of the subjects. Two of the studies[6,7] provided descriptive statistics on a large number of cephalometric measurements at consecutive ages for both males and females. Data presented on a yearly basis are of great value to those orthodontists interested in the detailed study of facial growth, yet such information presents the clinician with an overwhelming number of cephalometric standards at various ages for both males and females. As a result, the use of such data in the everyday practice of orthodontics has been rather limited and substituted by one set of cross-sectional values often obtained on adolescents or adults. This is in spite of the fact that the longitudinal studies have demonstrated that various cephalometric linear and angular measurements differ between males and females and also change significantly with age.[6-8] Accordingly, the use of normative cephalometric standards obtained for subjects at one age in the diagnosis of persons who might be of a completely different age or a different sex could adversely influence both the diagnosis and the treatment plan. As a result, six cephalometric standards, which can be used by the clinician for diagnostic purposes for males or females between 5 years of age and adulthood, were developed.

IOWA CEPHALOMETRIC STANDARDS

The Iowa cephalometric standards are specific by sex and applicable within an age range. For the vast majority of cases, only one of these standards needs to be used by the orthodontist to evaluate the patient before, during, and following orthodontic treatment.[8]

The original University of Iowa Facial Growth Study was started in March, 1946, by Howard V. Meredith and L. Bodine Higley. There were 89 boys

Text continued on p. 133

IOWA LONGITUDINAL CEPHALOMETRIC ANALYSIS
S.E. Bishara, D.D.S., M.S.
Values for *Males* and *Females* between *4 and 7* years of age*
--The values for 5 years of age are used—

NAME_____   NUMBER_____ BIRTH DATE_____   SEX_____

MEASUREMENTS	MIN.	AVG.	MAX.	S.D					
Skeletal Anteroposterior									
SNA°	74	**80**	88	3.7					
SNB°	68	**76**	82	3.4					
ANB°	-1	**4**	9	1.4					
Wits mm	-4	**0**	3	1.5					
NAPog°	2	**11**	17	3.8					
SNPog°	66	**75**	82	3.5					
FH:NPog°	56	**83**	88	5.5					
Skeletal Vertical									
N-Ans' mm°	25	**38**	43	3.1					
N-Me mm	58	**91**	101	7.0					
N:Ans' / N:Me %	28	**42**	48	3.0					
Ar'-Go mm	20	**39**	48	4.4					
S:Go mm	42	**60**	71	5.1					
Ar' : Go / S:Go %	47	**65**	69	3.7					
S : Go / N : Me %	60	**65**	75	3.9					
MP : SN°	18	**36**	42	5.2					
MP : FH°	16	**27**	34	4.4					
NSGn°	62	**68**	74	2.8					
FH : SGn°	40	**59**	66	4.5					
Dental Angular									
$\underline{1}$: $\overline{1}$ °	97	**142**	169	12.6					
$\underline{1}$: SN°	64	**91**	107	7.8					
$\overline{1}$: FH°	44	**64**	80	7.6					
$\overline{1}$: MP°	61	**88**	103	8.2					
Dental Linear									
$\underline{1}$: APog mm	0	**3**	7	1.3					
$\overline{1}$: NB mm	0	**2**	6	1.3					
Pog : NB mm	-3	**-1**	2	1.4					
Soft Tissue Profile									
Holdaway STA°	3	**15**	25	3.9					
Angle of Convexity°	160	**170**	178	4.0					
E-Plane LS mm	4	**0**	-5	1.9					
E-Plane : LI mm	4	**0**	-4	1.8					

Remarks_____

*The values were obtained from cephalograms of 20 male and 15 female normal Caucasians. All individuals were participants in the Iowa Growth Study from 4 years of age to adulthood.

All linear measurements are corrected for magnification.

Figure 11-1 Standard 1 for males and females between 4 and 7 years of age.

IOWA LONGITUDINAL CEPHALOMETRIC ANALYSIS

S.E. Bishara, D.D.S., M.S.

Values for *Males* between *5 and 10* years of age and for *Females* between *5 and 12* years of age*

--The values for 8 years of age are used--

NAME_____ NUMBER_____ BIRTH DATE_____ SEX_____

MEASUREMENTS	MIN.	AVG.	MAX.	S.D					
Skeletal Anteroposterior									
SNA°	74	80	90	4.0					
SNB°	70	76	83	3.4					
ANB°	1	4	8	1.6					
Wits mm	-4	0	3	1.8					
NAPog°	1	9	16	3.8					
SNPog°	68	76	84	3.5					
FH:NPog°	76	83	90	2.8					
Skeletal Vertical									
N-Ans' mm°	38	43	49	2.4					
N-Me mm	89	99	108	4.7					
N:Ans' / N:Me %	40	44	48	1.6					
Ar'-Go mm	35	42	52	3.4					
S:Go mm	55	66	76	4.6					
Ar' : Go / S:Go %	61	64	68	2.1					
S : Go / N : Me %	61	65	69	2.3					
MP : SN°	25	35	42	4.6					
MP : FH°	19	27	36	4.3					
NSGn°	62	68	74	2.8					
FH : SGn°	55	61	66	2.6					
Dental Angular									
$\underline{1} : \overline{1}$ °	117	131	143	7.3					
$\underline{1}$: SN°	93	101	109	4.6					
$\overline{1}$: FH°	49	59	69	4.7					
$\overline{1}$: MP°	83	94	104	5.1					
Dental Linear									
$\underline{1}$: APog mm	2	4	8	1.6					
$\overline{1}$: NB mm	1	4	6	1.2					
Pog : NB mm	-3	0	3	1.5					
Soft Tissue Profile									
Holdaway STA°	5	14	23	5.0					
Angle of Convexity°	159	168	174	3.5					
E-Plane LS mm	3	0	-5	1.9					
E-Plane : LI mm	3	0	-4	1.6					

Remarks_____

*The values were obtained from cephalograms of 20 male and 15 female normal Caucasians. All individuals were participants in the Iowa Growth Study from 4 years of age to adulthood.

All linear measurements are corrected for magnification.

Figure 11-2 Standard 2 for children and early adolescent males between 5 and 10 years of age and females between 5 and 12 years of age.

IOWA LONGITUDINAL CEPHALOMETRIC ANALYSIS

S.E. Bishara, D.D.S., M.S.

Values for *Males* between *10 and 17* years of age*

--The values for 12 years of age are used--

NAME_____ NUMBER_____ BIRTH DATE_____ SEX_____

MEASUREMENTS	MIN.	AVG.	MAX.	S.D					
Skeletal Anteroposterior									
SNA°	75	**81**	88	3.8					
SNB°	71	**78**	83	3.3					
ANB°	1	**3**	6	1.7					
Wits mm	-4	**-1**	3	1.9					
NAPog°	-1	**7**	12	4.3					
SNPog°	70	**78**	85	3.7					
FH:NPog°	74	**83**	90	3.7					
Skeletal Vertical									
N-Ans' mm°	42	**48**	52	2.4					
N-Me mm	102	**108**	116	4.4					
N:Ans' / N:Me %	41	**44**	48	1.6					
Ar'-Go mm	42	**47**	55	3.5					
S:Go mm	66	**74**	83	4.9					
Ar' : Go / S:Go %	60	**63**	66	1.9					
S : Go / N : Me %	60	**69**	77	4.7					
MP : SN°	23	**32**	42	5.2					
MP : FH°	16	**28**	36	4.9					
NSGn°	62	**68**	74	3.2					
FH : SGn°	56	**63**	70	3.3					
Dental Angular									
$\underline{1}$: $\overline{1}$ °	114	**128**	136	6.7					
$\underline{1}$: SN°	90	**102**	109	4.9					
$\overline{1}$: FH°	48	**55**	67	5.7					
$\overline{1}$: MP°	85	**98**	104	5.2					
Dental Linear									
$\underline{1}$: APog mm	3	**5**	9	1.6					
$\overline{1}$: NB mm	2	**5**	7	1.2					
Pog : NB mm	-3	**1**	3	1.8					
Soft Tissue Profile									
Holdaway STA°	4	**14**	23	4.2					
Angle of Convexity°	161	**168**	174	3.7					
E-Plane LS mm	2	**-1**	-6	1.9					
E-Plane : Ll mm	2	**0**	-4	1.7					

Remarks_____

*The values were obtained from cephalograms of 20 male and 15 female normal Caucasians. All individuals were participants in the Iowa Growth Study from 4 years of age to adulthood.

All linear measurements are corrected for magnification.

Figure 11-3 Standard 3 for adolescent males between 10 and 17 years of age.

IOWA LONGITUDINAL CEPHALOMETRIC ANALYSIS
S.E. Bishara, D.D.S., M.S.
Values for *Females* between *12 years of age and Adulthood**
--The values for 14 years of age are used—

NAME_____ NUMBER_____ BIRTH DATE_____ SEX_____

MEASUREMENTS	MIN.	AVG.	MAX.	S.D				
Skeletal Anteroposterior								
SNA°	74	**80**	90	3.8				
SNB°	71	**77**	84	3.3				
ANB°	0	**3**	7	2.1				
Wits mm	-3	**0**	3	2.0				
NAPog°	-6	**6**	17	5.6				
SNPog°	72	**77**	84	3.3				
FH:NPog°	79	**84**	89	2.5				
Skeletal Vertical								
N-Ans' mm°	44	**47**	50	1.9				
N-Me mm	96	**107**	116	5.0				
N:Ans' / N:Me %	40	**44**	49	2.2				
Ar'-Go mm	39	**45**	51	3.4				
S:Go mm	61	**72**	78	3.7				
Ar' : Go / S:Go %	58	**63**	68	2.4				
S : Go / N : Me %	63	**68**	75	3.5				
MP : SN°	24	**34**	39	4.2				
MP : FH°	19	**28**	35	4.9				
NSGn°	62	**68**	73	3.0				
FH : SGn°	58	**62**	68	2.9				
Dental Angular								
$\underline{1}$: $\overline{1}$ °	111	**129**	142	9.0				
$\underline{1}$: SN°	96	**102**	110	5.4				
$\overline{1}$: FH°	46	**58**	65	6.5				
$\overline{1}$: MP°	86	**95**	106	5.5				
Dental Linear								
$\underline{1}$: APog mm	3	**6**	9	1.7				
$\overline{1}$: NB mm	2	**4**	8	2.0				
Pog : NB mm	-2	**1**	4	1.5				
Soft Tissue Profile								
Holdaway STA°	3	**11**	19	5.2				
Angle of Convexity°	158	**168**	177	4.8				
E-Plane LS mm	2	**-2**	-5	2.2				
E-Plane : Ll mm	4	**0**	-3	2.3				

Remarks_____

*The values were obtained from cephalograms of 20 male and 15 female normal Caucasians. All individuals were participants in the Iowa Growth Study from 4 years of age to adulthood.

All linear measurements are corrected for magnification.

Figure 11-4 Standard 4 for adolescent females between 12 years of age and early adulthood.

IOWA LONGITUDINAL CEPHALOMETRIC ANALYSIS
S.E. Bishara, D.D.S., M.S.
Values for *Males (older than 18 years)**
--The values at adulthood are used--

NAME_____ NUMBER_____ BIRTH DATE_____ SEX_____

MEASUREMENTS	MIN.	AVG.	MAX.	S.D				
Skeletal Anteroposterior								
SNA°	76	82	89	3.7				
SNB°	73	80	86	3.7				
ANB°	-2	2	6	2.4				
Wits mm	-6	-1	8	3.0				
NAPog°	-10	3	12	6.1				
SNPog°	72	81	88	4.2				
FH:NPog°	79	86	94	4.5				
Skeletal Vertical								
N-Ans' mm°	48	54	60	2.9				
N-Me mm	113	122	135	6.0				
N:Ans' / N:Me %	40	44	49	2.0				
Ar'-Go mm	47	58	70	6.0				
S:Go mm	80	90	102	6.8				
Ar' : Go / S:Go %	58	64	68	2.9				
S : Go / N : Me %	61	74	87	6.5				
MP : SN°	13	28	43	7.2				
MP : FH°	7	23	42	7.4				
NSGn°	60	67	74	3.8				
FH : SGn°	54	62	70	4.5				
Dental Angular								
$\underline{1}$: $\overline{1}$ °	115	134	152	9.8				
$\underline{1}$: SN°	89	102	115	6.3				
$\overline{1}$: FH°	48	62	85	10.9				
$\overline{1}$: MP°	78	96	108	9.2				
Dental Linear								
$\underline{1}$: APog mm	0	4	7	1.9				
$\overline{1}$: NB mm	-1	4	9	2.5				
Pog : NB mm	-2	2	6	2.3				
Soft Tissue Profile								
Holdaway STA°	-5	8	14	5.5				
Angle of Convexity°	164	173	182	6.0				
E-Plane LS mm	-1	-5	-12	2.9				
E-Plane : LI mm	0	-4	-9	2.3				

Remarks_____

*The values were obtained from cephalograms of 20 male and 15 female normal Caucasians. All individuals were participants in the Iowa Growth Study from 4 years of age to adulthood.

All linear measurements are corrected for magnification.

Figure 11-5 Standard 5 for adult males older than 18 years of age.

IOWA LONGITUDINAL CEPHALOMETRIC ANALYSIS
S.E. Bishara, D.D.S., M.S.
Values for *Adult Females (older than 18 years)**
--The values at adulthood of age are used--

NAME_____ NUMBER_____ BIRTH DATE_____ SEX_____

MEASUREMENTS	MIN.	AVG.	MAX.	S.D				
Skeletal Anteroposterior								
SNA°	74	81	89	3.7				
SNB°	72	78	84	3.4				
ANB°	0	3	6	2.0				
Wits mm	-4	0	3	2.3				
NAPog°	-7	6	17	5.6				
SNPog°	74	78	84	3.3				
FH:NPog°	79	84	90	2.9				
Skeletal Vertical								
N-Ans' mm°	46	49	52	2.0				
N-Me mm	104	112	120	4.3				
N:Ans' / N:Me %	39	44	49	2.2				
Ar'-Go mm	42	47	55	3.6				
S:Go mm	67	76	83	3.6				
Ar' : Go / S:Go %	57	62	67	2.9				
S : Go / N : Me %	61	72	87	6.1				
MP : SN°	23	33	40	2.7				
MP : FH°	17	28	36	5.6				
NSGn°	63	68	72	2.9				
FH : SGn°	57	63	69	3.5				
Dental Angular								
$\underline{\text{I}}$: $\overline{\text{I}}$ °	107	130	144	10.4				
$\underline{\text{I}}$: SN°	94	102	112	6.1				
$\overline{\text{I}}$: FH°	43	57	69	7.9				
$\overline{\text{I}}$: MP°	85	95	105	6.5				
Dental Linear								
$\underline{\text{I}}$: APog mm	3	6	10	1.9				
$\overline{\text{I}}$: NB mm	2	5	9	1.7				
Pog : NB mm	-2	1	5	1.7				
Soft Tissue Profile								
Holdaway STA°	0	9	21	6.0				
Angle of Convexity°	159	171	185	6.6				
E-Plane LS mm	0	-5	-9	2.3				
E-Plane : LI mm	1	-2	-6	2.2				

Remarks_____

*The values were obtained from cephalograms of 20 male and 15 female normal Caucasians. All individuals were participants in the Iowa Growth Study from 4 years of age to adulthood.

All linear measurements are corrected for magnification

Figure 11-6 Standard 6 for adult females older than 18 years of age.

and 86 girls originally enrolled in the study, all of whom were not younger than 3 years of age. Records including dental casts, lateral and frontal facial photographs, and full-mouth series of radiographs were taken semiannually. Lateral and anteroposterior cephalograms along with medical history, height, and weight were taken quarterly until age 5 years. Thereafter, all records were taken semiannually until age 12 years, annually during adolescence, and once during early adulthood.[9,10] Twenty years later, in mid-adulthood, 16 females and 15 males were located and reported for follow-up examination.

The children in the original study group were North American white children, predominantly of Northern European descent, and living in or near Iowa City, Iowa. Most were from families of "above average socioeconomic status."[10]

The present standards are related more closely to the patient's age and sex than a single standard used for all ages and both sexes.[11] Measurements were obtained on 20 males and 15 females between 5 and 25 years of age. All had clinically acceptable occlusion and no apparent facial disharmony, and none of the subjects had undergone orthodontic therapy.[10] Angular and linear measurements as well as ratios of face heights were obtained to systematically evaluate the following parameters:

1. Skeletal anteroposterior relationships
2. Skeletal vertical relationships
3. Dental angular relationships
4. Dental linear relationships
5. Soft tissue relationships

The definitions of the various landmarks used appear in Chapter 10.

All linear measurements reported in Figures 11-1 through 11-6 are true size (i.e., corrected for magnification) to enable each clinician to interpret the data from their own cephalogram after adjusting for the magnification of their particular cephalometric machine. It should be reemphasized that for most cases only one of the six standards illustrated in Figures 11-1 to 11-6 needs to be used for the diagnosis, treatment planning, and treatment of an individual patient.

REFERENCES

1. Downs WB: Variation in facial relationships: their significance in treatment and prognosis, *Am J Orthod* 34:812-840, 1948.
2. Krogman W, Sassouni V: *A syllabus in roentgenographic cephalometry*, Philadelphia, 1957, Philadelphia Center for Research in Child Growth.
3. Riedel RA: A cephalometric roentgenographic study of the relation of the maxilla and associated parts to the cranial base in normal and malocclusion of the teeth, master's thesis, 1948, Evanston, Ill, Northwestern University.
4. Steiner CC: Cephalometrics for you and me, *Am J Orthod* 39:729-755, 1953.
5. Wylie WL: Rapid evaluation of facial dysplasia in the vertical plane, *Angle Orthod* 22:165-182, 1952.
6. Broadbent B et al: *Bolton standards of dentofacial developmental growth*, St Louis, 1975, Mosby.
7. Riolo ML et al: *An atlas of craniofacial growth: cephalometric standards from the University School Growth Study*, Ann Arbor, Mich, 1974, The University of Michigan.
8. Walker GF, Kowalski CJ: The distribution of the ANB angle in "normal" individuals, *Angle Orthod* 41:332-335, 1971.
9. Higley LB: Cephalometric standards for children 4 to 8 years of age, *Am J Orthod* 40:51-59, 1955.
10. Knott VB: Longitudinal study of dental arch widths at four stages of dentition, *Angle Orthod* 42:387-394, 1972.
11. Bishara SE: Longitudinal cephalometric standards from 5 years of age to adulthood, *Am J Orthod* 1:35-44, 1981.

CHAPTER 12

Tooth Size-Arch Length Analysis

Robert N. Staley

KEY TERMS

In the assessment of a crowded dentition, the lower arch takes precedence over the upper arch and is the key to orthodontic diagnosis. This is because the buccolingually narrow alveolar ridge in the mandible limits the possibility of significant tooth movement in most patients. Moving mandibular molars distally with an orthodontic appliance to create additional arch length is not wise in patients who have symmetric Angle Class I and Class II molar relations because the distal movement makes the relationship between the upper and lower molars more of a Class II relationship. However, distal movement of a mandibular molar that has tipped mesially in response to the premature loss of a primary molar is appropriate treatment that creates arch length and corrects asymmetry in the lower arch. In addition, mandibular incisors cannot be expanded labially beyond their alveolar support and remain stable. In the maxillary arch, molars can be moved distally in growing patients with Class II malocclusions to obtain needed arch length, and the maxillary arch can be widened laterally with rapid palatal expanders. Thus an analysis of arch length requirements in the mandibular arch is more critical because of the treatment limitations encountered there.

The maxillary arch assumes more importance in patients with Class III malocclusions in which the treatment-limiting factors apply to a small, deficient maxilla. In these patients the maxillary tooth size-arch length analysis is an important issue that may determine whether or not the patient can be treated orthodontically or with a combined surgical-orthodontic approach.

MEASUREMENT OF TOOTH SIZE-ARCH LENGTH RELATIONSHIP IN THE ADULT DENTITION

In this context an acronym, TSALD, is used to describe the tooth size-arch length discrepancy associated with dental spacing and crowding. The acronym for the upper arch is UTSALD; the acronym for the lower arch is LTSALD. Crowding in an arch is denoted as a negative number; excess spacing in an arch is denoted as a positive number.

Arch Length Measurements

Arch length (perimeter) measurements are obtained with either a Boley gauge (sharpened tips) or with dial or digital calipers (Figure 12-1). For the purpose of the analysis, only the arch length mesial to the permanent first molars is measured. The tips of the measuring instrument are placed in the buccal embrasures near the contact points between the teeth or on the alveolar ridge where the teeth are expected to contact one another in ideal alignment. Measurements are done according to the following steps:

1. The posterior parts of the arch from the mesial contacts of the first molars to the distal contacts of the canines are measured.
2. The arch lengths around the canines are measured. These lengths are added to the lengths of the posterior segments.

3. The anterior segments extend from a point on the cast between the central incisors to the mesial contact points of the canines.
4. The sum of all these segments on both sides represents the arch length.

The placement of pencil points on the cast can help in measuring arch segments where canines are malpositioned or unerupted and where central incisors are separated by a diastema.

Tooth Size Measurements

The mesiodistal widths of the teeth are obtained by measuring the distance between the anatomically correct contact points of each tooth mesial to the first molars. The

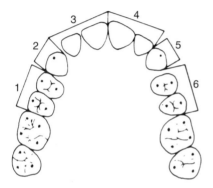

Figure 12-1 Segmental arch length measurements in the permanent dentition.

Boley gauge or calipers are usually positioned buccal to the teeth. However, the measuring device may need to be positioned occlusal to a rotated tooth.

Because of the number of measurements and the various positions in which the measuring instrument can be placed, errors can quickly multiply and produce a meaningless TSALD.

MEASUREMENT OF TOOTH SIZE-ARCH LENGTH RELATIONSHIP IN THE MIXED DENTITION

The permanent incisors of children are much larger in mesiodistal width than their corresponding primary incisors. Because of this incisor width difference, termed *incisor liability*, the alveolar arches must grow sufficiently in size to accommodate the larger erupting permanent incisors. In a longitudinal study of adolescents who had good alignment of their permanent teeth, Moorrees and Chadha[1] found that, during childhood, the permanent incisors erupted into either good or slightly crowded alignment in the mixed dentition. For many less fortunate children, eruption of the permanent incisors in the mixed dentition results in a marked crowding problem that attracts the attention of parents, children, and clinicians. For these children, a tooth size-arch length analysis can answer questions about future crowding and provide the basis for an appropriate treatment plan. A schema of the mixed dentition is shown in (Figure 12-2).

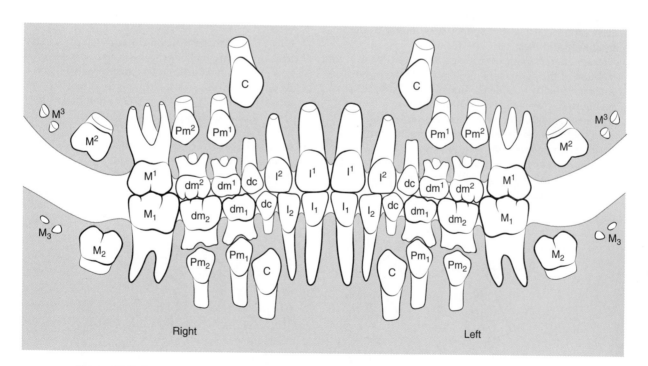

Figure 12-2 The mixed dentition after eruption of the permanent incisors and first molars. *I*, Permanent incisors; *C*, permanent canines; *Pm*, premolars; *M*, permanent molars; *dc*, primary canines; *dm*, primary molars.

Signs of Arch Length Deficiency

Children exhibit arch length deficiencies for two general reasons: (1) the arch length of some children is too small to accommodate the size of the teeth; and (2) a child may start with an adequate arch length but may develop a deficient arch length from a variety of environmental factors that affect the dentition (e.g., caries or loss of teeth) (Box 12-1).

MEASUREMENT OF THE AVAILABLE ARCH LENGTH IN THE MIXED DENTITION

The approach in measuring arch length in the mixed dentition is essentially the same as that described for the permanent dentition.

Measure arch length segments from the buccal and labial sides of the arch at the contact points between the teeth (Figure 12-3). Depending on whether or not the primary canines are present in the arch, the posterior arch length measurement between the molar and lateral incisor will have one or two components. If a space exists between the central incisors, the anterior arch length segments are measured from the distogingival surfaces of the lateral incisors to a midline point on the alveolar crest between the central incisors. The midline point is marked on the alveolar crest between the central incisors with a sharpened pencil to ensure that the two anterior segmental measurements are accurate.

The only difference between the permanent and mixed dentition tooth size-arch length analyses is the need to predict the mesiodistal widths of the unerupted permanent canines and premolars in the mixed dentition.

BOX 12-1	Ways the TSALD Can Be Expressed

1. When eruption of the permanent lateral incisors forces premature exfoliation of a primary canine, the child probably has permanent teeth that are too large to be accommodated by the available arch.
2. In patients with severe crowding, the permanent lateral incisors may actually come into contact with the mesial surfaces of the primary first molars.
3. After the unilateral forced exfoliation of a lower primary canine in a crowded mixed dentition, the permanent incisors drift toward the side of the lost primary canine causing discrepancy between the upper and lower midlines.
4. Another characteristic of crowded dentitions is the eruption of the permanent incisors, either too far lingually or labially outside the line of arch. These teeth are referred to as *blocked out* of the arch.
5. Lower incisors that are positioned too far labially often show noticeable labial gingival recession, another sign of crowding.
6. Premature loss of any of the primary teeth may result in an arch length deficiency. Premature loss of a primary second molar is usually followed by mesial migration of the permanent first molar, resulting in possible impaction of the adjacent second premolar. Following premature loss of a second primary molar, the adjacent permanent maxillary first molar tips forward and rotates around its large palatal root and the adjacent mandibular first molar tips forward. Environmental insults that prematurely reduce the mesiodistal size of the primary dentition include trauma, caries, poor restorations, extraction, and wear.
7. Other factors that may diminish arch length are ankylosis of primary molars, and delayed or ectopic eruption of permanent teeth. As an ankylosed primary second molar progresses farther into infraocclusion, arch length is lost as the permanent first molar tips forward after it loses proximal contact with the ankylosed molar.
8. Maxillary permanent canines can erupt buccally or palatally or they may become impacted, resulting in loss of arch length as posterior teeth migrate mesially.

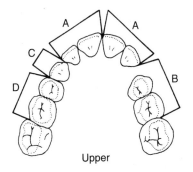
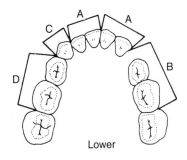

Figure 12-3 Segmental arch length measurements in the mixed dentition.

PREDICTION OF TOOTH WIDTHS OF UNERUPTED PERMANENT PREMOLARS AND CANINES IN THE MIXED DENTITION

Prediction of the mesiodistal widths of unerupted canines and premolars is an essential part of a tooth size-arch length analysis in the mixed dentition. Following the eruption of the permanent incisors, the mandibular arch length and width have, for all practical purposes, achieved adult dimensions. A meaningful mixed dentition tooth size-arch length analysis depends on an accurate prediction of the mesiodistal widths of the unerupted permanent canines and premolars.

Several prediction methods have been published. Some were developed from simple regression analysis, some from multiple regression analysis, and others from different approaches. All prediction methods have error. The error is described by a statistic called the *standard error of estimate.* The lower the standard error of estimate, the better the prediction method. The standard errors of estimate for several prediction methods vary from 0.2 mm to 0.86 mm.[2] The lowest standard errors of estimate among those reported are associated with prediction methods developed from multiple regression analysis.[3,4]

There are two approaches for predicting the size of the unerupted permanent canine and premolars in the mixed dentition, namely, with and without the use of radiographs.

RADIOGRAPHIC METHODS OF PREDICTION

Revised Hixon-Oldfather Prediction Method for the Mandibular Arch

Hixon and Oldfather[5] were the first to develop an equation to predict the mesiodistal widths of unerupted mandibular canines and premolars in children who participated in the Iowa Facial Growth Study. Staley and Kerber,[6] in a later study of Iowa

Facial Growth Study subjects, significantly reduced the standard error of estimate when they generated a revised Hixon and Oldfather prediction equation (Table 12-1). The coefficient of correlation (r) of the revised equation was higher than that of the original equation. The original equation was derived primarily from measurements of teeth on the left side of the arch of each subject, whereas the revised equation was derived from the means of measurements taken from both the right and left side teeth in each subject.

Records needed to perform the prediction include a cast of the lower arch and periapical radiographs of the unerupted lower premolars taken with a long-cone paralleling or right angle technique.

The addition of one standard error of estimate to the predicted sum would yield a predicted sum of widths

Steps for Predicting Tooth Size

1. Measure the mesiodistal widths of the lower right central and lateral incisors on a cast.
2. Measure the widths of the lower right first and second premolars on a periapical film.
3. Take the sum of these widths to the prediction graph (Figure 12-4) to determine the combined predicted widths of the lower right canine and premolars.
4. Add one standard error of estimate to the predicted sum as a hedge against underpredicting the true size of the teeth.
5. Use the same procedure with teeth on the left side of the arch to predict the lower left canine and premolar widths.
6. Add the predicted widths of the right and left canines and premolars to the widths of the erupted incisors to compute lower arch tooth size mesial to the permanent first molars.

A step-by-step chart for clinical use is shown in Figure 12-5.[7]

TABLE 12-1	A Comparison of the Original and Revised Hixon-Oldfather Prediction Equations[6]	
Variable	Original Equation N = 76	Revised Equation N = 57
Mean difference (mm)*	−0.4	−0.06
Mean absolute error (mm)	0.6	0.3
Standard error of estimate (mm)	0.57	0.44
Correlation coefficient (r)	0.87	0.92

From Staley RN, Kerber PE: *Am J Orthod* 78(3):296-302, 1980.
*Difference between predicted and actual means of the widths of the canine and premolars. A negative sign indicates that the predicted mean was smaller than the actual mean.

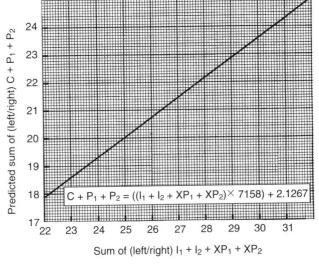

Figure 12-4 Prediction graph for the revised Hixon-Oldfather prediction method.

Predicted sum of (left/right) C + P₁ + P₂

$$C + P_1 + P_2 = ((I_1 + I_2 + XP_1 + XP_2) \times 7158) + 2.1267$$

Sum of (left/right) $I_1 + I_2 + XP_1 + XP_2$

Standard error of estimate = 0.44 mm

Patient _____

Date _____

	Left	Right	Both sides
Posterior arch			
1. Cast width of central incisor	___	___	
2. Cast of lateral incisor	___	___	
3. Radiograph width of first premolar	___	___	
4. Radiograph width of second premolar	___	___	
5. Sum of incisor and premolar widths	___	___	
6. Predicted sum of premolar and canine widths	___	___	
7. Add standard error of estimate (0.44 mm)	0.44	0.44	
8. Posterior tooth width sum (add lines 6 and 7)	___	___	
9. Posterior arch length (B or C + D)	___	___	
10. Arch length excess (+) or deficit (−) (line 9 minus line 8)	___	___	___
Anterior Arch			
11. Sum of cast widths of incisors	___	___	
12. Anterior arch length (A)	___	___	
13. Arch length excess (+) or deficit (−) (line 12 minus line 11)	___	___	___
Total Arch			
14. Arch length excess (+) or deficit (−) (line 10 plus line 13)			___
Adjustments			
15. Anteroposterior position of incisors			___
16. Other adjustments (curve of Spee, etc.)			___
17. Adjusted total arch length excess (+) or deficit (−)			___

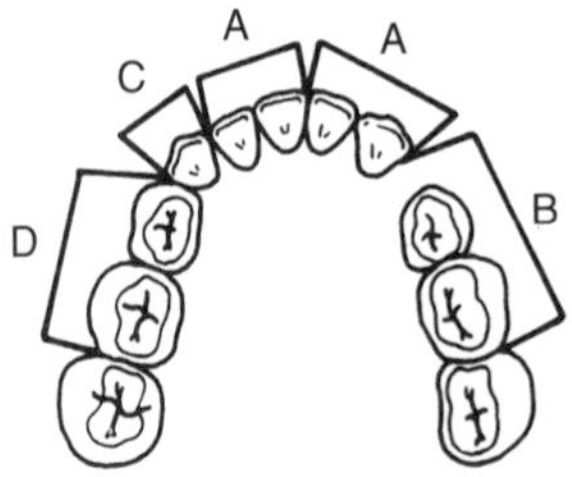

Figure 12-5 Clinical chart for the revised Hixon-Oldfather prediction method.

at the eighty-fourth percentile. This would provide assurance that the predicted sum of canine and premolar widths is as large or larger than the true sum in 84% of all possible patients.[8]

Iowa Prediction Method for Both Arches

Another prediction method using data from the Iowa Facial Growth Study was developed by Staley et al[9] to predict the mesiodistal widths of unerupted canines and premolars in both the upper and lower arches.

With this method, only measurements of the radiographic widths of unerupted canines and premolars are used as predictor variables. The standard errors of estimate are 0.48 mm in the upper arch and 0.47 mm in the lower arch.

Records needed for the complete analysis are casts of the upper and lower arches and periapical radiographs of the upper canines and premolars and lower premolars taken with a long-cone paralleling or right angle technique.

Upper Arch Prediction

1. Measure the mesiodistal widths of the upper right canine and second premolar on the radiographs.
2. Transfer the sum of these widths to the prediction graph (Figure 12-6) to obtain the predicted sum of the upper right canine and premolar widths.
3. For the most accurate prediction, measurements should be repeated for the left side.

Lower Arch Prediction

1. Measure the mesiodistal widths of the lower right premolars on the radiographs.
2. Transfer the sum of these widths to the prediction graph (Figure 12-7) to obtain the predicted sum of the lower right canine and premolar widths.
3. For the most accurate prediction, measurements should be repeated on the left side. NOTE: For various reasons, good measurable radiographic views of the unerupted premolars and canine on one side of the mouth may not be obtainable. Staley et al[9] found that a measurement from a satisfactory radiograph of a tooth on one side of the arch could be substituted for an unmeasurable antimere tooth without significantly altering the accuracy of the prediction.

How to Use the Graphs The sum of the radiographic tooth widths measurement is located on the horizontal axis at the bottom of each prediction graph and then projected vertically to intersect the prediction line. For example, the sum of the upper right canine

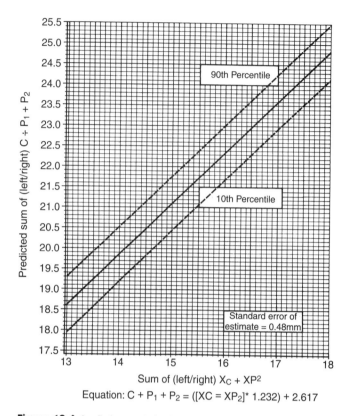

Equation: $C + P_1 + P_2 = ([XC = XP_2]^* \ 1.232) + 2.617$

Figure 12-6 Prediction graph for the maxillary arch of the Iowa prediction method.

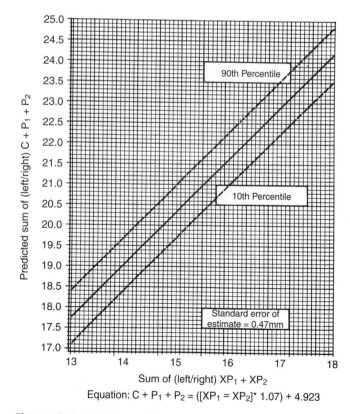

Equation: $C + P_1 + P_2 = ([XP_1 = XP_2]^* \ 1.07) + 4.923$

Figure 12-7 Prediction graph for the mandibular arch of the Iowa prediction method.

and second premolar widths as measured on the periapical film is 15 mm, which is located on the horizontal axis of the graph. Follow the vertical line from the 15-mm point on the bottom line of the prediction graph until it intersects with the solid prediction line (see Figure 12-6). Next, follow the horizontal line at the point of intersection to the left side of the chart to find the predicted sum of the canine and premolar widths (21.1 mm).

Step-by-step charts to calculate the TSALD were developed for the upper and lower arches for use by clinicians and are presented in Figures 12-8 and 12-9.

It is desirable that a prediction method be reasonably accurate, easily used, and cross-validated, that is, tested in a group of patients to determine how well it performs. The revised Hixon-Oldfather and Iowa prediction methods[6,9] described here have acceptably low standard errors of estimate, have easy-to-use prediction tables, and were successfully cross-validated on a sample of 53 orthodontic patients.

Patient _____

Date _____

	Left	Right	Both sides
Posterior arch			
1. Radiograph width of upper canine	_____	_____	
2. Radiograph width of upper second premolar	_____	_____	
3. Sum of radiograph widths	_____	_____	
4. Predicted sum of canine and premolar widths	_____	_____	
5. Add standard error of estimate (0.48 mm)	_____	_____	
6. Posterior tooth width sum (add lines 4 and 5)	_____	_____	
7. Posterior arch length (B or C + D)	0.48	0.48	
8. Arch length excess (+) or deficit (−) (line 7 minus line 6)	_____	_____	_____
Anterior Arch			
9. Cast width of upper central incisors	_____	_____	
10. Cast width of upper lateral incisors	_____	_____	
11. Sum of incisor widths	_____	_____	
12. Anterior arch length (A)	_____	_____	
13. Arch length excess (+) or deficit (−) (line 12 minus line 11)	_____	_____	_____
Total Arch			
14. Arch length excess (+) or deficit (−) (line 8 plus line 13)			_____
Adjustments			
15. Anteroposterior position of incisors			_____
16. Other adjustments (regain arch length, etc.)			_____
17. Adjusted total arch length excess (+) or deficit (−)			_____

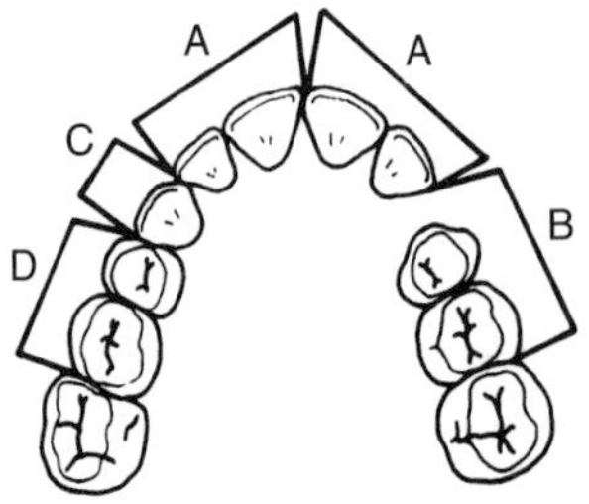

Figure 12-8 Clinical chart for the maxillary arch of the Iowa prediction method.

Proportional Equation Prediction Method

If most of the canines and premolars have erupted and if one or two succedaneous teeth are still unerupted, an alternative prediction method can be used to estimate the mesiodistal width of the unerupted permanent tooth. The widths of the unerupted teeth (e.g., a second premolar) and an erupted tooth (e.g., a primary second molar) are measured on the same periapical film.

The width of the erupted tooth, a primary second molar, is measured on a plaster cast. These three measurements comprise the elements of a proportion that can be solved to obtain the widths of the unerupted tooth on the cast:

If:
$$\frac{\text{Unerupted tooth width}}{\text{Unerupted tooth width (x-ray)}} = \frac{\text{Erupted tooth width (cast)}}{\text{Erupted tooth width (x-ray)}}$$

Then:
$$\text{Unerupted tooth width} = \frac{(\text{ETW Cast})(\text{UTW x-ray})}{(\text{ETW x-ray})}$$

Patient _____

Date _____

	Left	Right	Both sides
Posterior arch			
1. Radiograph width of lower first premolar	_____	_____	
2. Radiograph width of lower second premolar	_____	_____	
3. Sum of radiograph widths	_____	_____	
4. Predicted sum of canine and premolar widths	_____	_____	
5. Add standard error of estimate (0.47 mm)	0.47	0.47	
6. Posterior tooth width sum (add lines 4 and 5)	_____	_____	
7. Posterior arch length (B or C + D)	_____	_____	
8. Arch length excess (+) or deficit (−) (line 7 minus line 6)	_____	_____	_____
Anterior Arch			
9. Cast width of lower central incisors	_____	_____	
10. Cast width of lower lateral incisors	_____	_____	
11. Sum of incisor widths	_____	_____	
12. Anterior arch length (A)	_____	_____	
13. Arch length excess (+) or deficit (−) (line 12 minus line 11)	_____	_____	_____
Total Arch			
14. Arch length excess (+) or deficit (−) (line 8 plus line 13)			_____
Adjustments			
15. Anteroposterior position of incisors			_____
16. Other adjustments (curve of Spee, etc.)			_____
17. Adjusted total arch length excess (+) or deficit (−)			_____

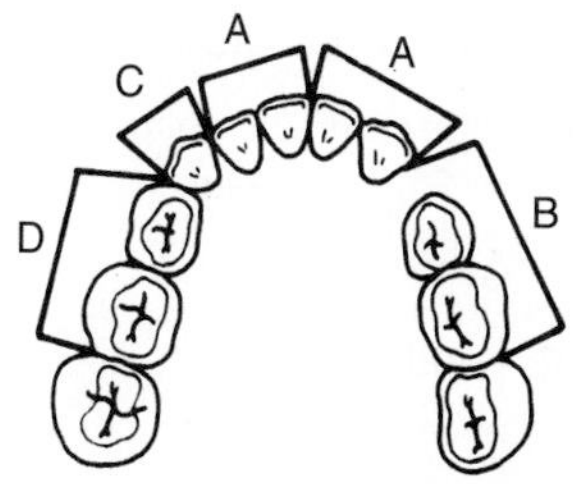

Figure 12-9 Clinical chart for the mandibular arch of the Iowa prediction method.

NONRADIOGRAPHIC PREDICTION METHODS

The main advantage of nonradiographic prediction methods is that they can be performed by measuring the erupted permanent lower incisors or primary teeth without the need of additional measurements from radiographs.[8,10,11] On the other hand, these methods are less accurate, as indicated by their larger standard errors of estimate as compared with the suggested radiographic methods.

Moyers[8] and Tanaka and Johnston,[10] in separate samples, correlated the sum of the mesiodistal widths of the four permanent lower incisors to the sum of the widths of the permanent canine, first premolar, and second premolar on one side of the arch in the maxilla and mandible. Moyers' prediction tables have been widely available, and his method has been used by many clinicians because the measurements are easily taken and the results can be obtained in a short time. No information is available concerning the correlation coefficients and error of his method. Tanaka and Johnston[10] developed prediction tables that were, essentially, similar to those of Moyers.[8] Their correlation coefficients were r = 0.63 for the maxillary teeth and r = 0.65 for the mandibular teeth. The standard errors of estimate were 0.86 mm for the maxillary teeth and 0.85 mm for the mandibular teeth. Unlike Moyers, who separated the sexes, Tanaka and Johnson combined the sexes in their study.

The prediction tables of Tanaka and Johnston in Box 12-2 contain the fiftieth percentile values. They recommended using the seventy-fifth percentile (higher) estimates as a hedge against underpredicting tooth size. However, evidence from other studies indicate that this method at the fiftieth percentile on average overpredicts the true size of the canine and premolars by 0.6 mm in

the upper arch,[3] 0.4 mm in the lower arch,[4] and in a third study, 1.1 mm in the lower arch.[11] Therefore the fiftieth percentile prediction most likely provides a desired hedge against underprediction of tooth size.

Other nonradiographic methods using primary teeth are available but are also less accurate than the previously discussed radiographic methods.[11]

APPLYING PREDICTION METHODS TO DIFFERENT RACIAL GROUPS

The radiographic and nonradiographic methods for predicting the mesiodistal widths of unerupted permanent canines and premolars in patients in the mixed dentition that are described in this chapter were developed in American white subjects of European ancestry. Evidence indicates that these methods would be acceptable in Egyptian and northern Mexican patients.[12] Lee-Chan et al[13] found that the nonradiographic method of Tanaka and Johnston[10] did not satisfactorily predict tooth size in Americans of Asian ancestry. Therefore they calculated more accurate prediction tables based on the correlation of lower incisor widths to canine and premolar widths in a sample of Asian Americans. Ferguson et al[14] developed a nonradiographic prediction method for a sample of American blacks by correlating lower incisor widths with the widths of canines and premolars. On average, the predicted values of canine and premolar width sums for each corresponding sum of incisor widths was larger in blacks by 0.2 mm in the maxilla and 0.6 mm in the mandible when compared with the values based on white Americans.[10] For these reasons it is recommended that clinicians use prediction methods in Asian-American and black patients that were developed in samples of these populations.

BOX 12-2	Prediction of the Widths of the Permanent Canines and Premolars in Millimeters in the Upper and Lower Arches

Sum of the mesiodistal widths of all four permanent mandibular incisors

20.5	21.0	21.5	22.0	22.5	23.0	23.5	24.0	24.5	25.0	25.5	26.0	26.5	27.0

Maxillary Arch
Predicted sum of the mesiodistal widths of the canine and premolars*

20.8	21.0	21.3	21.5	21.8	22.1	22.3	22.6	22.8	23.1	23.3	23.6	23.8	24.1

Mandibular Arch
Predicted sum of the mesiodistal widths of the canine and premolars*

20.2	20.5	20.7	21.0	21.3	21.5	21.8	22.1	22.3	22.6	22.9	23.1	23.4	23.7

*All predicted measurements are for one side of the arch.

OTHER FACTORS THAT INFLUENCE THE ESTIMATION OF THE TOOTH SIZE-ARCH LENGTH ANALYSIS

The primary and most important part of a tooth size-arch length analysis is the comparison of the size of the teeth to the size of the arch. This is the basic TSALD.

Clinicians also need to consider the impact of other factors on TSALD when developing the complete diagnosis of a patient. The other factors may not be readily quantified, therefore, clinicians have to make a qualitative judgment of how a particular factor may either increase or decrease the basic TSALD.

Incisor Inclination and Position

The inclination and anteroposterior position of the incisors affects the arch length analysis. Orthodontic movement of lingually inclined incisors in a labial direction increases arch length, and lingual movement of incisors decreases arch length. According to Tweed,[15] inclining the lower incisors 1 degree labially increases arch length by 0.8 mm. Conversely, inclining the lower incisors 1 degree lingually decreases arch length by 0.8 mm.

Orthodontists assess the inclination of the lower incisors by measuring the angle formed by the long axis of the mandibular incisor with both the mandibular and Frankfort horizontal planes on a cephalogram. Anteroposterior position can be determined by measuring the perpendicular distance from the incisal tip of the mandibular incisor to the nasion-B line. Further information about the normative values of these measurements is given in Chapters 10 and 11.

Curve of Spee

The curve of Spee is an important factor to consider in the overall space analysis because the curve is usually leveled during orthodontic treatment. During the leveling procedure, the incisors tip labially (Figure 12-10). If the lower incisors are in a satisfactory anteroposterior position or are inclined too far labially before treatment, leveling of the curve of Spee produces undesirable labial movement of the incisors unless there is excess arch length. In the latter cases, excess arch length (spacing) minimizes the movement of the

incisors during leveling. Baldridge[16] studied 30 patients who had an exaggerated curve of Spee in the mandibular arch and with all the permanent teeth erupted, excepting third molars. He found the mean additional arch length needed for leveling the curve of Spee without labial tipping of the incisors to be 3.5 mm ± 0.1 mm, with a minimum of 2.3 mm and a maximum of 5.2 mm depending on the degree of curve. As the curve of Spee becomes more exaggerated, the probability for an arch length deficiency increases.

To estimate the amount of additional arch length needed to level the curve of Spee for an individual patient, Balridge[16] suggested measuring the greatest depth of the curve on both sides of the arch, dividing the sum of both sides by 2, and adding 0.5 mm.

Position of the Permanent First Molars

If the primary second molars are intact and healthy before their physiologic exfoliation, the permanent first molars are probably well positioned between the premolars mesial to them and the second and third molars distal to them. Distal movement of well-positioned permanent first molars to create additional arch length in the mixed dentition may impact the permanent second molars. Distal movement of maxillary permanent molars in a Class II malocclusion is appropriate treatment that increases arch length; however, this movement is usually started in the early permanent dentition.

After a patient prematurely loses a primary second molar, the permanent first molar will move too far mesially unless arch length is held with a space maintainer. When a patient loses arch length for this reason, the permanent molar should be moved back with an orthodontic appliance to its original position in young patients. After the molars have been returned to an appropriate location, a space maintainer appliance is constructed to retain the regained arch length. Information about mesially tipped molars should be included in an arch length analysis.

Second and Third Molar Evaluation

The position of the unerupted molars in the alveolus is of importance. When unerupted second molar and third molar tooth buds are separated by spaces and the developing second molar is spatially separated from the erupted first molar, adequacy of posterior arch length is probable. When the unerupted second molar and the third molar buds are packed together tightly against the distal surface of the first molar, posterior arch length inadequacy is probable.

Impaction of second molars requires treatment. Orthodontists can usually correct second molar impaction. When the mandibular third molar bud is located closely behind and above the impacted lower

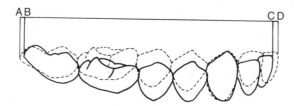

Figure 12-10 Leveling of the curve of Spee. Arch length before leveling (B-C) and after leveling (A-D).

second molar, an oral surgeon can remove the third molar—a procedure that may free the second molar to erupt. Impacted third molars are usually extracted, but extraction is commonly delayed until these molars have some root structure.

INTERPRETATION OF AN ARCH LENGTH ANALYSIS IN THE PERMANENT DENTITION

The factors discussed previously have an important impact on the interpretation of an arch length analysis. Therefore a precise threshold value for arch length deficiencies, above which extraction of teeth is required, does not exist. As an arch length deficiency exceeds 6 or 7 mm, careful consideration should be given to the factors that affect an extraction decision. Arch length deficiencies in excess of 10 mm have a high probability of requiring extraction.

When extractions are contemplated for a patient, their effect on the resulting occlusion must be considered. If two premolars must be extracted in the mandibular arch in patients with Class I or Class II malocclusions because of arch length deficiency, two premolars must also be removed from the maxilla to obtain Class I canine and molar relationships and normal overbite and overjet. The removal of two lower premolars without removal of two upper premolars produces a Class III molar relationship in which the upper second molars occlude with the lower third molars. If the lower third molars are not erupted or if they are not present, the upper second molars may become unopposed by lower teeth and could over-erupt and eventually will need to be extracted. Extraction of only two lower premolars is acceptable in some patients who have a Class III malocclusion and in some adult patients with Class II malocclusions who will undergo a mandibular advancement surgery. The extraction of only two maxillary premolars is acceptable for some patients who have no arch length deficiency in the mandible but who have either an arch length deficiency in the maxilla or a Class II malocclusion. This treatment results in Class II molar and Class I canine relationships, with normal overbite and overjet.

INTERPRETATION OF A MIXED DENTITION ARCH LENGTH ANALYSIS

1. If an analysis predicts that a child will have no crowding problem, continue routine care and periodic observation of the patient.
2. When an analysis predicts borderline crowding (1 mm to 4 mm), maintain arch length with an appliance and periodically examine the patient. If a permanent first molar moved mesially because of premature loss of a primary molar, use an appliance to regain the lost arch length before making a space maintainer. Prepare patients with borderline crowding for possible orthodontic treatment.
3. If an analysis predicts crowding in excess of 4 mm, the patient will likely develop crowding of the permanent teeth that will require orthodontic treatment following a comprehensive evaluation of the malocclusion.
4. If crowding in excess of 6 mm is predicted in the lower arch, the patient may benefit from serial extraction treatment (see Chapter 18).

Monitor all mixed dentition patients at regular intervals to follow tooth eruption and facial development.

REFERENCES

1. Moorrees CFA, Chadha JM: Available space for the incisors during dental development: a growth study based on physiologic age, *Angle Orthod* 35(1):12-22, 1965.
2. Staley RN et al: Prediction of the combined right and left canine and premolar widths in both arches of the mixed dentition, *Pediatr Dent* 5:57-60, 1983.
3. Staley RN, Hoag JF: Prediction of the mesiodistal widths of maxillary permanent canines and premolars, *Am J Orthod* 73(2):169-177, 1978.
4. Staley RN, Shelly TH, Martin JF: Prediction of lower canine and premolar widths in the mixed dentition, *Am J Orthod* 76(3):300-309, 1979.
5. Hixon EH, Oldfather RE: Estimation of the sizes of unerupted cuspid and bicuspid teeth, *Angle Orthod* 28(4):236-240, 1958.
6. Staley RN, Kerber PE: A revision of the Hixon and Oldfather mixed dentition prediction method, *Am J Orthod* 78(3):296-302, 1980.
7. Bishara SE, Staley RN: Mixed-dentition mandibular arch length analysis: a step-by-step approach using the revised Hixon and Oldfather prediction method, *Am J Orthod* 86:130-135, 1984.
8. Moyers RE: *Handbook of orthodontics for the student and general practitioner,* Chicago, 1973, Yearbook Medical.
9. Staley RN et al: Prediction of the widths of unerupted canines and premolars, *J Am Dent Assoc* 108(2):185-190, 1984.
10. Tanaka MM, Johnston LE: The prediction of the size of unerupted canines and premolars in a contemporary orthodontic population, *J Am Dent Assoc* 88(4):798-801, 1974.
11. Bishara SE, Jakobsen JR: Comparison of two nonradiographic methods of predicting permanent tooth size in the mixed dentition, *Am J Orthod Dentofacial Orthop* 113:573-576, 1998.
12. Bishara SE et al: Comparisons of mesiodistal and buccolingual crown dimensions of the permanent teeth in three populations from Egypt, Mexico, and the United States, *Am J Orthod Dentofacial Orthop* 96:416-422, 1989.

13. Lee-Chan S et al: Mixed dentition analysis for Asian-Americans, *Am J Orthod Dentofacial Orthop* 113:293-299, 1998.

14. Ferguson FS et al: The use of regression constants in estimating tooth size in a Negro population, *Am J Orthod* 73:68-72, 1978.

15. Tweed CH: The Frankfurt mandibular incisor angle in orthodontic diagnosis, treatment planning, and prognosis, *Angle Orthod* 24:121-169, 1954.

16. Baldridge DW: Leveling the curve of Spee: its effects on mandibular arch length, *J Pract Orthod* 3(1):26-41, 1969.

CHAPTER 13

An Approach to the Diagnosis of Different Malocclusions

Bronwen Richards

KEY TERMS

records	diagnostic parameters	anterior crossbite	moderate crowding
models	mild crowding	posterior crossbite	severe crowding
photographs	mild spacing	digit habit	significant spacing
pantomograph	diastema closure	Class II Division 1	skeletal posterior crossbite
space analysis	space maintenance	Class II Division 2	ectopic eruption
lateral cephalometric	serial extraction	Class III malocclusion	impacted tooth
radiograph	space regaining		

To evaluate a patient for potential orthodontic treatment, an objective set of **records** must be obtained. Using a systematic approach to assess these records enables the clinician to evaluate the complexity of the malocclusion. The records needed to assess a case for orthodontic treatment include a case history, photographs, models, a pantomograph, a space analysis, and a lateral cephalometric radiograph. Specific information can be obtained from each record to arrive at an orthodontic diagnosis; the details were presented in previous chapters. This section briefly describes each orthodontic record and reviews the information that should be gained from each record. To use this data efficiently, a set of 11 diagnostic parameters has been developed to guide the clinician to an orthodontic diagnosis. The same diagnostic parameters are used throughout the chapter to give the clinician a standardized method to evaluate a malocclusion and determine an orthodontic diagnosis. The primary goal of these parameters is to help the clinician distinguish between a case that requires limited orthodontic treatment versus one that requires comprehensive orthodontic treatment.

RECORDS

Plaster **models** are used to assess the Angle classification of molars and canines (see Chapter 9), the overbite and overjet, (Figure 13-1) the approximate amount of crowding or spacing in a particular dental arch, and the presence of an anterior or posterior crossbite. Because models are a three-dimensional representation of a patient's dentition, they may be used to demonstrate a malocclusion to both the parents and the patient.

Photographs include both intraoral and extraoral photographs. The extraoral photographs, which include a frontal view at rest, a frontal view smiling, and a profile view are used to assess a patient's profile, facial asymmetries, and the smile line. The extraoral photographs are not used to answer a specific diagnostic parameter on the list but, rather, are used to evaluate the facial appearance. The profile can be assessed as normal versus convex or concave on the lateral facial photograph. Conditions such as facial asymmetries, interlabial gap, or a high smile line may also be identified in extraoral photographs.

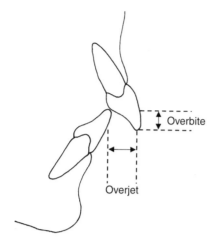

Figure 13-1 Overbite is the vertical overlap of incisors. Overjet is the horizontal overlap of incisors.

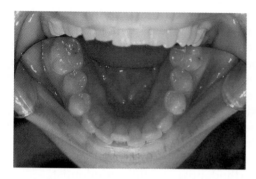

Figure 13-2 To estimate crowding, the amount of overlap may be assessed. When contacts are mildly overlapped or "slipped" such as between the left central and lateral, the amount of crowding can be estimated at 0.5 mm. When a contact is completely overlapped such as between the right central and lateral incisors, crowding should be estimated at 1 mm. The sum of crowding at each contact gives the total amount of crowding for the arch.

These facial findings may influence a treatment plan. A description other than normal may indicate a significant underlying skeletal discrepancy, which should be evaluated with a tracing of a lateral cephalometric radiograph. Intraoral photographs consist of a frontal view, right and left lateral views, and maxillary and mandibular occlusal views. Intraoral photographs provide a general overview of the malocclusion, the gingival condition, and any hypoplastic teeth.

A **pantomograph** or complete mouth survey is made before orthodontic treatment to assess the stage of dental eruption, missing supernumerary or impacted teeth, ectopically erupting teeth, and pathologic condition. The teeth must always be counted to determine if any are missing. The diagnostic parameter that correlates with the pantomograph asks the clinician to characterize eruption as either "within the range of normal" or "beyond the range of normal." A normal condition exists when all teeth are present and erupting in the appropriate location at an appropriate age.

A **space analysis** should be performed during the mixed dentition to determine if the permanent teeth have adequate space in which to erupt. Several different formulas may be used to determine if excessive crowding or spacing will be present in the permanent dentition. Knowing the amount of crowding or spacing in an arch helps the clinician determine the most appropriate treatment approach. The tooth size-arch length discrepancy (TSALD) in a patient with permanent dentition can be estimated by considering a mildly overlapped contact point to be 0.5 mm and an overlapped contact point to be 1 mm (Figure 13-2). However, this is only a rough estimate of a TSALD. To more accurately determine a TSALD of the permanent dentition, the cumulative mesiodistal width of the teeth on the models can be subtracted from the actual arch length present mesial to the first molars. The details of performing the space analysis are described in Chapter 12. The actual amount of crowding is given for each case in this chapter.

The **lateral cephalometric radiograph** is a tool used in orthodontics to evaluate the relationship of the jaws and teeth. Interpretation of lateral cephalometric tracings is also discussed in Chapters 10 and 11. As a brief overview, lateral cephalometric interpretation requires the clinician to evaluate the position of the maxilla and mandible to the cranial base and to one another

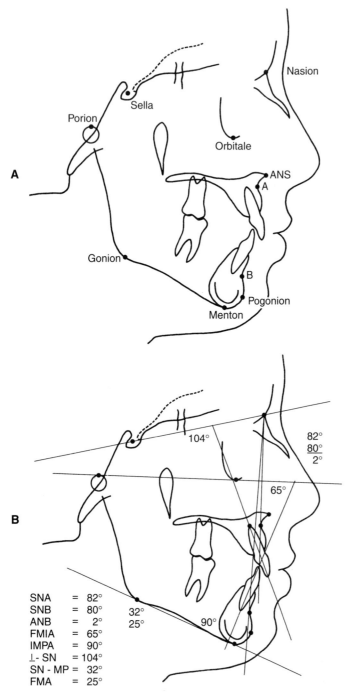

A

B

SNA	= 82°
SNB	= 80°
ANB	= 2°
FMIA	= 65°
IMPA	= 90°
⊥- SN	= 104°
SN - MP	= 32°
FMA	= 25°

Figure 13-3 A, Specific reproducible landmarks are labeled on a lateral cephalometric tracing. **B,** By connecting the landmarks, measurements can be made to compare the position of the teeth and jaws to "normal" measurements.

(Figure 13-3).[1] The angulation of the maxillary incisors, the mandibular incisors, and the mandibular plane angle is also evaluated.[2] If the position of the teeth and jaws varies greatly from the normal values, the malocclusion may require comprehensive orthodontic treatment instead of limited treatment. For a case to be considered for limited treatment, the

cephalometric findings must be within the range of normal values.

Patients with a skeletal discrepancy require a thorough evaluation and comprehensive orthodontic treatment. Once the problem has been identified, the decision regarding treatment options must be made. Options such as growth modification, camouflage of a malocclusion, and orthognathic surgery should be explored.

Before any orthodontic treatment is considered, the periodontium should be evaluated.[3] Periodontal disease can be an issue, particularly in adults. If periodontal disease is suspected, the patient should be referred to the periodontist for an evaluation before orthodontic treatment (see Chapter 24). Once the inflammation is under control and the periodontist approves the patient for orthodontic treatment, an orthodontic assessment may proceed. The treatment of patients with periodontal disease depends on the specific type of bone loss the patient demonstrates. Orthodontic forces that are well tolerated in a patient with healthy periodontium may exert excessive force on the teeth of a patient with generalized bone loss. Vertical bone defects, particularly mesial to molars that have tipped forward, also need to be carefully evaluated and treated. For example, molar uprighting can quickly identify the presence of a defect and therefore should be followed by both the orthodontist and the periodontist.

Using the information gathered from the clinical evaluation, photographs, models, pantomograph, space analysis, and lateral cephalometric tracing, the clinician should be able to assess the following diagnostic parameters in an attempt to determine the complexity of the malocclusion and its treatment.

DIAGNOSTIC PARAMETERS USED IN THE EVALUATION OF THE MALOCCLUSION

Limited vs. Comprehensive Treatment

The following **diagnostic parameters** have been designed to help the clinician efficiently use each record to gain pertinent data to distinguish between cases that require limited orthodontic treatment versus comprehensive treatment. Limited treatment cases may fall within the expertise of the general practitioner, depending on the individual practitioner's level of comfort in treating orthodontic cases. Comprehensive orthodontic cases should be referred to the orthodontic specialist for treatment.

A thorough evaluation of each diagnostic parameter helps the clinician distinguish between limited and comprehensive treatment needs. For a case to be con-

BOX 13-1	Diagnostic Parameters to Be Evaluated (Part 1 of 2)

1. Canine and molar relationships: right molar, right canine, left canine, left molar
   a. Class I
   b. Class II*
   c. Class III*
   d. Not fully erupted
2. Classification of malocclusion
   a. Class I malocclusion
   b. Class II Division 1 malocclusion*
   c. Class II Division 1, subdivision*
   d. Class II Division 2 malocclusion*
   e. Class II Division 2 malocclusion*
   f. Class III malocclusion*
   g. Class III, subdivision malocclusion*
3. Overbite
   a. Normal (5% to 20%)
   b. Moderate deep bite (20% to 50%)
   c. Severe deep bite (greater than 50%)*
   d. Edge to edge†
   e. Anterior open bite†
4. Overjet
   a. Normal (1 to 3 mm)
   b. Excessive (greater than 3 mm)*
   c. Edge to edge†
   d. Negative overjet or underjet
5. Stage of dental development
   a. Deciduous dentition
   b. Early mixed dentition
   c. Late mixed dentition
   d. Permanent dentition†
6. Presence of crossbite: with or without shift
   a. None
   b. Anterior†
   c. Posterior†
   d. Both†

7. Space analysis: tooth size-arch length discrepancy
   a. Adequate arch length (+1 to −1 mm)
   b. Mild crowding (−2 to −3 mm)
   c. Moderate or severe crowding (−4 to −6 mm, >−6 mm)*
   d. Mild spacing (1 to 3 mm)
   e. Moderate or severe spacing (4 to 6 mm, 6+ mm)*
8. Pantomograph interpretation
   a. Eruption within the normal range
   b. Eruption or radiographic findings beyond the range of normal (i.e., missing, supernumerary, ectopic eruption, impacted tooth*
   c. No pantomograph available
9. Lateral cephalometric radiograph interpretation
   a. Within the normal range (actual numbers close to the norms)
   b. Beyond the normal range (ANB is greater than 5 degrees or less than −1 degree)*
   c. No lateral cephalogram available
10. Scope of treatment
    a. Limited: within the range of treatment by a
    b. Comprehensive: should be referred to an orthodontic general dentist specialist
11. For limited treatment cases, designate case type (may be more than one)
    a. Mild crowding
    b. Mild spacing
    c. Diastema closure
    d. Space maintenance
    e. Space regaining
    f. Anterior crossbite
    g. Posterior crossbite
    h. Digit habit
    i. Not applicable (for comprehensive cases)

*Always a complicating factor, causing case to need comprehensive treatment
†Complicating factor under the condition mentioned, causing case to need comprehensive treatment (see text for details).

Continued

BOX 13-1   Diagnostic Parameters to Be Evaluated (Part 2 of 2)

Interpretation of the Diagnostic Parameters

Parameter 1: Canine and molar relationships

The first Parameter requires the clinician to determine the anteroposterior molar and canine relationships according to Angle classification (see Chapter 5 and 9). Plaster casts and lateral intraoral photographs should be used for this evaluation. If all canines and molars are Class I, the case may be considered as a limited treatment case. However, a Class II or Class III canine or molar relationship is a complicating factor that causes the case to be a comprehensive case.

Parameter 2: Classification of the malocclusion

The Angle classification is used to determine whether the case is a Class I, Class II Division 1, Class II Division 2, or a Class III malocclusion and if the problem is bilateral or unilateral. A unilateral malocclusion is classified as a subdivision case (see Chapter 9). A Class I malocclusion may be considered for limited treatment, but any other malocclusion is considered to be a complicating factor, leading to a comprehensive case diagnosis.

Parameter 3: Overbite

Overbite is the vertical overlap of the incisors and is recorded in percentage of overlap (see Figure 13-3). The overbite should be evaluated from the dental casts and the frontal intraoral photograph. A normal overbite ranges from 5% to 20%, a moderate overbite ranges from 20% to 50%, and a deep overbite exists when the maxillary anterior teeth overlap more than 50% of the lower teeth. A deep overbite is a complicating factor that requires comprehensive orthodontic treatment. If an edge-to-edge incisor relation or an anterior open bite exists, the patient should be evaluated for a thumb habit or a tongue habit. In the absence of a cause, an edge-to-edge overbite or an anterior open bite is considered a complicating factor. However, if the open bite is caused by a habit and the answers to all other parameters indicate a normal relationship, the edge-to-edge overbite or the anterior open bite may be addressed by the limited treatment approach of habit therapy.

Parameter 4: Overjet

Overjet, the horizontal overlap of the incisors is recorded in millimeters (see Figure 13-1). The overjet should be evaluated clinically as well as from plaster models and the lateral intraoral photograph. A normal overjet ranges from 1 to 3 mm. The presence of a functional shift between centric relation and centric occlusion, an excessive overjet, or a negative overjet (underjet) is considered to be a complicating factor requiring comprehensive treatment. The edge-to-edge overjet relationship requires evaluation to determine if it is a complicating factor. If the incisors can be tipped to correct the overjet, the malocclusion may be considered a limited treatment condition. A removable appliance may be considered in cases where tipping is the only movement desired. However, if more extensive treatment would be needed to correct the overjet, it should be considered a complicating factor.

Parameter 5: Stage of dentition

Primary dentition exists from the eruption of the first primary tooth until eruption of the first permanent tooth. Early mixed dentition occurs when the permanent incisors are erupting, but before the permanent canines and premolars erupt. Once the primary canines or molars exfoliate, the stage of the dentition is considered to be late mixed dentition. In general, the stage of dental development does not determine if a case requires limited versus comprehensive treatment. However, a patient with a segmental posterior crossbite in the permanent dentition requires a skeletal correction (i.e., comprehensive treatment). Thus the stage of dentition should be combined with the next parameter, which specifically addresses crossbites. The stage of dental development may be determined from the clinical examination, models, occlusal photographs, and the pantomograph.

Parameter 6: Presence of crossbite

The presence of a crossbite should be determined from the clinical examination, dental casts, and intraoral photographs. If an anterior crossbite can be corrected by a simple tipping movement and adequate space exists to correct the crossbite, the anterior crossbite may be corrected with limited treatment. However, if the tooth in crossbite is blocked out of the dental arch, the crossbite is a complicating factor requiring comprehensive treatment because space needs to be gained before the crossbite can be corrected.

A posterior crossbite may be caused by either an abnormal dental angulation or a maxillary skeletal constriction. Thus the treatment of the crossbite may involve either a skeletal or a dental correction. A multiple-tooth posterior crossbite in the primary or mixed dentition may often be corrected with a slow expansion appliance. Slow expansion is a limited treatment procedure that tips the maxillary posterior teeth facially and in the early mixed dentition may open the midpalatal suture. In the late mixed and early permanent dentition, however, rapid maxillary expansion is indicated. Thus a posterior crossbite in the permanent dentition is a complicating factor.

Parameter 7: Presence of spacing vs. crowding

In the mixed dentition an arch length analysis is used to determine the presence of either an excess or deficient arch length to accommodate the permanent dentition. Spacing or crowding may be estimated in the permanent dentition by summing spaces or overlapped contacts between teeth on the dental casts. Cases that are discussed in this chapter have the amount of crowding or spacing calculated for the reader. Cases with adequate arch length, mild spacing, or mild crowding may be considered for limited treatment. Significant crowding is sometimes addressed with extraction of permanent teeth. A cephalometric evaluation should be performed before the extraction of permanent teeth. Moderate crowding, severe crowding, and moderate or severe spacing are complicating factors that require comprehensive orthodontic treatment.

BOX 13-1	Diagnostic Parameters to Be Evaluated (Part 2 of 2)—cont'd

Parameter 8: Pantomograph interpretation

As discussed previously, the pantomograph is used to assess the stage of eruption, missing or supernumerary teeth, ectopically erupting teeth, and a pathologic condition. The teeth must always be counted to determine if any teeth are missing. To answer the diagnostic parameter, a normal condition exists when all teeth are present and erupting in the appropriate location at an appropriate age. When significant variance from normal eruption is identified, the condition needs a more comprehensive evaluation.

Parameter 9: Lateral cephalometric radiographic interpretation

The evaluation of lateral cephalometric radiographs was discussed in Chapters 10 and 11. This diagnostic parameter is needed to determine if a malocclusion has a skeletal component. Cases that have a skeletal malocclusion need a thorough evaluation. In general, an anteroposterior skeletal discrepancy may be present if the ANB angle is greater than 5.0 degrees or less than −1.0 degree. A skeletal malrelationship is a complicating factor requiring comprehensive treatment. The larger ANB angle relationship may be associated with a Class II malocclusion, whereas a negative ANB angle may be associated with a Class III relationship.

Cases with a Class II or Class III malocclusion are identified from the first two diagnostic parameters.

Parameter 10: Type of case

Based on responses to the previous parameter, a decision is made by the clinician on whether a specific case would benefit from limited orthodontic treatment versus comprehensive orthodontic treatment. If any of the previous parameters were answered with a complicating factor, the case would be most appropriately treated with comprehensive orthodontic treatment.

Parameter 11: Type of limited treatment case

To help categorize limited treatment cases, the final parameter lists a variety of cases that may be treated with limited treatment. Thus cases that do not have any complicating factors qualify for one or more of the case types listed.

In summary, possible complicating factors include the following: Class II or Class III malocclusion, deep overbite, open bite not associated with a habit, excessive overjet or underjet, moderate or severe spacing or crowding, a complex crossbite, or radiographic findings beyond the range of normal. In contrast, if a case had no complicating factors it may be a candidate for limited orthodontic treatment.

sidered as requiring limited treatment, the diagnostic parameters must not have a complicating factor. Complicating factors are described for each parameter and noted as either an asterisk (*) (i.e., definite complicating factor) or a dagger (†) (i.e., acts as a complicating factor under certain conditions) (Box 13-1). The assumption is that a case needs limited treatment until the answer for one or more parameters indicate that a complicating factor is present. In such a situation, the diagnosis indicates that the malocclusion will benefit from comprehensive treatment.

LIMITED ORTHODONTIC TREATMENT CASES

Mild Crowding

Diagnosis Once orthodontic records have been taken, the clinician should examine the dental casts, photographs, and radiographs to evaluate the various diagnostic parameters. The patient in Figure 13-4 has a Class I malocclusion in the permanent dentition with normal overjet and no crossbite. TSALD (crowding) is estimated to be 1.5 mm. The parameters that were not normal were moderate overbite and mild crowding.

Because moderate overbite and mild crowding are not complicating factors, the case is considered to be a limited treatment case. A summary of the findings to the diagnostic parameters is presented in Box 13-2. The orthodontic diagnosis for this case is Class I malocclusion with mild crowding.

Treatment **Mild crowding** can be treated by several methods. Cases that require only a simple tipping movement may often be treated with a removable appliance such as a spring retainer (Figure 13-5).[4] The teeth on a dental cast are cut and individually repositioned in correct alignment before the fabrication of a spring retainer. The retainer improves the minor rotations of the teeth if the appliance is worn continuously. For maximum control of tooth movement, fixed appliances can be used to align the teeth. This patient had bands placed on the upper and lower first molars and brackets bonded on the upper and lower anterior teeth. The teeth were initially leveled with flexible nitinol wires and then the finishing details were made with rectangular stainless steel wires in an edgewise appliance. The final result shows an improved alignment of the maxillary and mandibular anterior teeth (Figure 13-6).

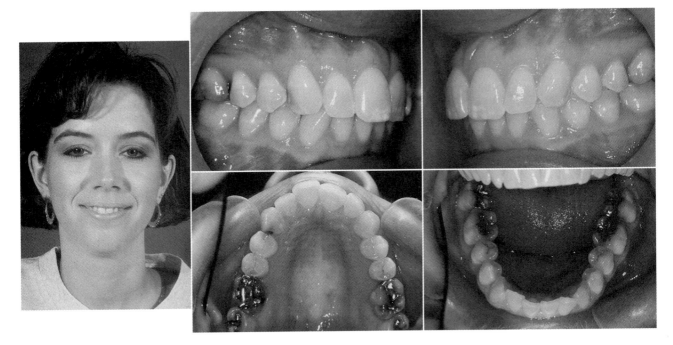

Figure 13-4 Pretreatment photographs showing mild crowding in a 20-year-old female with normal facial appearance. Dental findings show a Class I malocclusion with mild crowding.

BOX 13-2	Limited Treatment: Mild Crowding

Diagnostic Parameter	Answer	Mild Crowding
1	a, a, a, a	Class I molars and canines
2	a	Class I malocclusion
3	b	Moderate overbite (20% to 50%)
4	a	Normal overjet
5	d	Permanent dentition
6	a	No crossbite
7	b	Mild crowding (1 to 3 mm)
8	c	No pantomograph available
9	c	No lateral cephalometric radiograph needed
10	a	Limited treatment case
11	a	Mild crowding

A   B   C

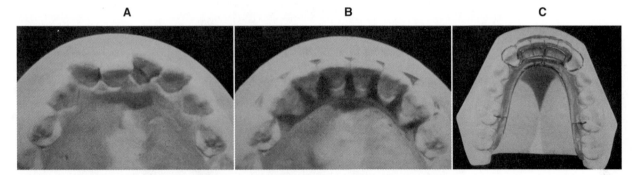

Figure 13-5 Spring retainer used to correct mild crowding. **A,** Model of crowded arch is made. **B,** Incisors are sectioned and realigned on a model. **C,** Spring retainer is designed on model with aligned teeth. The retainer will place pressure on the teeth to align them to the position of the model.

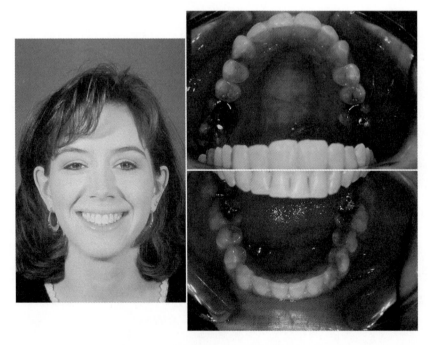

Figure 13-6 Mild crowding (posttreatment) following alignment with bands on first molars and brackets on the anterior teeth.

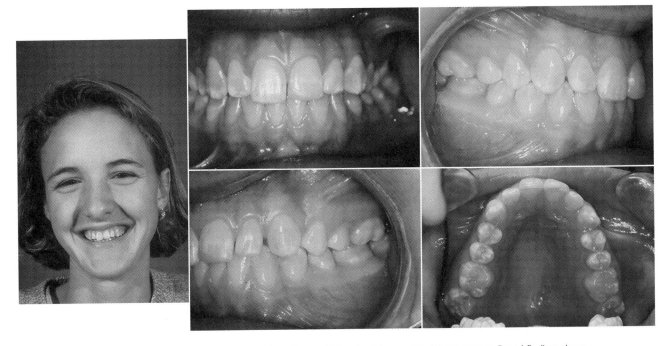

Figure 13-7 Mild spacing (pretreatment) in a 17-year-old female with normal facial appearance. Dental findings show Class I malocclusion with mild spacing.

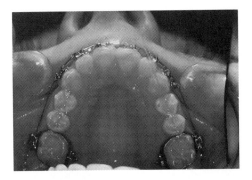

Figure 13-8 Maxillary partial arch bonding.

BOX 13-3	Limited Treatment: Mild Spacing	

Diagnostic Parameter	Answer	Mild Spacing
1	a, a, a, a	Class I molars and canines
2	a	Class I malocclusion
3	b	Moderate overbite (20% to 50%)
4	a	Normal overjet
5	d	Permanent dentition
6	a	No crossbite
7	d	Mild spacing (1 to 3 mm) (maxillary arch)
8	c	Pantomograph within normal limits
9	c	No lateral cephalometric radiograph needed
10	a	Limited treatment case
11	b	Mild spacing

Mild Spacing

Diagnosis The patient in Figure 13-7 has a Class I malocclusion in the permanent dentition with a normal overjet, a moderate overbite, and no crossbite. TSALD (spacing) is estimated to be 1.5 mm for the maxillary arch. The mandibular arch has mild crowding. Because moderate overbite and **mild spacing** are not considered to be complicating factors, the case is considered to be a limited treatment case. A summary of the findings to the diagnostic parameters is presented in Box 13-3. The orthodontic diagnosis for this limited treatment case is Class I malocclusion with mild spacings.

Treatment Generalized spacing is best treated with fixed appliances so elastometric power chains can be used to uniformly close the spaces (Figure 13-8). This patient was not concerned with the mild crowding in her lower incisors. Bands were placed on the maxillary first molars and brackets bonded on the maxillary anterior teeth. A nitinol wire was used to align the teeth, followed by a stainless steel wire. A power chain was used to close the spaces. The final result shows improved alignment and space closure in the maxillary anterior teeth (Figure 13-9). Once the spaces are closed, prolonged retention is essential to ensure that the spaces remain closed.

Diastema Closure

Diagnosis The patient in Figure 13-10 has a Class I malocclusion in the permanent dentition with normal overbite, overjet, and no crossbite. An evaluation of the overjet is essential in a patient with a diastema. If the maxillary incisors are in contact with the mandibular incisors, **diastema closure** cannot simply occur by tipping the maxillary incisors lingually. This factor is important in the treatment of the diastema. TSALD (spacing) is estimated to be 2 mm for the maxillary arch. This spacing is present as a midline diastema. The mandibular arch has adequate space. Radiographic findings are within the range of normal. Because mild spacing is not considered to be a complicating factor, the case is considered to be a limited treatment case. A summary of the findings to the diagnostic parameters is presented in Box 13-4. The orthodontic diagnosis for this case is a Class I malocclusion with a midline diastema.

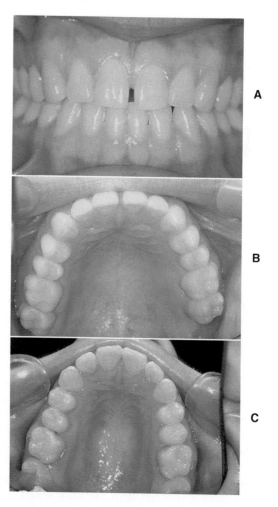

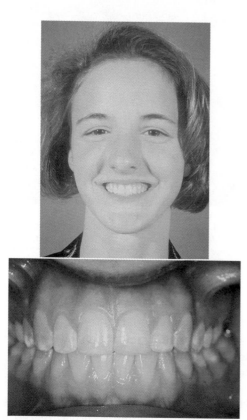

Figure 13-9 Mild spacing (posttreatment) following alignment with maxillary appliances only.

Figure 13-10 A and **B,** Diastema closure (pretreatment) in a 24-year-old male with a midline diastema. The decision to close space by tipping the incisors lingually depends on the amount of overjet present. **C,** Central incisors moved together orthodontically, and composite buildups were done on lateral incisors.

BOX 13-4	Limited Treatment: Diastema Closure

Diagnostic Parameter	Answer	Diastema Closure
1	a, a, a, a	Class I molars and canines
2	a	Class I malocclusion
3	a	Normal overbite (5% to 20%)
4	a	Normal overjet
5	d	Permanent dentition
6	a	No crossbite
7	d	Mild spacing (1 to 3 mm) (maxillary arch)
8	a	Pantomograph findings within normal limits
9	c	No lateral cephalometric radiograph needed
10	a	Limited treatment case
11	c	Diastema closure

Treatment Before closing a diastema, the clinician must assess the overjet. If adequate overjet exists (meaning that the maxillary incisors do not touch the mandibular incisors), the central incisors can be tipped lingually toward the mandibular incisors to close the space. Without an overjet the teeth cannot be tipped back to close the space.

Cases with no overjet can have the diastema closed by moving the central incisors toward the midline, creating spaces distal to the central incisors. Composite buildups on the lateral incisors provide an esthetic smile and maintain space closure (see Figure 13-10, C). Another approach is to place composite buildups on the mesial surfaces of the central incisors without moving them orthodontically so that the results will be esthetically acceptable.

Space Maintenance

Diagnosis In a mixed dentition case, even if most diagnostic parameters yield no complicating factors, a mixed dentition TSALD analysis needs to be performed (see Chapter 12). The analysis may indicate excess spacing, excess crowding, or adequate arch length. In mixed dentition cases in which just adequate space exists, the pattern of eruption should be evaluated. In the cases shown, the tooth size-arch length analysis indicated adequate arch length. Because the primary canines were prematurely lost, it is important to prevent any future loss of arch length by placing a space maintainer to ensure that the permanent molars will not drift mesially when the primary molars exfoliate and the permanent teeth erupt (Figure 13-11). Because of the absence of complicating factors and an arch length analysis indicating adequate space in the mixed dentition, this case is considered to be a limited treatment case requiring **space maintenance.**

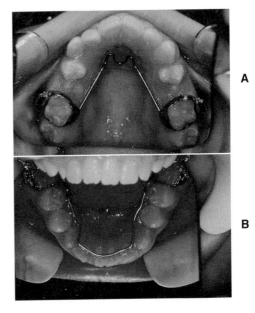

Figure 13-11 Space maintenance of the maxillary and mandibular arches. An arch length analysis indicated just adequate space in the arches shown. To prevent mesial drift of molars, space maintainers were placed. **A,** Nance holding arch. **B,** Lower lingual holding arch.

Treatment Because adequate arch length was present, a lower lingual holding arch was placed to prevent the permanent first molars from drifting mesially when the primary molars exfoliate. Because first permanent molars tend to drift mesially when proximal

BOX 13-5	Limited Treatment: Space Regaining

Diagnostic Parameter	Answer	Space Regaining
1	d, a, a, d	Class I right molar and canines; the left molar has drifted forward following premature loss of the maxillary left second deciduous molar
2	c	Class II Division 1 Subdivision malocclusion
3	a	Normal overbite (5% to 20 %)
4	a	Normal overjet
5	c	Late mixed dentition
6	a	No crossbite
7	b	Mild crowding (1 to 3 mm) (maxillary arch)
	d	Mild spacing (1 to 3 mm) (mandibular arch)
8	a	Pantomograph findings within normal limits
9	c	No lateral cephalometric radiograph needed
10	a	Limited treatment case
11	a	Space regaining

contact is absent, the premature loss of a second primary molar becomes a concern when adequate arch length exists before exfoliation or extraction. As a result, space maintenance is indicated when a primary tooth is lost prematurely because of caries or ectopic eruption of a permanent tooth (see Chapter 17).[5] There are various types of space-maintaining appliances, including a lower lingual holding arch, a band and loop space maintainer, and a Nance holding arch (see Figure 13-11, B).[6] If space maintenance is required but the molars are not Class I, the patient will need comprehensive orthodontic treatment. If the arch length analysis indicated mild crowding, space would need to be regained before the placement of a space maintainer. With severe crowding a **serial extraction** procedure should be contemplated (see Chapter 18).

Space Regaining

Diagnosis   The patient in Figure 13-12 presented in the mixed dentition with Class I canines, a Class I right molar, normal overjet and overbite, and no crossbite. The left maxillary second primary molar was prematurely extracted because of caries. Because no space maintainer was placed, the permanent first molar drifted mesially.[7] A mixed dentition space analysis of the maxillary arch indicated mild crowding. Further analysis of the maxillary arch showed that the crowding present in this arch is caused by the maxillary left first permanent molar that has drifted forward into a Class II relationship. The case classification is Class II Division 1, subdivision left. However, the evaluation of this case indicates that it is basically a Class I mal-

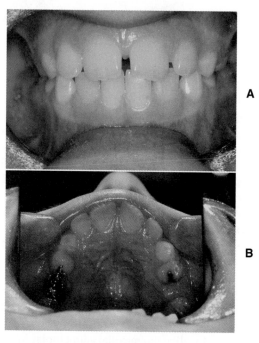

Figure 13-12 Space regaining (pretreatment). **A,** A 9-year-old male with premature loss of deciduous second molar and mesial drift of permanent first molar. **B,** Mesial drift is best seen on maxillary occlusal image.

occlusion case with mesial drift of the left maxillary first permanent molar secondary to premature loss of a second primary molar. As a result, tipping the molar distally regains the necessary arch length for the eruption of the premolars. Radiographic findings indicate that the sequence of eruption is within normal limits. The parameter that was not normal in this case was the

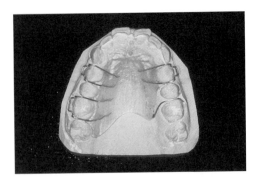

Figure 13-13 Shammy appliance used to distalize a mesially drifted first molar. Several Adam's clasps are placed for retention. A spring is used to move a mesially tipped tooth distally.

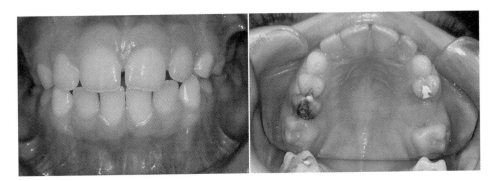

Figure 13-14 Space regaining (posttreatment). The first molar was moved distally to allow eruption of premolars.

crowding caused by the premature loss of a primary molar, leading to mesial drift of a permanent first molar in the mixed dentition. A summary of the findings to the diagnostic parameters is presented in Box 13-5. The orthodontic diagnosis for this limited treatment case is **space regaining.**

Treatment According to the space analysis, inadequate space exists for the permanent canine and premolars to erupt in the upper left quadrant. As a result, a removable maxillary appliance with a spring similar to that in Figure 13-13 was used to distalize the first permanent molar and regain adequate arch length for the permanent teeth to erupt. The spring was activated monthly to distalize the maxillary first molar into a Class I relationship (Figure 13-14). A Hawley retainer was worn as a space maintainer to hold the molar in the new position until the premolars erupted. Another option to retain the molar position is to use a Nance holding arch. A fixed orthodontic appliance should also be considered for space regaining if patient compliance is a concern.

Anterior Crossbite

Diagnosis When a case is identified as having an anterior or posterior crossbite, it must be determined whether a functional shift exists between centric rela-

tion (CR) and centric occlusion (CO) (see Chapter 9). As a patient closes the mandible in centric relation, tooth interferences cause the mandible to shift either laterally or anteriorly to allow the patient to bring the teeth together in a more comfortable position.

The patient in Figure 13-15 has an **anterior crossbite.** In such cases, the presence of a functional shift must be evaluated. In centric occlusion the incisors show negative overjet. However, in centric relation the incisors touch edge to edge. The anteroposterior difference between centric relation and centric occlusion is known as a functional shift. The goal of treatment is to make centric occlusion equal to centric relation and thus eliminate the functional shift. The presence of a shift might indicate that the malocclusion is dental in nature and may be considered for limited treatment, whereas the lack of a shift may indicate an underlying skeletal problem.

In centric relation, this patient has a Class I malocclusion in the early mixed dentition with normal overbite. The overjet is edge to edge. By evaluating the maxillary arch, it can be seen that the edge-to-edge overjet is caused by the central incisors being tipped lingually. Because the incisors could be tipped facially to correct the overjet, the condition of edge to edge is not considered to be a complicating factor. A space analysis indicated a TSALD of mild spacing in both arches.

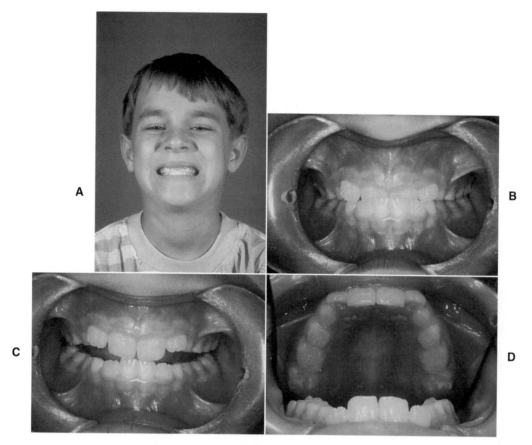

Figure 13-15 Anterior crossbite (pretreatment) in an 8-year-old male with an anterior crossbite. Patients with an anterior crossbite should be evaluated in **A,** centric occlusion, and **B,** centric relation, to determine if a functional shift exists. If the incisors can be contacted edge to edge and adequate space exists in the arch, the tooth in crossbite can be tipped forward to correct the malocclusion. **C** and **D,** View of occlusion.

BOX 13-6	Limited Treatment: Anterior Crossbite

Diagnostic Parameter	Answer	Anterior Crossbite
1	d, a, a, a	Class I molars and canines
2	a	Class I malocclusion
3	c	Deep overbite (greater 50%) in centric occlusion
	a	Normal overbite (5% to 20%) in centric relation
4	d`	Negative overjet in centric occlusion
	c	Edge to edge overjet in centric relation
5	b	Early mixed dentition
6	b	Anterior crossbite
7	d	Mild spacing (1 to 3 mm)
8	a	Pantomograph findings within normal limits
9	c	Lateral cephalometric radiograph needed
10	a	Limited treatment case
11	f	Anterior crossbite

Radiographic findings were within the range of normal. The parameters that were not ideal were the edge-to-edge overjet, anterior crossbite with functional shift, and mild spacing. As discussed previously, these findings are not considered to be complicating factors, thus the case is considered to be a limited treatment case. A summary of the findings to the diagnostic parameters is presented in Box 13-6. The orthodontic diagnosis for this limited treatment case is a Class I malocclusion with an anterior crossbite and anterior functional shift.

Treatment The patient in Figure 13-15 was able to bring the incisors edge to edge in centric relation, indi-

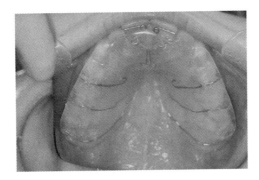

Figure 13-16 Hawley with finger spring. A Hawley retainer was constructed with a posterior bite plate to hold the bite open while the crossbite was corrected by activating the finger springs.

cating an anterior shift from CR to CO. In general, anterior crossbites with or without a functional shift should be corrected as soon as detected. Because this patient has upright maxillary incisors causing an anterior crossbite, the central incisors were tipped forward using a removable appliance with two finger springs (Figure 13-16). Once the incisors were slightly tipped forward, the patient could occlude with positive overjet (Figure 13-17). Correction of the crossbite and the functional shift allowed the dentition to erupt in a normal relationship.

Posterior Crossbite

Diagnosis As with an anterior crossbite, patients with a **posterior crossbite** must be evaluated for a functional shift. A posterior crossbite in the primary or mixed dentition is frequently associated with a bilateral maxillary constriction. Such a bilateral maxillary constriction may be accompanied with a lateral functional shift. A lateral functional shift may occur because closure of the mandible in centric relation causes the opposing cusp tips to contact in a cusp-to-cusp position. Because the patient is unable to occlude with the teeth in such a position, the mandible is shifted laterally to allow contact of more occlusal surfaces and to improve function. The identification of a lateral functional shift during diagnosis influences the prognosis and treatment of a crossbite.

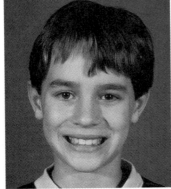
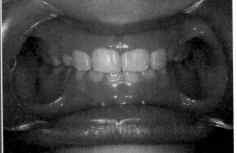

Figure 13-17 Anterior crossbite (posttreatment). Correction of the crossbite in the mixed dentition allows the clinician to restore a patient's dentition to normal for this stage of eruption.

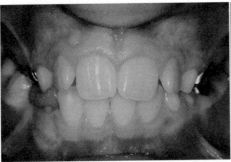
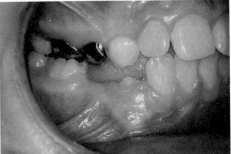

Figure 13-18 Posterior crossbite (pretreatment) in a 9-year-old female with posterior crossbite.

The patient in Figure 13-18 has a posterior crossbite. To determine the presence of a functional shift, the mandibular midline is evaluated in both centric relation and centric occlusion. A functional shift exists if the following conditions are present: (1) the mandibular and maxillary midlines coincide in centric relation and the posterior teeth contact cusp to cusp, and (2) the mandibular midline shifts toward the same side of the posterior crossbite in centric occlusion. In this case the mandibular midline is shifted to the right side in centric occlusion. A posterior crossbite is present on the patient's right side. Because the midline is shifted to the same side as the crossbite in centric occlusion, a functional shift to the right is present. Radiographic findings are within the range of normal. TSALD is estimated to be mild spacing in the mandibular arch. The parameters that were not normal were moderate overbite, mild spacing, and the posterior crossbite. A summary of the findings to the diagnostic parameters is presented in Box 13-7. This patient has a Class I malocclusion in the late mixed dentition, a normal overjet, a moderately deep overbite, and a posterior crossbite with a right lateral functional shift. Because moderate overbite, mild spacing, and posterior crossbite with functional shift in the mixed dentition are not considered to be complicating factors, the case is considered to need limited treatment.

Treatment If the maxillary arch constriction is bilateral in the primary or mixed dentition an expansion appliance can be used to correct the crossbite. The expansion appliance corrects the crossbite by a combination of dental tipping and opening of the midpalatal suture. Skeletal expansion is much easier to treat in the mixed dentition period than in the permanent dentition period because the midpalatal suture is less integrated. The patient wore a quad helix appliance to expand her maxillary arch (Figure 13-19). This was followed by the placement of a palatal arch as a retainer (Figure 13-20). Expansion should be corrected early to allow proper development of the dentition. Posterior crossbites have a tendency to relapse, so a Hawley retainer is often used for retention until the permanent teeth have erupted.[8] A true unilateral crossbite or a crossbite in the permanent dentition needs comprehensive treatment (see Chapter 23).

BOX 13-7	Limited Treatment: Posterior Crossbite	
Diagnostic Parameter	**Answer**	**Posterior Crossbite**
1	a, d, a, a	Class I molars and canines
2	a	Class I malocclusion
3	b	Moderate overbite (20% to 50%)
4	a	Normal overjet
5	c	Late mixed dentition
6	c	Posterior crossbite
7	d	Mild spacing (1 to 3 mm)
8	a	Pantomograph findings within normal limits
9	c	No lateral cephalometric radiograph needed
10	a	Limited treatment case
11	g	Posterior crossbite

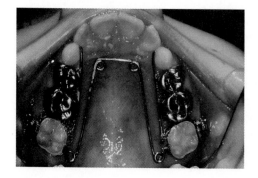

Figure 13-19 The Quad Helix is a slow expansion appliance that corrects bilateral posterior dental constrictions by tipping the teeth buccally and may have a small component of skeletal expansion in patients whose midpalatal suture is not well integrated.

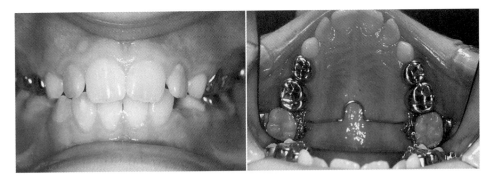

Figure 13-20 Posterior crossbite (posttreatment). The posterior crossbite was corrected to restore the patient's dentition to a normal relationship for this stage of eruption.

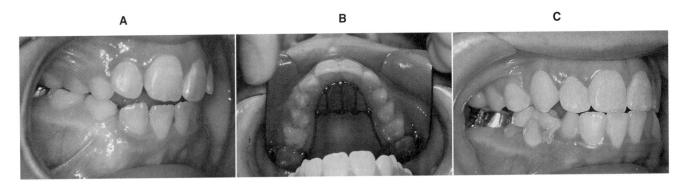

Figure 13-21 A, Digit habit in a 9-year-old male with anterior open bite secondary to thumb habit. **B,** Palatal crib habit appliance acts as a reminder to discourage this habit. **C,** Spontaneous closure of the open bite within a few months.

Digit Habit

Diagnosis The patient in Figure 13-21, *A* has a Class I malocclusion with normal overjet, no crossbite, and adequate arch length. The overbite appears normal on the left side with an open bite on the right side. The patient's history indicated an active thumbsucking habit in which the right thumb was placed in the right anterior part of her mouth, preventing the maxillary incisors from fully erupting. When no other complicating factors exist, an anterior open bite with a specific cause is considered a limited treatment case. Thus the diagnosis of this limited treatment case is a Class I malocclusion with an anterior open bite caused by a **digit habit.**

Treatment In cases that present with no complicating factors other than a mild anterior open bite associated with a digit habit, it is important to determine the duration and intensity of the sucking habit. Before attempting treatment, the patient should express a desire to stop the habit. Without patient cooperation, treatment of a digit habit may not be successful. This patient's digit habit was eliminated with a combination

of positive reinforcement and the placement of a palatal crib (see Figure 13-21, *B*).[4] This leads to the spontaneous closure of the open bite (see Figure 13-21, *C*).[9] The appliance should not be designed to cause pain or discomfort, but rather to serve as a reminder to the patient. The feeling of satisfaction from the finger touching the palate is disrupted with the appliance (see Chapter 17).

COMPREHENSIVE ORTHODONTIC TREATMENT CASES

Orthodontic cases requiring comprehensive treatment should be carefully evaluated to determine an appropriate diagnosis, treatment plan, and treatment regimen. Orthodontists trained in the management of dental and skeletal discrepancies in both growing and nongrowing patients should be involved in the treatment of these malocclusions. Such clinicians should have a thorough knowledge of all treatment options required to efficiently and appropriately treat these malocclusions (see Chapters 20 and 21).

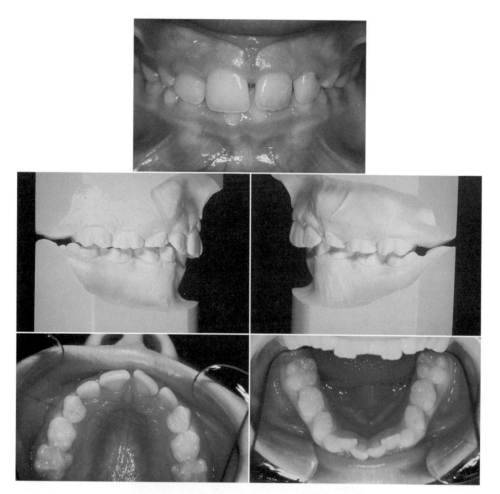

Figure 13-22 Class II Division 1 (pretreatment) in a 12-year-old male with normal facial appearance and Class II Division 1 malocclusion.

Class II Division 1 Malocclusion

Diagnosis An evaluation of the patient in Figure 13-22 indicated the presence of a Class II molar and canine relationships, leading to a diagnosis of a **Class II Division I** malocclusion. Additional answers to the diagnostic parameters included excessive overbite and overjet, both complicating factors that further designate the case as requiring comprehensive treatment. The stage of eruption is late mixed dentition and there was no crossbite present. The amount of crowding in the mixed dentition was determined by using the mixed dentition space analysis. The analysis indicated a crowding of 2.6 mm in the mandibular arch. This finding falls under mild crowding. The maxillary crowding was considerably larger at 8 mm. This moderate to severe crowding is a complicating factor. Radiographic findings were within normal limits because all teeth were present and erupting in a normal pattern. The lateral cephalometric tracing showed a retrusive maxilla and mandible with an ANB of 4.0 degrees. The difference between the two jaws falls

within the normal limits as defined in the lateral cephalometric standards (see Chapters 10 and 11). Thus this case has the following complicating factors: Class II malocclusion, excessive overbite, excessive overjet, and maxillary arch crowding. A summary of the findings to the diagnostic parameters is presented in Box 13-8. When a Class II malocclusion exists, the clinician must distinguish between a Division 1 and Division 2 situation. This is done by evaluating the inclination of the maxillary incisors and the overjet. Excessive overjet with normal or protrusive incisor angulation indicates a Division 1 situation. Normal overjet with Class II molars and upright maxillary incisors indicates a Class II Division 2 situation (see Chapter 8). The diagnosis of this case is a Class II Division 1 malocclusion.

Treatment Class II Division 1 cases can be treated by several approaches. Growing patients may wear an extraoral appliance headgear to restrict forward growth of the maxilla and allow the mandible to

BOX 13-8 Comprehensive Treatment: Class II Division 1 Malocclusion

Diagnostic Parameter	Answer	Class II Division 1 Malocclusion
1	b, b, b, b	Class II molars and canines
2	b	Class II malocclusion
3	c	Excessive overbite (greater than 50%)
4	b	Excessive overjet
5	c	Late mixed dentition
6	a	No crossbite
7	b	Mild crowding (1 to 3 mm) mandibular arch
8	a	Pantomograph findings within normal limits
9	a	Lateral cephalometric radiograph findings within normal limits
10	b	Comprehensive treatment case
11	i	Class II Division 1

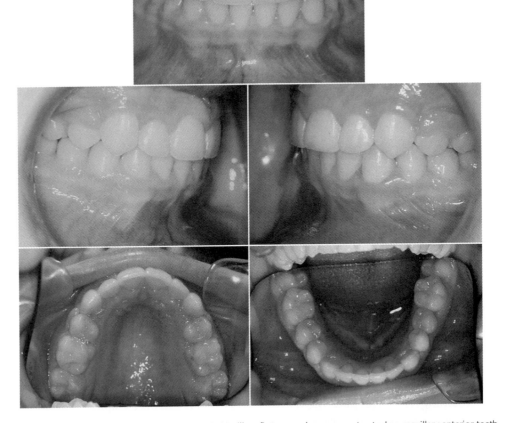

Figure 13-23 Class II Division 1 (posttreatment). Maxillary first premolars were extracted so maxillary anterior teeth could be retracted. Canines were finished in Class I occlusion, but the molars were finished in a Class II relationship.

grow forward and obtain a Class I occlusion. This is called *growth modification* or *differential jaw growth.* Nongrowing patients do not benefit from growth modification and thus are more likely to have teeth extracted or to undergo orthognathic surgery to correct the malocclusion. This patient was treated with extraction of maxillary first premolars. The extraction spaces were closed during treatment by retracting the maxillary anterior segment. At the end of treatment the canines were finished in a Class I relationship, whereas the molars were finished in a Class II relationship (Figure 13-23). The important factor for a clinician to realize is that several approaches are available to treat a Class II malocclusion and are detailed in Chapter 20. Most of these cases would benefit from undergoing orthodontic treatment during the late mixed dentition stage or early permanent dentition stage while the patient is still growing.

Class II Division 2 Malocclusion

Diagnosis An evaluation of the patient in Figure 13-24 indicates a Class II molar and right canine relationship and an unerupted left canine, leading to a

diagnosis of a Class II malocclusion (see Figure 13-24, A-C). The overjet is normal. A Class II malocclusion with normal overjet and upright maxillary incisors is described as **Class II Division 2.** Additional answers to the diagnostic parameters include excessive overbite, a complicating factor that further designates the case as a comprehensive case. The stage of eruption is late mixed dentition and there is no crossbite present. The mixed dentition space analysis indicated adequate space in the mandibular arch. Pantomographic findings are within normal limits because all teeth are present and erupting in a normal pattern. The lateral cephalometric tracing indicates an ANB difference of 6.5 degrees, which is beyond the range of normal (see Figure 13-24, D). In summary, this case has the following complicating factors: Class II malocclusion, excessive overbite, and a maxillary-mandibular skeletal discrepancy. A summary of the findings to the diagnostic parameters is presented in Box 13-9. The diagnosis of this case is a comprehensive case with a Class II Division 2 malocclusion that needs comprehensive orthodontic treatment.

Treatment Class II Division 2 cases are often treated by, first, tipping the maxillary incisors labially to cor-

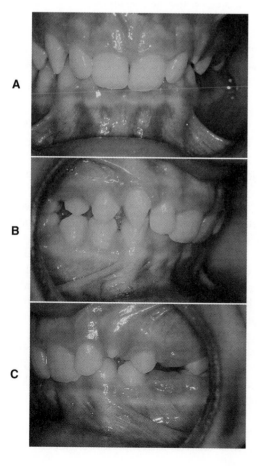

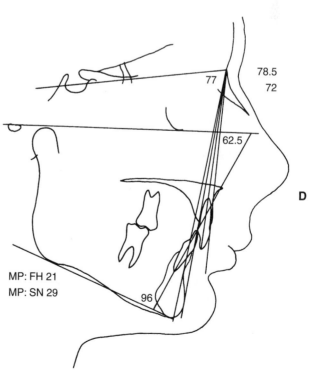

Figure 13-24 Class II Division 2 (pretreatment) in a 13-year-old male with retrusive mandible and Class II Division 2 malocclusion.

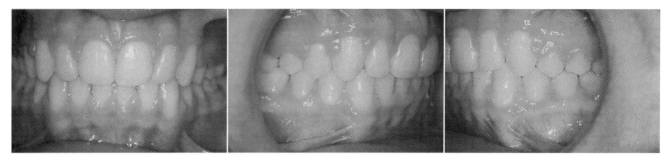

Figure 13-25 Class II Division 2 (posttreatment) following correction with full fixed appliance, headgear, and Class II elastics.

BOX 13-9	Comprehensive Treatment: Class II Division 2 Malocclusion

Diagnostic Parameter	Answer	Class II Division 2 Malocclusion
1	b, b, d, b	Class II molars and right canine
2	b	Class II Division 2 malocclusion
3	c	Excessive overbite (greater than 50%)
4	a	Normal overjet
5	c	Late mixed dentition
6	a	No crossbite
7	b	Mild crowding (1 to 3 mm)
8	a	Pantomograph findings within normal limits
9	b	Lateral cephalometric radiograph findings beyond normal limits
10	b	Comprehensive case
11	i	Class II Division 2

rect their inclination. The treatment that follows depends on the severity of the case and amount of growth remaining, as explained in the previous case. For this patient the maxillary incisors were tipped labially and intruded to eliminate the deep overbite. This patient wore a headgear and Class II elastics to improve the jaw discrepancy and achieve a Class I relationship (Figure 13-25).

Class III

Diagnosis An evaluation of the patient in Figure 13-26 indicates the presence of a Class III molar and canine relationship, leading to a diagnosis of a **Class III malocclusion.** This finding is a complicating factor causing this case to be a comprehensive case. The stage of dentition is permanent dentition. Additional answers to the diagnostic parameters include normal overbite, no overjet, and no crossbite. Severe Class III malocclusions are often associated with anterior and posterior crossbites because either the maxilla is too far back or the

mandible is too far forward (see Chapter 21). Because arch width gets larger toward the posterior part of the arch, a change in the jaw relationship toward a Class III relationship can cause both anterior and posterior crossbites. The amount of TSALD in the mandibular arch is 5 mm and is considered to be moderate crowding. The maxillary arch has 3 mm of crowding. The mandibular arch crowding is a complicating factor. Radiographic findings are within normal limits because all teeth are present and erupting in a normal pattern. The lateral cephalometric tracing shows a normal skeletal relationship because the ANB relationship is within the normal range. In summary, this case has the following complicating factors: Class III malocclusion and moderate mandibular arch crowding. A summary of the findings to the diagnostic parameters is presented in Box 13-10. The diagnosis of this case is a Class III malocclusion, which requires comprehensive treatment.

Treatment Class III malocclusions can be difficult to treat. If a skeletal discrepancy exists in a growing

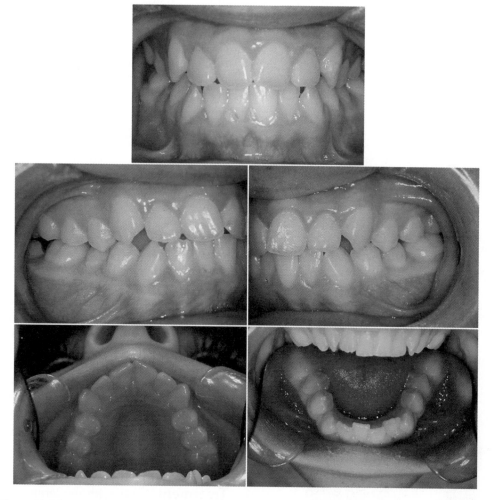

Figure 13-26 Class III (pretreatment) in a 13-year-old male with normal facial appearance, a mild Class III malocclusion.

BOX 13-10	Comprehensive Treatment: Class III Malocclusion

Diagnostic Parameter	Answer	Class III Malocclusion
1	c, c, c, c	Class III molars and canines
2	c	Class III malocclusion
3	a	Normal overbite (5% to 20%)
4	a	Normal overjet
5	d	Permanent dentition
6	a	No crossbite
7	c	Moderate crowding (4 to 6 mm) mandibular arch
8	a	Pantomographic findings within normal limits
9	a	Lateral cephalometric radiograph findings within normal limits
10	b	Comprehensive case
11	i	Class III malocclusion

patient, the patient must cooperate to achieve a skeletal correction. Growing patients may be treated by a reverse pull headgear if the maxilla is deficient or by a chin cup if the lower jaw is prognathic (see Chapter 21). A normal skeletal relationship with Class III molars and canines can be managed with orthodontic treatment alone. On the other hand, in nongrowing patients a significant Class III malocclusion may require extraction of teeth or orthognathic surgery. This patient was treated with nonextraction Class III elastics (Figure 13-27). Extrusion of upper molars by the Class III elastics must be closely monitored, particularly in cases with minimal overbite to avoid creating an anterior open bite.

Moderate Crowding

Diagnosis The patient in Figure 13-28, *A-F,* has a Class I malocclusion with excessive overjet and overbite in the permanent dentition. The diagnostic consideration included excessive overjet and excessive overbite. An overjet of greater than 3 mm and deep overbite are both complicating factors. Mandibular TSALD (crowding) was estimated to be 5 mm and considered to be **moderate crowding.** Radiographic findings are within normal limits because all teeth are present and erupting in a normal pattern. The lateral cephalometric tracing shows a slightly protrusive maxilla and a normal mandible with an ANB difference of 3.5 degrees, which is within the normal range (see Figure 13-28, *G*). In summary, this case has the following complicating factors: excessive overjet, excessive overbite, and moderate mandibular crowding. A summary of the findings to the diagnostic parameters is presented in Box 13-11. These complicating factors lead to a diagnosis of Class I malocclusion with excessive overbite and overjet as well as moderate crowding.

Treatment Cases with moderate crowding may be treated with either extraction or nonextraction of permanent teeth. A thorough evaluation of the cephalometric data and dental casts is necessary to determine if extraction is indicated. Because the mandibular inci-

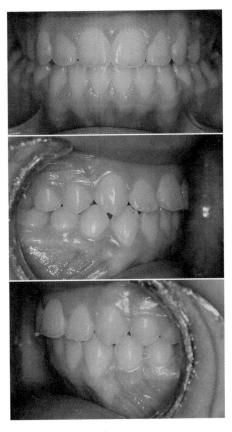

Figure 13-27 Class III posttreatment following correction with full fixed appliances and elastics.

BOX 13-11	Comprehensive Treatment: Moderate Crowding	

Diagnostic Parameter	Answer	Moderate Crowding
1	a, a, a, a	Class I molars and canines
2	a	Class I malocclusion
3	c	Excess overbite (greater than 50%)
4	b	Excessive overjet (greater than 3 mm)
5	d	Permanent dentition
6	a	No crossbite
7	c	Moderate crowding (4 to 6 mm)
8	a	Pantomograph findings within normal limits
9	a	Lateral cephalometric radio graph findings within normal limits
10	b	Comprehensive treatment case
11	i	Moderate crowding

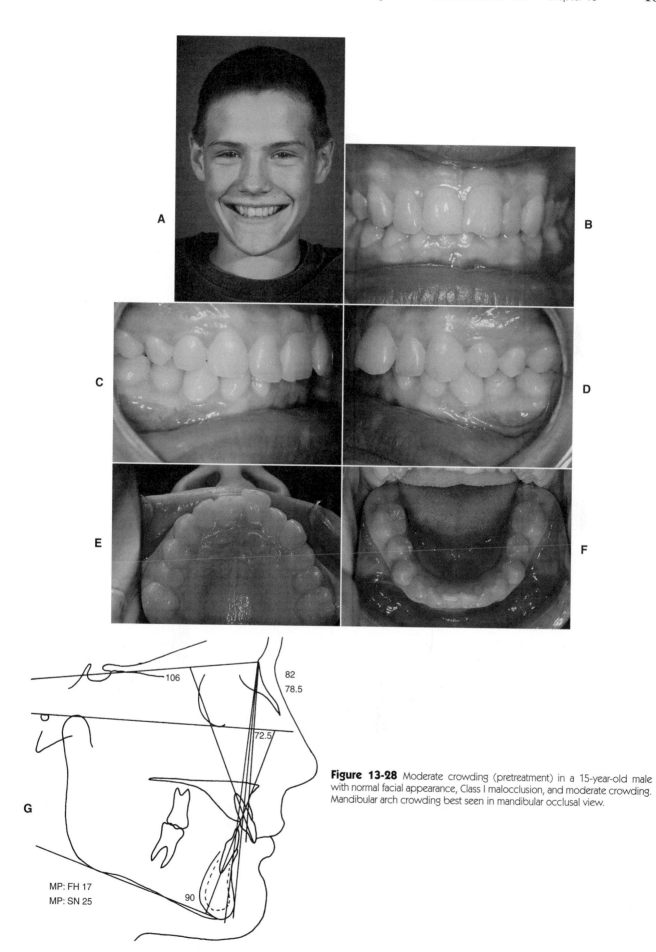

Figure 13-28 Moderate crowding (pretreatment) in a 15-year-old male with normal facial appearance, Class I malocclusion, and moderate crowding. Mandibular arch crowding best seen in mandibular occlusal view.

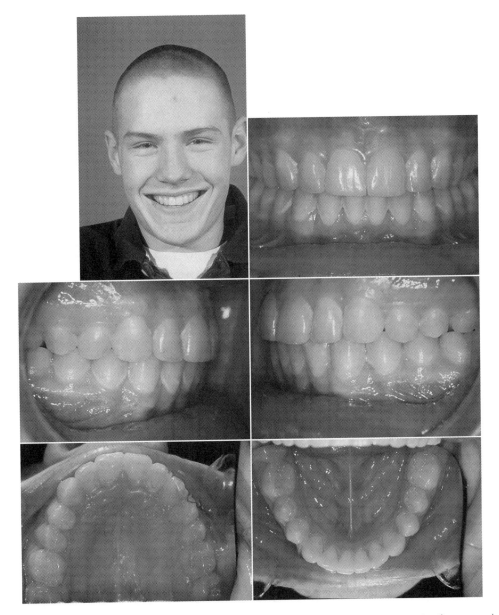

Figure 13-29 Moderate crowding (posttreatment) following alignment with full braces; a nonextraction approach was selected to avoid retraction of the lips. Retraction of the lips should be avoided in patients with a strong nose and chin, particularly in female patients.

sors were diagnosed as being upright in the cephalogram, the decision was made to relieve the crowding by tipping the mandibular incisors labially. The overall profile of this patient was taken into consideration. His strong chin and prominent nose would be better balanced by a nonextraction approach to avoid the retraction of the lips that might occur if permanent teeth were extracted. The arches were initially leveled and aligned with nitinol wires. Artistic bends were placed in stainless steel wires to detail the final occlusion (Figure 13-29). Because of the crowding that was initially present, retainer wear is important to prevent relapse of the rotated and crowded teeth.

Severe Crowding

Diagnosis The patient in Figure 13-30, *A-F,* has a Class I molars and a Class I left canine relationship, a normal overjet, permanent dentition, and no crossbite. Because the right canine had a Class II relationship, the malocclusion is described as Class II Division 1, subdivision right. The Division 1 was determined from the presence of protrusive maxillary incisors with an incisor angulation of 112 degrees on the lateral cephalogram (see Figure 13-30, *G*). There are additional complicating factors, which include a deep overbite and severe crowding of 14 mm in both arches. Radiographic findings are within

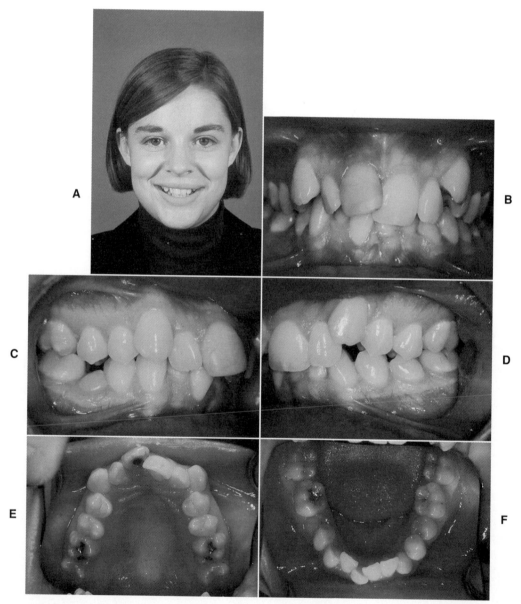

Continued

Figure 13-30 Severe crowding (pretreatment) in a 22-year-old female with normal facial appearance and severe dental crowding. The decision of which teeth to extract is based on the existing canine and molar relationship as well as the site of crowding.

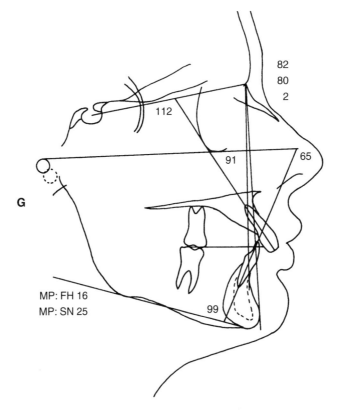

82
80
2

112

91   65

G

MP: FH 16
MP: SN 25   99

Figure 13-30, cont'd For legend see p. 171.

BOX 13-12	Comprehensive Treatment: Severe Crowding	

Diagnostic Parameter	Answer	Severe Crowding
1	a, b, a, a	Class I molars and left canine, Class II right canine
2	a	Class II Division 1 Subdivision malocclusion
3	c	Deep overbite (greater than 50%)
4	a	Normal overjet
5	d	Permanent dentition
6	a	No crossbite
7	c	Severe crowding (greater than 6 mm)
8	a	Pantomograph findings within normal limits
9	a	Lateral cephalometric radiograph findings within normal limits
10	b	Comprehensive treatment case
11	i	Severe crowding

normal limits because all teeth are present and erupted in a normal pattern. The lateral cephalometric tracing shows a normal position of the maxilla, the mandible, and protrusive incisors. A summary of the findings to the diagnostic parameters is presented in Box 13-12. This case is an example of a Class II Division 1, subdivision right malocclusion with a deep bite and severe crowding.

Treatment **Severe crowding** is generally considered when the TSALD is greater than 6 to 8 mm. It may seem that, in such cases, teeth would need to be extracted to create adequate space. However, as in moderately crowded cases, a thorough evaluation of cephalometric data and study models is necessary to determine if extractions are indicated. The patient shown in this case had severe crowding, protrusive lips, and a normal skele-

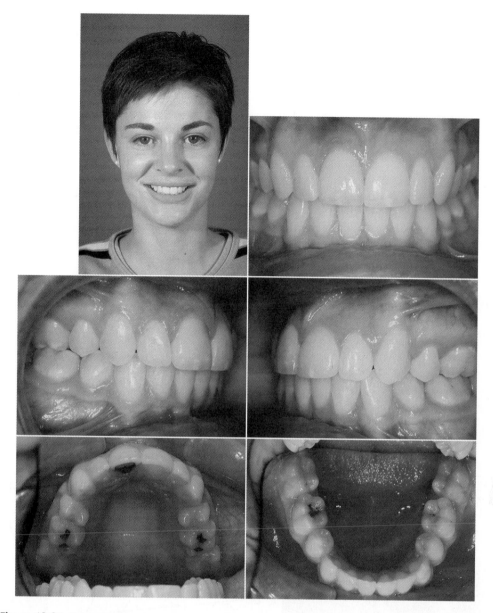

Figure 13-31 Severe crowding (posttreatment) following extraction of four first premolars and alignment. Permanent restoration of the central incisor with a crown should be delayed until orthodontic treatment is complete.

tal relationship but protrusive incisors. Four first premolars were extracted to create space for the alignment of the other teeth (Figure 13-31). The maxillary right central incisor has a dark crown, failing root canal treatment, amalgam lingual restoration, and a composite buildup. Final restorative treatment such as crowns or buildups should always be done after orthodontic treatment is completed to ensure proper occlusion and anatomy.

Serial Extraction in Severely Crowded Cases in the Mixed Dentition

When a patient is diagnosed with a Class I malocclusion and a severe TSALD of 8 to 10 mm or greater during the early mixed dentition, a decision may be made by the orthodontist that the patient would ultimately require extraction of four premolars to allow space for the proper alignment of the remaining teeth. Delaying the extraction of premolars until all permanent teeth erupt may lead to severely displaced teeth that may require prolonged orthodontic treatment at a later stage.[4,10] A different approach, serial extraction, may be considered when several other conditions are met.[11] If the lips and incisors are protrusive and the first premolars are radiographically erupting ahead of canines and second premolars, the primary canines and first molars may be extracted to allow the incisors more space to align themselves and to encourage the first premolars to erupt early. Once the first premolars are visible, they are extracted. This provides the erupting canines and second premolars with adequate arch length in which to erupt.[4] Following serial extraction the alignment of the erupting teeth is usually not ideal and requires orthodontic treatment to establish proper occlusion. However, total orthodontic treatment time is usually minimized when serial extraction is indicated and properly executed (see Chapter 18).

Significant Spacing

Diagnosis The patient in Figure 13-32, *A-D*, has a Class I malocclusion in the permanent dentition with no crossbite and mild spacing in the mandibular arch. The parameters that were not normal were excessive over-

jet, excessive overbite, and **significant spacing** in the maxillary arch. An overjet of greater than 3 mm and deep overbite are both complicating factors causing the case to require comprehensive orthodontic treatment. A maxillary TSALD of 8 mm indicates the presence of excessive spacing—a complicating factor. Radiographic findings are within normal limits because all the teeth are present and erupting in a normal pattern. The lateral cephalometric tracing shows normal positioning of the maxilla and mandible but with relatively retrusive lips in relation to the strong chin (see Figure l3-32, *E*). In summary, this case has the following complicating factors: excessive overjet, excessive overbite, and excessive maxillary spacing. A summary of the findings to the diagnostic parameters is presented in Box 13-13. This

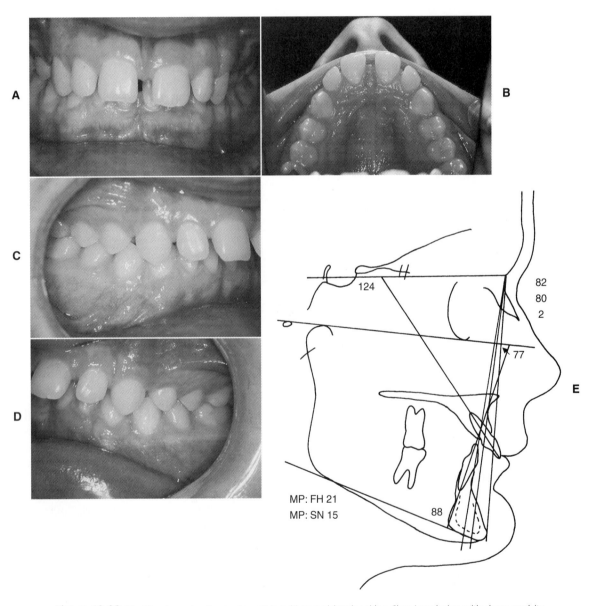

Figure 13-32 Significant spacing (pretreatment) in a 16-year-old male with a Class I occlusion with deep overbite and excessive overjet. Cephalometric findings include protrusive upper incisors, strong chin, and retrusive lower lip.

case is an example of a Class I malocclusion with excessive spacing, excessive overjet, and excessive overbite that is in need of comprehensive orthodontic treatment.

Treatment In a case with significant spacing it is sometimes difficult to accomplish space closure and retraction of the maxillary anterior teeth without losing anchorage (i.e., the maxillary canines and molars may move forward into a Class II relationship—an undesirable outcome). In addition, the deep bite and deep curve of Spee are complicating factors that require comprehensive treatment. Both arches were leveled and the maxillary canines were retracted. The incisors were then brought together and retracted as one unit. Class II elastics between maxillary canines and mandibular first molars were used to maintain the Class I canine relationship during incisor retraction (Figure 13-33). Cases with excessive spaces need prolonged retention to minimize relapse tendencies.

BOX 13-13	Comprehensive Treatment: Severe Spacing	

Diagnostic Parameter	Answer	Severe Spacing
1	a, a, a, a	Class I molars and canines
2	a	Class I malocclusion
3	c	Severe overbite (greater than 50%)
4	b	Excessive overjet (greater than 3 mm)
5	d	Permanent dentition
6	a	No crossbite
7	e	Severe spacing (greater than 6 mm) upper arch
	d	Mild spacing mandibular arch
8	a	Pantomograph findings within normal limits
9	a	Lateral cephalometric radiograph findings not within normal limits
10	b	Comprehensive treatment case
11	i	Severe spacing

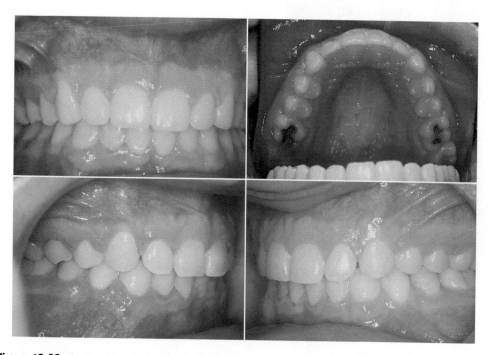

Figure 13-33 Significant spacing (posttreatment) following correction with full fixed appliances and Class II elastics. A frenectomy or supracrestal fibrotomy may be recommended to maintain space closure.

Anterior Crossbite with Space Loss

Diagnosis The patient in Figure 13-34, *A-D*, has a Class I malocclusion in the permanent dentition. The canines are Class I and the molars, although not clearly seen in the photographs, are also Class I. Additional findings include a normal overjet. The overbite is moderately deep at approximately 50%. The maxillary right lateral incisor is in crossbite. The TSALD indicated the presence of mild crowding, which must be taken into account with the anterior crossbite. The maxillary right lateral incisor is blocked lingually with inadequate space. Because it cannot be simply tipped forward, this is a complicating factor. Radiographic findings are within normal limits because all teeth are present and erupting in a normal pattern. The lateral cephalometric tracing shows a tendency for retrusive position of the maxilla and mandible, but the ANB angle of 2.5 degrees is within normal limits (see Figure 13-34, *E*). In summary, this case has the following complicating factors: anterior crossbite with inadequate space for the lateral incisors. A summary of the findings to the diagnostic parameters is presented in Box 13-14. This complicating factor leads to the diagnosis of a Class I malocclusion with an anterior crossbite with space loss.

Treatment Simple anterior crossbites can be corrected by tipping the affected tooth into available space in the arch. This is often possible in the early

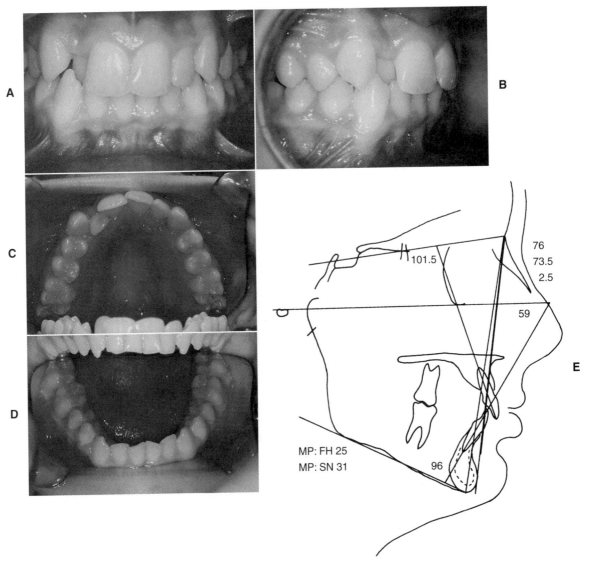

Figure 13-34 Anterior crossbite with space loss (pretreatment) in a 15-year-old male with a Class I occlusion. The right maxillary incisor in lingual crossbite cephalometric measurements are within normal limits.

mixed dentition. Once the permanent canines erupt, it is more likely that an incisor in crossbite will get blocked out of the arch. This case shows a lateral incisor that erupted lingually and was later blocked out of the arch by the erupting maxillary canine. Space must be gained to create adequate arch length for the lateral incisor before it can be moved labially to correct the crossbite. After placing fixed orthodontic appliances to align the teeth, a compressed open coil spring was used to create space for the lateral incisor. Once adequate space was present, the patient was provided with a maxillary bite plate with a finger spring. The bite plate held the bite open while the lateral incisor crossbite was corrected. The crossbite correction was simultaneously accomplished by the forces from a flexible 0.016 nitinol wire on the labial side and the finger spring pushing the tooth from the lingual side. The occlusion at the end of treatment is illustrated in Figure 13-35.

Skeletal Posterior Crossbite

Diagnosis The patient in Figure 13-36, *A-B*, has a Class I canine and molar relationships leading to a diagnosis of a Class I malocclusion. Other findings include normal overjet and overbite in the permanent dentition with adequate arch length in both arches. Crossbites are present in both the anterior and posterior arch segments. Because the anterior tooth in crossbite has adequate space for it to be moved labially, it is not considered to be a complicating factor. On the other hand, this patient has a bilateral posterior crossbite with a functional shift to the right. This is shown by the lower dental midline, which shifted toward the same side of the posterior crossbite. A posterior crossbite in the permanent dentition involving multiple teeth requires expansion of the maxilla. A skeletal crossbite is a complicating factor causing this case to require comprehensive treatment. Radiographic find-

BOX 13-14	Comprehensive Treatment: Anterior Crossbite with Space Loss

Diagnostic Parameter	Answer	Anterior Crossbite with Space Loss
1	d, a, a, d	Class I canines (molars not seen, but Class I)
2	a	Class I malocclusion
3	b	Moderate overbite (20% to 50%)
4	a	Normal overjet
5	d	Permanent dentition
6	a	No crossbite
7	b	Mild crowding (1 to 3 mm)
8	a	Pantomograph findings within normal limits
9	a	Lateral cephalometric radiograph findings within normal limits
10	b	Comprehensive treatment case
11	I	Anterior crossbite with space loss

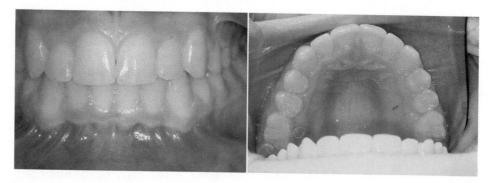

Figure 13-35 Case treated for anterior crossbite with space loss. Posttreatment treatment results following space regaining and crossbite correction with full fixed appliances.

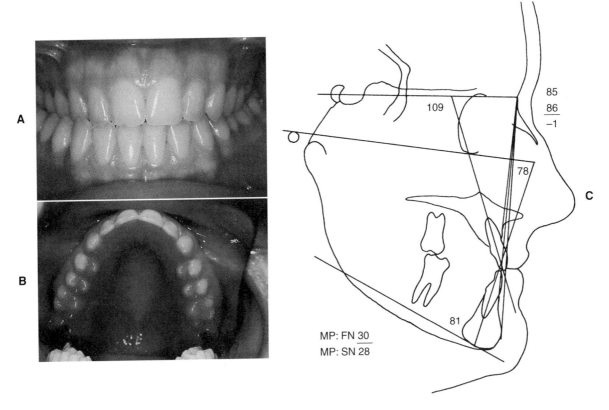

Figure 13-36 Case with skeletal posterior crossbite (pretreatment) in a 15-year-old female. **A** and **B,** Intraoral photographs indicate Class I occlusion with a skeletal posterior crossbite in the permanent dentition. **C,** Tracing indicates a prognathic tendency and dental compensations.

BOX 13-15	Comprehensive Treatment: Skeletal Posterior Crossbite

Diagnostic Parameter	*Answer*	*Skeletal Posterior Crossbite*
1	a, a, a, a	Class I molars and canines
2	a	Class I malocclusion
3	a	Normal overbite (5% to 20 %)
4	a	Normal overjet
5	d	Permanent dentition
6	d	Anterior and posterior crossbites
7	a	Adequate arch length
8	a	Pantomograph findings within normal limits
9	a	Lateral cephalometric radiograph findings within normal limits
10	b	Comprehensive treatment case
11	i	Skeletal posterior crossbite

ings are within normal limits because all teeth are present and erupting in a normal pattern. The lateral cephalometric tracing shows a protrusive mandible with an ANB angle of −1.0 degree (see Figure 13-36, *C*). Although the angle is less than the average relationship of 2.0 degree, it is still within the normal

range. The presence of dental compensations to accommodate the skeletal relationships should also be noticed. A summary of the findings to the diagnostic parameters is presented in Box 13-15. The diagnosis of this case is a Class I malocclusion with a **skeletal posterior crossbite.**

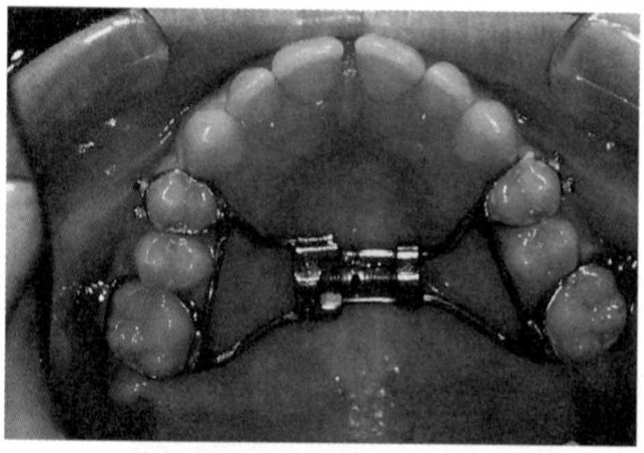

Figure 13-37 A rapid maxillary expander is used to open the midpalatal suture in patients who have a skeletal constriction, indicated by a high, narrow palate accompanying a posterior crossbite. When the suture is opened, a midline diastema will be created temporarily.

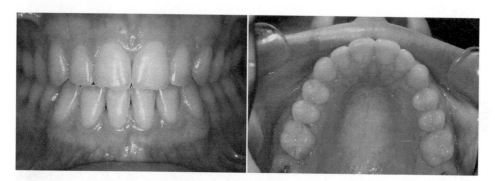

Figure 13-38 Intraoral photographs of a case with skeletal posterior crossbite after correction of the crossbite with rapid maxillary expander followed by fixed appliances and elastics.

Treatment A skeletal posterior crossbite must be corrected by opening the midpalatal suture. Removable appliances are only able to tip the teeth but not open the midpalatal suture for skeletal expansion. Slow expanders, such as the quad helix and W-arch, are more likely to tip teeth than open the suture.[12] A rapid maxillary expander (RME) is a rigid appliance that can open the midpalatal suture.[13] An RME was used to accomplish the needed skeletal expansion (Figure 13-37). Opening the suture is relatively easier and stability is more predictable in the adolescent patient. Figure 13-38 illustrates the final results. In adults the suture is more difficult to open and the relapse tendencies are greater. Treatment planning of skeletal posterior crossbites in adults may involve the possibility of surgical expansion or finishing cases in crossbite. Relapse is common in adults, so retention must also be prolonged.[8]

Ectopic Eruption

Diagnosis The patient in Figure 13-39 had a Class I malocclusion, normal overjet, no crossbite, and minimal spacing in the permanent dentition. Because the overbite is only moderately deep, it is not considered to be a complicating factor. The pantomograph shows that the maxillary canines are erupting between the premolars (see Figure 13-39, *D*). Such transposed teeth are beyond the range of normal eruption and

serve as a complicating factor, which causes this case to be designated as a comprehensive case with **ectopic eruption.** A summary of the findings to the diagnostic parameters is presented in Box 13-16.

Treatment This example is unusual because the maxillary canines erupted in a transposed position between the premolars. The decision was made to maintain the teeth in their transposed positions as seen in the post-treatment photographs (Figure 13-40). Cases with unusual eruption are often best treated with a multi-disciplinary approach combining input from both the orthodontist and the restorative dentist. If function or esthetics is a concern at the end of treatment, the canines may have crowns placed that resemble premolars and the transposed premolar crowns may be reshaped to look like canines.

Impacted Tooth

Diagnosis The patient in Figure 13-41, *A-E*, has Class I molars, a Class II left canine, and an unerupted right canine (Figure 13-41, *F*) leading to a diagnosis of a Class II Division 2, subdivision left malocclusion. The Division 2 categorization was determined by the presence of upright maxillary incisors, as shown on the lateral cephalometric tracing (see Figure 13-41, *G*). Other findings include normal overjet and moderate overbite. Mild crowding is present in both arches.

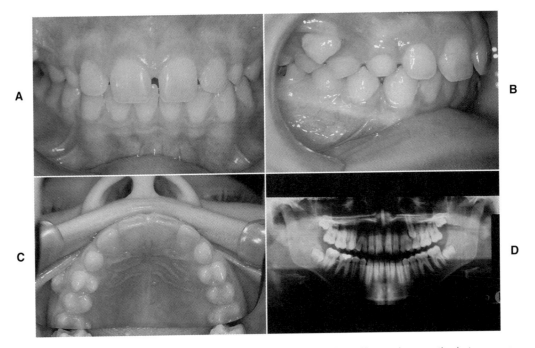

Figure 13-39 Ectopic eruption (pretreatment) in a 12-year-old male with maxillary canines erupting between premolars. Pantomograph shows position of ectopically erupting canines. Primary canines were extracted and first premolars moved mesially to maintain a transposed position with the canines.

BOX 13-16	Comprehensive Treatment: Ectopic Eruption

Diagnostic Parameter	Answer	Ectopic Eruption
1	a, a, a, a	Class I molars and canines
2	a	Class I malocclusion
3	b	Moderate overbite (20% to 50%)
4	a	Normal overjet
5	c	Late mixed dentition
6	a	No crossbite
7	d	Mild spacing (1 to 3 mm)
8	b	Eruption beyond the range of normal (canines between the premolars)
9	c	Lateral cephalometric radiograph within normal limits
10	b	Comprehensive treatment case
11	i	Ectopic eruption/transposed canines with premolars

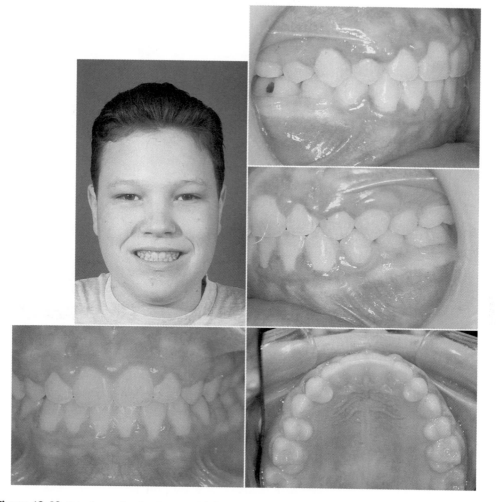

Figure 13-40 Ectopic eruption (posttreatment) following alignment of transposed maxillary canines and first premolars.

Because this patient is still in the late mixed dentition stage, a modified Hixon-Oldfather space analysis was used to calculate the TSALD. Although the anterior crowding appears to be more severe, it must be remembered that the primary second molars are larger than the second premolars. Thus anterior crowding is minimized by the space gained when the primary second molars are exfoliated.

An anterior crossbite is present, but the lateral incisor appears to have adequate space to be tipped forward. Therefore this is not considered to be a complicating factor. Evaluation of the pantomograph shows an impacted maxillary right canine (see Figure 13-41, *F*). The management of an **impacted tooth** will always require a multidisciplinary approach between a number of specialists. The lateral cephalometric tracing shows a normal position of the maxilla and mandible. The ANB relationship of 3.0 degrees is within the normal range (see Figure 13-41, *G*). A summary of the findings to

the diagnostic parameters is presented in Box 13-17. The complicating factor in this case is the presence of an impacted canine. The diagnosis is a Class II Division 2, subdivision left with an impacted maxillary right canine.

Treatment As teeth erupt, a general guideline is that contralateral teeth will erupt within 6 months of one another. When a patient has a delay in the eruption of a contralateral tooth for more than 6 months, a periapical or panoramic radiograph should be made to assess the condition. The radiograph may show no permanent successor, a tooth that is close to eruption, or a tooth that is ectopically erupting. Often these teeth need to be surgically exposed, have a bracket bonded to the impacted tooth, and be brought down into the arch with orthodontic forces (Figure 13-42). Posttreatment results following comprehensive orthodontic treatment is shown in Figure 13-43.

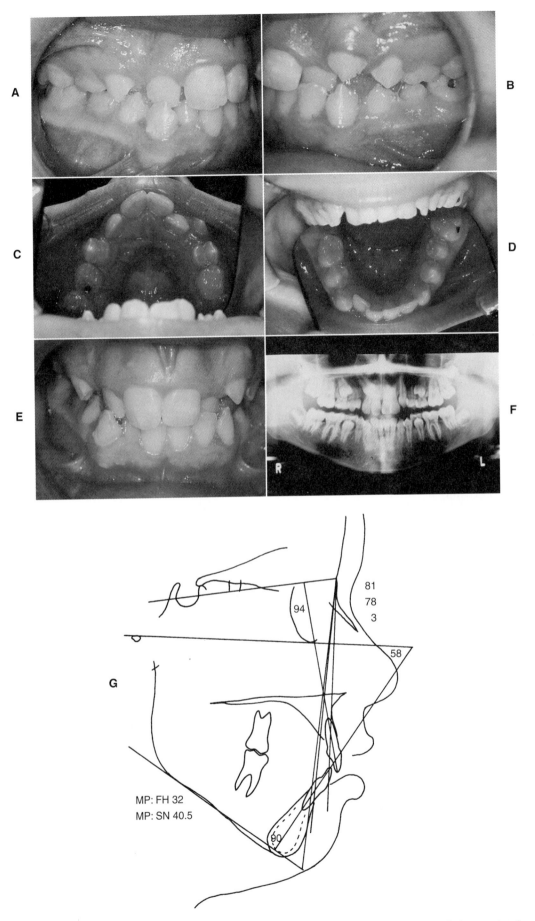

Figure 13-41 Case with an impacted tooth (pretreatment) in a 13-year-old female. **A** to **E,** Intraoral photographs of the dentition. **F,** Pantomograph shows position of impacted canine. **G,** Tracing of the lateral cephalogram of the patient.

BOX 13-17	Comprehensive Treatment: Impacted Tooth

Diagnostic Parameter	Answer	Impacted Tooth
1	a, d, b, a	Class I molars, Class II left canine, right canine not visible
2	e	Class II Division 2 Subdivision malocclusion
3	b	Moderate overbite (20% to 50%)
4	a	Normal overjet
5	c	Late mixed dentition
6	b	Anterior crossbite
7	b	Mild crowding (1 to 3 mm) both arches
8	b	Impacted maxillary right canine
9	a	Lateral cephalometric radiograph findings within normal limits
10	b	Comprehensive treatment case
11	i	Impacted tooth

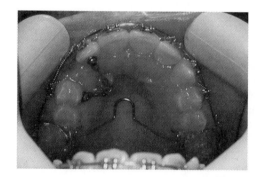

Figure 13-42 Impacted tooth was surgically exposed; elastics were changed to move the tooth from the palate toward the dental arch.

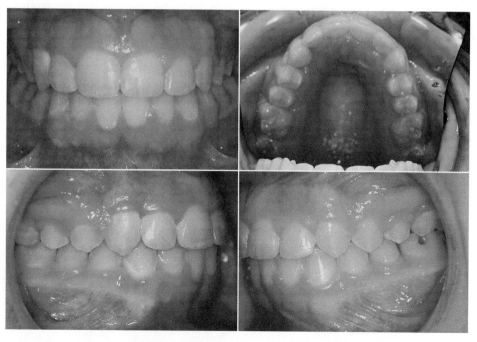

Figure 13-43 Case with impacted tooth. Intraoral photographs at the end of treatment following movement of impacted tooth into the dental arch.

SUMMARY

This chapter has focused on a series of diagnostic parameters that were designed to simplify and standardize the evaluation of a malocclusion to arrive at a proper orthodontic diagnosis. Specific information on different parameters must be obtained to systematically distinguish between cases that require limited versus comprehensive orthodontic treatment. The different diagnostic parameters listed are intended to help the clinician assess the malocclusion and determine whether the treatment is within the scope of the general practitioner or whether referral to an orthodontic specialist is indicated. As a result, treatment of the different malocclusions is determined by the knowledge and experience of the clinician. The most important factor in treatment of malocclusions is an appropriate diagnosis. The various complicating factors in the diagnostic parameters help the clinician distinguish between cases requiring limited treatment and those that benefit from and require comprehensive treatment. A thorough understanding of the treatment options is necessary to tailor the treatment plan to each individual patient.

REFERENCES

1. Ricketts RM: Perspectives in the clinical application of cephalometrics: the first fifty years, *Angle Orthod* 51(2):115-150, 1981.
2. Popovich F, Thompson GW: Craniofacial templates for orthodontic case analysis, *Am J Orthod* 71:406-420, 1977.
3. Claffey N: Decision making in periodontal therapy: the reevaluation, *J Clin Periodontol* 18:117-125, 1991.
4. Proffit WR, Fields HW Jr: *Contemporary orthodontics,* ed 3, St Louis, 2000, Mosby.
5. Cameron AC, Widmer RP: *Handbook of pediatric dentistry,* London, 1997, Mosby-Wolfe.
6. Haryett RD, Hansen FC, Davidson PO: Chronic thumb sucking, *Am J Orthod* 5(7):467-470, 1970.
7. Richardson ME: Mesial migration of lower molars in relation to facial growth and eruption, *Australian Orthod J* 14(2):87-91, 1996.
8. Storey E: Tissue response to the movement of bones, *Am J Orthod* 64:229-247, 1973.
9. Villa NL, Cisneros GJ: Changes in the dentition secondary to palatal crib therapy in digit-suckers: a preliminary study, *Pediatr Dent* 19(5):323-326, 1997.
10. Dale JG: Guidance of occlusion: serial extraction. In Graber TM, Vanarsdall RL (eds): *Orthodontics: current principles and techniques,* ed 3, St Louis, 2000, Mosby.
11. Moskowitz E: Serial extractions in orthodontic therapy: a literature review, *Int J Orthod* 11(3):89-96, 1973.
12. Bell RA: A review of maxillary expansion on relation to rate of expansion and patient's age, *Am J Orthod* 81:32-37, 1982.
13. Bishara SE, Staley RN: Maxillary expansion: clinical implications, *Am J Orthod Dentofacial Orthop* 91:3-14, 1987.

SUGGESTED READINGS

1. Angle EH: *Treatment of malocclusion of the teeth and fractures of the maxillae, Angle's system,* ed 6, Philadelphia, 1900, SS White Dental Mfg.
2. Brickbauer GP: Preventive and interceptive orthodontics for the growing child, *Intern J Orthod* 26(l-2):19-22, 1988.
3. Graber TM, Vanarsdall RL: *Orthodontics: current principles and techniques,* ed 3, St Louis, 2000, Mosby.
4. Hicks EP: Slow maxillary expansion: a clinical study of the skeletal vs. dental response to low magnitude force, *Am J Orthod* 73:121-141, 1978.
5. Krebs AA: Expansion of the midpalatal suture studied by means of metallic implants, *Eur Orthod Soc Rep* 34:163-171, 1958.

SECTION III

Appliances

CHAPTER 14

Fixed Edgewise Orthodontic Appliances and Bonding Techniques

Pramod K. Sinha and Ram S. Nanda

KEY TERMS

edgewise bracket system
straight wire appliance

preadjusted appliance
edgewise appliances

preformed bands
separators

direct bonding
indirect bonding

The orthodontic profession has gone through an evolving process to reach the current bracket systems used in clinical practice. In 1928 Dr. Angle[1] came up with the edgewise system, which has served as the blueprint for all subsequent **edgewise bracket systems.**

Another popular system developed in the 1920s by Dr. P.R. Begg in the 1920s was a modification of the ribbon arch appliance created by Angle (Figure 14-1).[2] Dr. Begg was a student at Angle's school where he was taught how to use the ribbon arch appliance. On his return to Australia Dr. Begg modified the appliance and created the Begg system.

For many years orthodontists used the standard edgewise and Begg systems with great success. During this period practitioners made their own modifications on the appliances to provide more desirable features. However, it was not until Dr. Lawrence Andrews developed the fully programmed straight-wire appliances that this concept became commercially available.

 Historic Milestones in Orthodontics

Dr. Edward Angle
Dr. Edward Angle is considered the father of modern orthodontics. His contributions to orthodontics between the late 1800s and his death in 1930 at 75 years of age are many and include the development of the modern edgewise appliance, the Angle classification of malocclusion, and the Angle School of Orthodontia to train dental specialists (1900).

Dr. P.R. Begg
In the mid 1950s Dr. P.R. Begg, an Australian orthodontist, adopted the light wire technique for the treatment of var-

ious malocclusions. The technique is based on differential force application and the use of the pin and tube appliances to move teeth.

Dr. Larry Andrews
In the early 1970s Dr. Larry Andrews introduced the **straight wire appliance** based on his concepts of normal occlusion. He incorporated the details of the final tooth position in the bracket itself to minimize the need by the clinician to place the bends in the arch wire. A number of modifications in the angulation and torque were later introduced based on his concepts.

Dr. Andrews conducted studies to determine the amounts of tip (mesial or distal), step (in-out or vertical), and torque (twisting facial or lingual) for each tooth (Box 14-1).[3] The results were incorporated into the fabrication of the straight-wire appliances. The aim was to incorporate individual tooth movements into the appliance, minimizing the need for wire bending. However, individual variations in jaw relationships, tooth size, and tooth shape do exist. Therefore wire bending and adjustments are still necessary to idealize the position of teeth in the finishing stages to optimally treat each case. Brackets combining the edgewise and Begg slots are also available.

BOX 14-1	The Six Keys to Normal Occlusion

1. Molar relationship
2. Crown tip
3. Crown torque
4. Absence of rotations
5. Absence of spaces
6. Flat plane of occlusion

From Andrews LF: *Am J Orthod* 63:296-309, 1972.

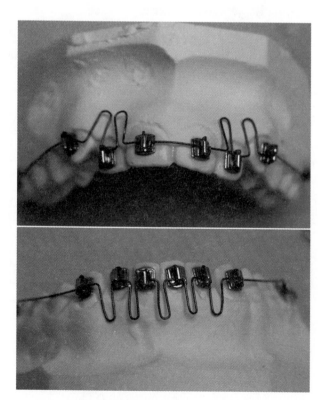

Figure 14-1 The Begg appliance system.

This modified system attempts to combine the mechanics of the two different systems.[4,5] In contemporary orthodontic practices the preadjusted edgewise appliance is the most popular among practicing clinicians.[6]

PREADJUSTED ORTHODONTIC APPLIANCES VS. THE STANDARD EDGEWISE SYSTEMS

The **preadjusted appliance** was designed to achieve high-quality orthodontic results with minimal wire bending and simplified mechanics. However, individual variations in skeletal, soft tissue and dental relationships as well as in dental morphology have to be considered in treating each case. Therefore the preadjustment incorporated in the appliance serves as an average from which variations need to be made to idealize the position of teeth for most orthodontic patients.

Although the preadjusted appliance affords certain advantages over the standard edgewise system (Box 14-2), some disadvantages become apparent with the initial use of these appliances. Box 14-3 presents a summary of the differences between these two systems during the different stages of treatment.

Preadjusted Prescriptions

Bracket angulations in different planes of space were established to position teeth properly without too much wire bending. Hence the term *straight wire* or *preadjusted* appliances. However, clinical experience has demonstrated that individual anatomic variations and different malocclusion types more often than not require additional adjustments in the arch wires to properly position the teeth.

The prescription in the built-in bracket adjustments suggested by the manufacturers and clinicians are based on the individual practitioner's preference. Therefore numerous variations exist in the market. Examples of two common bracket prescriptions are presented in Table 14-1.

MATERIALS USED TO FABRICATE ORTHODONTIC BRACKETS

Orthodontic appliances are made up of three types of materials: metals, plastics, and ceramics.

Contemporary Metal Brackets

Metal brackets made from stainless steel are the most commonly used in orthodontic practice,[6] but the color

BOX 14-2   Appliance Design

The preadjusted appliance is designed to provide the following features:

1. *Rotational control:* Rotational control is provided by the twin wing design (see Figure 14-2) of the modern appliances or by the incorporation of rotational arms in single-wing bracket systems (see Figure 14-3).
2. *Horizontal control:* Variations in the relative thickness of the bracket bases provide corrective movement for varying thickness of teeth and therefore align teeth in the horizontal plane of space. Different bracket systems should not be used in the same patient because of this feature. With earlier edgewise brackets, bends in the arch wire were necessary to accomplish these movements. The preadjusted appliance does not totally eliminate this requirement because of individual variations in tooth size and shape.
3. *Vertical control:* The appliance provides control in the vertical plane of space.
4. *Mesiodistal tip control:* The edgewise slot is angulated relative to the base of the bracket to provide appropriate mesiodistal tipping movement for each individual tooth.

5. *Torque control:* The edgewise slot is angulated in the labiolingual plane of space to provide appropriate root and crown movements in the process of tooth alignment.
6. *Other features:* A variety of modifications have been made in appliance design to accommodate desirable features. These features are not incorporated in all appliances.

   One such feature is a self-ligating system in which a clip has been incorporated in the bracket design for wire engagement (see Figure 14-4). This design lowers friction during sliding mechanics and therefore has the potential to allow for light forces to move teeth. Another feature that has the potential to reduce friction is incorporated in appliances that allow modifications in the ligation method (see Figure 14-5). This is accomplished by removal of the pressure of ligation on the wire, allowing easier sliding mechanics.

   The addition of a vertical slot in the edgewise bracket is another modification that increases the versatility of the force system that can be applied.

BOX 14-3   Differences Between Preadjusted and Standard Edgewise Systems

Initial Stages

During the initial stages of treatment, practitioners reported that anchorage loss was greater with the use of the new preadjusted appliances. This was because of the increased tipping of the anterior teeth during the initial stages. In an attempt to control anchorage, appropriate force systems should be used in the initial stages. A study of the anchorage requirements in the case is essential and needs to be addressed at the initial stages.

Intermediate Stages

During the intermediate stages of treatment, the increased emphasis on anchorage control with the preadjusted appliances also helps with overbite control and correction.

In addition, the leveling of the bracket slots during the initial stages allows the use of sliding mechanics to close spaces. On the other hand, with the standard edgewise system, if tips or torque is placed in the arch wires it may not allow effective sliding mechanics.

Finishing Stages

The major benefit of the preadjusted appliance system is evident in the finishing stages of treatment. Proper bracket positioning is critical to take full advantage of the preadjustments in the finishing stages. Because individual tooth positions are defined during the initial stages, only minor adjustments are required in most cases to idealize tooth positions. Therefore after the intermediate stages, final settling is generally all that is necessary.

TABLE 14-1	Bracket Prescriptions in Degrees for Two Commonly Used Appliance Adjustments			
	Original Straight Wire		*Roth*	
	Tip	Torque	Tip	Torque
Maxillary Teeth				
Central incisors	5.0	7.0	5.0	12.0
Lateral incisors	9.0	3.0	9.0	8.0
Canines	11.0	−7.0*	13.0	−2.0*
Premolars	2.0	−7.0*	0.0	−7.0*
Molars	5.0	−9.0*	0.0	−14.0*
Mandibular Teeth				
Central incisors	2.0	−1.0*	2.0	−1.0*
Lateral incisors	2.0	−1.0*	2.0	−1.0*
Canines	5.0	−11.0*	7.0	−11.0*
First premolars	2.0	−17.0*	−1.0†	−17.0*
Second premolars	2.0	−22.0*	−1.0†	−22.0*
First molars	2.0	−30.0*	−1.0†	−30.0*
Second molars	2.0	−30.0*	−1.0†	−30.0*

*Negative torque refers to the intended movement of the roots of teeth toward the buccal side.
†Negative tip refers to distal crown tip.

of the metal and its visibility may be objectionable to some adult patients (Figures 14-2 to 14-5). Manufacturers have tried to reduce the size of the bracket and hence its visibility by continuously redesigning the appliance. Another relatively recent introduction is a bracket made of titanium. A titanium bracket has the potential of working well in the small number of patients who experience nickel hypersensitivity from traditional metal brackets.[7]

Another variant of the metal bracket is a stainless steel bracket coated with a microthin layer of zirconia-nitride to impart a gold color (Figure 14-6). Along with this bracket, gold arch wires are available to complement the color.

Esthetic Orthodontic Appliances

Metal Lingual orthodontic appliances were introduced in the 1970s to overcome the esthetic disadvantages of conventional labial appliances. These appliances introduced new challenges to orthodontists and patients. Orthodontists found that day-to-day practice with these appliances is more time consuming and required altered dexterity. The most probable reason for this difficulty is the lingual placement of the orthodontic attachments making direct visualization impossible. Further, the treatment results achieved were often less than desirable when compared with those obtained with the use of conventional appliances.

Also, patient discomfort increases significantly because of constant irritation to the tongue. Lingual appliances have declined in their popularity over the years in the United States.[6]

Plastic Brackets Plastic brackets to be bonded directly to enamel were initially made of polycarbonate and plastic molding powder (Plexiglas).[8,9] Plexiglas brackets did not last long because of their discoloration, fragility, and breakage under stress.[10-13] Also, much of the energy in the wire was expended in distorting the brackets because of the poor integrity of the arch wire slot, and therefore forces were not transmitted to the tooth.[14-16] In recent years there have been several improvements to reinforce plastic brackets, such as precision-made stainless steel slot inserts (Figure 14-7) and ceramic material fillers (15% to 30%). Metal slot reinforcement of plastic brackets appears to strengthen the matrix adequately so that torque can be applied at the same level as with metal brackets.[17] Ceramic-reinforced composite brackets without a metal slot insert have been shown to have fairly low frictional characteristics compared with ceramic and metal brackets.[18] Hence the newly introduced ceramic-reinforced plastic brackets are suitable for clinical use because they are color stable, have lower friction,[18] and have the structural integrity to transmit orthodontic forces without distorting.[17]

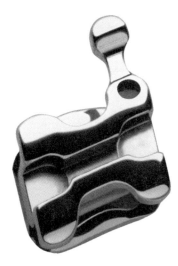

Figure 14-2 Mini Uni-Twin bracket showing a contemporary twin-wing design bracket. (Courtesy Unitek Corporation/3M, Monrovia, Calif.)

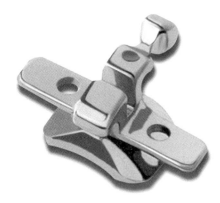

Figure 14-3 A single-wing bracket with rotational arms. (Courtesy Unitek Corporation/3M, Monrovia, Calif.)

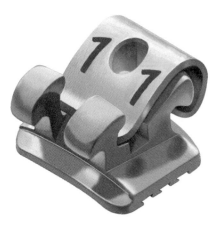

Figure 14-4 A self-ligating bracket in which a clip has been incorporated in the bracket design for wire engagement. (Courtesy American Orthodontics, Sheboygan, WI.)

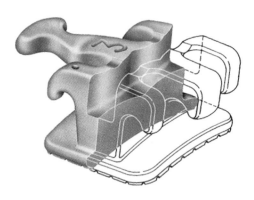

Figure 14-5 A bracket design that allows modifications in the ligation method. (Courtesy GAC International, Inc, Islip, NY.)

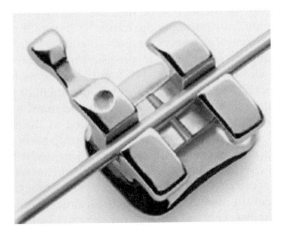

Figure 14-6 Another variant of the metal bracket is a stainless steel bracket coated with a micro-thin layer of zirconia-nitride to impart a gold color. (Courtesy Unitek Corporation/3M, Monrovia, Calif.)

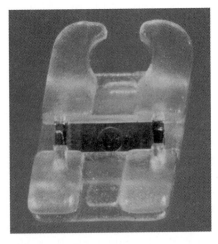

Figure 14-7 A plastic bracket with a stainless steel slot insert. (From Sinha PK, Nanda RS: *Dent Clin North Am* 41:89-109, 1997.)

Ceramic Brackets   During the last decade, ceramic brackets have become the esthetic alternative to plastic brackets. The monocrystalline and polycrystalline ceramic materials used in manufacturing these brackets provide excellent color fidelity and stain resistance. However, clinicians may be inhibited from using ceramic brackets because of their reported fracture tendencies and, more importantly, their reported tendency to damage enamel during the debonding procedure.[19-22] The manufacturers of these brackets have tried to improve bracket characteristics to facilitate easier debonding.[29,30] These changes have included a shift from the purely chemical retention mechanism of resin bonding to the bracket base to a totally mechanical mode of bonding for the polycrystalline bracket.[19-22]

Investigations have found that debonding with sharp-edged pliers applies a bilateral force at the bracket base-adhesive interface and is the most effective method for debonding both polycrystalline and monocrystalline orthodontic brackets.[31-33] Therefore forces applied at the interface rather than the bracket itself may prevent breakage on debonding. Brackets bonded by indirect techniques, which create a resin interlayer, facilitate debonding at the interface formed between this interlayer and the filled resin.[31-33]

Ceramic brackets may fracture during torsional and tipping movements,[34-36] cause abrasion of opposing teeth, and have increased frictional resistance in sliding mechanics compared with plastic and metal brackets.[37-42] Ceramic brackets have limitations and caution must be exercised in their use. Ceramic brackets should not be bonded to teeth that have cracks or signs of physical defects.

A new design of the ceramic bracket is borrowed from the design of the metal reinforced plastic bracket. This bracket system incorporates a metal slot in the ceramic bracket, reducing the friction to levels experienced by stainless steel brackets. Another feature of this appliance is the ease of debonding via a vertical scribe line placed in the base of the bracket (Figure 14-8).[43]

BANDING IN THE CONTEMPORARY ORTHODONTIC PRACTICE

The original **edgewise appliances** involved the banding of all teeth. These bands were customized for each patient. Hence bands were prepared by stretch molding the band material around the tooth, creating a joint, and then the brackets were welded to the bands. This involved a long appointment to fit the bands and cement the appliance in place. The introduction of preformed bands changed this procedure significantly. **Preformed bands** are available in a variety of sizes and follow the average anatomy for each tooth type. Minor tooth variations require band adaptation by the clinician to ensure a proper fit.

The development of the bonding procedure revolutionized the use of fixed orthodontic appliances. Some practitioners exclusively bond all fixed appliances, including molars. However, banding molar teeth is commonly done in clinical practice. Before banding, space is created to allow band fitting and cementation via **separators** that are placed between teeth (Figure 14-9).

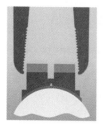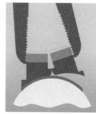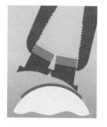

Figure 14-8 A ceramic bracket design showing a vertical scribe line placed in the base of the appliance for ease of removal or debonding. (Courtesy Unitek Corporation/3M, Monrovia, Calif.)

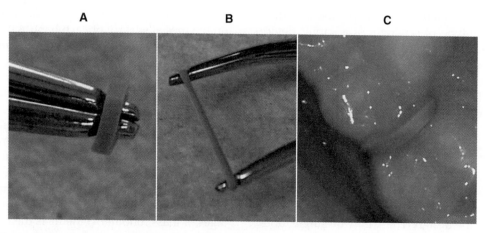

Figure 14-9 A, Alastik separators on the beaks of the separating pliers. **B,** Separators stretched on the beaks of the separating pliers. **C,** Separators placed between teeth before banding.

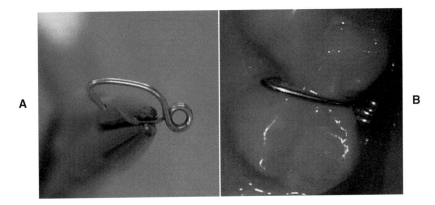

Figure 14-10 A, Metal separating springs held by a hemostat. **B,** Metal separators placed between teeth before banding.

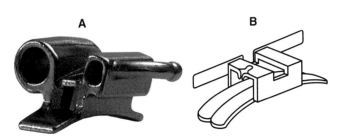

Figure 14-11 A, A triple-tube molar attachment for bands. **B,** A transpalatal bar sheath that may be attached to the palatal side of the molar bands. (Courtesy American Orthodontics, Sheboygan, WI.)

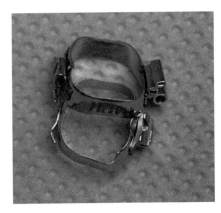

Figure 14-12 Band sizes scribed on the mesial surface of bands with a laser device.

Commonly used separators are made of an elastomeric material and are placed with the help of an instrument that spreads the elastomeric module to allow threading the separator between the contact points of neighboring teeth. Pieces of floss can be used to apply this separator as well. Another type of separator is a spring device made of stainless steel, which can be applied using hemostat-type pliers (Figure 14-10). The separator is placed between the teeth in such a manner that the ends of the spring lie above and below the contact area between two teeth.

Band Selection

Orthodontic bands are made exclusively from stainless steel material. The buccal attachments on the molar bands vary as to the number of tubes and hooks incorporated in the design. These may be single, double, or triple tubes (Figure 14-11, *A*), depending on the

practitioner's philosophy and requirements. A variety of lingual attachments are also available and can be preselected by the clinician (see Figure 14-11, *B*). These attachments are generally cast separately and then welded to the preformed bands. Band sizes are scribed on the mesial surface of each band with a laser device (Figure 14-12 and Box 14-4). The proper placement of the band is illustrated in Figure 14-13.

Band Cementation

Different types of band cements are used for cementing the selected bands (Box 14-5). The most commonly used material in contemporary practice is a type of glass ionomer cement. These cements can be resin based or nonresin based and may or may not require light activation for curing purposes. One of the advantages of glass ionomer cements is their release of fluoride to minimize decalcification.

BOX 14-4   Sequence for Band Size Selection

1. The patient's casts can be used to decide the approximate size of the band for each tooth. Also, a study of the anatomy of the tooth on the models and the presence of restorations are helpful in determining variations from the norm and the need for further adjustments. Examples of other variations include extra cusps and tapered crowns.
2. The fitting procedure is started by selecting a size that may seem larger than the one that may fit the tooth. This method prevents wasteful distortion of the bands.
3. The mandibular bands are fit by first applying finger pressure only to seat on the mesial and distal sides (see Figure 14-13, *A*). An amalgam plugger or band pusher is used to seat the band further on the mesial and distal sides (see Figure 14-13, *B*). Once the band is seated two thirds of the way as shown in Figure 14-13, *C,* the patient should apply the force via biting pressure on a bite stick to seat the band on the facial and the lingual sides (see Figure 14-13, *D*). The fitting for both maxillary and mandibular bands follows identical steps. The difference in banding the mandibular teeth vs. the maxillary teeth is that the final seating pressure should be on the buccal/facial side of the tooth for the mandibular band and on the palatal side of the tooth for the maxillary band.
4. A measuring gauge can be used to determine the correct height of the buccal attachments.
5. The bands should fit such that all cusps on the banded tooth are equally visible, the band margins are just below the marginal ridge and above the contact points, and the buccal slot is accurately positioned mesiodistally and occlusogingivally (see Figure 14-13, *E*). Open occlusal margins should be crimped toward the tooth using a band pusher to enhance fitting and eliminate plaque traps.

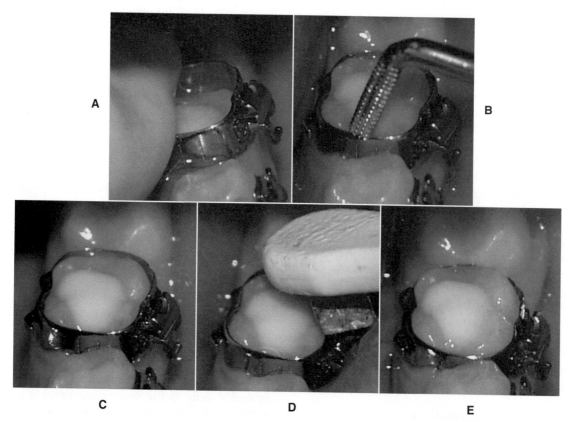

Figure 14-13 A, Starting the band-fitting procedure by placing the band on the tooth and applying finger pressure to seat the band. **B,** An amalgam plugger or band pusher may be used to seat the band further on the mesial and distal sides. **C,** The band can be seated two thirds of the way using the pusher. **D,** A bite stick is used to seat the band to its final position. **E,** All cusps on the banded tooth are equally visible, the band margins are just below the marginal ridge and above the contact points, and the buccal slot is accurately positioned mesiodistally and occlusogingivally.

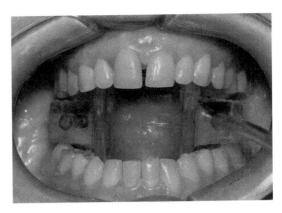

Figure 14-14 *Devices used for isolation during bracket bonding. (From Sinha PK, Nanda RS: Bonding in clinical orthodontics. In Hardin JF [ed]: Clark's clinical dentistry, vol 2, St Louis, 1998, Mosby.)*

BOX 14-5   Three-Steps of Band Cementation

1. Wax is applied in the tubes before placing the cement to prevent clogging of the tubes and attachments. The teeth being banded are isolated.
2. The occlusal end of the selected bands is taped to hold the cement. A cement spatula is used to carry the cement to the bands. An even layer is applied around the inside of the band.
3. The band is placed on the tooth and positioned via finger pressure. A band pusher is required to finally seat the band. Excess cement is wiped off the occlusal surface. The cement material is either cured using a light or allowed to set before violating the isolation.

ORTHODONTIC BONDING

The Basic Mechanism of Bonding Teeth

In dentistry, *bonding* is a term conventionally used to describe the attachment of the bracket using bonding resins to the enamel surfaces. Both physical and chemical forces play a role in the process; however, the mechanical interlocking of the low viscosity polymer bonding agent and the enamel surface is the principal mechanism of attachment between the enamel and resin-bonding systems.[44-47]

The adhesion of orthodontic attachments to enamel can be classified into direct and indirect techniques based on the method of placement.

No matter which technique is used, the basic mechanism of bonding has remained the same and involves prophylaxis, enamel surface preparation-enamel etching, and bonding the bracket to the enamel surface.

Prophylaxis Enamel prophylaxis before etching has been shown to result in maximum bond strengths.[48] This procedure removes the pellicle, accentuates the irregularities present in natural enamel and enhances the wetting of the enamel surface by the acid.[49] A rubber cup prophylaxis and a thin slurry of medium grain pumice powder and water on a slow speed hand piece is recommended.[50] The prophylaxis should be done before the placement of moisture control and retraction devices, thus allowing the patient to rinse after the procedure.

Enamel Surface Preparation

Isolation and Moisture Control The prepared enamel surface requires proper isolation and moisture control for successful bonding. It is important that contamination of the surface by moisture or saliva should be prevented (Figure 14-14) by using cheek retractors and a plastic bite block to open the bite and restrain the tongue.

Enamel Etching Following proper isolation and moisture control with saliva ejectors (see Figure 14-14), the tooth or segments of teeth to be etched are dried using an oil and moisture-free air source. The etching agent is usually 35% unbuffered phosphoric acid, which may be in the form of a gel or a liquid.[51] The authors prefer the use of a gel dispensed from a syringe. The advantage of the gel is that the placement of this agent can be controlled, whereas the liquid etchant has a tendency to spread beyond the area to be bonded. The etching time should be between 15 to 30 seconds. The etching time should be increased with age with primary teeth and in cases where the enamel has a higher fluoride content.[52-56] A low-pressure water spray combined with high volume suction is used to thoroughly flush out the etchant from the tooth or teeth. After a thorough cleansing of the enamel surface an oil-free and moisture-free air source should be used to completely dry the etched surface. The etched surface should have a lightly frosted, matte, dull, or whitish appearance.[57]

Bracket Positioning Preadjusted appliances have built-in adjustments in the bracket slot required to facilitate achieving the proper position of individual teeth. These adjustments include mesiodistal tip, labiolingual torque, and in-out horizontal movements. However, these built-in adjustments work as intended only if the individual bracket position is accurate and the tooth is of average size and shape. Further, each bracket should be positioned in specific relative arrangements with the teeth in the same arch. This sequential arrangement ensures the proper relative positions of teeth at the completion of treatment.

Individual Bracket Positioning on the Tooth Brackets should be positioned on individual teeth such that they are at the center of the clinical crown mesiodistally. The angulation of the bracket slot or base should be based on the long axis of the tooth. Guides used for proper placement of the bracket could be either used as the base of the bracket or a built-in long-axis line, which is scribed in some brackets.

Relative Position of Brackets within an Arch Several methods have been used for proper positioning of brackets on teeth relative to each other in the same arch. These have been based on the average size of crowns of teeth or by placing the brackets at the center of the clinical crowns. Both techniques have inherent problems because crown shapes and sizes have innumerable variations.

The authors have used the following scheme with significant clinical success based on measurements made from the incisal edge or crown tip to the center of the bracket slots.

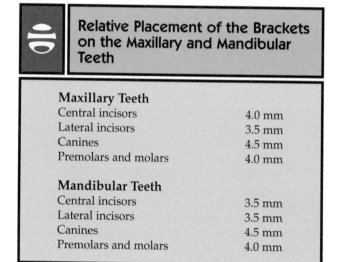

Relative Placement of the Brackets on the Maxillary and Mandibular Teeth	
Maxillary Teeth	
Central incisors	4.0 mm
Lateral incisors	3.5 mm
Canines	4.5 mm
Premolars and molars	4.0 mm
Mandibular Teeth	
Central incisors	3.5 mm
Lateral incisors	3.5 mm
Canines	4.5 mm
Premolars and molars	4.0 mm

Different malocclusion types may require adjustments in these measurements. Deep bite patients may require decreasing the measurements on the central and lateral incisors and increasing measurements on the premolars and molars. Open bite patients require increasing the measurements on the central and lateral incisors and decreasing the measurements on the premolars and molars. Further, individual crown shapes and sizes may further influence the relative positioning of the brackets on the teeth.

Bonding Materials

There are three types of filled acrylic- (BIS-GMA) based composite resins available for orthodontic bonding depending on the mode of polymerization or curing (chemically cured, light-cured, and a combination of thermal- and chemically cured). Resins with formulations containing fluoride are available in all of the previously mentioned polymerization modes. Resin-reinforced glass ionomer cements have also been used for bonding in clinical orthodontics.

ORTHODONTIC BONDING TECHNIQUES
Direct Bonding

The **direct bonding** technique refers to the direct attachment of orthodontic appliances to etched teeth using chemically and light-cured adhesives. All types of orthodontic bonding adhesives used with the direct technique can reliably attach orthodontic appliances to teeth (Figure 14-15). The direct technique is the most popular method with clinicians because of its simplicity and reliability (Box 14-6).

The initial steps with the direct technique involve prophylaxis, isolation of the arches to be bonded, cheek retraction with tongue restraint, and enamel etching. On obtaining all of the above, the etched teeth are ready to receive the bonding adhesive to attach orthodontic appliances.

Indirect Bonding

The **indirect bonding** technique, in which the brackets were first positioned on study casts with a water-soluble adhesive and then transferred to the mouth with a custom tray, was introduced in 1972 (Box 14-7).[58] Now the bracket is positioned on the patient's study cast with the filled resin (Figure 14-16).[31-33,59] The bracket is then transferred to the mouth with a custom tray, and bonding is facilitated by applying an unfilled liquid sealant to the prepared tooth surface and the precured resin at the bracket base. The advantage of this technique is that the excess resin or "flash," which consists of the unfilled liquid sealant, can be easily removed. This technique has also been shown to create an interlayer of unfilled resin between the enamel and the filled resin, which facilitates the debonding of brackets.[31-33] This technique can be performed using any type of commercially available orthodontic bonding resin. This section describes a slight modification of the Thomas technique[59] and a new indirect bracket bonding method using a thermal-cured resin.[60]

Direct vs. Indirect Bonding Techniques

Two major advantages of the indirect bonding technique over the direct bonding technique are the accuracy of placement of orthodontic appliances[61-63] and easier debonding of brackets, specifically the ceramic brackets.[31-33]

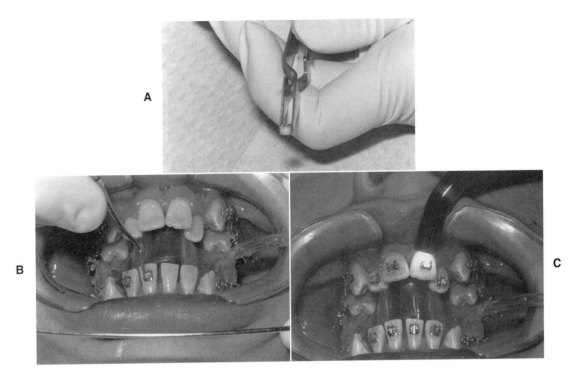

Figure 14-15 **A,** Filled resin paste (a mixture of base and catalyst paste for the two-paste or paste resin for the no-mix or light-cured resins) is applied on the base of the bracket. **B,** The bracket is positioned using a composite instrument. **C,** Light-cured resins require a light source to initiate curing. (From Sinha PK, Nanda RS: Bonding in clinical orthodontics. In Hardin JF [ed]: *Clark's clinical dentistry,* vol 2, St Louis, 1998, Mosby.)

BOX 14-6	Step-by-Step Direct Bonding Procedure

1. Enamel surface preparation is performed.
2. Unfilled liquid sealant is applied to the bracket base (if indicated) and the etched tooth surface.
3. Filled resin paste is applied on the base of the bracket (see Figure 14-15, *A*).

4. The resin-loaded bracket is placed on the tooth surface, and the excess resin is removed before setting the material (see Figure 14-15, *B*). The desired bracket position is confirmed, and the bracket slot height is verified using a gauge. Light-cured resins require a light source to initiate curing (see Figure 14-15, *C*).

The resin thickness between the bracket base and the tooth surface can be better controlled using the indirect technique; hence the programmed appliance can express the built-in prescription more accurately. The indirect procedures described in this chapter have been shown to create a resin interlayer that forms between the filled resin on the bracket base and the enamel surface. This interlayer creates a weak interface between the filled and the unfilled resin layers, which is helpful during the debonding procedures. This has been shown to be helpful during the debonding of ceramic brackets by eliminating bracket fracture and enamel damage.

Other advantages include reduced chairside time, patient comfort related to reduced chairside time and easier cleanup during the bonding and debonding procedures.[59,61,62] The major disadvantage of the indirect bonding technique is that it involves laboratory time required to set brackets and make the transfer tray in addition to the chairside time.[62] The indirect bonding technique is more complex and technique sensitive hence extra precautions have to be taken during the bonding procedures. Failures with the indirect bonding technique require additional time to rebond.

BOX 14-7

Step-by-Step Indirect Bonding Procedure

1. An accurate alginate impression of the arch to be bonded is obtained and poured in orthodontic model stone.
2. After drying, vertical lines are drawn on the teeth to aid in positioning the brackets accurately (see Figure 14-16, *A*). Panoramic radiographs should be used as guides to aid in the process. The models are then painted with a thin coat of separating medium and allowed to dry.
3. The bracket base is loaded with the filled resin paste, which is placed on the plaster model, and the excess resin is removed before the setting of the material for the chemically cured resins (see Figure 14-16, *A*). The light-cured materials need a light source, and thermal-cured resins require the models with the brackets to be placed in an oven at 375° F for 20 minutes.
4. Following the initial set of the resin material, individual silicone/polyvinyl Siloxane positioning trays are formed for each arch by manipulating the impression material over the brackets and a portion of the clinical crowns (see Figure 14-16, *B*).
5. After the impression material has set, the model-positioner complex is placed in warm water for 20 minutes to allow the dissolution of the separating medium.
6. The positioner with the embedded brackets is separated from the model (see Figure 14-16, *C*), and the bracket pads are cleaned with a soft-bristle brush under running water.
7. Enamel surface preparation is performed.
8. Unfilled liquid sealant is applied to the cured resin on the bracket base and to the etched tooth surface.
9. The positioner is placed over its corresponding teeth and held with light pressure until the liquid resin material has obtained its initial set (see Figure 14-16, *D*).
10. The positioner is removed after an additional 5 minutes (see Figure 14-16, *E*).

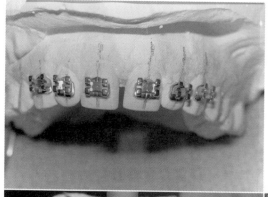
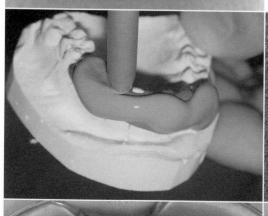
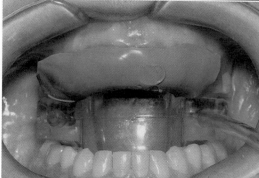
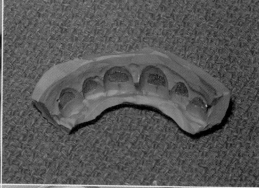
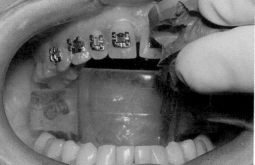

A

B

C

D

E

Figure 14-16 **A,** Brackets are positioned on the dry models following the placement of orientation vertical lines and separating medium. **B,** Individual silicone/polyvinyl Siloxane positioning trays are formed by manipulating the impression material over the brackets and a portion of the clinical crowns. **C,** A cleaned positioner with embedded brackets. **D,** The positioner in place following the initial set of the liquid resin. **E,** The positioner is removed after the final set of the material. (**A, D,** and **E** From Sinha PK, Nanda RS: Bonding in clinical orthodontics. In Hardin JF [ed]: *Clark's clinical dentistry,* vol 2, St Louis, 1998, Mosby. **C** From Sinha PK, Nanda RS: *Dent Clin North Am* 41:89-109, 1997.)

DEBONDING ORTHODONTIC ATTACHMENTS
(Figures 14-17 to 14-19)

The successful use of the bonded appliance also includes the safe removal of the brackets and the adhesive without altering the enamel surface of the tooth (Box 14-8). Reports have shown that improper debonding techniques can lead to significant enamel damage.[64-73]

Debonding Ceramic Brackets

Ceramic brackets require special attention during debonding; hence the practitioner is advised to follow the instructions provided by the manufacturer. A few general guidelines for ceramic brackets employing mechanical retention and those that rely on chemical bonding are outlined in the following paragraph. During the process of debonding, if the bracket fractures, it may be safer to grind the remnants. Should this situation arise, the clinician should reduce the size of the bracket by using a pin and ligature cutter or similar pliers followed by grinding off the remaining bracket material using a high-speed hand piece with a diamond bur. The residual composite can be removed by a scaler or a finishing bur. Bonding ceramic brackets by the indirect bonding methods described previously facilitates debonding.[31-33]

Ceramic Brackets Using Chemical and Mechanical Retention
Ceramic brackets that use chemical or mechanical retention as their mechanism of attachment should be debonded by careful removal of excess resin if present, using a finishing bur before the use of debonding pliers. Different methods have been shown to be effective in debonding these brackets.[31-33]

1. The first method employs a pistol grip debonding instrument (Unitek/3M, Monrovia, CA) that is positioned over the brackets with its jaws

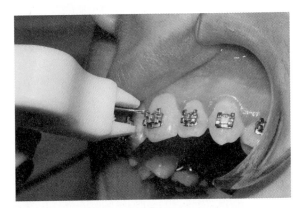

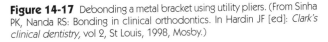

Figure 14-17 Debonding a metal bracket using utility pliers. (From Sinha PK, Nanda RS: Bonding in clinical orthodontics. In Hardin JF [ed]: *Clark's clinical dentistry*, vol 2, St Louis, 1998, Mosby.)

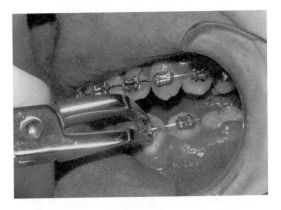

Figure 14-18 Debonding a metal bracket using the sharp-edged blades of the debonding pliers at the enamel-composite or the bracket-composite interface.

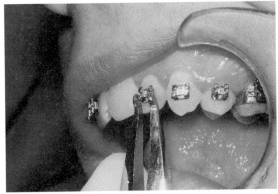

Figure 14-19 Debonding a metal bracket using specially designed pliers that exerts a tensile type of force by engaging a wing of the bracket. (Courtesy Unitek Corporation/3M, Monrovia, Calif. From Sinha PK, Nanda RS: Bonding in clinical orthodontics. In Hardin JF [ed]: *Clark's clinical dentistry*, vol 2, St Louis, 1998, Mosby.)

aligned horizontally over the bracket in an occlusogingival direction over the tie wings (Figure 14-20). Debonding of the bracket occurs when the handles are squeezed, the jaws contact the tie wings, and the bracket is pulled away from the tooth surface. Bracket failure often occurs.

2. The second method employs a sharp-edged instrument, ETM pliers #346 (Ormco Corporation, Glendora, CA), that is placed at the enamel-adhesive interface (Figure 14-21). The application of force produces a wedging effect of the sharp edge to separate the enamel and adhesive surfaces and has been shown to eliminate bracket failures when used on brackets bonded by the indirect bonding techniques described previously. This technique minimizes the amount of force applied and its detrimental effect on the tie wings of the bracket.[31-33] The reduced force application may also be less harmful to the enamel. Therefore this technique is the one recommended to the clinician.

BOX 14-8   **Techniques Used to Debond Metal Brackets**

1. The first method employs *utility pliers* like the Wiengart or Howe pliers to squeeze the mesial and distal wings of the brackets as shown in Figure 14-17. This technique exerts a pinch-and-peel effect on the brackets and debonds the attachment with a large amount of the resin left on the tooth surface, which can be removed using a finishing bur or scaler.[73]
2. The second method employs a shearing force delivered by the *sharp-edged blades* of the debonding pliers at the enamel-composite or the bracket-composite interface as shown in Figure 14-18. The bracket is debonded, leaving minimal amounts of resin on the tooth surface.

Brackets bonded by the direct bonding technique may have the potential for enamel damage when this technique is employed.[73] A finishing bur or scaler can remove any remaining resin residue on the debonded tooth.
3. The third method uses specially designed pliers that exert a *tensile-type force* that lifts the bracket off the enamel surface by engaging a wing of the bracket and braces the beak against the tooth as shown in Figure 14-19. This technique leaves almost all the resin on the tooth surface with minimal bracket distortion.[73] The remaining resin can be cleaned using a finishing bur or scaler.

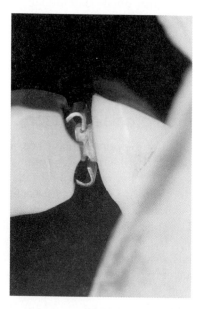

Figure 14-20 Debonding a ceramic bracket using a pistol grip debonding instrument. (Courtesy Unitek Corporation/3M, Monrovia, Calif. From Sinha PK, Nanda RS: *Dent Clin North Am* 41:89-109, 1997.)

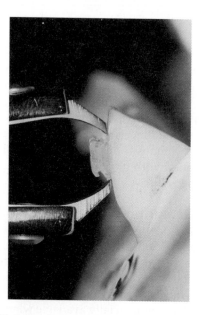

Figure 14-21 Debonding a ceramic bracket using a sharp-edged instrument that is placed at the enamel-adhesive interface. (Courtesy Ormco Corporation, Glendora. From Sinha PK, Nanda RS: *Dent Clin North Am* 41:89-109, 1997.)

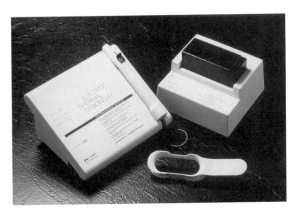

Figure 14-22 An electrothermal debonder. (Courtesy A-Company, San Diego, CA. From Sinha PK, Nanda RS: *Dent Clin North Am* 41:89-109, 1997.)

3. Using an ultrasonic scaler or an electrothermal debonder as shown in Figure 14-22 can also debond these brackets. The tip of the electrothermal debonder engages the slot running occlusogingivally in the bracket and, with a mild torsional force, detaches the bracket from the tooth surface. The procedure using the ultrasonic scaler can mutilate the working tip and involves more clinic time.

4. A new ceramic bracket introduced in the market allows easier debonding via a vertical scribe line placed in the base of the appliance (see Figure 14-8).[43] Pliers are used to apply forces in a mesiodistal grip of the bracket ears, allowing the bracket to fold on the vertical line.

BONDING IN SPECIAL SITUATIONS

Bonding Lingual Attachments and Lingual Retention Wires

Lingual attachments including lingual buttons, lingual brackets, hooks, and lingual sheath are bonded using similar techniques as that used for buccal and labial attachments. For isolated buttons or hooks the direct technique of bonding is preferable using any type of orthodontic composite resin. Lingual appliances can also be bonded with greater accuracy using the indirect bonding technique.

Lingual Retention Wires Wires in solid or braided forms are bonded on the lingual surfaces of the lower anterior teeth for retaining the alignment after orthodontic treatment. A variety of prefabricated lingual retention wires are commercially available; however, some clinicians prefer fabricating the wire in their laboratory. The commercially available wires may have meshed pads attached to the ends that bond to the lingual surfaces of the mandibular canines. Either direct or indirect methods of bonding can be used to bond these wires (Box 14-9 and Figure 14-23).

Bonding to Porcelain Veneer Crowns and Cast Gold

Agents Used Bonding orthodontic attachments to single unit crowns has distinct advantages over banding. These include improved esthetics in the anterior region, improved oral hygiene, and, consequently, a reduction of soft tissue irritation.[74] Bonding can sometimes be done in areas where banding is difficult or physically impossible. Orthodontic practice today includes an increasing number of adults who may have crown and bridge restorations fabricated from porcelain and gold. Silane treatment for porcelain and mechanical abrasion of cast gold surfaces have been conventionally used in clinical orthodontics with some success. Recently introduced materials and techniques claim to enhance the bond strength of composite materials to porcelain and metal surfaces.[75] These materials use different resin systems like 4-META, PENTA-UDMA, NTG-GMA-BPDM, and HEMA-BIS-GMA. These systems have not been evaluated in clinical studies, and hence the description of techniques in this chapter is limited to the use of silane-coupling agents.

Surface Preparation Surface preparation of the crown to be bonded is important before treatment with the silane agent. Electron microscopy reveals that the roughness created by abrading the metal surface with a green stone is far inferior to that created by an intraoral sandblaster.[76] Further, adhesion of metal to composite was shown to be enhanced by 300% using intraoral sandblasting.[77,78] The abrasive aluminum oxide powder strips away contaminants along with creating microscopic retention tags to enhance bonding. The evolution of methods to bond orthodontic attachments effectively to cast gold and porcelain veneer surfaces without creating irreversible surface alterations will be an important advance.

Bonding to Porcelain Veneer Crowns

Silane treatment of the porcelain surface before bonding orthodontic attachments is commonly used. The process relies on the hydrolysis of the silane-coupling agent, which results in a chemical interaction between silane and the porcelain surface. Hydrolyzed and non-hydrolyzed coupling agents are commercially available; however, hydrolyzed silane is unstable and, consequently, has a shorter shelf life. Box 14-10 describes the technique employed.

Bonding to Cast Gold

Bonding orthodontic attachments to cast gold surfaces has had limited success. Reports indicate that roughening the surface and the use of commercially available

BOX 14-9 | Indirect Lingual Wire Method

1. An accurate alginate impression of the arch is made and poured in orthodontic stone.
2. A wire is bent so that it conforms to the lingual arch of the lower anterior teeth and touches the cingulum area of each tooth. These wires are also commercially available, in which case the arch has to be adjusted.
3. The wire is positioned on the cast at the desired level using utility wax. A positioner is made by molding a medium to heavy bodied elastomeric impression material over the labial, occlusal, and lingual surfaces of the central incisors and part of the lateral incisors as shown in Figure 14-23, *A* and *B*. The excess material is trimmed using a scalpel blade on a holder.
4. The lingual surfaces of the lower anterior teeth are pumiced, cleaned, and isolated.
5. The lingual surface of the canine tooth is etched.
6. The etched surface is painted with the unfilled liquid sealant and cured with a light source.
7. The wire using the silicone index as a guide is held at an ideal position as shown in Figure 14-23. A small amount of the filled paste is applied on the ends of the wire resting on the lingual surfaces of the canines. The paste is manipulated on the wire using a flat-ended composite instrument. All excess resin is removed and the resin is then cured with light.
8. Any excess composite is trimmed using a finishing bur, and, if required, flexible finishing disks may be used to smooth the contour of the composite to allow easy access while brushing (Figure 14-23, *C*). On recall visits, checking for loose wires, hygiene, and decalcification in the immediate vicinity of the wire and composite is recommended.

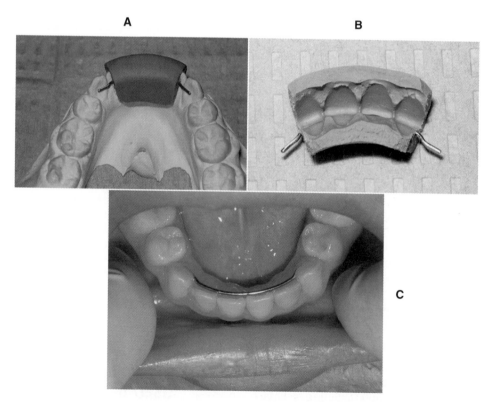

Figure 14-23 A, The positioner on the model following trimming. **B,** The positioner-wire complex before bonding. **C,** The lingual retainer in place following the curing of the composite resin. (From Sinha PK, Nanda RS: *Dent Clin North Am* 41:89-109, 1997.)

BOX 14-10   Porcelain Veneer Bonding and Debonding Techniques

Bonding Technique

1. The surface is prepared by abrasion using pumice or an intraoral sandblaster with 50-micron aluminum oxide particles. A high-volume suction should be positioned adjacent to the area being sandblasted.

2a. If using a *nonhydrolyzed silane*, thoroughly dry the area and apply 37% phosphoric acid etchant to the prepared area for 1 minute. Do not rinse. Apply the nonhydrolyzed silane-coupling agent to the porcelain without rinsing the surface. The etchant hydrolyzes the coupling agent to interact with the nonhydrolyzed coupling agent. Allow an additional minute for its action. Rinse thoroughly with a water spray using high-volume evacuation.

2b. If using a *hydrolyzed silane*, apply the solution to a clean dry porcelain surface for 2 to 3 minutes, and dry this layer using warm air. Do not rinse.

3. Use a highly filled composite resin system for bonding, which includes the application of the unfilled resin primer to the prepared porcelain surface.

4. Load the base of the orthodontic attachment with the highly filled paste, and position this attachment on the prepared area.

5. Apply firm pressure on the attachment and clean the excess resin before setting.

Debonding Technique

1. To debond orthodontic attachments from porcelain surfaces a tensile pull- or pinch-and-peel–type force is recommended.[79] This type of force can be generated by using Weingart utility pliers or sharp-edged debonding pliers. This method ensures that the composite fracture fails at the bracket-composite interface.

2. Remove almost all of the remaining composite with a finishing bur. Do not touch the porcelain surface with the bur, hence leaving a thin layer of the resin on the surface.

3. Scale the remaining composite using a scaler. The porcelain surface can be polished using commercially available kits.

BOX 14-11   Bonding to Cast Gold Using Conventional Methods of Surface Roughening and Highly Filled Composite Resin

1. Proper isolation and moisture control along with a high-volume evacuant should be placed before starting the procedure.

2. The surface should be roughened with an intraoral sandblaster using 50-micron aluminum oxide particles. This method of roughening significantly increases bond strength of composite to metal.

3. Etch the surface of the gold using 35% phosphoric acid for 1 minute.

4. Rinse thoroughly and dry the area.

5. Apply the unfilled resin primer to the prepared surface.

6. Apply the highly filled resin to the back of the attachment and position this on the prepared surface of the crown. Position the attachment as desired and apply firm pressure to express the excess resin from underneath the bracket.

7. Remove the excess resin before the material obtains its initial set.

primers can result in clinically acceptable bond strength (Box 14-11).[79,80] New materials and techniques have been reported,[75] but these have not been tested with respect to bonding orthodontic attachments.

Debonding these attachments involves little or no risk compared to the attachments bonded to porcelain or even enamel. The wings of the attachment are pinched and peeled with Wiengart utility pliers or a pin and ligature cutter. The brackets generally detach at the composite-gold interface. The resultant surface can be polished using commercially available polishing kits.

ARCH FORM AND ARCH WIRES USED IN CONTEMPORARY ORTHODONTIC PRACTICE

Arch Form

The search for the elusive "ideal" arch form to suit every individual has been the focus of several reports.[81-85] However, dental arch form and shape varies in individuals based on anatomic dimensions of the craniofacial skeleton.

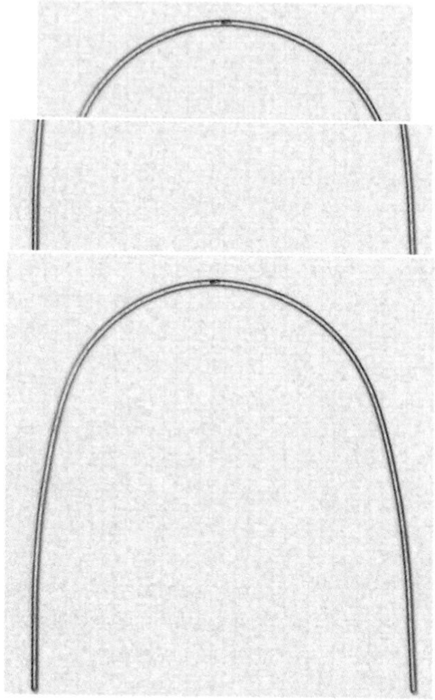

Figure 14-24 A, The anterior curvature and intercanine width of an arch wire. **B,** The posterior curvature and intermolar width of an arch wire. **C,** An arch form commonly used in orthodontic practice.

BOX 14-12   Selection of Arch Form for Each Individual Patient

The preformed arch wire can be customized for each individual patient by adhering to the following protocol:
1. Select the appropriate arch form using the patient's lower model (i.e., tapered, ovoid, or square).
2. Adjust anterior curvature and intercanine dimensions if necessary.
3. Adjust posterior curvature and intermolar width if necessary.
4. Coordinate the upper arch wire to lie passively immediately outside the lower arch wire.
5. Photocopy the corrected arch wires to serve as a template for the patient's treatment and place it in the chart for future reference.

Arch form in individuals generally falls within three clinically described shapes: tapered, ovoid, and square.[85] Further, these forms vary in their dimensions in two different areas: the anterior curvature and intercanine width (Figure 14-24, A and C) and posterior curvature and intermolar width (see Figure 14-24, B and C). A change in intercanine width during treatment has been shown to be a significant predictor of orthodontic relapse.[85,86] Therefore it is imperative to maintain the patient's original arch form, including its width, throughout treatment (Box 14-12). These findings do not imply that preformed arch wires should not be used in clinical orthodontics.

Arch Wire Types and Rationale for Use

The discussion on arch wires can be a complex issue because of such things as different alloy types, shapes, sizes, and forces. The rationale behind the use of different arch wires by different practitioners varies according to the ingrained philosophy of treatment of each clinician. The main questions have centered around rapid vs. slow movements, continuous vs. intermittent, and light vs. heavy forces.

This state of incomplete understanding of bone biology as well as the physiology of tooth movement has led to differences in arch wire selection and in force systems used during orthodontic treatment. In light of the present state of knowledge, bone biology research may be interpreted to imply that light contin-

uous or intermittent forces may be best suited for optimal orthodontic movement.[87] This conclusion is based on two important facts: (1) light forces create minimal hyalinized tissue and therefore avoid undermining resorption thus allowing quick tooth movements and (2) continuous forces create a constant system for continued effect. Periods of rest are required for the tissues to recover and, therefore, intermittent application of forces is preferred.[87]

Historical Perspective Arch wire selection has gone through an historic evolution concurrent with the introduction of different alloy systems and arch wire configurations.

In the early part of this century gold was the only material used to manufacture orthodontic appliances and arch wires. Dr. Edward Angle used a rigid arch wire termed the *E arch (expansion arch).*[88] Teeth were aligned by forces directed via ligature wires to draw them toward the rigid wire.[88] Stainless steel was introduced to orthodontics in 1929 and shortly after replaced gold as the commonly used arch wire.[89] Since then, different alloy types and configurations have been developed to broaden the selection of arch wire types (Box 14-13). These include cobalt-chromium, nickel-titanium, beta-titanium, and multistrand wires.

The introduction of stainless steel provided the option of varying the load deflection rates by changing the size and shape of the wires. In other words, flexibility of the wires was modified by varying (1) the cross-sectional dimensions, (2) the length, and (3) the shape.

The conventional method of arch wire progression was to start with increased flexibility to engage all the

BOX 14-13   Choice of Arch Wire Materials in an Orthodontic Practice[94]

1. *Stainless steel:* Stainless steel replaced gold as the arch wire material of choice because of its improved properties and lower costs. A typical composition would include about 71% iron, 18% chromium, 8% nickel, and less than 0.2% carbon. Stainless steel is still considered the main arch wire material in most orthodontic practices. Practitioners can modify the size, shape, and length of the stainless steel wire and can use it at the various stages of orthodontic treatment. Multistrand stainless steel wires have been developed and are used in different stages of treatment. The braided nature increases the flexibility of the wire to the extent that it compares very favorably with nickel titanium wires in laboratory tests.[92,94]

2. *Cobalt chromium:* A typical composition consists of about 40% cobalt, 20% chromium, 15% nickel, 15% iron, 7% molybdenum, and 2% manganese. These wires have similar properties to stainless steel with the additional feature of first providing easy formability (i.e., bending) modified by heat treatment, which causes the wire to become stiff.[94]

3. *Nickel titanium:* A typical composition of nickel titanium wire consists of almost 50% nickel and 50% titanium. In today's practice three types of nickel titanium wires are used.[94]
   a. *Conventional:* The conventional wire was introduced to the orthodontic profession by Dr. George Andreason.[91] These wires possessed the property of shape memory in which the deflected portion returns to its original shape. One important property of nitinol wires is that they are not very stiff. Therefore the force applied with large deflections is extremely low when compared with stainless steel wires.
   b. *Pseudoelastic:* The pseudoelastic wires have the capability of phase transformation on applied stress to maintain the same force of activation.[94] The wire undergoes a transformation from the active austenitic phase to martensitic and then back to austensitic based on the stress applied.[94] This feature gives these wires the property of longer periods of light continuous forces compared with the conventional nickel titanium wires.[94]
   c. *Thermoelastic:* The third type of nickel titanium wire undergoes phase transformation at oral temperature to produce the active austenitic phase.[94] This wire can be distorted at lower temperatures and undergoes a thermally induced shape memory effect to return to an active austenitic phase.[94]

4. *Beta titanium:* A typical composition of the beta titanium wire includes 79% titanium, 11% molybdenum, 6% zirconium, and 4% tin. These wires have the property of delivering half the force levels for the same deflection compared with stainless steel. Therefore these wires can be used in clinical situations where force levels lower than stainless steel and higher than nickel titanium are necessary.

bracket slots and end up with rigid unyielding wires to maintain the position of teeth.

In the 1970s nickel-titanium wires were introduced to the orthodontic profession.[90] This wire was flexible compared to conventional stainless steel. Therefore flexibility could now be modified using a different alloy type in addition to the factors mentioned in the previous paragraph. Burstone[91] coined the term *variable modulus orthodontics,* where the intrinsic property of stiffness (modulus of elasticity) could be modified to influence wire selection and progression. Nickel-titanium arch wires deliver lighter forces for large deflections compared with stainless steel wires of the same dimension.[91-93] Therefore arch wire progression could be modified by changing the alloy type rather than the conventional size, shape, and length of wire.[91] Newer modifications of the nickel titanium wires have further widened the spectrum for clinicians.[94]

Arch Wire Selection

The introduction of newer wires to the profession has allowed significant clinical changes in orthodontic arch wire progression and use. These include the use of larger cross-section wires during the initial stages of treatment with the newly introduced titanium wires instead of the earlier routine of progressing arch wire size gradually. Further, upon proper bracket engagement, the new wires can be left in the mouth for longer periods to produce the desired movements. To take advantage of the desirable properties of these newer alloy wires a rational approach should be employed based on the particular case (Box 14-14).

The wire selection protocol is the one used by the authors and does not represent all of the possibilities used in clinical practice. Wire selection is based on the treatment philosophy of each clinician.

REFERENCES

1. Angle EH: The latest and best in orthodontic mechanisms, *Dent Cosmos* 70:1143-1158, 1928.
2. Begg PR, Kesling PC: *Begg orthodontic theory and technique,* ed 3, Philadelphia, 1977, WB Saunders.

BOX 14-14   Arch Wire Selection during the Different Phases of Orthodontic Treatment

Initial stages: During the initial phase, intraarch leveling and alignment are of prime importance. Therefore an arch wire that allows complete bracket engagement is desirable. Arch wire options may include nickel titanium, multistrand stainless steel or multilooped stainless steel.

Intermediate stages: Stainless steel or beta titanium wires are the wires of choice during the intermediate phase because greater control of tooth movement is required to allow for interarch corrections while providing stability to intraarch units. Further, space closure is one of the features of this phase and requires a controlled force system with stiff wires.

Finishing stages: Flexibility is of essence during the finishing phase to allow settling of the occlusion following space closure and idealization of tooth positions during the intermediate and early finishing stages. Sectioning the stainless steel or beta titanium wire and using light titanium wires and multistrand stainless steel wires are appropriate options during this phase.

3. Andrews LF: The six keys to normal occlusion, *Am J Orthod* 63:296-309, 1972.

4. Kesling PC: Expanding the horizons of the edgewise arch wire slot, *Am J Orthod Dentofacial Orthop* 94:26-37, 1988.

5. Kesling PC: Dynamics of the tip-edge bracket, *Am J Orthod Dentofacial Orthop* 96:16-25, 1989.

6. Gottlieb EL, Nelson AH, Vogels DS: 1996 JCO Study of orthodontic diagnosis and treatment procedures. Part 1. Results and trends, *J Clin Orthod* 30:615-629, 1996.

7. Kapur R, Sinha PK, Nanda RS: Comparison of frictional resistance in titanium and stainless steel brackets, *Am J Orthod Dentofacial Orthop* 116(3):271-274, 1999.

8. Newman GV: Adhesion and orthodontic plastic attachments, *Am J Orthod* 56:573-588, 1969.

9. Newman GV: First direct bonding in orthodontia, *Am J Orthod Dentofacial Orthop* 101:190-191, 1992.

10. Aird JC, Durning P: Fracture strength of polycarbonate edgewise brackets: a clinical and SEM study, *Br J Orthod* 14:191-195, 1987.

11. Miura F, Nakagawa K, Mashuara E: New direct bonding system for plastic brackets, *Am J Orthod* 59:350-361, 1971.

12. Dooley WD, Hembree JH, Weber FN: Tensile and shear strength of Begg plastic brackets, *J Clin Orthod* 9:694-697, 1975.

13. Pulido LG, Powers JM: Bond strength of orthodontic direct bonding cement plastic systems in vitro, *Am J Orthod* 83:124-130, 1983.

14. Dobrin RJ, Kamel IL, Musich DR: Load-deformation characteristics of polycarbonate orthodontic brackets, *Am J Orthod* 67:24-33, 1975.

15. Rains MD et al: Stress analysis of plastic bracket configurations, *J Clin Orthod* 11:120-125, 1977.

16. Goldstein MC, Burns, MH, Yurfest P: Esthetic orthodontic appliances for the adult, *Dent Clin North Am* 33:183-193, 1989.

17. Feldner JC et al: Torque-deformation characteristics of polycarbonate brackets, *Am J Orthod Dentofacial Orthop* 106:265-272, 1994.

18. Bazakidou E et al: Evaluation of frictional resistance in esthetic brackets, *Am J Orthod Dentofacial Orthop* 112:138-144, 1997.

19. Letter of the President of the AAO Re: *Ceramic bracket survey,* April 7, 1989.

20. American Association of Orthodontics: *Summary of AAO ceramic bracket survey,* Bulletin suppl 7, 1989.

21. Jeiroudi MT: Enamel fractures caused by ceramic brackets (case reports), *Am J Orthod Dentofacial Orthop* 99:97-99, 1991.

22. Storm ER: Debonding ceramic brackets, *J Clin Orthod* 24:91-94, 1990.

23. Swartz ML: Ceramic brackets, *J Clin Orthod* 22:82-88, 1988.

24. Swartz ML: *A technical bulletin on the issues of bonding and debonding ceramic brackets,* Glendora, Calif, 1988, Ormco Corporation.

25. Scott GE: Fracture toughness and surface cracks: the key to understanding ceramic brackets, *Angle Orthod* 58:5-8, 1988.

26. Kusy RP: Morphology of polycrystalline alumina brackets and its relationship to fracture toughness and strength, *Angle Orthod* 58:197-203, 1988.

27. Kusy RP: Commentary: ceramic brackets, *Angle Orthod* 61:291-292, 1991.

28. Ghafari J: Problems associated with ceramic brackets suggest limiting use to selected teeth, *Angle Orthod* 62:145-152, 1992.

29. Unitek Corporation/3M: *Transcend series 2000-instructional manual,* Monrovia, Calif, 1991, Unitek Corporation/3M.

30. Unitek Corporation/3M: *Transcend Series 2000: technical topics,* vol 3, no 1 and vol 2, no 5, Monrovia, Calif, 1991, Unitek Corporation/3M.

31. Sinha PK et al: Interlayer formation and its effect on debonding polycrystalline ceramic orthodontic brackets, *Am J Orthod Dentofacial Orthop* 108:455-463, 1995.

32. Sinha PK et al: Evaluation of hard tissue sections of bonded and debonded teeth, *J Dent Res* 75:339 (abstr no 2569), 1996.

33. Sinha PK, Nanda RS: The effect of different bonding and debonding techniques on debonding ceramic orthodontic brackets, *Am J Orthod Dentofacial Orthop* 112:132-137, 1997.

34. Holt MH: Fracture strength of ceramic brackets during archwire torsion, masters thesis in orthodontics, Norman, Okla, 1989, University of Oklahoma.

35. Rhodes RK et al: Fracture strengths of ceramic brackets subjected to mesial-distal arch wire tipping forces, *Angle Orthod* 62:67-75, 1992.

36. Aknin P et al: Fracture strength of ceramic brackets during arch wire torsion, *Am J Orthod Dentofacial Orthop* 109:22-27, 1996.

37. Pratten DH et al: Frictional resistance of ceramic and stainless steel orthodontic brackets, *Am J Orthod Dentofacial Orthop* 98:398-403, 1990.

38. Bednar JR, Gruendeman GW, Sandrik JL: A comparative study of frictional forces between orthodontic brackets and arch wires, *Am J Orthod Dentofacial Orthop* 100:513-522, 1991.

39. Ireland AJ, Sherriff M, McDonald F: Effect of bracket and wire composition on frictional forces, *Eur J Orthod* 13:322-328, 1991.

40. Kusy RP, Whitley JQ: Coefficients of friction for arch wires in stainless steel and polycrystalline alumina bracket slots. I. The dry state, *Am J Orthod Dentofacial Orthop* 98:300-312, 1990.

41. Springate SD, Winchester LJ: An evaluation of zirconium oxide brackets: a preliminary laboratory and clinical report, *Br J Orthod* 18:203-209, 1991.

42. Tanne K et al: Wire friction from ceramic brackets during simulated canine retraction, *Angle Orthod* 61:285-290, 1991.

43. Bishara SE, Olsen ME, Von Wald L: Evaluation of debonding characteristics of a new collapsible ceramic bracket, *Am J Orthod Dentofacial Orthop* 112:552-559, 1997.

44. Matasa CG: Adhesion and its ten commandments, *Am J Orthod Dentofacial Orthop* 95:355-356, 1989.

45. Craig RG: *Restorative dental materials,* ed 10, St Louis, 1997, Mosby.

46. Buonocore MG, Matsui A, Gwinnet AJ: Penetration of resin dental materials into enamel surfaces with reference to bonding, *Arch Oral Biol* 13:61-70, 1968.

47. Gwinnett AJ: The scientific basis of the sealant procedure, *J Prev Dent* 3:15-28, 1976.

48. Miura F, Nakagawa K, Massuhara E: New direct bonding systems for plastic brackets, *Am J Orthod* 59:350-361, 1971.

49. Newman GV, Facq JM: The effect of adhesive systems on tooth surfaces, *Am J Orthod* 59:67-75, 1971.

50. Gwinnett AJ: Acid etching for composite resins, *Dent Clin North Am* 25:271-289, 1981.

51. Gorelick L: Bonding metal brackets with a self-polymerizing sealant-composite: a 12-month assessment, *Am J Orthod* 71:542-553, 1977.

52. Brannstrom M, Nordenvall KJ, Malmgren O: The effect of various pretreatment methods of the enamel in bonding procedures, *Am J Orthod* 74:522-530, 1978.

53. Nordenvall KJ, Brannstrom M, Malmgren O: Etching of deciduous teeth and young and old permanent teeth: a comparison between 15 and 60 seconds of etching, *Am J Orthod* 78:99-108, 1980.

54. Brannstrom M, Malmgren O, Nordenvall KJ: Etching of young permanent teeth with an acid gel, *Am J Orthod* 83:379-383, 1982.

55. Surmont P et al: Comparison in shear bond strength of orthodontic brackets between five bonding systems related to different etching times: an in vitro study, *Am J Orthod Dentofacial Orthop* 101:414-419, 1992.

56. Gourley J: A one year study of fissure sealant in two Nova Scotia communities, *J Can Dent Assoc* 40:549-552, 1974.

57. Buonocore MG: Retrospections on bonding, *Dent Clin North Am* 25:241-253, 1981.

58. Silverman E et al: A universal direct bonding system for both metal and plastic brackets, *Am J Orthod* 62:236-244, 1972.

59. Sinha PK et al: Bond strengths and adhesive remnant adhesive on debonding for orthodontic bonding techniques, *Am J Orthod Dentofacial Orthop* 108:302-307, 1995.

60. Sinha PK, Nanda RS, Ghosh J: A thermal-cured, fluoride-releasing indirect bonding system, *J Clin Orthod* 29:97-100, 1995.

61. Thomas RG: Indirect bonding: simplicity in action, *J Clin Orthod* 13:93-105, 1979.

62. Aguirre MJ, King GJ, Waldron JM: Assessment of bracket placement and bond strength when comparing direct bonding to indirect bonding techniques, *Am J Orthod* 82:269-276, 1982.

63. Newman GV: Direct and indirect bonding of brackets, *J Clin Orthod* 8:264-272, 1974.

64. Zachrisson BU, Artun J: Enamel surface appearance after various debonding procedures, *Am J Orthod* 75:121-137, 1979.

65. Pus MD, Way DC: Enamel loss due to orthodontic bonding with filled and unfilled resins using various cleanup techniques, *Am J Orthod* 77:269-283, 1980.

66. Thompson RE, Way DC: Enamel loss due to prophylaxis and multiple bonding/debonding of orthodontic attachments, *Am J Orthod* 79:282-295, 1981.

67. Diedrich P: Enamel alterations from bracket bonding and debonding: a study with the scanning electron microscope, *Am J Orthod* 79:500-522, 1981.

68. Meister RE: A comparison of enamel detachments after debonding between Unitek's Dynalock bracket and a foil-mesh bracket: a scanning electron microscope study, *Am J Orthod* 88:266, 1985.

69. Bennett CG, Sheen C, Waldron JM: The effects of debonding on the enamel surface, *J Clin Orthod* 18:330-334, 1984.

70. Gwinnett AJ, Gorelick L: Microscopic evaluation of enamel after debonding, *Am J Orthod* 71:651-665, 1977.

71. Newman GV, Facq JM: The effects of adhesive systems on tooth surfaces, *Am J Orthod* 59:67-75, 1971.

72. Howell S, Weekes WT: An electron microscopic evaluation of the enamel surface subsequent to various debonding procedures, *Aust Dent J* 35:245-252, 1990.

73. Oliver RG: The effect of different methods of bracket removal on the amount of residual adhesive, *Am J Orthod* 93:196-200, 1988.

74. Boyd RL, Baumrind S: Periodontal considerations in the use of bonds or bands on molars in adolescents and adults, *Angle Orthod* 62:117, 1992.

75. Zachrisson BU, Buyukyilmaz T: Recent advances in bonding to gold, amalgam, and porcelain, *J Clin Orthod* 27:12:661-675, 1993.

76. Burgess JO, Nourian L, Summit JB: Shear bond strength of six bonding agents to four metal alloys, *J Dent Res* 73 (abstr no 2475), 1994.

77. Barzilay I et al: Mechanical and chemical retention of laboratory cured composite to metal surfaces, *J Prosthet Dent* 59:131-137, 1988.
78. Matsumura H et al: Adhesive bonding of titanium with a titanate coupler and 4-META/MMA-TBB opaque resin, *J Dent Res* 69:1614-1616, 1990.
79. Wood DP et al: Bonding to porcelain and gold, *Am J Orthod* 89:194-205, 1988.
80. Andreasen GF, Stieg MA: Bonding and debonding brackets to porcelain and gold, *Am J Orthod* 93:341-345, 1988.
81. Chuck GC: Ideal arch form, *Angle Orthod* 4:312-327, 1934.
82. Musich DR, Ackerman JL: The catenometer: a reliable device for estimating dental arch perimeter, *Am J Orthod* 63:366-375, 1973.
83. Brader AC: Dental arch form related to intraoral forces: PR = C, *Am J Orthod* 61:541-561, 1972.
84. Sampson PD: Dental arch shape: a statistical analysis using conic sections, *Am J Orthod* 79:535-548, 1981.
85. Felton JM et al: A computerized analysis of the shape and stability of mandibular arch form, *Am J Orthod Dentofacial Orthop* 92:478-483, 1987.
86. De La Cruz AR et al: Long-term changes in arch form after orthodontic treatment and retention, *Am J Orthod Dentofacial Orthop* 107:518-530, 1995.
87. Reitan K, Rygh P: Biomechanical principles and reactions. In Graber TM, Vanarsdale RL Jr (eds): *Orthodontics: current principles and techniques*, ed 3, St Louis, 2000, Mosby.
88. Proffit WR: Contemporary fixed appliances. In Proffit WR, Fields HW Jr (eds): *Contemporary orthodontics*, ed 3, St Louis, 2000, Mosby.
89. Wilkinson JV: Some metallurgical aspects of orthodontic stainless steel, *Angle Orthod* 48:192-206, 1962.
90. Andreasen GF, Hileman TB: An evaluation of 55-cobalt substituted wire for orthodontics, *J Am Dent Assoc* 82:1373-1375, 1971.
91. Burstone CJ: Variable-modulus orthodontics, *Am J Orthod* 80:1-16, 1981.
92. Kusy RP: Comparison of nickel-titanium and beta-titanium wire sizes to conventional orthodontic arch wire materials, *Am J Orthod* 79:625-629, 1981.
93. Kusy RP, Greenberg AR: Comparison of the elastic properties of nickel-titanium and beta-titanium arch wires, *Am J Orthod* 82:199-205, 1982.
94. Kusy RP: A review of contemporary archwires: their properties and characteristics, *Angle Orthod* 67:197-208, 1997.

SUGGESTED READINGS

1. McLaughlin RP, Bennett JC: The transition from standard edgewise to preadjusted appliance systems, *J Clin Orthod* 23:142-153, 1989.
2. Kapur R, Sinha PK, Nanda RS: The effect of a self-ligating bracket design on frictional resistance, *J Clin Orthod* 32:485-489, 1998.
3. Shivapuja PK, Berger JL: A comparative study of conventional ligation and self-ligation bracket systems, *Am J Orthod Dentofacial Orthop* 106:472-480, 1994.
4. Ogata RH et al: Frictional resistances in stainless steel bracket wire combinations with effects of vertical deflections, *Am J Orthod Dentofacial Orthop* 109:535-542, 1996.
5. Kapila S, Sachdeva R: Mechanical properties and clinical applications of orthodontic wires, *Am J Orthod Dentofacial Orthop* 96:100-109, 1989.
6. Kusy RP, Stevens LE: Triple-stranded stainless steel wires: evaluation of mechanical properties and comparison with titanium alloy alternatives, *Angle Orthod* 57:18-32, 1987.
7. Goldberg AJ, Burstone CJ: Status report on beta titanium orthodontic wires: council on dental materials, instruments and equipment, *J Am Dent Assoc* 105:684-685, 1982.

CHAPTER 15

How Orthodontic Appliances Work

A. Denis Britto and Robert J. Isaacson

KEY TERMS

orthodontic appliances	center of rotation	elastic properties of wires	utility arches
forces	moment of the couple	stress-strain curve	palatal expanders
moments	moment of the force	load deflection curve	transpalatal arches
couples	one-couple force system	headgear	2 × 6 appliance
moment-to-force ratio	two-couple force system	functional appliance	2 × 4 appliance
tooth movement	V-bend principle	intrusion arches	lip bumpers
center of resistance			

The purpose of this chapter is to demonstrate the similarity of all **orthodontic appliances** in terms of their fundamental mechanics and engineering statics. The principles of mechanics and engineering statics are universal to all orthodontic appliances and do not change over time. When the physical principles of appliance systems are understood, it is then possible to move beyond the technical training necessary to construct and place a given appliance. One who is armed with an understanding of how appliances function is able to rationally design, select, and use orthodontic appliances in an efficient manner for the patient.

New orthodontic appliance systems appear regularly. However, each new appliance is simply a different application of the same physical principles reinvented under a new name. They all must operate using the principles described here, no matter what new marketing campaign might accompany them. A clinician can always be retrained in a new appliance system, but the training is worthless and potentially dangerous if the principles underlying its mechanism of action are not understood. A good understanding of fundamental principles gives the clinician the education necessary to understand all appliance systems and the ability to select the best one for any given patient.

Most patients with dental facial problems appear in a dentist's office for routine general dental care. Good general care of patients includes recognizing dental facial problems and being knowledgeable regarding the treatment alternatives that exist. All dentists must determine for themselves which treatment options they will elect to perform and which treatment option they will refer for treatment by others. The important point is that the patient becomes aware of all the treatment options available. The only criteria determining what care is delivered and where it is delivered should be what is in the best interest of the patient.

The increase in frequency and complexity of adult treatments today makes integration of orthodontic treatment with restorative and periodontal treatments increasingly common (see Chapter 28). The best interest of the patient demands that these treatments be done with consultation and coordination. Regardless of who ultimately does the actual treatment, the patient's best interest requires that everyone involved have a thorough understanding of and agreement on the diagnosis and the type of appliance design necessary to reach the agreed treatment goals.

GOALS AND OBJECTIVES OF ORTHODONTIC APPLIANCES

The design of efficient orthodontic appliances does not occur by trial and error. Instead, an approach based on sound biologic and physical principles leads to development of appliances with predictable actions. Orthodontists and dentists should be able to define and quantify what engineers call the **forces, moments, couples,** and equilibriums associated with appliances. If the force systems acting on a tooth cannot be defined, their effects on cells and tissues will be difficult to understand. In the field of orthodontics, biomechanics analyzes the reaction of dental and facial structures to orthodontic or orthopedic forces.

Many variables affect the outcome of orthodontic treatment. Some of these variables are partially or totally out of the clinician's control such as growth, bone-periodontal-gingival responses, and neuromuscular adaptation to changes in jaw and tooth position. Factors that are within the control of the clinician are the magnitude and direction of the forces, couples, moments, and the **moment-to-force ratio** exerted by an appliance. A thorough understanding of the physical principles operating in orthodontic appliances eliminates appliances as an uncontrolled variable affecting the final result.

Orthodontic appliances are analogous to the role of drugs in medicine. Both require an accurate diagnosis to define the right treatment plan to achieve clearly defined treatment goals. In medicine, the physician first makes a diagnosis and then selects the best medication to achieve the desired treatment goals. In orthodontics, the clinician must first make a diagnosis and then select the best appliance design to achieve the desired treatment goals (Box 15-1). In pharmacology, medications are used to act on specific cells, tissues, or organs. In orthodontics, moments and forces are used to act on specific cells or tissues supporting teeth or bones. Side effects from drugs are inevitable and must be managed. Side effects occur during tooth movement as well, and these, too, must be recognized and managed. When the side effects are known in advance, measures can be instituted to counter unwanted effects or sometimes the side effects can be used to the clinician's advantage. Finally, appliances, like medications, are only as effective as the level of patient compliance.

The original edgewise appliance was a unique development because of its abilities to control rotational tooth movement in three planes of space. Today there are multiple modifications of the original edgewise appliance such as Straight Wire, Tweed-Merrifield, Bioprogressive, Tip-Edge, and others. No mechanical principles are available to one technique that are not available to another. The differences among techniques are simply the ingenuity incorporated in

each technique to apply the principles found in the sciences of mechanics and engineering statics. A good understanding of fundamental principles demystifies each system, making it easy to obtain predictable tooth movement as defined by physical principles.

| BOX 15-1 | **Desirable Characteristics of an Orthodontic Appliance** |

Although the ideal orthodontic appliance has yet to be designed, the following goals and objectives are desirable in all appliances:
1. Simple and easy to fabricate
2. Hygienic
3. Inexpensive
4. Esthetic
5. Easy to place, adjust, and remove
6. Biologically compatible: minimal alveolar bone loss and root resorption
7. Move teeth efficiently, expeditiously, and predictably in three dimensions at force magnitudes that are optimal for tooth movement
8. Built-in safety factors to prevent unwanted side effects if the patient misses several appointments
9. Require minimal patient cooperation
10. Cause minimal discomfort or pain to the patient
11. Does not affect mastication or speech

COMMON PROPERTIES OF ALL FORCE SYSTEMS

First the basic, well-established physical science terms and concepts that are common in biomechanics and appliance design are defined. The basic building block is the application of a force to teeth or bones. A force is defined as a vector with both a magnitude and a direction. The correct units used to express forces are Newtons (N). However, in orthodontics forces have been commonly expressed in grams (g).[1] The conversion factor for grams to Newtons is $1 g = 0.00981 N$ or $1 N = 101.937 g$.

Center of Resistance

Forces Acting at the Center of Resistance
Imagine a tooth as a free body in space. Such a free body can be considered to have a single point within it where all of its mass is centered. Any force that is directed through this center of mass in any direction causes all points on the body to move the same amount in the same direction as the line of force. When all points on a body move the same amount in the

same direction the movement is called *translation.* In orthodontics this same movement where all points on the tooth move the same amounts in the same direction is also called *bodily movement* (Figure 15-1).

A tooth in the oral cavity is not a free body because its supporting periodontal tissues restrain it. The analogous center of mass for an *in vivo* tooth is referred to as the **center of resistance** of the tooth. Any force acting through a tooth's center of resistance causes the tooth to translate (see Figure 15-1).[2] Because brackets can only be bonded to the crowns of teeth, limited opportunities exist in orthodontics where it is possible to apply a force at a bracket that also acts through the tooth's center of resistance. The precise location of a tooth's center of resistance is determined by the root's attachment, root length, root morphology, number of roots, and the level of alveolar bone height.

Forces Not Acting at the Center of Resistance

If a force is applied to a free body and the force does not act through the center of resistance, the force causes the body to rotate. *Rotation,* by definition, is the movement of a body whereby no two points on the body move the same amount in the same direction. Tendencies to rotate are termed moments, and the tendency to rotate resulting from a force not acting through the center of resistance is termed the *moment of the force* (Figure 15-2).

The total tooth movement resulting from forces not acting through the center of resistance is a combination of rotation and translation occurring simultaneously (Figure 15-3, *C*). In other words, the tooth is viewed as rotating around its center of resistance (see Figure 15-3, *B*) while the center of resistance is simultaneously translating in the direction of the line of force (see Figure 15-3, *A*). The resulting tooth movement must show rotation around the center of resistance and translation of the center of resistance in the direction of the line of force.

Center of Rotation

When a body rotates, there is another point located either internal or external to the body around which the body turns. This point is termed the **center of rotation** (Figure 15-4). A single force, applied not at the center of resistance, must cause the body to rotate around the center of resistance while the center of resistance simultaneously moves in the direction of the line of force. The center of rotation is located at variable points depending on how far the force is applied from the center of resistance. The center of rotation can approach, but it can never reach the center of resistance. If the force is applied at the center of resistance, the body translates and the center of rotation is at infinity.

In terms of tooth movement, forces applied at the bracket can almost never act through the center of resistance in all three planes of space, and the tooth rotates when a force is applied to it. In orthodontics, when the process of rotation is around the long axis of the tooth it is termed *rotation,* or *first-order tooth movement.* When the rotation occurs around a faciolingual axis it is termed *tipping,* or *second-order tooth movement.* When the rotation occurs around a mesiodistal axis, it is termed *torque,* or *third-order rotation* (see Figure 15-2).

Few forces can be applied to teeth through the center of resistance because the center of resistance is located in the root of the tooth. Therefore almost all tooth movements result in a rotational movement with the center of resistance moving in the same direction as the line of applied force (see Figure 15-3).

Couples: All Rotation and No Translation

A pure force can be applied either at or away from the center of resistance of a tooth. The only other force system that can be applied to a tooth is termed a *couple.* The control that couples provide in three planes of space was the unique feature of the original edgewise bracket and is the fundamental characteristic of most fixed appliances today.

A couple is a pair of equal and opposite non-collinear forces acting on a body (Figure 15-5). The action of a couple is the sum of the action of two equal and opposite single-force systems. Each force of the couple tends to move the center of resistance in the direction of the force as described for the single-point force. Because the two forces are equal and opposite, each force tends to move the center of resistance in an equal and opposite direction. As a result, no net movement of the center of resistance ever occurs from a couple. A couple is a special system because the result of its action produces a rotation that is always located at the center of resistance. When the center of rotation is coincident with the center of resistance, no movement of the center of resistance can ever occur regardless of where the couple is applied on the tooth. The rotational tendency of the couple is termed a *moment* and is referred to as the **moment of the couple** (M_C).

Clinically, this means that whenever a couple is applied to an edgewise bracket in any plane, the center of resistance cannot move in any direction and the tooth will always rotate around the center of resistance. More important, the tooth movement is always the same and unaffected by the location of the bracket on the tooth. The movement is also independent of any torque or angulation built into the bracket. The only function of the preangulation built into the bracket is to activate a straight wire in the last few degrees of final tooth movement.

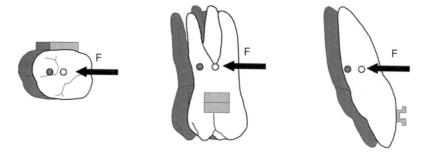

Figure 15-1 White circles indicate the center of resistance at the starting tooth position. Shaded circles show the center of resistance moved in the direction of the force. A force through the center of resistance causes all points of the tooth to move the same amount in the same direction. This type of movement is called *translation* or *bodily movement.*

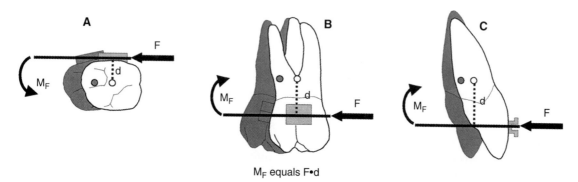

M_F equals F•d

Figure 15-2 A force, applied at a bracket that does not act through the center of resistance, causes rotation of a tooth. This tendency to rotate is measured in moments and is called the *moment of the force (M_F)*. The magnitude of the M_F is measured as the magnitude of the force times the perpendicular distance from the line of force to the center of resistance (i.e., $M_F = F \times d$). Rotations are shown in the first **(A)**, second **(B)**, and third **(C)** order.

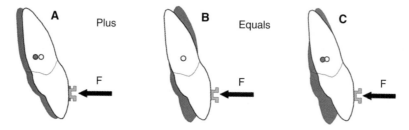

Figure 15-3 Rotational movement caused by a force not acting through the center of resistance is best visualized as the simultaneous process of tooth translation, **A,** that moves the center of resistance in the direction of the force and tooth rotation, **B,** around the center of resistance. The result is a combination of translation and rotation around the center of resistance **(C).**

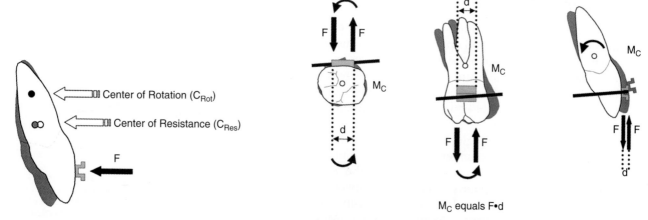

M_C equals F•d

Figure 15-4 Center of rotation is an arbitrary point about which a body appears to have rotated as determined from its initial and final position. It is the result of the relative amounts of translation and rotation occurring during tooth movement.

Figure 15-5 This illustration shows diagrammatic representation of couples in the first, second, and third order. The forces acting on the teeth are equal and opposite *(straight arrows)*. The rotational tendency *(curved arrows)* is called the *moment of the couple (M_C)*. The moment of the couple is measured as the magnitude of one of the forces *(F)* of the couple times the perpendicular distance between the two forces of the couple *(d)* (i.e., $M_C = F \times d$).

Moments: a Measure of the Tendency to Rotate by Single Forces or Couples

A moment is a measure of the tendency to rotate. A moment, or the tendency for a body to rotate, is produced in one of two separate ways. If a single force is applied to a body that does not act through the center of resistance, the force causes a tendency for the body to rotate. This moment, the **moment of the force** (M_F), is quantitatively equal to the magnitude of the applied force times the perpendicular distance between the line of the applied force and the center of resistance (see Figure 15-2). The magnitude of the tendency to rotate created by a force, M_F, is increased equally by either applying a larger force to the tooth or applying the force further away from the center of resistance.

A moment can also be applied to a tooth with a couple (M_C). The magnitude of the tendency to rotate produced by a couple is equal to the sum of the moment created by each of the two forces making up the couple. Because the forces are equal and opposite, they act to rotate the body in the same direction. The values for each force of a couple times its perpendicular distance to the center of resistance can be mathematically reduced to the value of one of the forces of the couple times the perpendicular distance between the two parallel forces of the couple (see Figure 15-5). The magnitude of the tendency to rotate created by a couple, M_C, is increased by either increasing both of the forces of the couple or increasing the distance between the two forces of the couple.

M_C is unique because the rotation it produces is independent of where the couple is applied on the tooth. Therefore a couple applied to a bracket attached anywhere on the tooth rotates the tooth in exactly the same way—around its center of resistance. Finally, rotation is the only tooth movement possible with a couple.

System Equilibrium

Newton's third law of motion states that for every action there is an equal and opposite reaction. The single forces and couples of orthodontic appliances are no exception. Static equilibrium requires that the sum of both the forces and the moments acting on an appliance in any plane must be equal to zero to maintain the system in equilibrium.

Equilibrium for a single force, as an equal and opposite force, is easy to understand. The equilibrium of a couple, however, is probably one of the most important and most poorly understood aspects of appliance design and use. It is also responsible for many unwanted and surprise tooth movements. Most dentists probably once understood the equilibrium of a couple when they took college physics. Orthodontic appliances are the practical application of the theoretic concept of the equilibrium of a couple.

The important point in understanding the equilibrium of a couple is that the sum of the forces and the moments must both be equal to zero. The tendency to rotate (i.e., each moment) must also be opposed by an equal and opposite tendency to rotate in the opposite direction.

Equilibrium of the One-Couple Force System

Equilibrium demands that a system with a couple and its associated tendency to rotate must have an equal and opposite tendency to rotate the system in the opposite direction. A **one-couple force system** inherently must have two equal and opposite couples present because it is in equilibrium.

For example, as an intrusion arch is pulled down anteriorly to place an intrusive point force on the incisor, the wire inserted into the molar tube creates a second equal and opposite extrusive force at the molar tube. These two equal and opposite forces form a couple, creating a tendency to rotate the whole system in one direction (F_1 and F_1 with counterclockwise rotation) (Figure 15-6).

Inherent in this system is a second simultaneous couple resulting from the same activation of the intrusion arch. The second couple is at the molar tube and

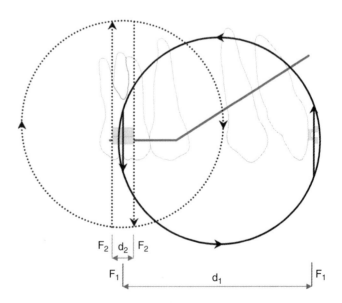

Figure 15-6 Equilibrium in a one-couple system. The first circle (*solid*) shows a passive intrusion arch. It is activated by tying it down anteriorly at the level of the bracket. This causes an intrusive force at the incisor and an extrusive force at the molar. This circle shows the direction of the couple associated with this extrusive and intrusive force. The second circle (*dotted*) shows a second couple at the molar bracket (M_C) that is equal and opposite in direction to the first couple.

results from a pair of equal and opposite forces at the interface of the wire and the molar tube as the intrusion arch is activated. These forces are at each end of the molar tube and create an equal and opposite tendency for the bracket and attached tooth to rotate in the opposite direction from the system rotation described in the previous paragraph (F_2 and F_2 with clockwise rotation) (Figure 15-6).

These two couples with their equal tendencies to rotate in opposite directions create the equilibrium of a couple. It is impossible to alter the wire in any way or to change any part of this equilibrium without affecting the other parts of the equilibrium. Additional force systems may be superimposed on the system, but the equilibrium of a couple must be equal and opposite. A change in part of the wire results in a change in the equilibrium of the whole system.

More recently, Lindauer and Isaacson[3] described the mechanics of an inverted intrusion arch (i.e., the extrusion arch). An extrusion arch is simply the intrusion arch with all of its force systems inverted.

The Equilibrium of the Two-Couple Force System

An old commonly accepted rule for determining the actions of an arch wire was to place one end of an arch wire in a bracket and view the position of the other end of the wire as an indicator of the direction of the resulting forces. This rule holds true for the one-couple system but often does not hold true for the **two-couple force system** (Figure 15-7).

When an arch wire is inserted into two consecutive brackets, activation of the wire creates a couple at each bracket. The couple at each bracket exists with an associated equilibrium just as if they were two one-couple force systems acting together. Therefore the two-couple force system's equilibrium is equivalent to the algebraic sum of the two one-couple force systems present (Figure 15-8). It is easy to see why the two-couple force system is more difficult to understand.[4-7]

In practice, the rotational tendency of the couple at each bracket exists unaffected by the couple at the other bracket. However, the equilibrium forces associated with each of the couples at the two brackets act on the same two teeth, and net action of these forces on each tooth is the sum of their combined individual actions.

For example, with the one-couple intrusion arch, the two forces acting at each end of the wire (extrusion at the molar and intrusion at the incisor) make up the vertical pair of forces comprising the equilibrium associated with the couple at the molar bracket (see Figure 15-6). If the wire is also inserted into the incisor bracket, the couple at the incisor bracket will also have vertical equilibrium forces acting at the incisor and molar. If the direction of rotation of the couple at the incisor bracket is the same as the direction of the rotation at the molar bracket, the associated pair of equilibrium

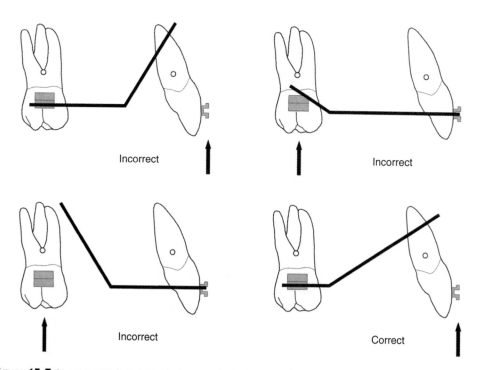

Incorrect

Incorrect

Incorrect

Correct

Figure 15-7 In a two-couple system, placing an archwire into one of the brackets and observing the position of the other end of the wire to determine the direction of force is not a reliable method.

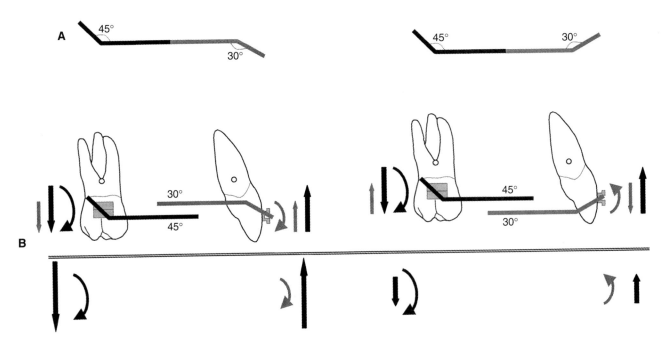

Figure 15-8 Two types of wire bends. **A,** Step bend. **B,** V bend. To determine the equilibrium in a two-couple system, the bracket slot with the larger angle of entry indicates the direction of the associated net equilibrium forces acting at each bracket. The larger angle of entry is at the molar bracket (45 degrees), and the moments and forces associated with it are shown *(solid arrows)*. Moments and forces from the incisor bracket (30 degrees) are also shown *(open arrows)*. The cumulative effect from this two-couple system is additive **(A)** because both couples are in the same direction (clockwise) and the associated equilibrium forces are in an equal and opposite direction (counterclockwise), making them extrusive at the molar and intrusive at the incisor. The direction of the couple in at the incisor bracket **(B)** is in a direction opposite from the couple in the molar bracket. Therefore the greater clockwise couple (45 degrees), which is at the molar, determines the direction of the equilibrium forces, which are extrusive at the molar and intrusive at the incisor. Note that the magnitude of the vertical equilibrium forces in **B** is less than it is in **A.**

forces at the molar and incisor will be additive in amount (see Figure 15-8, *A*). This type of bend is called a step bend. However, if the direction of rotation of the couple at the incisor bracket is in the opposite direction as the direction of the rotation of the couple at the molar bracket, the associated equilibrium forces at the molar and incisor will also be in opposite directions and thus reduced or even eliminated (see Figure 15-8, *B*). This type of bend is called a *V bend.*

One test for the direction of movement caused by a wire inserted into two brackets is to place the wire passively over the slots of the two brackets where it will be inserted and note the angle of entry of the wire with the bracket slots (see Figure 15-8). Think of the bracket moving to the wire to recognize the direction of the rotation. The bracket slot with the larger angle of entry creates the greatest couple at that bracket and therefore has the larger moment. This direction of the larger moment of the couple is important because, irrespective of the direction of the moment at the second bracket, the larger moment dictates the direction of the associated net equilibrium forces acting at each bracket.

V-Bend Principle

Assume two collinear brackets spanning a segment of a dental arch with each end of a wire inserted in each bracket—a two-bracket system (Figure 15-9). Various positions of placement of the V bend change the moments experienced at the two brackets.[9,10] This is called the **V-bend principle.** It should be noted that this is a two-dimensional view of force systems. Although several relationships are possible, the central tendency is as follows:

1. If the bend is centered between the two teeth, the M_C on the two adjacent teeth is equal. The system is in equilibrium because the associated equilibrium forces are equal and opposite and cancel each other out (see Figure 15-9, *A*).
2. If the bend is moved off center toward one tooth, that tooth has the greater M_C with larger associated vertical equilibrium forces. The equilibrium forces are extrusive or intrusive, depending on the direction of the V bend, at that tooth. The second tooth has a couple with a moment often in the opposite direction (see Figure 15-9, *A-E*). Be-

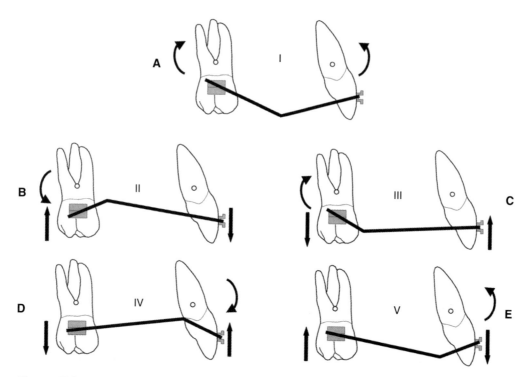

Figure 15-9 **A,** A centered V bend, which produces equal and opposite couples and therefore equal and opposite equilibrium forces that cancel each other out. **B-E,** The tooth with the greater M_C (greater angle of entry) and direction of rotation is shown with curved arrows. The associated equilibrium forces are shown with straight arrows.

cause the second tooth has a smaller M_C in the opposite direction, the magnitude of its equilibrium forces is smaller and in the opposite direction. A special situation is present when the moment of the smaller couple is less than half of the moment of the larger couple, but this detail only affects the direction of the smaller moment and the magnitude of the associated equilibrium forces.[2,4,9]

Figure 15-10 shows ways the equilibrium forces from moments in a two-couple system with two V bends impact each other.

1. Symmetric V bends with equal and opposite moments obtained by combining Figure 15-9, *C* and *E*.
2. Same as 1 with directions reversed (see Figures 15-9, *B* and *D*).
3. Two moments acting in the same direction (called *step bends*) create associated equilibrium forces acting in the same direction which are additive (see Figures 15-9, *B* and *E*). This is a useful procedure if greater vertical forces at the incisors or molars are needed.
4. Same as 3 with directions reversed (see Figures 15-9, *C* and *D*).

All appliance systems including those currently in existence and those yet to come must obey these physical principles.

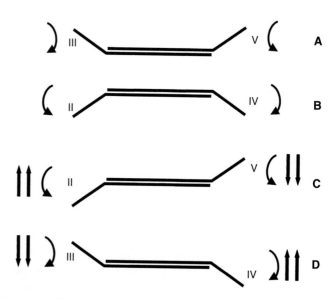

Figure 15-10 Combinations of two V bends shown in Figure 15-9. **A,** A combination of III and V. **B,** A combination of II and IV. It can be seen that **A** and **B** are symmetric V bends with equal and opposite couples and no associated equilibrium forces. **C,** A combination of II and V. **D,** A combination of III and IV. **C** and **D** are step bends with couples acting in the same direction and therefore equilibrium forces that are additive.

TOOTH MOVEMENT RESULTING FROM FORCE SYSTEMS

The Biologic Signal

The purpose of an orthodontic appliance is to physically displace a tooth (or bone) to stimulate the cells present at all of the involved articulations. The goal is to remodel bone and create a new homeostasis or equilibrium between the tooth and its supporting structures. The mechanism of how this is accomplished is still under investigation and remains unclear. What is the problem and why is the question unresolved?

If the amount of displacement is important in provoking the stimulus that causes the cellular response, an ideal amount of displacement should be able to make the processes proceed faster and more efficiently. This view is consistent with the **tooth movement** descriptions that set up an ideal appliance as one that can displace the tooth in a translatory fashion such that all points on the tooth root-bone surface are equally and optimally displaced and stimulated. Such a goal is unrealistic with the appliances in common use today.

Translatory displacement of a tooth requires that either a force is placed to act through the center of resistance or the root and the crown are caused to rotate in the same direction at the same rate. The goal of a force acting through the center of resistance is usually unattainable because brackets are placed at the crown of the tooth and hence the force cannot be directed through the center of resistance.

The idea of rotating the crown of the tooth and the root of the tooth in the same direction to obtain parallel or translatory movement is another way of describing the goal of most orthodontic appliances. If a force is put on the crown of a tooth to tip the crown in a clockwise direction, it will move the center of resistance of the tooth in the same direction as the line of force while simultaneously rotating the tooth in a clockwise direction around its center of resistance. This is the only way the center of resistance of a tooth can be moved. The result of this rotation, which orthodontists call a *tipping movement,* is a center of rotation somewhere between the center of resistance and the apex of the tooth. Such a tooth displacement necessarily results in a gradient of compression and tension along the root surface that is inconsistent with the goal of a constant degree of compression to obtain the ideal biologic response.

If some ideal displacement exists to get an ideal biologic response, rotational tooth movement alone cannot be ideal. If the biologic response moves the tooth equally well with rotational tooth displacement, the differential in compression and the magnitude of load applied may not matter. In this way of thinking, tooth movement is a matter of a force just being present or absent. If this is true, tooth movement cannot be differentially titrated biologically.

Based on the concept that some optimal level of load does exist, the goal of appliances is to rotate the root the same amount in a counterclockwise and opposite direction as the crown. This conceptually requires making the root move in the same direction and at the same rate as the crown. This is a good theoretic goal, but the reality is that it is not yet possible to apply a force and a couple that displaces the tooth equally and results in a parallel displacement of the tooth for any extended period.[8]

The goal of applying a force to rotate the crown and a couple to rotate the root is referred to as a *moment-to-force ratio* (Figure 15-11). The moment is the M_C applied at the bracket to cause the root to tip counterclockwise. The force is the force at the bracket that causes the crown to rotate clockwise.

An ideal moment-to-force ratio is often thought of as being about 10:1 because the force that causes clockwise rotation is applied about 10 mm from the center of resistance. For example, a force of 80 g makes the tendency to rotate clockwise equal to 80 g × 10 mm or 800 g-mm (see Figure 15-8). The couple applied to cause rotation of the root must be equal and opposite, or 800 g-mm, in a counterclockwise direction. This results in a moment-to-force ratio of 800 ÷ 80 = 10:1.

A moment-to-force ratio greater than 10 g-mm means that a larger counterclockwise moment of the couple exists where the tipping of the root exceeds the tipping of the crown. A moment-to-force ratio less than 10:1 means a larger force exists and means tipping but this time in the opposite direction with the crown movement exceeding the root movement. Either of these rotations results in unequal compression of the periodontium and a variation in the degree of stimulation of the cells producing the desired biologic changes. A moment-to-force ratio of about 10 g-mm equals translation and a parallel displacement of the tooth in the sagittal plane (see Figure 15-11).

It is also obvious that a tooth is a three-dimensional object and displacement of the tooth can never be totally equal on all sides of the root as the tooth is displaced. Thus the concept of differential forces to cause differential tooth movement is a complex question that has not been satisfactorily resolved in theory or in practice.

ELASTIC PROPERTIES OF WIRES

Elastic properties of wires are explained based on their stress-strain or a load deflection curve (Figure 15-12). Stress-to-strain relationships are associated with intrinsic properties of the wire related to its composition. The

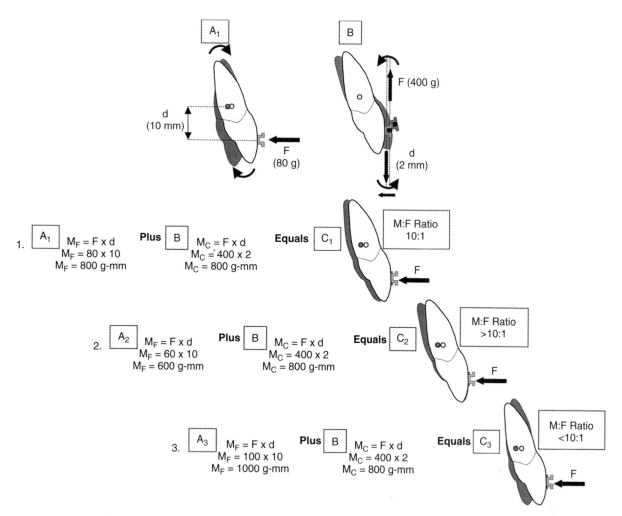

Figure 15-11 Representation of how changing the moment-to-force ratio can affect the type of tooth movement obtained. In the first example a lingual force of 80 g (A_1) applied 10 mm from the CRes with a counterclockwise M_C of 800 g-mm and an M:F ratio of 10:1 leads to translation. In the second example a smaller force of 60 g (A_2) applied at the same point of the tooth with the same counterclockwise M_C of 800 g-mm and an M:F ratio of greater than 10:1 leads to greater root movement. In the third example a greater force of 100 g (A_3) applied at the same point on the tooth with the same countermoment of 800 g-mm and an M:F ratio of less than 10:1 leads to greater crown movement.

ratio of stress to strain in the elastic portion of the curve defines the modulus of elasticity of the wire (ϵ). The modulus of elasticity is constant for the wire as it reflects the intrinsic properties of the wire. Load, or force, deflection rate refers to the amount of force produced for every unit of activation of an orthodontic wire.

The slope of a **stress-strain curve** within its elastic limit is an indicator of the stiffness or flexibility of a wire. The flatter the slope, the more flexible the wire. A flexible wire has a flatter slope, and a rigid wire has a steeper slope.

There are three points on the **load deflection curve** that are of clinical importance in appliance design: elastic limit, ultimate tensile strength, and failure point. The elastic limit (proportional limit, or yield strength) is the point at which any greater force leads to permanent deformation of the wire. The amount of deflection

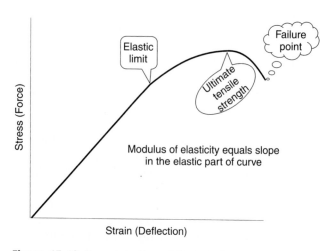

Figure 15-12 Stress-strain (force-deflection) diagram. (See text for a description of desirable characteristics for materials and appliances.)

that a wire can withstand before permanent deformation reflects an appliance's elastic range. A high elastic range in a wire enables activation of a wire to a greater extent with a lesser chance of it undergoing permanent deformation. On the other hand, the ability to permanently deform a material beyond its elastic limit enables the clinician to place bends in the wire.

The ultimate tensile strength is the maximum force a wire can withstand before the material begins to weaken. It corresponds to the peak of the force deflection curve. The portion of the force deflection curve from the elastic limit to the ultimate tensile strength is the plastic range of the wire. The extent to which an appliance returns to its original form when deflected into its plastic range determines its springiness. A wire with an extended plastic range is more formable, which means it can be bent several times without undergoing failure. If a wire is deflected past its ultimate tensile strength, it will eventually fail by breaking.

Wires with a low-load deflection are preferred in orthodontics in areas where large tooth movements are required because they maintain a fairly constant force as the tooth moves and the appliance is deactivated. In areas where minimal tooth movement is desired, such as in maximum anchorage extraction cases or during finishing, a high load deflection rate is desirable.

Factors That Influence the Load Deflection Rate of an Appliance

There are four factors that the clinician has control over that can reduce the load deflection rate: use of low modulus wires, reducing the wire cross section, increasing interbracket distance, and placing loops in the arch wire.

1. Changing the wire material: Stainless steel is the stiffest material used in orthodontics. Burstone[11,12] compared the stiffness of modern orthodontic wire materials. If steel were given an arbitrary modulus of elasticity of 100, titanium/molybdenum alloys would be 35% as stiff as steel and nitinol would be 17% as stiff as steel. The advantage and, sometimes, disadvantage of nickel/titanium alloys is that they cannot be easily permanently deformed.
2. Decreasing the cross section of the wire-load deflection rate varies directly as the fourth power of the diameter of a round wire. Decreasing the diameter of the wire by half decreases the stiffness of a wire by 16 times. The limiting factor in reduction of the diameter of a wire is the elastic limit of the wire so as to prevent it from undergoing permanent deformation. Multistrand steel wires make use of small diameter wires. This increases the springiness and elastic range of these wires without significantly affecting their strength.
3. Increasing interbracket length
   a. Increasing interbracket distance[13]: The load deflection rate is inversely proportional to the third power of the length of the wire. An example using this principle is an intrusion arch that bypasses the teeth that are not involved in deep bite correction (see Figure 15-16).
   b. Placing loops in the arch wire: Loops increase the amount of interbracket wire length and thereby reduce the load deflection rate created.[14] With the introduction of new low modulus wires, the need for placing loops in orthodontic appliances has decreased considerably.

CLINICAL APPLICATION OF FORCE SYSTEMS

This section of the chapter introduces some of the common appliances that are used to treat malocclusions. The force systems associated with each of these appliances are briefly discussed. Appliances should be designed to meet specific treatment goals for a particular patient and certainly not vice versa.

Appliances to Modify Jaw Growth

Appliances that are used to modify jaw growth can be broadly divided into headgear and functional appliances.

Headgear Headgear is used in orthodontics to modify growth of the maxilla, to distalize and protract maxillary teeth, or to reinforce anchorage. When headgear is used for skeletal modifications, heavier forces are recommended.[15] Such heavier forces bring about actions on the sutures of the maxilla, changing the magnitude and direction of their growth. There are several studies to document orthopedic changes in the maxilla.[16] Some combination of skeletal and dental changes occur, and, in most instances, tooth movement changes exceed skeletal changes. There are several types of headgear that can be used to bring about a desired effect. The type of headgear and desired force level should be selected according to the specific treatment objectives for a patient.

Headgear should usually be worn for at least 8 to 14 hr/day to achieve successful results. For orthopedic changes forces used are in the range of 250 to 500 g per side, and for dental movements they are in the range of 100 to 200 g per side. As with functional appliances the success of headgear therapy is dependent on compliance obtained from the patient.

Biomechanics of Headgear The use of biomechanical principles enables the operator to control the direction and magnitude of the forces produced by different headgear designs and determines the type of clinical changes that can be expected. An important principle in analyzing the force system from a headgear is the relationship between the line of force action and its relationship to the center of resistance of the maxilla or the first molar. A force passing through the center of resistance causes pure translation in the direction of the line of the force. Any other force produces translation and a rotation with a moment.

To analyze force systems on an upper first molar, first draw an imaginary line connecting the point of attachment on the strap and the outer bow of the headgear when the appliance is in place. Drop a perpendicular line from the center of resistance of the upper first molar to the line of force. The magnitude of the moment of the force is the product of the magnitude of the force and the perpendicular distance from the center of resistance to the line of force. Although the position of the inner bow cannot be changed, the position of the outer bow can be bent up or down and length adjusted. This changes the direction of the force to obtain the desired results.

Cervical Headgear (Figure 15-13) The force systems for a headgear must follow the same rules as applies to other orthodontic force systems. It is possible to align the outer bow of the facebow such that when the neck strap is attached, the line of force passes through the center of resistance of the molar. This force system translates the molar in the direction of the line of force. This description of the force system is accurate if the facebow is not deformed. More commonly, cervical headgear used for the correction of Class II malocclusions results in a line of force acting occlusal to the center of resistance, and the tooth movement resulting is a rotation with a distal tip of the molar crown.

To counteract the distal crown tip a distal root tip is needed. This is accomplished by bending the outer bows of the headgear upward such that they are lowered when attaching the bow to the neck strap. This results in a deformation of the facebow. This downward deformation of the facebow results in a counterclockwise couple at the molar tube. The moment of this couple causes the molar root to rotate distally. The equilibrium associated with this couple is extrusive at the molar and upward at the neck strap. The headgear tooth movement can be adjusted to be effectively the same as the intrusion arch described previously.

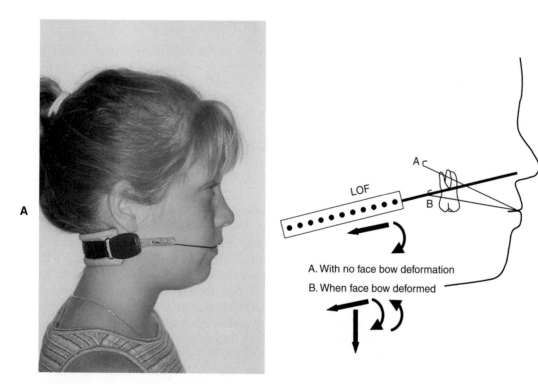

Figure 15-13 A, Cervical headgear. **B,** A line of force *(LOF)* passing through the center of resistance translates the tooth in the direction of the force. *A,* With no facebow deformed. *B,* If the facebow must be deformed and lowered to attach to the neck strap, a couple is created at the headgear tube.

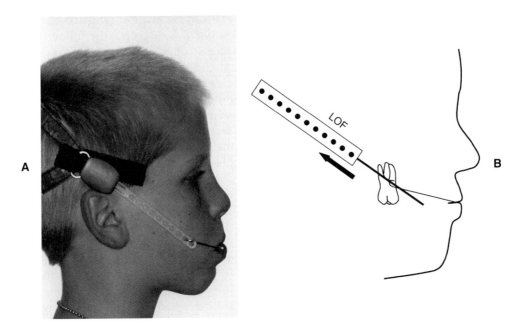

Figure 15-14 A, Occipital headgear. **B,** When the occipital strap and the facebow result in a line of force *(LOF)* acting through the center of resistance, the tooth is translated in the direction of the line of force.

Because of the extrusive force placed on the molar there is a tendency to open the bite. Hence cervical headgear should be used with care on patients with open bite tendencies.

Occipital and High Pull Headgear (Figure 15-14)

Occipital headgear is commonly used in Class II correction in which controlling anterior open bite tendencies is part of the problem (see Chapter 20). An occipital headgear is constructed with the outer bow cut short at a position adjacent to the first molar. This results in a line of force that acts vertically and posteriorly through the center of resistance. This line of force acts to intrude and retract the molar. This appliance does not deform the facebow as readily as the longer cervical outer bow, reducing the tendency for a large couple at the molar tube.

Protraction Headgear

Protraction headgear is used for skeletal and dental protraction of the maxilla in Class III malocclusions caused by a maxillary deficiency (see Chapter 21). The forces and moments associated with a protraction headgear are illustrated in Figure 15-15. Protraction headgear exerts a mesial force on the maxilla below the center of resistance with an equal and opposite reciprocal force on the chin and forehead. The force on the chin may cause a change in the posture of the mandible that may affect its direction of growth. The counterclockwise moment on the maxilla and dentition caused by the line of force acting below the center of resis-

tance leads to a tendency for extrusion of the maxillary posterior teeth with an associated opening of the bite.

Functional Appliances

The term **functional appliance** means that when the appliance is fully seated in the mouth, the mandible is forced into an eccentric/noneccentric relation position. Any such mandibular posture causes the musculature to try to move the mandible toward a centric relation position. This results in force systems being exerted wherever the appliance is mounted on the teeth or soft tissues of the mouth.

Most commonly, functional appliances are used to hold the mandible in a protrusive position to effect a correction of Class II dental relationships (see Chapter 20). The correction has long been believed to result in advancing the condyle out of the fossa with a stimulation of condylar growth. Studies have been unable to verify the occurrence of significant additional growth from this approach, but the approach has clearly been used with successful empiric results.

Most functional appliances are partially or totally tooth mounted. Therefore when the musculature attempts to move the mandible toward centric relations, the teeth receive forces to advance the lower arch and to retract the upper arch. Studies of treated cases have documented these actions, but the amount of tooth movements observed has been insufficient to explain the Class II corrections that occurred. The rest

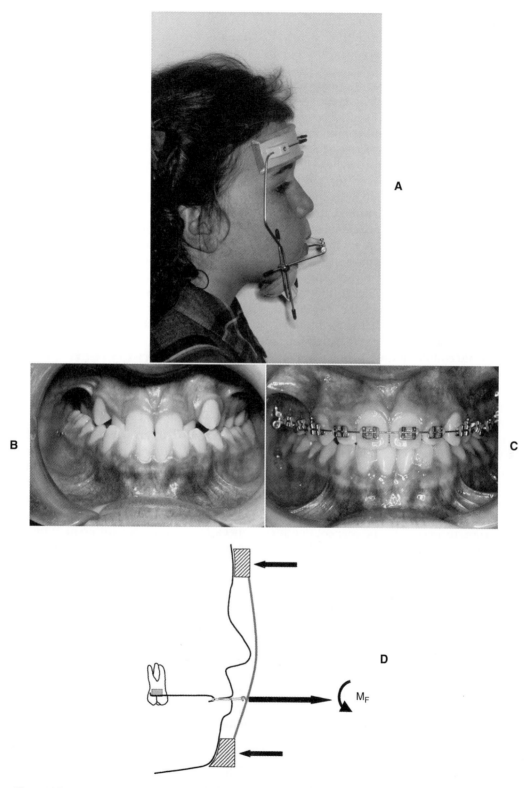

Figure 15-15 A, Protraction headgear. **B,** Teeth before orthodontic treatment including protraction headgear. **C,** After treatment. **D,** Force system with line of force below the center of resistance resulting in a counterclockwise moment.

of the change has been attributed to redirection of the growth of the maxilla and the mandible. The result is that considerable controversy has existed regarding the mechanism of action of removable functional appliances. For the same reason, no uniform agreement exists regarding the optimal way to construct or use these appliances.

Because most functional appliances are removable appliances, it is apparent that patient compliance plays a major role in their success. The absence of an ability to quantitatively assess patient compliance is one key element in the problem of assessing the efficacy of functional appliance therapy. When functional appliances are in place, however, the mechanism of action must follow the same principles of statics and engineering mechanics applied to fixed appliances. The functional displacement of the mandible is designed for the purpose of impacting growth of the jaws. This phenomenon is biologic and not defined in engineering terms as to direction and amount of outcome. The forces applied to the teeth are mostly forces not acting through the center of resistance and must result in a simultaneous rotation and a translation of the teeth affected. It is theoretically possible to create couples with functional appliances by creating equal and opposite forces, but this is difficult and rarely seen clinically. The result of most tooth movement with functional appliances is similar to tooth movement from any single force not acting through the center of resistance—the tooth tips with a center of rotation between the apex and the center of resistance.

It is apparent that, from the longitudinal work of Bishara et al[17] and from Bjork's and Skieller's implant studies,[18] Class II malocclusions in the mixed dentition remain Class II malocclusions in the permanent dentition even though the jaws are undergoing dissimilar amounts of vertical and anteroposterior growth. This tooth movement has been termed *dental compensation* and probably results, at least in part, from the intercuspation of the upper and lower teeth. Thus when mandibular growth is tending to grow the mandible anteriorly, the intercuspation of the teeth is providing a force system to perpetuate the dental Class II malocclusion by moving the upper teeth forward and the lower teeth distally. The result is that the skeleton is growing toward the correction of the Class II malocclusion, but the dentition is moving in the opposite direction, tending to preserve the dental Class II malocclusion.

Johnston[19] recently offered a new and creative explanation of the mechanism of action of functional appliances. He suggested that functional appliances act by holding the teeth out of occlusion and preventing dental compensations from taking place. In other words, the mandible and its dentition are placed in a

dental Class I relationship with the maxilla with the mandibular condyle displaced out of the fossa. Normal condylar growth is anticipated to allow the condyle to grow back into the fossa, whereas the dentition is prevented from undergoing the dental compensation usually associated with dissimilar jaw growth. Johnston[17] reviewed the functional appliance literature and concluded that evidence was lacking for the ability of functional appliances to grow mandibles any significantly greater amount than they would have grown without treatment. He also noted that the tooth movement observed is not sufficient to account for the Class II corrections seen.

It is likely that the mechanism of action of all functional appliances, whether they are fixed or removable, is to displace the mandible while allowing the normal amount of growth potential to express itself without the associated dental compensation taking place simultaneously. While the jaw is held in an eccentric position, the musculature can be expected to exert forces on the teeth supporting the appliance and the resulting tooth movement will be tipping with the center of rotation below the center of resistance.

Appliances to Correct Anteroposterior Variations

Class II   Class II malocclusions may be caused by a deficient mandible, maxillary excess or a combination of these. In growing patients with Class II malocclusions, correction often is obtained by growth modification using headgear or functional appliances (see Chapter 20). The choice between the selection of headgear therapy or functional appliances is not easy or always clear. Although these two appliances seem to target different types of jaws, posttreatment results seem to show that they bring about similar changes.

In growing patients with crowding, Class II correction sometimes is achieved by extraction and differential space closure combined with growth modifications. Class II problems in nongrowing patients are usually corrected either by surgery or by single-arch extractions.

Several appliances such as pendulum appliances and Jones' Jigs have been introduced that obtain correction of Class II dental relationships using force systems to distalize maxillary posterior teeth.

Class III   Class III malocclusions can be caused by a deficient maxilla, mandibular excess, or a combination of these. These patients usually present with anterior crossbites. It is important for the clinician to assess whether there is a functional shift into an anterior crossbite. Also the amount of dental compensation in terms of retroclined lower incisors and excessively proclined maxillary incisors should be determined to evaluate the feasibility of dental vs. skeletal correction (see Chapter 21).

A protraction headgear places a forward force on the maxilla and its dentition, encouraging improvement of Class III relationships. The case in Figure 15-15 was a Class III relationship caused by a hypoplastic maxilla. Slow maxillary skeletal expansion and protraction of the maxillary complex was carried out. A protraction headgear was used to place an anterior force on the sutures of the maxilla and the maxillary teeth. The line of action of force of a protraction headgear lies below the center of resistance of the maxilla (see Figure 15-15, *D*). The moment of the force rotates the maxillary complex and molar counterclockwise, moving the center of resistance in a downward and forward direction. For maximum skeletal effect, patients are best treated using protraction headgear in the early mixed dentition, preferably before 8 years of age.

Anterior crossbites in the mixed dentition are an indication for early treatment to minimize the potential for marginal skeletal Class III malocclusion from growing into a more severe skeletal Class III malocclusion. Figure 15-16 shows a case of a 9-year-old child who was congenitally missing a maxillary left lateral incisor and had an anterior crossbite. The anterior crossbite was not a result of an anterior functional shift of the mandible. Cephalometric analysis revealed that the maxillary incisors could tolerate labial positioning. The anterior crossbite was corrected by flaring the incisors around the center of resistance using a couple created by a torquing arch (see Figure 15-16).[6]

Appliances Used to Correct Variations in the Vertical Dimension

Deep Bites Correction of deep bites can be brought about by intrusion of anterior teeth, modifying vertical growth of the dental alveolus, extrusion of posterior teeth or combinations of these. The method most suitable for a particular patient depends on the treatment objectives. When intrusion of anterior teeth is the goal, light forces should be used. Heavier forces are more likely to create a greater tendency for posterior teeth to erupt as a result of the equal and opposite extrusive force at the molar. Recommended forces for intrusion of lower incisors are in the range of 12.5 g per tooth and for maxillary incisors about 15 to 20 g per tooth.

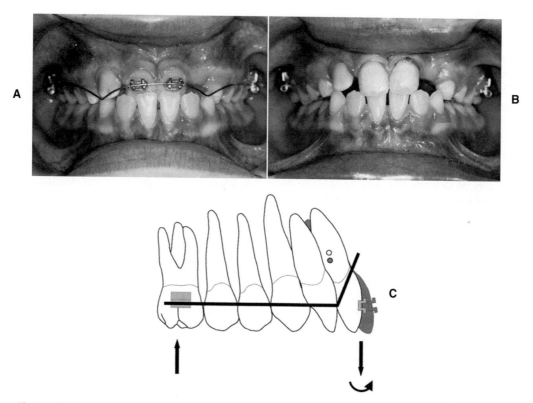

Figure 15-16 Correction of a true anterior crossbite using a torquing arch. **A,** Before treatment. **B,** Anterior crossbite corrected 4 months after the start of treatment. **C,** Force systems from a torquing arch.

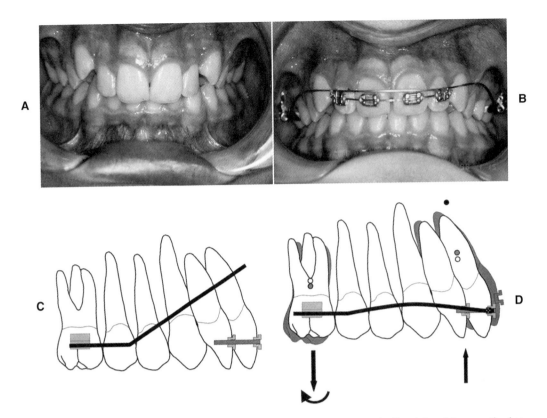

Figure 15-17 Intrusion arch. **A,** Before treatment. **B,** After 3 months of treatment, significant deep bite correction has occurred. **C,** A passive intrusion arch. **D,** Intrusion arch with a point contact tie at the incisors. NOTE: If the intrusive force does not pass through the center of resistance of the four incisors *(black circle),* a moment of the force moves the crowns labially *(shown in gray).*

Appliances used for deep bite correction are generically termed **intrusion arches** and variations include base arches, **utility arches,** and reverse curve of Spee wires. Figure 15-17 demonstrates an intrusion base arch and its associated force systems. An intrusion base arch is an example of a one-couple system that is capable of varying the direction of an intrusive force to ensure it acts through the center of resistance.[3] The point of application of force is within the control of the operator and the force system can be determined. The advantage of this appliance is that it has a large interbracket distance, which decreases the load deflection rate and thereby maintains a constant force throughout tooth movement. Therefore this appliance requires minimum adjustment during deep bite correction.

The utility arch is an example of a two-couple intrusion arch used for deep bite correction (Figure 15-18).[20] All utility arches used for deep bite correction have a tip back bend that creates a larger M_C at the molars in a clockwise direction. It is recommended that the same clockwise moment (facial root torque) be placed on the incisors. Because the M_C at both brackets are in the same direction, it can be seen how the equilibrium forces are additive. If counterclockwise lingual root torque is present on the incisors, it results in moments at the two teeth in opposite directions and a decrease in the intrusive force on the anterior segment (see Figure 15-8, *B*). If the moment for lingual root torque at the incisors is greater than the clockwise moment for molar tip back, the incisor equilibrium forces are greater and actually extrude the incisors.

A reverse curve of Spee wire on the lower arch acts mainly by tipping molars distally and incisors labially. As the incisors flare labially, angular changes contribute to overbite correction. If the wire is in place for a long enough period and vertical facial growth occurs, premolars extrude and, to a lesser degree, molars and incisors get intruded.

Open Bites Open bites are more difficult to correct and are more unpredictable in their prognosis than deep bites. Open bites are ideally corrected dentally by intrusion of posterior teeth, thereby permitting counterclockwise rotation of the mandible. Extrusion of anterior teeth represents a dental compensation and is achieved with vertical elastics or an extrusion arch wire. The lip-to-tooth and gingival displays on smiling are two factors that are important in the design of an appliance for correction of open bites. In some instances treatment cannot be accomplished by orthodontics alone, in which case a combined approach of orthodontics and surgery is necessary.

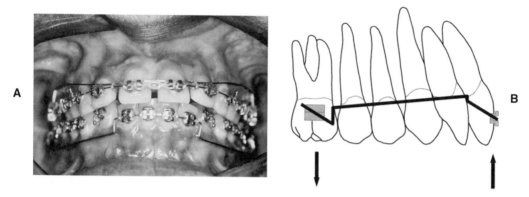

Figure 15-18 **A,** Utility arch in the maxillary dentition. **B,** Force systems from a maxillary utility arch with a tip back bend at the molar and facial root torque on the incisors. Note the similarity of this appliance design to Figure 15-10, *D.*

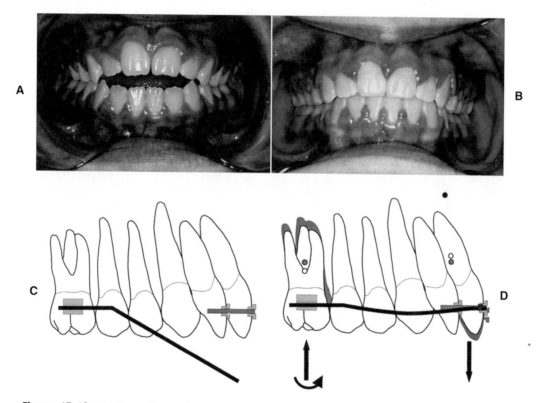

Figure 15-19 Extrusion arch. **A,** Before treatment. **B,** After open bite was corrected. **C,** Passive extrusion arch. **D,** Activated extrusion arch with associated force systems.

A one-couple extrusion arch may be used to dentally correct open bites (Figure 15-19).[3] Extrusion arches have all the advantages of an intrusion arch. Extrusion arches bring about a clockwise M_C at the molar bracket when activated. The equilibrium forces are extrusive at the incisors and intrusive on the molars. Extrusion occurs much more rapidly than intrusion, and treatment must be carefully watched to prevent overtreatment.

A two-couple utility arch that is inserted into the molars and the four incisors may be activated as an extrusion arch (see Figure 15-10, *C*). The normal V bend at the molar is made in the opposite direction as is used for intrusion of incisors. The third-order rotation or torque at the incisors must be lingual root torque. Such activation acts as a step bend with counterclockwise moments in the same direction at the molar and incisors and strong equilibrium forces that are extrusive at the incisors and intrusive at the molars.

Appliances to Correct Variations in the Transverse Dimension

Crossbites can present as lingual or buccal crossbites and may be of dental or skeletal origin. Lingual crossbites are seen far more commonly in clinical practice (see Chapters 16, 17, and 19).

Lingual crossbites are treated with several types of appliances, all of which attempt to expand the maxilla skeletally by exerting forces at the midpalatal suture or by moving maxillary teeth buccally. Some of the appliances used are maxillary rapid expanders, quadhelices, transpalatal arches, 2 × 4 appliances, and 2 × 6 appliances.

Palatal Expanders   Transverse skeletal expansion may be carried out either by rapid palatal expansion at the rate of 0.5 to 1 mm/day or by slow palatal expansion at the rate of about 1mm/wk using **palatal expanders** (Figure 15-20). The final expansion seen is usually a combination of skeletal and dental expansion. During skeletal expansion the orthodontist should realize that the rotation of the palatal bones and the rotation

of the teeth determine the final position of the teeth. Unless the center of resistance of each half of the maxilla is located at or near the level of the line of application of the expansion force, it would be incorrect to assume that the maxillary bones translate. Although the center of resistance of the palatal bones has not been precisely determined, it can safely be assumed that it lies above the line of application of force (which is at the cusps of the molar teeth). Hence during skeletal expansion there is a tendency for the palatal shelves to rotate buccally in the transverse dimension. In addition, all expansion appliances exert a lateral force on the teeth they are attached to below the center of resistance. Hence they create an M_F that tends to rotate the teeth. This rotation causes the lingual cusps of these teeth to drop occlusally and to increase the curve of Monson.

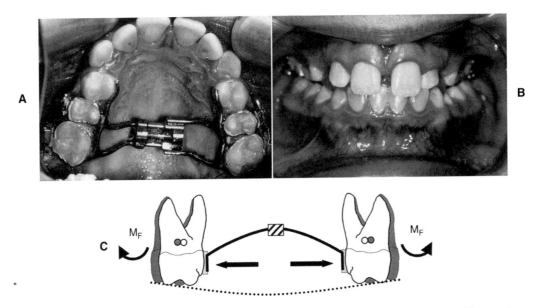

Figure 15-20 A, Hyrax expander. **B,** After palatal expansion. **C,** Illustration showing a horizontal force acting occlusally from the center of resistance. This force causes an M_F, which rotates the molar crown buccally and steepens the Monson curve.

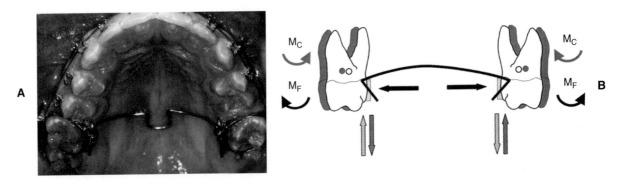

Figure 15-21 A, Transpalatal arch *(TPA)*. **B,** Illustration and associated force systems of a TPA used for molar expansion by translation.

Ultimate dental expansion is the sum of the expansion of the palatal halves of the bone and the expansion of the teeth.

Transpalatal Arches

Transpalatal arches, unlike many other expanders, are capable of generating an M_C in all three dimensions of space because they engage a bracket slot on both ends of the wire. Transpalatal arches are examples of two-bracket, two-couple systems and can be activated accordingly. Transpalatal arches are versatile appliances and are used for multiple purposes. They can be activated to establish and maintain arch widths, prevent molar rotations, perform symmetric and asymmetric rotations of either the molars or buccal segments, correct mesiodistal asymmetries, change the cant of the occlusal plane from the right to the left side, correct symmetric and asymmetric crossbites, and correct third-order axial inclinations. Using a transpalatal arch makes it possible to bring about translation, torque, tip, and rotations around the center of resistance (Figure 15-21). Rebellato[21] provides an excellent detailed review of the applications of transpalatal arches.

2 × 6 and 2 × 4 Appliances

A **2 × 6 appliance** has brackets on the first molars and the six anterior teeth (canine to canine). Using the principles of a one-couple, two-bracket appliance system discussed previ-ously in this chapter, asymmetric V bends, and step bends can be used to expand molars. Rebellato[22] provides an in-depth review on the applications of a **2 × 4 appliance** and a 2 × 6 appliance for the correction of transverse discrepancies.

Appliances to Correct Intraarch Variations

When teeth are malpositioned in an arch, it is often the result of a lack of space. Crowding in the mixed dentition or early permanent dentition is managed by holding the Leeway space, expanding the arches, distalizing posterior teeth, or extracting teeth.

Lip Bumpers

Lip bumpers gain intraarch space by removing the pressure of the buccal musculature permitting lateral and anterior dentoalveolar development. Lip bumpers act by holding the muscles and soft tissue away from the teeth with shields that are placed up to 3 mm away from the teeth (Figure 15-22, *A*). By reducing the pressure of the lips and cheeks on the teeth, the tongue applies an uncompensated lingual force on the teeth. This appliance has been shown to cause distal molar crown tipping, slight expansion of the buccal segments, and incisor proclination.[23] Using the principles of biomechanics discussed previously it can be seen that a lip bumper

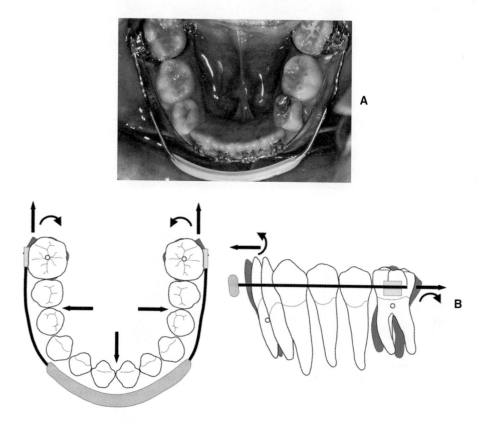

Figure 15-22 **A,** Lip bumper. **B,** The force systems from a lip bumper.

applies a distal force buccal and occlusal to the center of resistance of the tooth. This appliance causes distal crown tipping and distolingual rotation of the lower molars (see Figure 15-22, *B*).

Intraarch Spacing (Diastema) A *diastema* is defined as a space between two teeth (Figure 15-23, *A*). When the spacing is mainly the result of interarch and intraarch tooth size discrepancies it can be treated by orthodontic or restorative means. The spacing commonly has a sagittal or vertical component causing it. With a fixed appliance it is important for the operator to determine the cause of the diastema before designing an appliance to correct it. It is often necessary to place an intrusive and distal force during space closure. In addition, an M_C is often necessary to prevent the incisors from tipping lingually around a point between the center of resistance and the apex of the tooth (Figure 15-23, *C* and *D*).

Impacted Canines Palatally impacted canines have a poor prognosis for erupting into the oral cavity spontaneously. Figure 15-24 shows palatally impacted canines that were surgically exposed and guided into the oral cavity using a one-couple appliance. Analyzing the appliance in the sagittal plane shows that the M_C at the molar rotates it in a counterclockwise direction. The associated equilibrium forces with this M_C are to extrude the canine and intrude the molar. In the sagittal plane the M_C rotates the molar crown mesiolingually. The equilibrium forces are to move the canine labially and the molar lingually. A transpalatal arch was used to counteract the side effects at the molar. The increased bracket distance of this appliance design creates a low-load deflection rate, thereby maintaining force constancy over a large range of activation. The canines were brought into the arch in about 10 months. Tooth #8 was ankylosed and was treated later, surgically.

Minor Intraarch Tooth Movement Figure 15-25 is an example of a case where two central incisors had excessive distal root tip and caused the gingival embrasure between the maxillary incisors to be enlarged. A dark triangle was present when the patient smiled. Minor orthodontic treatment consisting of moving the roots mesially by rotating the tooth around its center of resistance corrected the problem. Proper appliance design to bring about the desired tooth movement and a normal papilla helped eliminate the dark triangle.

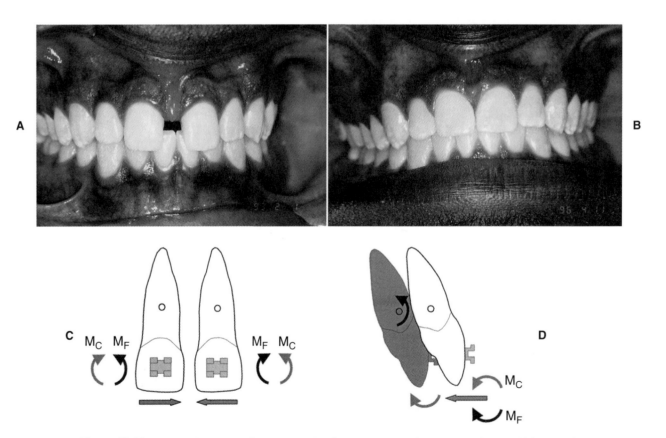

Figure 15-23 Diastema closure. **A,** Before treatment. **B,** After treatment. **C,** In the transverse plane mesial forces and a counterclockwise second-order couple were placed to enable translation of the incisors. **D,** In the sagittal plane intrusion and retraction forces were placed together with a counterclockwise third-order couple to permit translation.

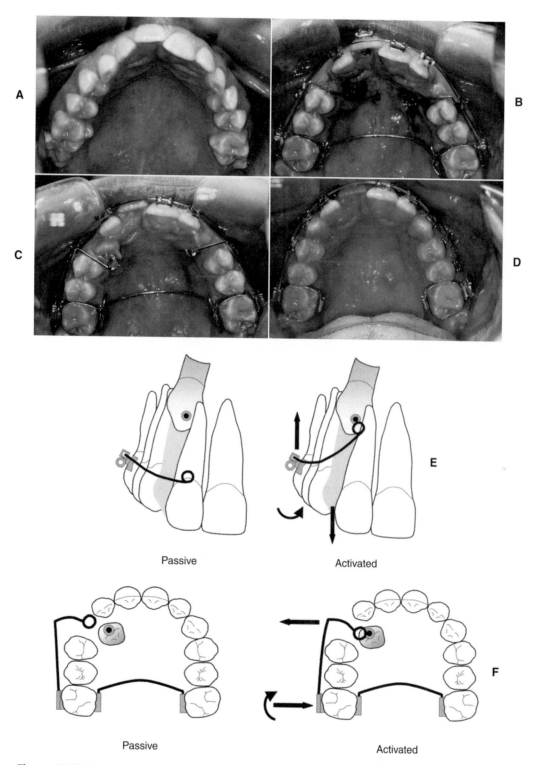

Figure 15-24 Eruption of palatally impacted maxillary canines. **A,** Before treatment. **B,** Immediately after surgical exposure and removal of primary canines. **C,** Appliance in place. **D,** After 1 year of treatment. **E,** Force systems in the frontal plane. **F,** Force systems in the transverse plane. Refer to text for explanation of force systems from this spring.

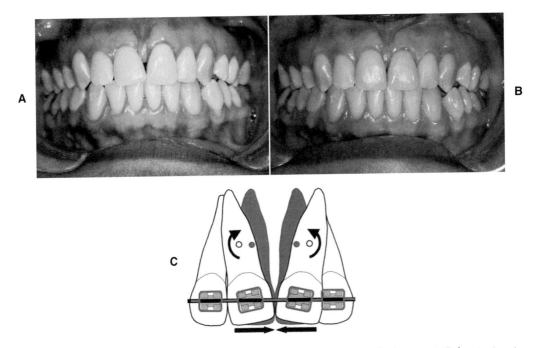

Figure 15-25 Second-order couple *(M_C)* on tooth #8 to place mesial root or distal crown. **A,** Before treatment. **B,** After 3 months. **C,** A couple that rotated the two central incisors around their center of resistance was placed using an arch wire. The crowns of the incisors were tied together to prevent distal movement of the crowns.

SUMMARY

Clinical application of biomechanical principles enhances the quality and efficiency of orthodontic appliances. During the career of a dental professional, appliance designs continually change and evolve. New appliances have to be based on the biomechanical principles described. It is important for the clinician not to be captivated by marketing claims when new appliances are introduced but to evaluate them scientifically, determine their true abilities, and select the ones that are best for each patient.

REFERENCES

1. Burstone CJ, Baldwin JJ, Lawless DT: The application of continuos forces to orthodontics, *Angle Orthod* 31:1-14, 1961.
2. Smith RJ, Burstone CJ: Mechanics of tooth movement, *Am J Orthod* 85:294-307, 1984.
3. Lindauer SJ, Isaacson RJ: Biomechanics and appliance design: one-couple orthodontic appliance systems, *Semin Orthod* 1(1):12-54, 1995.
4. Mulligan TF: *Common sense mechanics in everyday orthodontics,* Phoenix, 1998, CSM.
5. Isaacson RJ, Lindauer SJ, Davidovitch M: Biomechanics and appliance design: the ground rules for archwire design, *Semin Orthod* 1(1):3-11, 1995.
6. Isaacson RJ, Lindauer SJ, Rubenstein LK: Moments with the edgewise appliance-incisor torque control, *Am J Orthod Dentofacial Orthop* 103(5):428-438, 1993.
7. Isaacson RJ, Lindauer SJ, Rubenstein LK: Activating a 2 × 4 appliance, *Angle Orthod* 63(1):17-24, 1993.
8. Burstone CJ, Koenig HA: Creative wire bending: the force system for step and V bends, *Am J Orthod Dentofacial Orthop* 93:59-67, 1988.
9. Isaacson RJ: Biomechanics and appliance design: creative arch wires and clinical conclusion, *Semin Orthod* 1(1)55-56, 1995.
10. Isaacson RJ, Lindauer SJ, Davidovitch M: On tooth movement, *Angle Orthod* 63(4):305-309, 1993.
11. Kapila S, Sachdeva R: Mechanical properties and clinical applications of orthodontic wires, *Am J Orthod Dentofacial Orthop* 96(2):100-109, 1989.
12. Burstone CJ: Variable-modulus orthodontics, *Am J Orthod* 80(1):1-16, 1981.
13. Burstone CJ: The mechanics of the segmented arch technique, *Angle Orthod* 36(2):99-120, 1966.
14. Burstone CJ: Application of bioengineering to clinical orthodontics. In Graber TM, Vanarsdall RL Jr (eds): *Orthodontics: current principles and techniques,* ed 3, St Louis, 2000, Mosby.
15. Kloehn S: Guiding alveolar growth and eruption of the teeth to reduce treatment time and produce a more balanced denture and face, *Am J Orthod* 17:10-33, 1947.
16. Baumrind S et al: Quantitative analysis of the orthodontic and orthopedic effects of maxillary traction, *Am J Orthod* 83:384-398, 1983.

17. Bishara SE et al: Changes in the molar relationship between the deciduous and permanent dentitions: a longitudinal study, *Am J Orthod Dentofacial Orthop* 93:19-28, 1988.
18. Bjork A, Skieller V: Facial development and tooth eruption, *Am J Orthod* 62:339-383, 1972.
19. Johnston LE: Early and often: a critical examination of two-phase growth-modification treatments. In Jacob A: Salzman lecture. 98th annual meeting of the American Association of Orthodontics, Dallas, Tex, May 17, 1998.
20. Davidovitch M, Rebellato J: Biomechanics and appliance design: two-couple orthodontic appliance systems: utility arches, *Semin Orthod* 1(1):25-30, 1995.
21. Rebellato J: Biomechanics and appliance design: two-couple orthodontic appliance systems: transpalatal arches, *Semin Orthod* 1(1):44-54, 1995.
22. Rebellato J: Biomechanics and appliance design: two-couple orthodontic systems: activation in the transverse dimension, *Semin Orthod* 1(1):37-43, 1995.
23. Davidovitch M, McInnis D, Lindauer SJ: The effects of lip bumper therapy in the mixed dentition, *Am J Orthod Dentofacial Orthop* 111:52-58, 1997.

CHAPTER 16

Steps in Orthodontic Treatment

Andrew J. Kuhlberg

KEY TERMS

first-order plane	tip	maximum posterior anchorage	separate canine retraction
second-order plane	torque	reciprocal anchorage	root correction
dentofacial orthopedic treatment	preliminary alignment	maximum anterior anchorage	finishing details
interceptive treatment	intermaxillary growth space	extraoral appliances	retention phase
edgewise bracket	incisor intrusion	intermaxillary elastics	removable appliances
preadjusted appliances	posterior extrusion	Nance holding arch	bonded (fixed) retainers
	anchorage control	lip bumpers	

Contemporary orthodontic treatment is not simply the insertion of a sequence of arch wires. Orthodontic treatment involves the controlled application of mechanical forces to the teeth and periodontium producing a biologic response ending in tooth movement. These forces are generated by the activation of wires, springs, and elastics selected by the orthodontist and are consistent with an intended type and direction of tooth movement. The activation forces of the arch wire are transmitted via the orthodontic bracket to the tooth and, ultimately, the periodontal membrane. The mechanical stimulus on the cells of the periodontium determines the nature of the tooth movement. Effective, efficient, and patient-centered treatment requires the deliberate selection of treatment mechanics specific to each individual's problems (see Chapter 15).

Establishing specific treatment goals is an integral step in orthodontic treatment. These goals aid in determining the sequence of treatment for each patient. Because patients and their malocclusions come in so many shapes and ages, individualized treatment planning is necessary.[1,2] Determining specific objectives identifies the tooth movements that will correct each aspect of the malocclusion (Box 16-1). Planning tooth movement in all three planes of space requires taking a precise approach to orthodontic treatment. The three planes that describe orthodontic tooth movements are termed **first-order plane, second-order plane,** and **third-order plane** (Figure 16-1).

In the majority of cases, orthodontic therapy can be divided into stages or steps. The steps target interim objectives on the way to the final result. In many circumstances the stages of treatment merge or are accomplished simultaneously.

EARLY TREATMENT FOR MANAGEMENT OF DENTOSKELETAL PROBLEMS

In situations where significant skeletofacial changes are necessary, early **dentofacial orthopedic treatment** should be considered. Additionally, **interceptive treatments** directed at parafunctional habits or the premature loss of primary teeth are beneficial early procedures (see Chapter 17). Early treatment should be carefully selected and planned with clear, concise objectives for this intervention.

BOX 16-1	General and Specific Objectives for Orthodontic Treatment Planning

General objectives of comprehensive orthodontic treatment	Well-interdigitated occlusion, usually a Class I relationship
	Normal overjet
	Normal overbite
	Coincident midlines
	Coordinated dental arch forms
	Proper occlusal guidance
	Periodontal health
	Temporomandibular joint health
	Balanced facial and dental esthetics
	Normal function
Specific objectives identifiable for each individual orthodontic patient	Skeletofacial objectives
	Soft tissue profile
	Occlusal plane level and cant
	Midline position
	Transverse dimension
	Vertical incisor position
	Anteroposterior incisor position
	Vertical molar position
	Anteroposterior molar position (posterior occlusion)

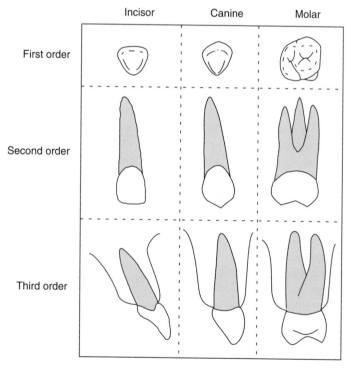

Figure 16-1 The first-order, second- order, and third-order planes commonly used in orthodontic terminology. The first-order plane represents the occlusal view, the second-order plane represents the labial (or buccal) view, and the third-order plane represents the transalveolar view.

The two primary methods of orthopedic approaches used in the treatment of malocclusions are extraoral headgear and intraoral functional appliances. Typically used for Class II treatment, each approach relies on the patient's growth for correction of the occlusal discrepancies (see Chapter 20). Many studies have analyzed the effects of these treatment approaches. These investigations have reported varying results.[3-7] The single, consistent finding has been that the patient's growth was necessary for effective treatment. Another crucial factor in treatment effectiveness is patient compliance; without cooperation, these treatment techniques cannot achieve the desired responses (see Chapter 25).

Another important early treatment stage is palatal expansion.[8] Frequently termed *rapid palatal expansion (RPE)*, this procedure is directed at skeletal crossbites caused by narrow maxillae. Heavy, orthopedic forces generated by the RPE screw broaden the maxilla through sutural expansion. The use of high loads results in separation of the sutures of the maxillary bones. The skeletal movements produced widen the transverse dimension of the maxillary dental arch. Young patients demonstrate more predictable skeletal changes because they have less interlocked sutures. Following RPE, a period of retention with the appliance itself, a palatal arch, or a removable retainer is necessary to allow remodeling and bony growth into the widened suture spaces.

SELECTION AND PLACEMENT OF FIXED APPLIANCES

Contemporary and comprehensive orthodontic therapy utilizes bonded or banded orthodontic appliances (see Chapter 14). For most orthodontists, the **edgewise bracket** is the central tool for treatment. The majority of edgewise orthodontic appliances available have specific design features that, when used properly, enhance the effectiveness and economy of treatment. Many variations of the orthodontic bracket are available. These designs are frequently termed **preadjusted appliances.** The bracket prescription describes the relationship of the bracket slot to the labial and buccal surfaces of the tooth and the long axis of the tooth. The primary differences between preadjusted bracket prescriptions are the amount of **tip** and **torque** incorporated into the bracket. Figure 16-2 contrasts differences in the second-order tip and the third-order torque between brackets with no preadjustment (zero degrees) and one with preadjustment. The central concept of the preadjusted appliance is the creation of an idealized occlusion with a rectangular arch wire that completely fills the bracket slot with minimal adjustments by the clinician.

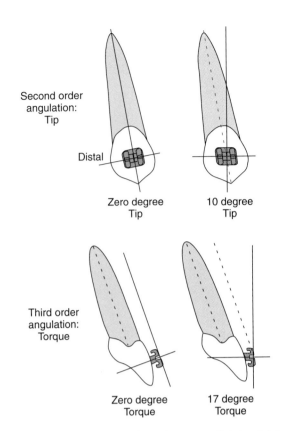

Figure 16-2 Tip and torque angulations incorporated into bracket design.

To capitalize on these design properties, accurate positioning of orthodontic brackets and bands is critical. Bracket placement is a major factor in efficient and successful treatment. Depending on the specific design, the bracket placement is determined either relative to the center of the crown or to the incisal edge/cusp tip (see Chapter 14). Whichever method is used, careful and accurate bracket placement permits the greatest amount of efficient tooth movement without excessive adjustments. Setting the bracket heights for the posterior teeth first helps minimize occlusal interferences on the attachments. The anterior brackets can be set based on the position of the molar and premolar slots.

STEPS IN THE BIOMECHANICAL MANAGEMENT OF ORTHODONTIC THERAPY

Initial Alignment

Achieving well-aligned arches is one of the first objectives in treatment (Figure 16-3). Eliminating rotations, occlusogingival and buccolingual displacements facilitate future treatment stages. **Preliminary alignment,** whether into complete arches or arch segments, simplifies future adjustments and tooth movements by eliminating significant interbracket discrepancies.

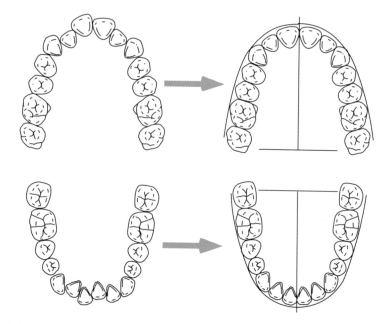

Figure 16-3 A major objective of initial alignment is the creation of well-aligned and coordinated dental arches.

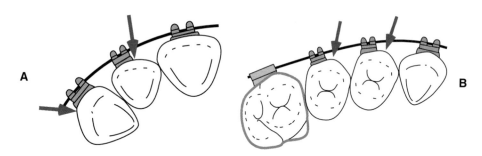

Figure 16-4 The effect of first-order bracket discrepancies on initial alignment. The brackets are aligned on the wire, but rotations of the teeth remain. **A,** The lateral incisor bracket has been placed too far distally, and the canine bracket has been placed too far mesially. **B,** Both premolar brackets are distal to the desired position. The arrows indicate the approximate position for proper bracket placement.

Initial alignment is usually obtained by the use of light, round arch wires. Common choices for arch wires at this stage are nickel/titanium alloys or braided steel wires.[9-11] Wire diameters frequently range from 0.012-inch to 0.020-inch diameter wires, depending on severity of the malalignment and bracket slot size. Nickel/titanium wires have the further advantage of superelasticity, providing a constant force on the teeth independent of the wire deflection.

Efficient clinicians avoid reflexively or automatically progressing through a sequence of arch wire sizes (i.e., arch wires should be changed purposefully). Specific clinical responses should be desired when replacing an arch wire. These early wires should be changed only if there is permanent deformation of the wire or if the wire is delivering inadequate force levels and treatment is progressing too slowly.

Toward the end of initial alignment, the brackets become well aligned on the arch wire. At this point, bracket placement discrepancies become apparent (Figure 16-4). The bracket position errors result in incorrect tooth positions even though the wire rests passively in the bracket slots. Further correction of tooth position with round wires could be obtained through placing bends in the wires to compensate for the faulty bracket position or by repositioning the bracket.

It is generally more efficient to remove and reposition brackets following initial alignment rather than placing bends in the arch wires. Both first-order and second-order bracket discrepancies should be identified and corrected at this stage by placing a new bracket more ideally on the tooth. The same light arch wire can be used until alignment is attained.

Vertical Occlusal Correction

Growth Considerations The most common vertical occlusal discrepancy is deep overbite (Figure 16-5). Correction of deep overbite is achieved through intrusion of the anterior teeth, extrusion of posterior teeth, or some combination of both.[12-13] Further, the correction can be made in the upper or lower arch. Finally, the tooth movement can be absolute or relative (i.e., associated with growth changes).

Viewed in the sagittal plane (i.e., the facial profile), normal maxillofacial growth occurs in a downward and forward direction (Figure 16-6). In general, growth in the vertical dimension (facial height) is the last to be completed. Orthodontists routinely capitalize on this growth to enhance their treatment mechanics. Relative to the correction of deep overbite, the key concern is the vertical growth of the dentoalveolar structures, which play a key role in this vertical facial growth. Differential growth of the mandible and maxilla creates a space for the vertical development of the dentoalveolus (Figure 16-7). In effect, this natural growth represents an **intermaxillary growth space** that the clinician can exploit for deep overbite correction. Differential tooth movement between the anterior and posterior teeth into this growth space allows correction of the deep overbite without changing the patient's profile features.

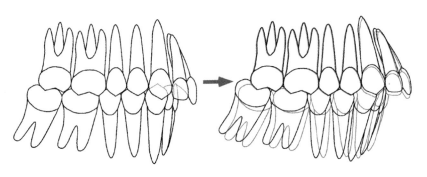

Figure 16-5 Deep overbite correction.

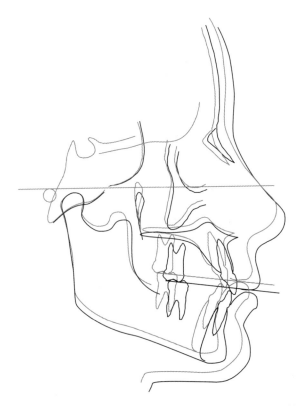

Figure 16-6 In the sagittal plane, normal facial growth occurs in a downward and forward direction.

Tooth Movements Associated with Overbite Correction Four types of tooth movement will correct a deep overbite: (1) maxillary anterior intrusion, (2) maxillary posterior extrusion, (3) mandibular anterior intrusion, and (4) mandibular posterior extrusion. Depending on the specific problems and treatment objectives for an individual patient, any or all of these movements may be used for overbite management.

Several approaches to the mechanics of overbite correction are available. **Incisor intrusion** is especially indicated in patients with excessive maxillary incisor display at rest or when smiling ("gummy smiles"). The intrusion arch (Figure 16-8) and utility arch are two techniques designed for this purpose. Both appliance designs rely on an activation of the wire at the molar tube to generate an intrusive force on the incisors. These appliances bypass the premolars and typically have activations larger than the desired tooth movement (see Chapter 15).[14-16]

Arch wires, bite plates, and occlusal wedges are common means of **posterior extrusion** (Figure 16-9). Bite plates prevent the posterior teeth from contacting, thus

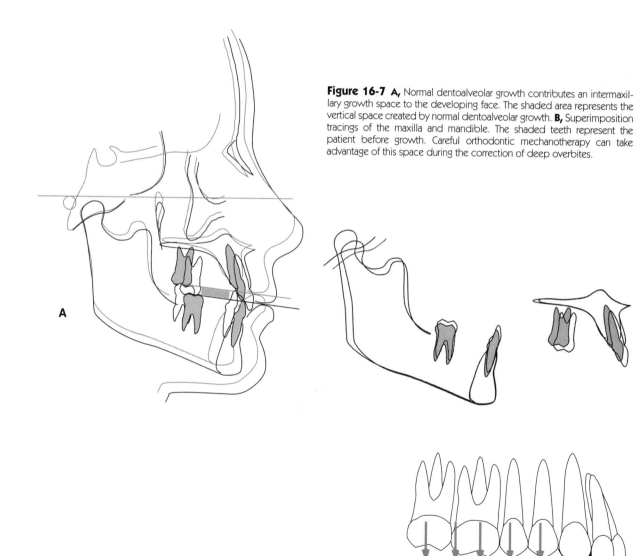

Figure 16-7 A, Normal dentoalveolar growth contributes an intermaxillary growth space to the developing face. The shaded area represents the vertical space created by normal dentoalveolar growth. **B,** Superimposition tracings of the maxilla and mandible. The shaded teeth represent the patient before growth. Careful orthodontic mechanotherapy can take advantage of this space during the correction of deep overbites.

A

B

Figure 16-8 The intrusion arch.

Figure 16-9 Bite plates for facilitating posterior eruption.

they allow an accelerated development of the posterior dentoalveolar area. Vertical elastics are frequently combined with bite plates to quickly obtain bite opening.

The use of a reverse curve arch wire is another common approach to the management of deep overbite (Figure 16-10). These wires provide both an intrusive force on the anterior teeth and an eruptive force on the posterior teeth. As the forces created by these arch wires suggest, this mode of overbite cor-

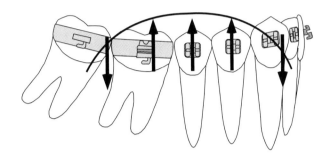

Figure 16-10 A reverse curve of Spee arch wire.

rection typically results in a combination of both tooth movements.

Relative vs. Absolute Tooth Movements It is important to emphasize the concepts of relative and absolute tooth movements. In growing patients, "holding" the anterior teeth against normal vertical growth appears to intrude the incisors, thereby normalizing the overbite. Relative to the growing posterior dentoalveolar structures, these incisors appear to be intruded (Figure 16-11). On the other hand, in non-growing patients, any vertical tooth movements result in absolute intrusion or extrusion of the teeth. The teeth are repositioned relative to each other and to their skeletal support structures.

Effect of Posterior Tooth Extrusion on the Face Finally, the effect of the vertical tooth position must be considered in relation to the patient's vertical facial dimensions. Excessive eruption of the posterior teeth increases the patient's vertical dimension with a

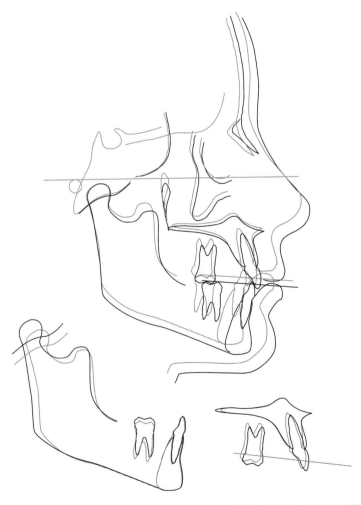

Figure 16-11 Relative intrusion occurs when the anterior teeth are maintained in their vertical position within a growing face. Notice that deep overbite is corrected but that the incisor position is unchanged in the regional superimpositions of the maxilla and mandible.

resultant backward mandibular rotation (Figure 16-12). Indiscriminate extrusion of posterior teeth on a non-growing patient hinges the mandible open, increasing the vertical dimension of occlusion, the lower face height, the mandibular plane angle, and the convexity of the profile. In cases with a steep mandibular plane and an open bite tendency, extrusion of the posterior teeth may adversely affect the patient's appearance and may be detrimental to the long-term stability of the treatment. Extrusion of the posterior teeth may be indicated in growing patients with deep overbite and a flat mandibular plane.

Anteroposterior Correction

The major objective in malocclusions involving the anteroposterior relationship between the upper and lower arches is obtaining a normal overjet and a Class I canine relationship. In most cases, a Class I molar relationship is also a goal (Figure 16-13). However, in uniarch extraction treatments the molar occlusion may be either Class II or Class III, depending on the location of the extractions. Extraction of only upper premolars aims to achieve a Class II molar relationship and Class I canine relationship (see Chapter 20).

Anchorage Control The principle factor determining the success of treatment is **anchorage control.** Essentially, anchorage control involves the ability to achieve differential tooth movement, most frequently the relative mesiodistal movement of the anterior and posterior teeth (Figure 16-14).

Maximum posterior anchorage involves retraction of the incisors and canines without mesial movement of the premolars and molars (see Figure 16-14, A). **Reciprocal anchorage** is equal movement of the posterior teeth mesially and the anterior teeth distally (see Figure 16-14, B). **Maximum anterior anchorage** requires protraction of the posterior teeth mesially without retraction of the incisors and canines (Figure 16-14, C).

Anchorage control is established in a variety of ways.[17] **Extraoral appliances,** such as headgear, are frequently prescribed for anchorage control. Headgear is used as an attempt to secure the posterior teeth to extraoral structures. Additionally, the forces delivered from most headgears should exceed the mesiodistal force levels of the elastics or springs used for retraction of the anterior segment.

Intermaxillary elastics pit the upper teeth to the lower teeth and are another common means of gaining differential tooth movement. The direction of the

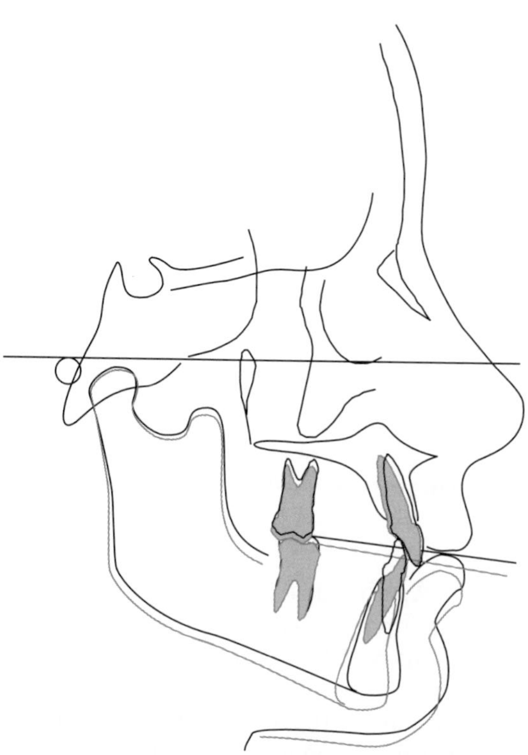

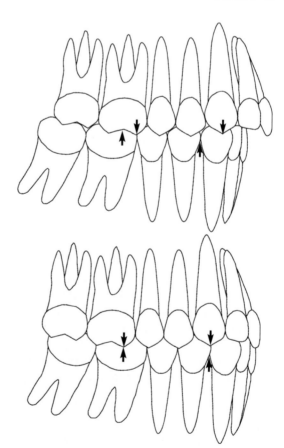

Figure 16-12 Inappropriate extrusion of the posterior teeth results in a backward rotation of the mandible. Backward rotation results in an increase in vertical facial height and an increase in facial convexity.

Figure 16-13 Anteroposterior correction of the occlusion focuses on improving the overjet, canine, and molar relationships.

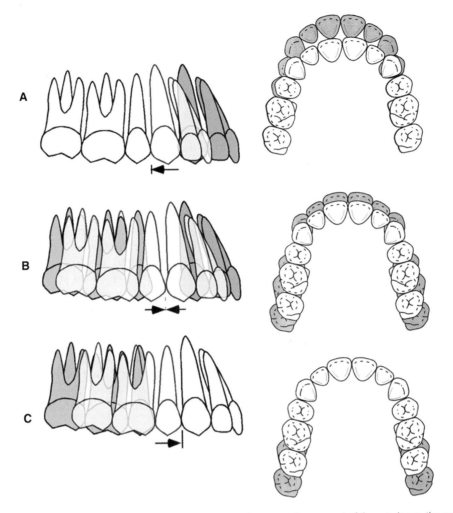

Figure 16-14 Orthodontic anchorage describes the desired amount of movement of the anterior vs. the posterior teeth. Maximum posterior anchorage holds the molar and premolar teeth in position while retracting the anterior teeth. Maximum anterior anchorage holds the incisor position while protracting the posterior teeth.

elastic defines its force vector and the terminology used to describe it. Class II elastics attach to the anterior maxillary teeth and the posterior mandibular teeth (Figure 16-15, *A*). Thus a Class II elastic acts to correct a Class II relationship by providing a retraction force to the upper anterior teeth and a simultaneous protraction force to the lower molars. Alternatively, a Class III elastic hooks from the lower anterior teeth to the upper posterior teeth, creating a force for lower anterior retraction and upper posterior protraction for the resolution of a Class III occlusion (Figure 16-15, *B*).

The major limitation in the use of either headgear or elastics as an anchorage technique is their dependence on patient compliance. Without patient cooperation these methods are incapable of influencing the treatment results. Many approaches have been devised to eliminate patient compliance as a crucial factor in anchorage control. Ultimately, these techniques attempt to establish anchorage with intraarch appliance designs.

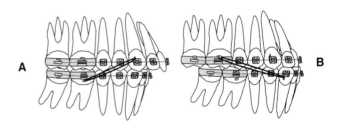

Figure 16-15 A, Class II elastics. **B,** Class III elastics.

Intraarch Anchorage   Two simple techniques used to augment intraarch anchorage include the use of palatal buttons and lip bumpers. The **Nance holding arch** attaches a small acrylic pad to a palatal arch that rests on the palatal rugae. This method relies on the palatal structures to aid in resisting mesial migration of the molars during anterior retraction. **Lip bumpers** extend from the lower molar forward (anterior) to the labial vestibule. Inserted into headgear tubes on the

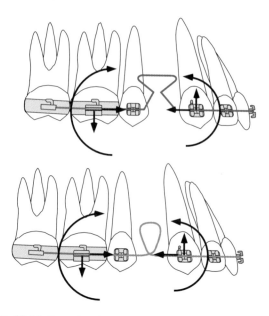

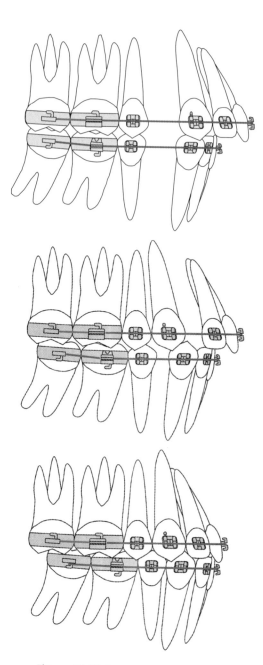

Figure 16-16 Examples of loop designs created for space closure and anchorage control.

Figure 16-17 Separate canine retraction.

molars, these designs depend on lip pressure to either cause distal molar movement or prevent mesial molar movement (see Chapter 15).

Rather than basing anchorage on anatomic features, orthodontic spring and loop designs are aimed to produce differential tooth movement by controlling the force system applied to the teeth.[18-22] By producing a force system that applies different pressures to the anterior vs. the posterior teeth, various spring designs have been suggested to provide anchorage control during treatment (Figure 16-16). The cardinal feature of each is the production of an anchorage-enhancing force system. The selection of any individual design is generally at the discretion and experience of the operator.

Another approach to enhance posterior anchorage control during space closure is by the separate canine retraction (Figure 16-17). Some orthodontists prefer this technique because it is perceived to be beneficial in preserving the position of the posterior teeth. Conceptually, **separate canine retraction** is seen as being less taxing on anchorage because two canine teeth are opposed by several posterior teeth in the anchor unit. Another indication for initial canine retraction is creating space between the two canines to allow for incisor alignment when there is severe crowding.

As the anteroposterior treatment objectives are achieved by the retraction of the canines and incisors, a careful evaluation of the results of this phase of treatment is in order. Three types of undesirable tooth movements need to be evaluated toward the end of this stage of treatment (Figure 16-18): (1) mesial-in rotation of the molars, (2), tipping of the canine or premolar into

the extraction space (in cases with premolar extraction) and (3) excessive lingual inclination of the incisors.

Because of the mechanical force acting on the molars during this stage of treatment, these teeth tend to rotate mesially. The effect of this rotation is to move the mesiobuccal cusp of an upper molar toward a Class II relationship. Precise analysis of the tooth position may reveal that proper occlusion can be reestablished with correcting the rotation of the molar rather than moving it distally.

Closure of the extraction spaces should not be considered complete until root alignment of the adjacent teeth is accomplished. The correction of axial inclination

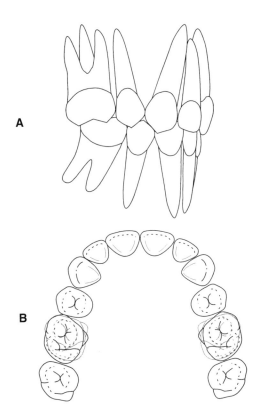

Figure 16-18 Common tooth movement side effects following space closure. **A,** Tipping of the canine and premolar into the extraction space and excessive lingual inclination of the incisors. **B,** Mesial-in rotation of the molars.

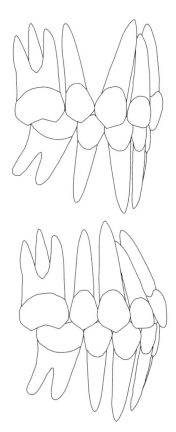

Figure 16-19 Correction of the axial inclination and root position of the teeth.

problems marks the beginning of the next stage of orthodontic treatment. A panoramic film would be helpful for such an evaluation.

Torque and Axial Inclination Correction

Root correction, or paralleling the long axes of the roots of the teeth, and establishing the proper inclination of the teeth within their basal bone are major objectives of this stage of treatment (Figure 16-19). This stage is directed at second-order root movement of the teeth adjacent to the extraction sites as well as the third-order correction of the inclination of the teeth, especially the incisors.

The clinical observation of tooth contact between the canine and the second premolar is not the sole criterion signaling the end of space closure. If the teeth have tipped toward one another, the root apices may be widely divergent (see Figure 16-19). The root parallelism must be evaluated. Clinically, root alignment can be assessed by examining the tip of the crowns of the canine and premolar, checking for marginal ridge discrepancies, and palpating the root prominence of

these teeth especially at the apices. As stated previously, a radiographic evaluation may be useful.

Third-order correction of the incisors creates the proper position of the teeth over the supporting alveolar bone. Retraction of the incisors may tip them lingually creating a large interincisal angle. Lingual movement of the incisor roots to obtain an ideal occlusion is termed *torque.*

Third-order plane correction, or torque control, is the major emphasis of this stage of treatment. Rectangular wires in a preadjusted edgewise bracket are used in an attempt to automate these tooth movements. The angulation of the bracket slot relative to the long axis of the tooth provides a means for a rectangular arch wire to achieve the desired buccolingual root movement (Figure 16-20).

With ideal bracket positions and large rectangular arch wires, the brackets are designed to produce normal occlusal relationships and to reduce the potential for occlusal interferences. The promoters of each bracket prescription believe that their designs reduce the need for too many individualized bends in an arch wire. Unfortunately, the wide variation in the individual anatomy of each tooth makes such an objective dif-

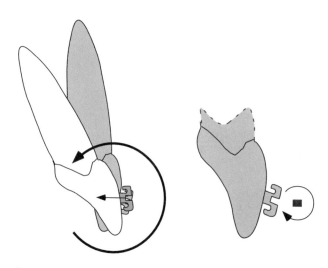

Figure 16-20 Inserting rectangular wires into rectangular bracket slots produces torque or rotational movements of the teeth.

ficult, if not impossible, to accomplish for any given individual. As a result, the clinician regularly needs to incorporate bends in the arch wires to obtain proper tooth alignment.

Finishing and Occlusal Detailing

If each of the previous steps in treatment were perfectly executed, orthodontic finishing and occlusal detailing should be minimized. However, most cases require specific attention to **finishing details** (Figure 16-21). This fine-tuning of individualized tooth position and occlusion optimizes the treatment result.[23] As in many disciplines, these refinements require a concerted commitment by the clinician to obtain the best results.

A systematic examination of all aspects of the outcome of treatment will identify any remaining discrepancies.[24-26] The first-, second-, and third-order positions of each tooth should be assessed relative to their ideal positions. The actual results obtained should be evaluated relative to both the specific objectives of the treatment plan and the general objectives of all well-treated orthodontic cases (see Box 16-1).

A wide array of finishing techniques may be used to complete orthodontic treatment. Small-diameter, formable arch wires (i.e., 0.016-inch stainless steel) that easily allow fine, precise bends in the wire are frequently used in detailing. Alternatively, rectangular beta-titanium wires are sufficiently flexible to be used for finishing when third-order control is necessary. Subtlety to finishing bends is critical because these tooth movements tend to be small. Another key is awareness of the undesirable side effects of

introducing interbracket bends in an arch wire such as V bends and step bends that produce predictable tooth movements. Careful attention to the size and position of these bends can minimize any potential problems.[27,28]

Another approach is to use vertical elastics to aid occlusal settling. Interlacing elastics between the upper and lower posterior teeth can direct and speed the interdigitation of the occlusion. These elastics can also be angled either in a Class II or a Class III vector, depending on the specific needs during finishing.

Retention

Active orthodontic treatment ends with the removal of the bands and brackets. The **retention phase** of treatment typically is followed by the insertion of either fixed (bonded) or removable retainers. During retention the objective is to maintain the corrections made while monitoring the continuing maturation and development of the patient. Much of this stage of treatment is observational to ensure the long-term stability.

No one appliance or approach to retention is indicated for all patients. **Removable appliances** (Hawley retainers) have certain advantages over bonded retainers, including (1) variability of design, especially the option of incorporating springs for minor tooth movement, (2) better oral hygiene, and (3) flexibility in the amount of time the patient wears the retainers. Compliance is a major issue during retention. Failing to follow retainer wear guidelines may result in relapse of the malocclusion. Another disadvantage of removable retainers is the propensity for breaking or losing the appliance.

Bonded (fixed) retainers are especially popular for the lower anterior teeth. These teeth have the greatest probability of postorthodontic treatment movement and continue to confound many orthodontists with their predilection for misalignment. The use of fixed retainers may minimize this problem. Fixed retainers come in many varieties, from heavy steel bars bonded to the lingual surface of the lower canines to light braided wires bonded to all six lower anterior teeth. Bonded retainers effectively eliminate the possibility of undesirable tooth movement, but they present alternative concerns. Oral hygiene in the area of the bonded retainer can be a major problem. Care must be taken during the placement of the bonded retainers to avoid creating overhangs or plaque traps. Also, breakage of fixed retainers requires considerable time and effort to repair. Finally, the permanence of the retainer is an issue. Whether these retainers should be considered lifetime appliances remains controversial.

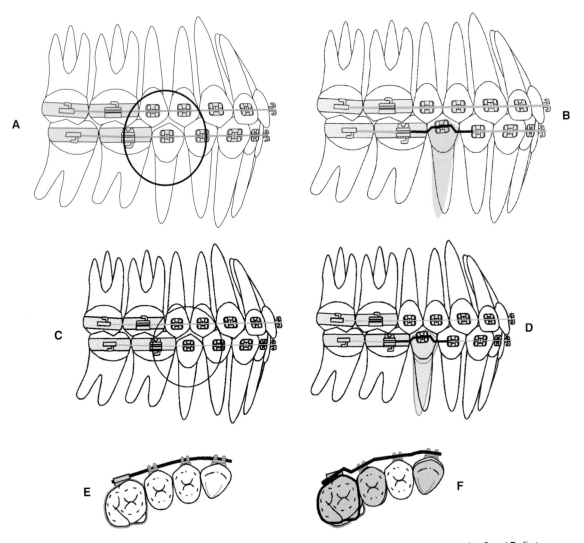

Figure 16-21 Finishing details. **A** and **B,** Occlusal step to upright and elevate the second premolar. **C** and **D,** First-order details depicting mesial-out rotation of second premolar and first molar and improving canine prominence. **E** and **F,** Occlusal view detailing the correction of the molar rotation with an offset, toe-in bends, and premolar bends.

SEQUENCING MECHANICS

Because patients and their individual problems vary widely, orthodontic treatment generally cannot be properly delivered with a few simple standardized formulas. Every patient must be individually evaluated and the treatment plan appropriately specific. This requires critical analysis of the patient's problems and thoughtful treatment planning to allow the selection of alternative treatment strategies. Thus the sequence of treatment for orthodontic patients may vary greatly between individuals.

The specific sequence of treatment mechanics should be selected to maximize treatment efficiency. When possible, treatment may be "telescoped" (i.e., multiple problems addressed simultaneously). Ideally, all tooth movements proceed consistently toward the treatment goal; one stage of treatment should not undo the results of a prior stage. Avoiding the repetition of treatment stages has a significant impact on the efficiency of care and the overall treatment time. Therefore considering alternative treatment mechanisms, selecting appropriate treatment mechanics, and sequencing them appropriately for each specific patient will maximize the benefits, efficiency, and effectiveness of treatment.

One of the attractive challenges of orthodontics is the problem solving required in planning treatment. Imagination and creative thinking expand the means available for patient-centered care. Innovations developed for unique problems frequently lead to superior methods of providing efficient treatment.

SUMMARY

The steps of orthodontic treatment should not be viewed as an inviolate protocol. Certain aspects of orthodontic treatment follow common paths with similar interim objectives but the particular sequence of tooth movements and the tactics used to achieve them may vary widely between patients as well as between orthodontists.

Early treatment best addresses severe skeletofacial problems or intercepts potential problems such as those associated with premature loss of teeth or parafunctional habits. Efficient, comprehensive orthodontic treatment requires careful analysis and coordination between diagnosis and treatment. Fixed appliance treatment depends on a systematic understanding of various approaches for the correction of various malocclusions. In general, the steps of treatment include (1) preliminary alignment to establish coordinated and regular arch forms; (2) the resolution of vertical discrepancies, especially the correction of deep overbites, to prepare the dentition for anterior tooth retraction; (3) reducing the overjet through anterior retraction, which requires careful posterior anchorage control; (4) third-order tooth movements to provide optimal tooth inclination over the basal bone; (5) occlusal detailing and finishing, which require a critical examination of the patient and an exacting approach to the final tooth movements to provide an esthetic and functional occlusion; and (6) retention aims to maintain the treatment effects and improve the long-term stability of the results.

REFERENCES

1. Kuhlberg AJ, Glynn E: Treatment planning considerations for adult orthodontic patients, *Dent Clin North Am* 41:17-27, 1997.
2. Lindauer SJ: *Orthodontic treatment planning: biomechanics in clinical orthodontics*, Philadelphia, 1996, WB Saunders.
3. Bishara SE, Ziaja RR: Functional appliances: a review, *Am J Orthod Dentofacial Orthop* 95:250-258, 1989.
4. Ghafari J et al: Headgear versus function regulator in the early treatment of Class II, division 1 malocclusion: a randomized clinical trial, *Am J Orthod Dentofacial Orthop* 113:51-61, 1998.
5. Gianelly AA: One-phase versus two-phase treatment, *Am J Orthod Dentofacial Orthop* 108:556-559, 1995.
6. Johnston LE: Growth and the Class II patient: rendering unto Caesar, *Semin Orthod* 4:59-62, 1998.
7. Pancherz H: The effects, limitations and long-term dentofacial adaptations to treatment with the Herbst appliance, *Semin Orthod* 3:232-243, 1997.
8. Haas AJ: Palatal expansion: just the beginning of dentofacial orthopedics, *Am J Orthod* 57:219-255, 1970.
9. Burstone CJ, Qin B, Morton JY: Chinese NiTi wire, *Am J Orthod* 87:445-452, 1985.
10. Burstone CJ: Variable modulus orthodontics, *Am J Orthod* 80:1-16, 1981.
11. Lopez I, Goldberg AJ, Burstone CJ: Bending characteristics of nitinol wire, *Am J Orthod* 75:569-574, 1979.
12. Schudy FF: The control of vertical overbite in clinical orthodontics, *Angle Orthod* 38:19-38, 1968.
13. Ricketts R: Bioprogressive therapy as an answer to orthodontic needs: Part I, *Am J Orthod* 70:241-268, 1976.
14. Burstone CJ: Deep overbite correction by intrusion, *Am J Orthod* 72:1-22, 1977.
15. Shroff B et al: Simultaneous intrusion and retraction using a three-piece base arch, *Angle Orthod* 67:455-456, 1997.
16. Nanda R, Marzban R, Kuhlberg A: The Connecticut intrusion arch, *J Clin Orthod* 32:708-715, 1998.
17. Nanda R, Kuhlberg AJ: *Biomechanics of extraction space closure: biomechanics in clinical orthodontics*, Philadelphia, 1996, WB Saunders.
18. Burstone CJ: The segmented arch approach to space closure, *Am J Orthod* 82:361-378, 1982.
19. Kuhlberg AJ, Burstone CJ: "T"-loop position and anchorage control, *Am J Orthod Dentofacial Orthop* 112:12-18, 1997.
20. Firouz T, Kuhlberg AJ, Nanda R: Efficacy of extraction space closure by precalibrated T-springs, *IOK* 3:663-674, 1998.
21. Thompson WJ: Combination anchorage technique, *Am J Orthod Dentofacial Orthop* 93:363-379, 1988.
22. Root TL: Level anchorage system for correction of orthodontic malocclusions, *Am J Orthod* 80:395-410, 1981.
23. Andrews LE: The six keys to normal occlusion, *Am J Orthod* 62:296-309, 1972.
24. Poling A: A method of finishing the occlusion, *Am J Orthod Dentofacial Orthop* 115:476-487, 1999.
25. Zachrisson BU: Excellence in finishing, Part I, *J Clin Orthod* 20:460-468, 1986.
26. Zachrisson BU: Excellence in finishing, Part II, *J Clin Orthod* 20:536-559, 1986.
27. Burstone CJ, Koenig HA: Creative wire bending: the force system from step and V bends, *Am J Orthod Dentofacial Orthop* 93:59-67, 1988.
28. Burstone CJ, Koenig HA: Force systems from an ideal arch, *Am J Orthod* 65:270-289, 1974.

SECTION IV

Treatment and Treatment Considerations

CHAPTER 17

Orthodontic Treatment in the Primary Dentition

Michael J. Kanellis

KEY TERMS

primary dentition
orthodontic intervention
space management
root development
primary incisors
primary molars

primary canines
unilateral
digit and pacifier habits
psychoanalytic theory
learning theorists

prolonged habit
digit habits
Class II malocclusions
distal step
Class III malocclusions

functional shift
anterior open bite
deep bites
posterior crossbites
crowding and spacing

The primary objective of managing orthodontic problems in the **primary dentition** is to intercept or correct malocclusions that would otherwise be maintained or become progressively more complex in the permanent dentition or result in skeletal anomalies. **Orthodontic intervention** in the primary dentition does not always prevent orthodontic problems from occurring in the permanent dentition; however, there can be significant advantages to early intervention. By identifying and treating certain problems at an early age it is often possible either to prevent more serious orthodontic problems from developing or to redirect skeletal growth and improve the occlusal relationship. The purpose of this chapter is to identify common situations and malocclusions in the primary dentition that lend themselves to early intervention.

SPACE MANAGEMENT IN THE PRIMARY DENTITION

Space management is necessary when a child loses a primary tooth prematurely, either from caries or trauma. Placement of a space maintainer should be considered. The premature loss of primary teeth can lead to orthodontic problems later if the resulting space is not adequately maintained. However, not all teeth lost prematurely require space maintenance. The potential for orthodontic problems depends on multiple factors, including the age at which tooth loss occurs and which teeth are involved. Many factors should be considered in decision making: (1) root development, (2) the distance between the permanent tooth and the alveolar crest, and (3) the position of the tooth in the dental arch.

Root Development

When a primary tooth is lost prematurely, radiographic examination can assist the clinician in determining whether a space maintainer is necessary. If it is determined that the eruption of the permanent tooth is imminent, no space maintenance is required. The amount of **root development** on the succedaneous tooth can help predict how much longer it will be until the permanent tooth will erupt. The extent of root development is believed to be the most reliable predictor of readiness for eruption. Tooth eruption generally occurs when root development is 75% of the future total root length.[1] Regardless of the chronologic age of the patient, if sufficient root development exists on the succedaneous tooth, space maintenance may be needed for just a short period or not at all.

248

Distance between the Permanent Tooth and the Alveolar Crest

Another factor to consider in predicting how long it will be until the permanent tooth erupts is the amount of bone overlying the succedaneous tooth (as measured on bitewing or periapical radiographs). It has been demonstrated that erupting premolars generally move through bone at the rate of 1 mm every 4 to 5 months.[2]

Position of the Tooth in the Dental Arch

When **primary incisors** are prematurely lost, either from caries or from trauma, space maintenance is generally not a concern as long as the primary canines have already erupted into occlusion. Although premature loss of an incisor at this stage of development may still result in the adjacent teeth tipping into the space available from the tooth loss, overall arch length and width generally remain unchanged.[3] When the loss of a primary incisor occurs before the complete eruption of the primary canine, however, space maintenance is recommended to prevent loss of arch space. Space maintenance in these instances is difficult because of the age of the patient and because of esthetic concerns. Maintaining the space of an incisor is often best accomplished by fabricating a fixed appliance bilaterally anchored to the first **primary molars** and including prosthetic teeth to replace the missing incisors (Figure 17-1).

The premature loss of **primary canines** either from trauma or caries is relatively rare. More common is the premature loss of primary canines from the eruption of permanent incisors in cases with inadequate arch length. If the canine loss is **unilateral,** there is often a shift in the position of the permanent incisors toward the side of the loss, creating a midline deviation. The extraction of the contralateral primary canine and the placement of a fixed lower lingual holding arch can prevent undesired drifting of the teeth from occurring (Figure 17-2). In these cases, a mixed dentition space analysis should be conducted to determine the extent of the space discrepancy (see Chapter 12).

The early loss of a first primary molar in the primary dentition is always of concern; space maintenance is routinely recommended. Without adequate space maintenance, eruption of the permanent first molar can cause mesial drifting of the second primary molar. In addition, the eruption of the permanent lateral incisors can cause distal drifting of the primary canines. These movements reduce the space available for the unerupted first premolar. The space maintainer of choice in this situation would be either a band and loop space maintainer or a crown and loop space maintainer (Figures 17-3 and 17-4).

The decision regarding space maintenance following the loss of a first primary molar in the mixed dentition is not as straightforward. It has been suggested that the space loss resulting from early loss of first primary molars is caused by the mesial migration of the second primary molars during the eruption of the first permanent molars. If the permanent first molars are fully erupted, however, and they are in a solid Class I relationship (cuspal interlock), there is controversy regarding whether or not space maintenance is necessary at all.[4] Cuspal interlock is believed to minimize the mesial shifting of permanent molars following early loss of primary molars. Much of the space loss in this situation, however, is attributed to the distal drifting of the primary canines.[5] For this reason, strong consideration should be given to the placement of a space maintainer following the premature loss of a first primary molar, even in situations with good Class I interdigitation of the first permanent molars.

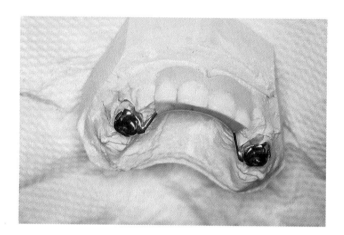

Figure 17-1 Cosmetic space maintainer replacing maxillary incisors extracted because of caries.

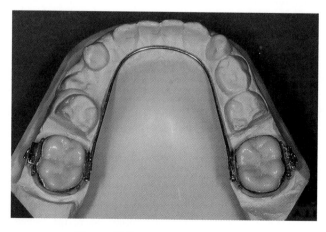

Figure 17-2 Lower lingual holding arch.

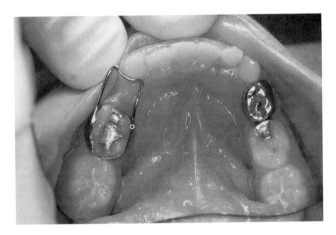

Figure 17-3 Band and loop space maintainer.

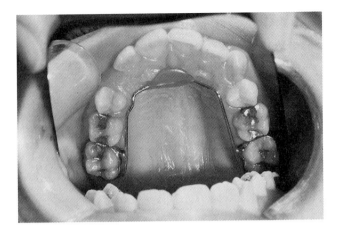

Figure 17-5 Nance holding arch.

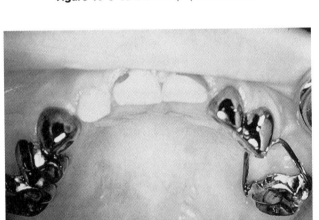

Figure 17-4 Crown and loop space maintainer.

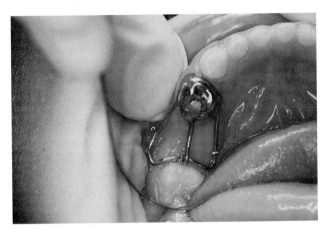

Figure 17-6 Distal shoe space maintainer following eruption of the permanent first molar.

If the premature loss of a first primary molar in the mixed dentition is unilateral, the space maintainer of choice is still either a band and loop or a crown and loop space maintainer. If the loss is bilateral, however, and the first permanent molars and permanent incisors have sufficiently erupted, either a lingual holding arch (mandibular arch) or a Nance holding arch (maxillary arch) can be the space maintainer of choice (see Figures 17-2 and 17-5).

When a second primary molar is lost prematurely, space maintenance is almost always recommended. When the loss occurs before the eruption of the first permanent molar, the space maintainer of choice is the distal shoe appliance (Figure 17-6). This appliance is designed to guide the unerupted permanent molar into position and, if properly constructed, can adequately maintain space following its eruption. Some authors have discouraged the use of the distal shoe appliance because of concerns about infection and potential breakage and have instead recommended allowing the first permanent molar to erupt before

placing a space maintainer.[6] This scenario, however, often leads to space loss and a need for active orthodontic treatment following eruption. Occasionally there are cases when distal shoe appliances may be medically contraindicated and alternative pressure appliances (fixed or removable) have been described in the literature.[7] These fixed or removable appliances put pressure on the soft tissues just forward of the unerupted permanent molars without penetrating the soft tissue. They are preferred over fixed appliances in the primary dentition when both first and second primary molars have been prematurely lost.

DIGIT AND PACIFIER HABITS

Considerable controversy exists on the topic of thumb, finger, and pacifier sucking (nonnutritive sucking) regarding the potential harm these **digit and pacifier habits** present to the developing occlusion and treatment recommendations. In infancy and early childhood, nonnutritive sucking is considered a normal condition.[8] Most children outgrow the need for nonnutritive sucking by 3 years of age. **Psychoanalytic theory** suggests that children who continue much beyond this age have some "underlying psychologic disturbance." **Learning theorists,** however, consider nonnutritive sucking to be a learned habit and do not believe it is necessarily a sign of psychologic problems. In their review of the literature, Johnson and Larson[8] concluded that there is significant evidence supporting the learning theory over the psychoanalytic theory, but that in some patients a prolonged habit may be the result of underlying psychologic or emotional problems. Therefore it is important for the clinician to distinguish children with potential psychologic disturbances and those that have "empty" habits.

Prolonged habits can have deleterious effects on the occlusion. The extent of these effects varies from case to case, depending on a wide range of variables including the actual habit employed, the duration and intensity of the habit, and the inherent dental and skeletal relationship. Some of the negative sequelae associated with prolonged digit-sucking habits include a higher incidence of anterior open bite, maxillary incisor protrusion, Class II canine relationship, distal step molar relationship, posterior crossbites, lip incompetence, increased tongue thrust, and speech defects.[8-10]

Following habit cessation, there is generally some spontaneous correction of the malocclusion. The extent to which malocclusions self-correct varies depending on the age of the patient at the time of habit cessation as well as the severity of the malocclusion resulting from the habit. In general, there is a reduction of the dental open bite and a decrease in maxillary incisor proclination.[8] Anteroposterior dental and skeletal changes associated with or caused by prolonged **digit habits** (e.g., Class II malocclusion) are much less likely to self-correct than are the anterior dental changes.

The decision regarding whether or not to interfere with a nonnutritive sucking habit in the primary dentition should be guided by the following factors: (1) if the digit sucking is associated with a distal step molar relationship (developing Class II malocclusion), the skeletal malocclusion generally worsens the longer the habit continues; (2) if the child is developing a Class III malocclusion or is prognathic, digit-sucking habits are believed to be less deleterious and may in fact be beneficial for dental development[11]; and (3) anterior open bites secondary to digit sucking do not generally need to be treated because spontaneous correction generally occurs following habit cessation, especially if the habit ceases before 9 years of age.[12]

Several additional factors should be taken into consideration before deciding whether to treat thumbsucking or digit-sucking habits: (1) extent of the malocclusion—if there is no malocclusion associated with a prolonged digit habit, there seems to be little dental rationale for intervening; (2) potential for self-correction of malocclusion—even if self-correction is not likely, it is important to realize that subsequent orthodontic treatment will have greater stability once the causative habit ceases; and (3) attitude of the child—in all instances it is important for the child to be involved in the decision making so that the child does not view the intervention as a punishment.

When habit treatment is recommended, it has been suggested that timing of treatment be determined on a case-by-case basis.[13] In most cases, treatment for a prolonged nonnutritive sucking habit should be initiated between the age of 4 years and the eruption of the permanent incisors.[13]

Treatment options can include relaxation and mental imagery, behavior modification (using rewards, encouragement, and reminders), and appliance therapy.[13-16] Davidson et al[17] found that appliance therapy using a palatal crib (see Figure 17-14) was more effective than psychologic treatment in a study of 65 thumbsucking subjects between the ages of 4 and 12 years. Of the 22 children who received palatal crib therapy in Davidson's study, 100% were successfully able to break their habit within a 10-month period.

CLASS II MALOCCLUSIONS

Developing **Class II malocclusions** in the primary dentition are typically associated with a **distal step** terminal plane relationship of the second primary molars (Figure 17-7). Other identifying factors include an end-to-end or Class II primary canine relationship and excessive overjet or overbite. The causes of Class II molar relationships can be either genetic or environmental. As mentioned previously, children with persistent digit-sucking habits have a higher incidence of Class II molar and canine relationships and larger overjets than do children without sucking habits.[18-19]

The association between distal step malocclusions in the primary dentition and Class II malocclusions in the mixed and permanent dentition is well documented. Baccetti et al[20] have shown that all Class II features in the primary dentition are maintained or worsen during the transition to the mixed dentition. Class II malocclusions in the primary dentition should, therefore, be considered highly predictive of Class II malocclusions in the mixed and permanent dentitions (see Chapter 5).

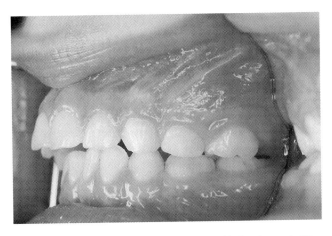

Figure 17-7 Distal step terminal plane relationship in primary dentition (highly predictive of Class II malocclusion in the permanent dentition).

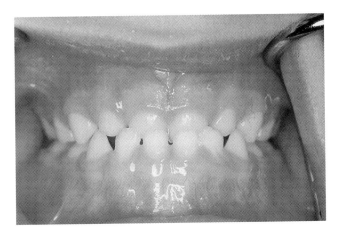

Figure 17-8 Anterior crossbite in the primary dentition.

Treatment to correct Class II malocclusions can be initiated in the primary dentition, although there is little documentation in the literature regarding the long-term effectiveness of treating this type of malocclusion in children this young. The vast majority of treatment decisions for Class II malocclusions are made in the mixed and early permanent dentitions (see Chapter 20).

Occasionally, severe Class II malocclusions can accompany certain genetic or congenital disorders including Pierre Robin syndrome, where the Class II malocclusion results from a micrognathic mandible.

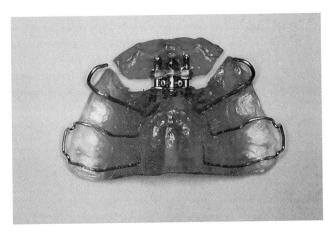

Figure 17-9 Maxillary removable appliance designed to correct anterior crossbite.

CLASS III MALOCCLUSIONS

Developing **Class III malocclusions** are clinically expressed as anterior crossbites in the primary dentition. They can be dental, functional, or skeletal in origin. Cephalometric radiographs can be helpful in making the distinction between dental and skeletal problems, and cephalometric norms for this age group are available (see Chapter 11).[21-23] To aid in diagnosis the clinician should evaluate the following parameters: the patient's profile, the inclination of the maxillary and mandibular incisors, and the presence of a **functional shift** between centric relation and centric occlusion. Dental anterior crossbites often present with end-to-end incisor interference, resulting in a functional shift of the mandible in a forward direction. With skeletal Class III malocclusions it is often impossible to manipulate the mandible into an end-to-end incisor relationship.

Several authors have recommended that dental anterior crossbites in the primary dentition be corrected when identified to allow for normal dental development and a more favorable skeletal growth.[24-26] Inclined planes and removable acrylic appliances

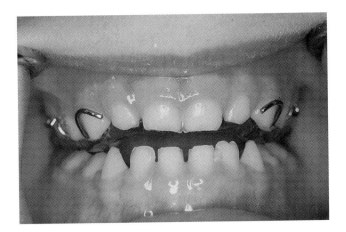

Figure 17-10 Acrylic coverage of occlusal surfaces "unlocks" anterior crossbite while appliance is being worn.

can be used for the correction of dental anterior crossbites (Figures 17-8 through 17-11). Chin cups and reverse-pull face masks (Figure 17-12) can be used to treat skeletal Class III malocclusions (see Chapter 21).[27-30]

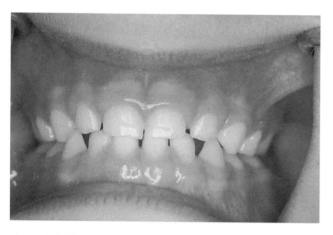

Figure 17-11 Following correction of anterior crossbites, positive overbite and overjet often make retention unnecessary.

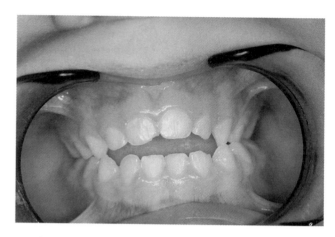

Figure 17-13 Anterior open bite associated with pacifier use.

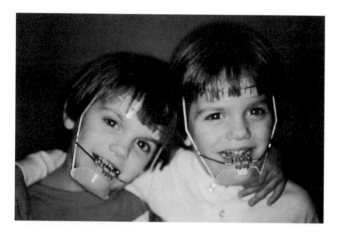

Figure 17-12 Identical twins with skeletal Class III malocclusions wearing reverse-pull face masks.

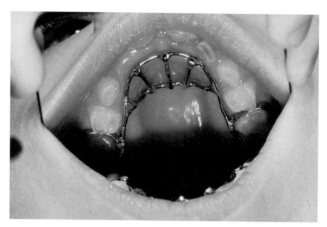

Figure 17-14 Fixed palatal crib appliance designed to discourage digit habit.

ANTERIOR OPEN BITE

Anterior open bite in the primary dentition is the most frequent malocclusion associated with persistent digit and pacifier sucking (Figure 17-13).[31] Fukuta et al[31] reported an increased tendency for malocclusions to occur in the permanent dentition in children who continue digit-sucking habits past the age of 4 years.

Many interventions are available for the treatment of anterior open bites caused by a digit or pacifier habit. As stated previously, treatment options range from giving the child more time to discontinue the habit, offering behavioral therapy for habit cessation, and placing an inactive fixed appliance to discourage the habit. The habit appliance generally consists of two orthodontic bands on the second primary molars and a palatal crib covering the anterior part of the palate (Figure 17-14). Active orthodontic treatment of open bites in the primary dentition usually involves a removable appliance. The long-term clinical outcomes of such treatment are not well documented.

DEEP BITE

Anterior **deep bites** in the primary dentition are fairly common but are rarely treated. They may be associated with the presence of developing Class II malocclusions. As with Class II malocclusions, treatment decisions are typically postponed until the mixed dentition. Indications for treatment in the primary dentition include impingement on the palatal mucosa, excessive grinding, clenching, and headaches if they are believed to be secondary to the deep bite (Figures 17-15 to 17-18).

POSTERIOR CROSSBITE

Posterior crossbites are relatively common in the primary dentition with incidences ranging from 7% to 17%.[32] They are believed to be genetic or hereditary in nature or to be caused by prolonged digit or pacifier habits. From a clinical perspective, the majority of

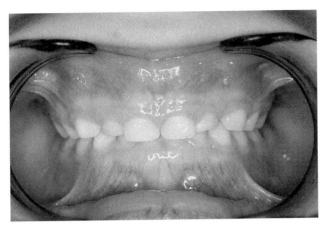

Figure 17-15 A 4-year-old patient presenting with deep bite and chief complaint of clenching, grinding, and headaches.

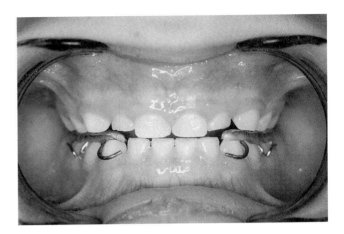

Figure 17-17 Patient with appliance in place.

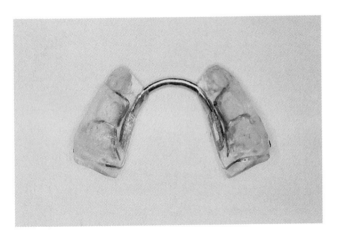

Figure 17-16 Removable mandibular splint appliance designed to increase vertical dimension.

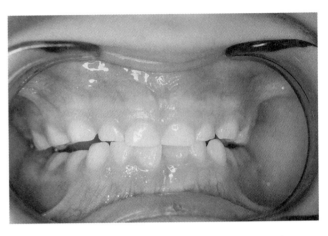

Figure 17-18 Increased vertical dimension has been achieved. As permanent teeth erupt, appliance continues to be worn until occlusion of permanent molars is achieved.

crossbites are unilateral when the teeth are in centric occlusion. But, in reality, the vast majority of unilateral crossbites in the primary dentition are the result of a bilaterally constricted maxillary arch with a functional shift.[33] Bilateral constriction of the maxillary arch leads to premature contacts on closure (typically in the canine area) and a functional shift to one side, which allows for maximum interdigitation of the arches. One important diagnostic feature of unilateral posterior crossbites resulting from bilateral maxillary constriction and a functional shift is that they typically have a midline discrepancy in centric occlusion (Figure 17-19).

Some authors believe that unilateral posterior crossbites with functional shifts should be treated in the primary dentition to prevent asymmetric positioning of the condyles and asymmetric growth.[34] The goal of early treatment in these cases is to establish skeletal symmetry that allows for a more normal growth and dental development.

When left untreated, rarely do posterior crossbites in the primary dentition self-correct.[35,36] On the other hand, when correction is achieved in the primary dentition, it is less likely that the permanent teeth will erupt into a posterior crossbite. However, there can be no guarantees for the outcome because functional disturbances in the permanent dentition may occur.[32,34,37] Parents need to be made aware of this possibility.

Treatment of posterior crossbites in the primary dentition is relatively simple and predictable. Crossbites can be corrected in some cases by selective grinding of the primary canines. A longitudinal study by Kurol and Berglund[38] demonstrated that 64% of identified posterior crossbites in the primary dentition could be corrected with selected grinding. However, Thilander, Wahlund, and Lennartsson[36] found that complete correction of posterior crossbites using selective grinding could only be achieved in 27% of children. Belanger[39] has described the rationale and indi-

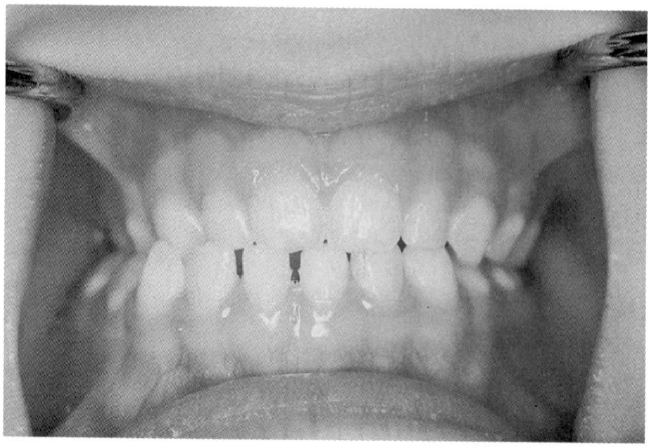

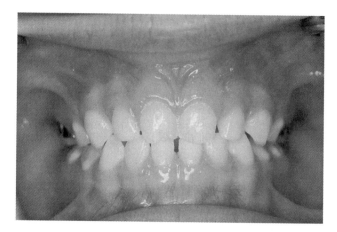

Figure 17-19 Unilateral posterior crossbite caused by bilateral maxillary constriction and functional shift (note midline discrepancy).

Figure 17-21 Following correction of posterior crossbite (note improvement in midlines).

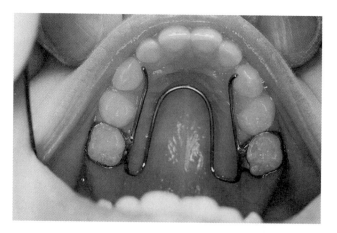

Figure 17-20 Porter arch appliance (W-arch appliance).

cations for equilibration in the primary dentition, specifically when the maxillary arch width is equal to or greater than the mandibular width. The technique Belanger[39] advocates involves "fairly aggressive enamel removal" on the primary canines on the affected side and the primary molars, if necessary, using a diamond bur.

Another option for treatment involves the use of either a fixed or removable appliance. Fixed appliances capable of correcting posterior crossbites in the primary dentition include the porter arch (W-arch) (see Figures 17-19 to 17-21), quad helix, or a removable appliance with an expansion screw (see Chapters 13 and 19).

CROWDING AND SPACING

Crowding and spacing concerns in the primary dentition should be noted. However, it is generally impossible to accurately predict the tooth size-arch length relationships in the permanent dentition from the findings in the primary dentition.[40] In a longitudinal study designed to explore the relationship between tooth size-arch length relationships in the primary and permanent dentitions, Bishara, Khadivi, and Jakobsen[40] found that there is a correlation between the mesiodistal diameter of the primary and permanent teeth and between available arch length in the primary and permanent dentitions. However, the accuracy with which one can predict the permanent tooth size-arch length relationships in individual patients is relatively low. Based on this finding, mechanical intervention in the primary dentition for correction of tooth size-arch length relationship problems is generally not recommended.[40]

REFERENCES

1. Grøn AM: Prediction of tooth emergence, *J Dent Res* 41:573-585, 1962.
2. Dean JA, McDonald RE, Avery DR: Managing the developing occlusion. In McDonald RE, Avery DK (eds): *Dentistry for the child and adolescent*, ed 7, St Louis, 2000, Mosby.
3. Christensen JR, Fields HW: Space maintenance in the primary dentition. In Pinkham JR et al: *Pediatric dentistry: infancy through adolescence*, ed 3, Philadelphia, 1999, WB Saunders.
4. Taylor LB, Full CA: Space maintenance: is it necessary with cuspal interlock? *J Dent Child* 61:327-329, 1994.
5. Lin YT, Chang LC: Space changes after premature loss of the mandibular primary first molar: a longitudinal study, *J Clin Pediatr Dent* 22(4):311-316, 1998.
6. Ngan Peter, Wei SH: Management of space in the primary and mixed dentition, *Update Pediatr Dent* 3(4):1-7, 1990.
7. Carroll CE, Jones JE: Pressure-appliance therapy following premature loss of primary molars, *J Dent Child* 49:347-351, 1982.
8. Johnson ED, Larson BE: Thumb-sucking: literature review, *J Dent Child* 60:385-391, 1993.

9. Nanda RS, Khan I, Anand R: Effect of oral habits on the occlusion in preschool children, *J Dent Child* 39:449-452, 1972.

10. Larsson E: Artifical sucking habits: etiology, prevalence and effect on occlusion, *Int J Orofacial Myology* 20:10-21, 1994.

11. Larsson E: Dummy- and finger-sucking habits with special attention to their significance for facial growth and occlusion. 7. The effect of earlier dummy- and finger-sucking habit in 16-year-old children compared with children without earlier sucking habit, *Swed Dent J* 2:23-33, 1978.

12. Larsson E: Dummy- and finger-sucking habits with special attention to their significance for facial growth and occlusion. 4. Effect on facial growth and occlusion, *Sven Tandlak Tidskr* 65:605-634, 1972.

13. Johnson ED, Larson BE: Thumb-sucking: classification and treatment, *ASDC J Dent Child* 60:392-398, 1993.

14. Kohen DP: Applications of relaxation and mental imagery (self-hypnosis) for habit problems, *Pediatr Ann* 20:136-144, 1991.

15. Haskell BS, Mink JR: An aid to stop thumb sucking: the "Bluegrass" appliance, *Pediatr Dent* 13:83-85, 1991.

16. Viazis AD: The triple-loop corrector (TLC): a new thumbsucking habit control appliance, *Am J Orthod Dentofacial Orthop* 100:91-92, 1991.

17. Davidson PO et al: Thumbsucking: habit or symptom, *J Dent Child* 34:252-259, 1967.

18. Adair SM et al: Effects of current and former pacifier use on the dentition of 24- to 59-month-old children, *Pediatr Dent* 17(7):437-444, 1995.

19. Farsi NM, Salama FS: Sucking habits in Saudi children: prevalence, contributing factors and effects on the primary dentition, *Pediatr Dent* 19(1):28-33, 1997.

20. Baccetti T et al: Early dentofacial features of Class II malocclusion: a longitudinal study from the deciduous through the mixed dentition, *Am J Orthod Dentofacial Orthop* 111(5):502-509, 1997.

21. Vann WF, Dilley GJ, Nelson RM: A cephalometric analysis for the child in the primary dentition, *ASDC J Dent Child* 45(1):45-52, 1978.

22. Bugg JL, Canavati PS, Jennings RE: A cephalometric study for preschool children, *ASDC J Dent Child* 40(2):19-20, 1973.

23. Tollaro I, Baccetti T, Franchi L: Floating norms for the assessment of craniofacial pattern in the deciduous dentition, *Eur J Orthod* 18:359-365, 1996.

24. Grimm SE: Treatment of a pseudo-class III relationship in the primary dentition: a case history, *ASDC J Dent Child* 58(6):484-488, 1991.

25. Campbell PM: The dilemma of Class III treatment: early or late? *Angle Orthod* 53(3):175-191, 1983.

26. Merwin D et al: Timing for effective application of anteriorly directed orthopedic force to the maxilla, *Am J Orthod Dentofacial Orthop* 112(3):292-299, 1997.

27. Croll TP, Riesenberger RE: Anterior crossbite correction in the primary dentition using fixed inclined planes. I. Technique and examples, *Quintessence Int* 18(12):847-853, 1987.

28. Croll TP, Riesenberger RE: Anterior crossbite correction in the primary dentition using fixed inclined planes. II. Further examples and discussion, *Quintessence Int* 19(1):45-51, 1988.

29. Major PW, elBadrawy HE: Maxillary protraction for early orthopedic correction of skeletal Class III malocclusion, *Pediatr Dent* 15:203-207, 1993.

30. Ngan P, Fields H: Orthodontic diagnosis and treatment planning in the primary dentition, *ASDC J Dent Child* 62(1):25-33, 1995.

31. Fukuta O et al: Damage to the primary dentition resulting from thumb and finger (digit) sucking, *ASDC J Dent Child* 63(6):403-407, 1996.

32. Vadiakas GP, Roberts MW: Primary posterior crossbite: diagnosis and treatment, *J Clin Pediatr Dent* 16(1):1-4, 1991.

33. Lindner A, Modeer T: Relation between sucking habit and dental characteristics in preschool children with unilateral crossbite, *Scand J Dent Res* 97:278-283, 1989.

34. De Boer M, Steenks MH: Functional unilateral posterior crossbite: orthodontic and functional aspects, *J Oral Rehabil* 24(8):614-23, 1997.

35. Kutin G, Hawes RR: Posterior cross-bites in the deciduous and mixed dentitions, *Am J Orthod* 56:491-504, 1969.

36. Thilander B, Wahlund S, Lennartsson B: The effect of early interceptive treatment in children with posterior crossbite, *Eur J Orthod* 6:25-34, 1984.

37. Schroder U, Schroder I.: Early treatment of unilateral posterior crossbite in children with bilaterally contracted maxillae, *Eur J Orthod* 6:65-69, 1984.

38. Kurol J, Berglund L: Longitudinal study and cost-benefit analysis of the effect of early treatment of posterior crossbites in the primary dentition, *Eur J Orthod* 14(3):173-179, 1992.

39. Belanger GK: The rationale and indications for equilibration in the primary dentition, *Quintessence Int* 23(3):169-174, 1992.

40. Bishara SE, Khadivi P, Jakobsen JR. Changes in tooth size-arch length relationships from the deciduous to the permanent dentition: a longitudinal study, *Am J Orthod Dentofacial Orthop* 108(6):607-613, 1995.

CHAPTER 18

Mixed Dentition Guidance of Occlusion: Serial Extraction Procedures

T. M. Graber

KEY TERMS

guided extraction
noniatrogenic treatment
  philosophy
stomatognathic systems
crestal bone loss

gingival recession
root resorption
tooth size-arch length
  discrepancy
homeostasis

neuromuscular balance
incisor liability
leeway space
flush terminal plane

ectopic eruption
curve of Spee
total space analysis
knife-edging

HISTORY OF MIXED DENTITION GUIDANCE OF OCCLUSION

There has been an increasing tendency to confine orthodontic management to as narrow a time frame as possible. Never was the old adage, "Rush, rush, rush, Orange Crush!" more apparent than now. New, efficient light force appliances with reduced friction, greater emphasis on tooth movement, less emphasis on growth guidance, and strong admonishments from financially oriented practice consultants to confine patient care to as short a period as possible have been used as reasons to mitigate against any approach that would add more than one phase of treatment. Inevitably, such an approach stresses the biomechanical aspects and downplays the biologic aspects of orthodontics.

Even with the massive knowledge of and continuing research on the growth of the dentofacial structures, individual variation makes any absolute projections of the development of the skeleton and dentition more an approximation than an exact template. We have been enamored with so-called cephalometric norms for too long. Literally, the mythical innkeeper, Procrustes, has been emulated, fitting all patients into the same diagnostic and mechanical straitjackets.

There is no question that the orthodontist should examine most children by the age of 7 years and make a determination on what is best and if and when treatment is indicated for that particular galaxy of problems (Figure 18-1).

Sage advice can be taken from one of the greatest mechanical geniuses and orthodontists of all time, Charles Tweed[1]:

As we learn more about growth and its potentials, the influences of function on the developing denture, and the normal mesiodistal position of the denture in its relation to basal jawbones and head structures, we will acquire a better understanding of when and how to intervene in the guidance of growth processes so that nature may better approximate her growth plan for the individual patient. In other words, knowledge will gradually replace harsh mechanics, and in the not too distant future the vast majority of orthodontic treatment will be carried out during the mixed dentition period of growth and development and before the difficult age of adolescence.

Charles Tweed[1] was influenced by two of the same researchers and clinicians that helped establish my practice philosophy early in my career—Birger Kjellgren[2] of Sweden and Rudolph Hotz[3] of Switzerland. No one

257

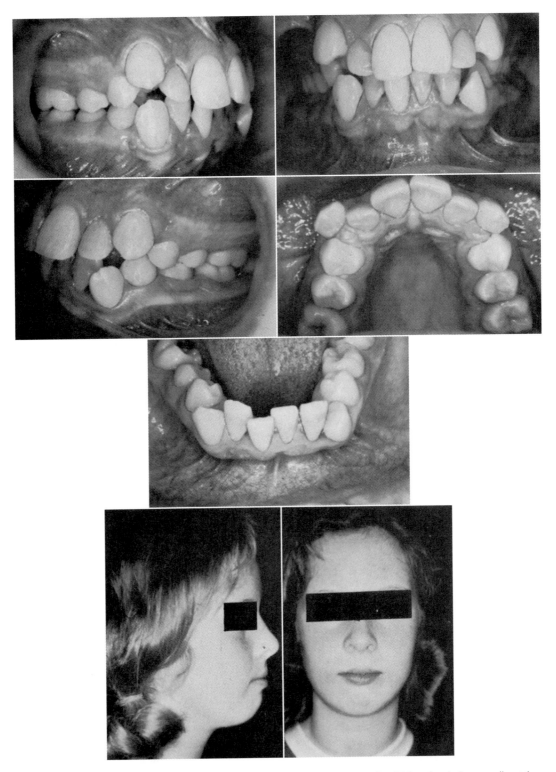

Figure 18-1 An excellent example of a severe tooth size/jaw discrepancy case in which malocclusion was allowed to progress to maturity without the benefits of early extraction intervention. Serial extraction could have reduced needed appliance therapy by 50% and prevented a muscular system from developing under highly unfavorable conditions. This is the type of case in which serial extraction makes its greatest contribution not only to dental health and facial balance, but also by substantially reducing the amount of necessary tooth movement. (From Graber TM: *Current orthodontic concepts and techniques,* Philadelphia, 1969, WB Saunders.)

can do justice to **guided extraction** procedures without reading their publications. Their long-term records are as valid and their conclusions as appropriate as when they were written. I introduced Tod Dewel[4-8] to them in the 1950s and he, too, became a disciple of properly managed serial extraction. Concurrently, Hayes Nance,[9] John Heath,[10] and Z. Bernard Lloyd[11] followed much the same route for their mixed dentition guidance. The serial extraction diagnostic and therapeutic procedures, which were important chapters in earlier textbooks, were further amplified by Warren Mayne.[12,13]

The works of Karl Sandstedt[14] of Sweden in 1904, Noyes[15] in 1912, Oppenheim[16] of Germany in 1911, and Weinmann and Sicher[17] of Austria in the 1920s allow one to realize that their biologically founded research was the basis for the current emphasis on a **noniatrogenic treatment philosophy**. This does not minimize the contributions of Noyes' detailed analysis of tissue changes[15] associated with tooth movement in 1912 nor of that of Albert Ketcham,[18] whose pioneer work on root resorption is still valid. Right behind these orthodontic giants is Axel Lundström[19] of Sweden. Although Benno Lischer[20] had delineated the role of the neuromusculature in his 1912 text on orthodontics, it remained for Lundström[19] to stress the relationships between the three systems—tooth, muscle, and bone. This brought him into conflict with Angle[21] and his followers who resorted to expansion to preserve all teeth, regardless of the amount of crowding. Occlusion was the primary objective, as shown on those beautiful anthropologic remains illustrating their writings (i.e., Broomell's skull and the Ravenscroft-Summa-Angle skull in the seventh edition, referred to as *Old Glory*).[21]

If this neglect of a proper balance of the **stomatognathic systems** was history, it could be excused. However, the renaissance of expansionist mechanotherapy with newer and more efficient appliances ignores the bitter lessons that long-term studies have shown—teeth moved off their apical base into excessive neuromuscular force are unlikely to be stable in the long run. Of even more concern, iatrogenic sequelae are likely (i.e., **crestal bone loss, gingival recession,** and **root resorption**).[7,12,13,22-33] Litigious challenges in court are not necessary to remind us of the potential deleterious consequences.

Rationale of Serial Extraction

Dale's detailed treatise on the ramifications and techniques of serial extraction,[34] or guidance of eruption, covers all types of malocclusion. On the other hand, this chapter deals mainly with Class I malocclusions. The essential elements of the stomatognathic system are in balance, but there is a malocclusion present caused by a **tooth size-arch length discrepancy**. The objective is to correct the dental irregularities while maintaining the multisystem balance and the best possible facial harmony.

With all the current emphasis on invisible braces, ceramic attachments, and esthetically acceptable appliances for adult patients, the best way to hide appliances is to use them over as short a period as possible with minimum iatrogenic potential. Properly managed serial extraction achieves that objective (Figure 18-2).*

In common vernacular, the malocclusion is akin to having a five-room house on a four-room foundation. Knowledge of growth and development assists in achieving a proper diagnosis and intercepting therapeutically at the right time. The decision is always based on what is best for the patient, has the least potential of producing damage, makes use of that fundamental phenomenon called **homeostasis** or spontaneous adaptation, and is not confined to an arbitrary treatment schedule based on practice efficiency considerations. In no way is this a compromise approach. The demands for a comprehensive diagnosis are as great or greater than for the conventional single-phase multiattachment treatment. Continuing diagnostic reassessment, particularly estimation of the tooth size-arch length discrepancy (see Chapter 12) is essential during the occlusal guidance phase. Also a thorough knowledge of tooth formation and development is vital for timing of interceptive procedures.

At first glance, serial extraction seems deceptively simple and financially rewarding. This is hardly the case.[34,45-49] Much of the criticism of this approach in the past was based on inadequate diagnosis, both in the beginning and during the 3- to 5-year period of observation and interceptive guidance, followed by comprehensive therapy. On the contrary, this approach is efficient, noniatrogenic, and esthetically satisfying mechanotherapy to produce the best possible and most stable result.[47-50]

ADVANTAGES OF SERIAL EXTRACTION

In the orofacial region the stomatognathic system is comprised of several components that can affect morphogenetic pattern and facial development and that include the dynamic neuromuscular envelope (including all contiguous muscles), the respiratory structures and function, the osseous structures, and the teeth themselves. The dynamic implications cannot be overstressed. Dentists are accustomed to looking at teeth on an articulator, ignoring the associated elements of the craniofacial and cervical areas and their potential influence of ultimate morphology. In patients with Class I malocclusions, nature has achieved a **neuro-**

Text continued on p. 266

---

*References 1-7, 10, 11, 13, 23-27, 30, 35-44.

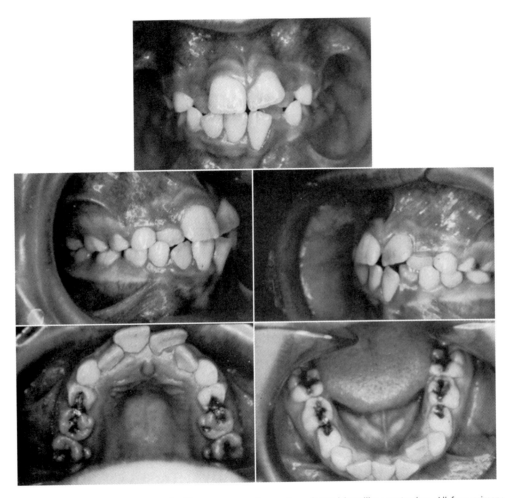

Figure 18-2 Case first seen at age 8 with severe crowding and moderate bimaxillary protrusion. All four primary canines were extracted followed by removal of first primary molars and first premolars. The high Frankfurt horizontal-mandibular plane angle should be noted as well as the less than average unraveling of lower incisors during the extraction sequence. Nine months of appliance therapy were required to achieve final result. It is interesting to compare this case to the mother's untreated malocclusion. (From Graber TM: *Current orthodontic concepts and techniques,* Philadelphia, 1969, WB Saunders.)

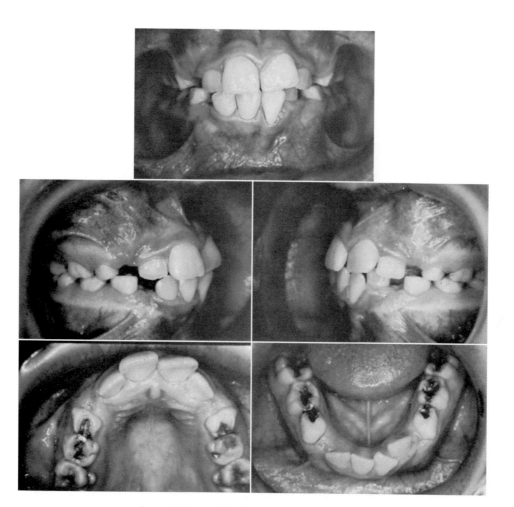

Figure 18-2, cont'd For legend see opposite page.

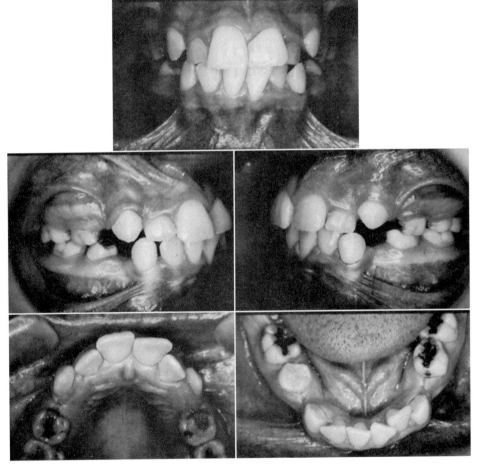

Figure 18-2, cont'd For legend see p. 260.

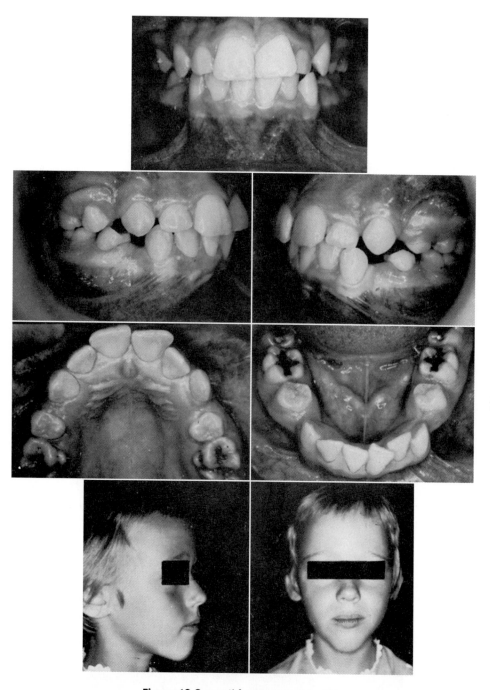

Figure 18-2, cont'd For legend see p. 260.

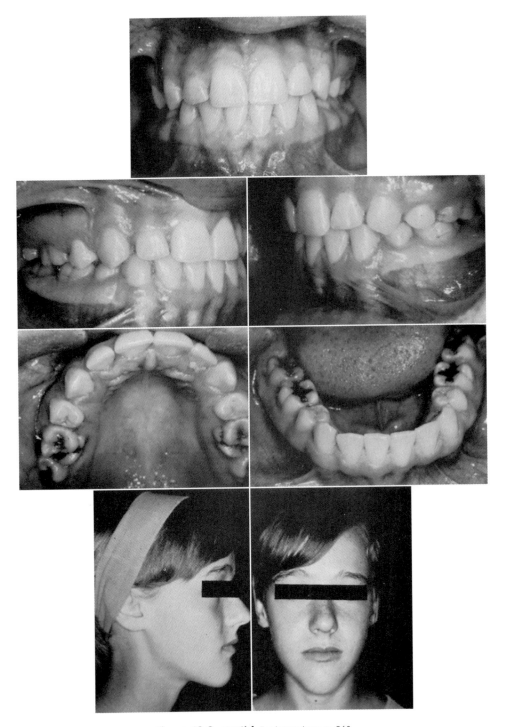

Figure 18-2, cont'd For legend see p. 260.

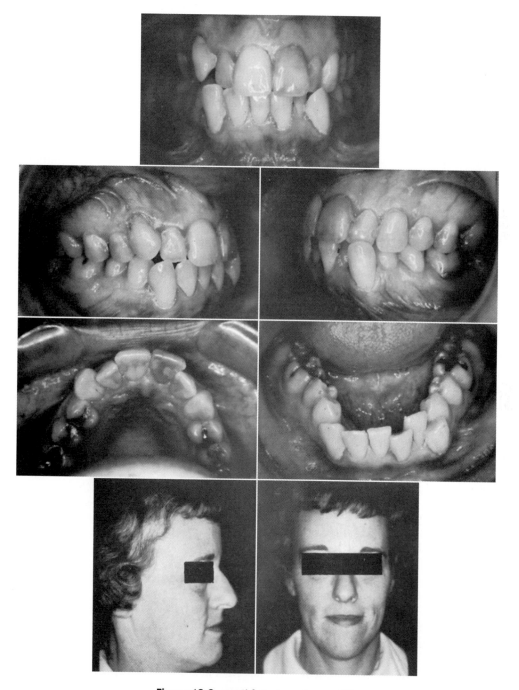

Figure 18-2, cont'd For legend see p. 260.

muscular balance at that particular time. In serial extraction procedures, this normal balance is accepted and the dentist tries to maintain it. A mechanistic, articulator-oriented approach is to ignore all but the tooth system and to align the teeth.

Chief Benefits of Extraction Guidance

1. Naturally induced movement and alignment of seriously crowded anterior teeth
2. Improved health of investing tissues
3. Improved psychologic state and better patient compliance as a result of the improved alignment
4. Reduction of the total workload and treatment effort by the clinician and, likely, the patient's financial investment
5. Less potential iatrogenic damage

Although guided extraction procedures can be of benefit in properly selected patients with Class II and Class III malocclusions, it is beyond the purview of this chapter. In patients with these types of malocclusions, abnormal and adaptive functional patterns exist and they must be altered. On the other hand, in most patients with a Class I malocclusion, the neuromuscular envelope is normal and it should stay that way. The primary concern is the tooth system.

DENTAL DEVELOPMENT, OCCLUSION, AND MALOCCLUSION

In a comprehensive study jointly conducted by the University of Toronto and the Burlington Study group, the findings indicated that only 34% of all 3-year-old children have a normal occlusion. This drops to only 11% at 12 years of age. Local environmental factors are blamed for the 23% reduction. Of the remaining ⅔ of the 3-year-old children without normal occlusion, 41% had Class I malocclusion, 23% had Class II malocclusion, and only 2% had Class III malocclusion. By 12 years of age the percentage of patients with Class I occlusion had risen to 55%, whereas 32% had Class II occlusion and 2% had Class III occlusion.[51] It is estimated that ⅔ of all malocclusions are hereditary at 3 years of age. Thus those most likely to benefit from serial extraction, which is directed at tooth size-arch length discrepancies, are those who have dominant Class I malocclusions. Before embarking on a description of the diagnostic discipline, a discussion of dental development is essential as a scientific background for interpreting diagnostic records. The seminal study by

Hurme[52] on eruption age and sequence is still state of the art (Figure 18-3). A more detailed description of the dental changes from the primary to the mixed and permanent dentitions is presented in Chapter 5.

Incisor Liability and the Associated Changes in the Dental Arches

The increase in anterior tooth mass during the mixed dentition, following the eruption of the permanent teeth could not be accommodated in the available arch length unless nature makes some adjustments to achieve the fit and maintain the dynamic balance. According to Black,[53] the four maxillary permanent incisors are, on the average, 7.6 mm larger than the primary predecessors. For the mandibular incisor segment, the permanent successors are 6.0 mm larger (Figures 18-4 to 18-6). This difference was termed the **incisor liability** by Warren Mayne,[36] and it varies greatly from person to person. This is just one reason why the American Association of Orthodontists recommends that a child should be seen by 7 years of age–not to place appliances but to perform a diagnostic assessment of potential problems and to determine the optimal treatment timing and regimen (Figure 18-7). Incisor liability illustrates in a dramatic fashion the challenge of trying to fit larger teeth into a smaller anterior alveolar support.

Factors That Allow for or Prevent Proper Alignment of Erupting Permanent Teeth

1. Interdental spacing of the primary incisor teeth
2. Intercanine arch width change
3. Arch length increase via more labial/buccal placement of the permanent successors
4. Favorable variation in the ratios between the size of the primary and permanent teeth[36,54,55]

Interdental Spacing Interdental spacing of the primary teeth, whether present or not present, essentially does not change from the time of the completion of the primary dentition until the permanent incisors start erupting.* Interdental spacing may range from 0 to 10.0 mm in the maxillary arch, but averages about 5.0 mm. In the mandibular arch interdental spacing can range from 0 to 6.0 mm, averaging 3.0 mm. This is one of the first observations to be made on the young patient. Lack of sufficient interdental spacing (Figure 18-8) must

---

*References 1, 6, 23-25, 36, 37, 54, 56-62.

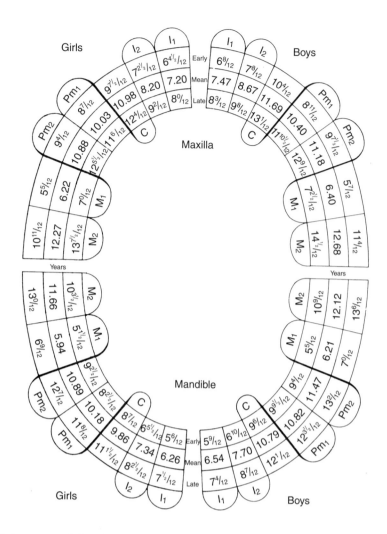

Figure 18-3 Assessment of dental age by means of tooth emergence (±1 SD). (From Hurme VO: *J Dent Child* 16:11, 1949.)

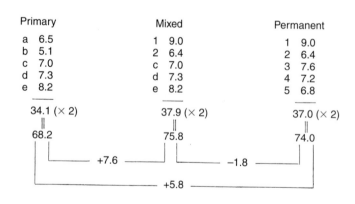

Primary		Mixed		Permanent	
a	6.5	1	9.0	1	9.0
b	5.1	2	6.4	2	6.4
c	7.0	c	7.0	3	7.6
d	7.3	d	7.3	4	7.2
e	8.2	e	8.2	5	6.8
34.1 (× 2)		37.9 (× 2)		37.0 (× 2)	
68.2		75.8		74.0	

+7.6   −1.8

+5.8

Figure 18-4 Width (in millimeters) of teeth in the maxillary arch. (From Graber TM: *Current orthodontic concepts and techniques*, Philadelphia, 1969, WB Saunders.)

Primary		Mixed		Permanent	
a	4.2	1	5.4	1	5.4
b	4.1	2	5.9	2	5.9
c	5.0	c	5.0	3	6.9
d	7.7	d	7.7	4	6.9
e	9.9	3	9.9	5	7.1
30.9 (× 2)		33.9 (× 2)		32.2 (× 2)	
61.8		67.8		64.4	

+6.0   −3.4

+2.6

Figure 18-5 Width (in millimeters) of teeth in the mandibular arch. (From Graber TM: *Current orthodontic concepts and techniques*, Philadelphia, 1969, WB Saunders.)

Maxillary Arch
Mesiodistal Diameters

Permanent centrals	(9.0 mm)	18.0 mm
Permanent laterals	(6.4 mm)	12.8 mm
	Total width	30.8 mm
Deciduous centrals	(6.5 mm)	13.0 mm
Deciduous laterals	(5.1 mm)	10.2 mm
	Total width	23.2 mm
	Liability (Mayne)	−7.6 mm

Mandibular Arch
Mesiodistal Diameters

Permanent centrals	(5.4 mm)	10.8 mm
Permanent laterals	(5.9 mm)	11.8 mm
	Total width	22.6 mm
Deciduous centrals	(4.2 mm)	8.4 mm
Deciduous centrals	(4.1 mm)	8.2 mm
	Total width	16.6 mm
	Liability (Mayne)	−6.0 mm

Figure 18-6 Mesiodistal diameters of the maxillary and mandibular incisors showing crown size differential between primary and permanent incisors (liability [Mayne]). (From Graber TM: *Current orthodontic concepts and techniques*, Philadelphia, 1969, WB Saunders.)

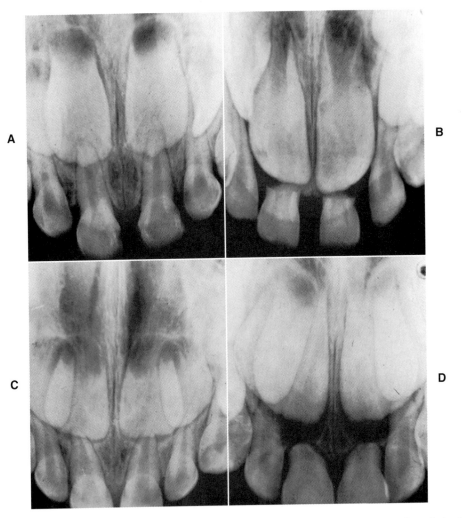

Figure 18-7 Incisor liabilities. **A,** Very favorable. **B,** Typical. **C,** In trouble. **D,** Very unfavorable. (From Graber TM: *Current orthodontic concepts and techniques*, Philadelphia, 1969, WB Saunders.)

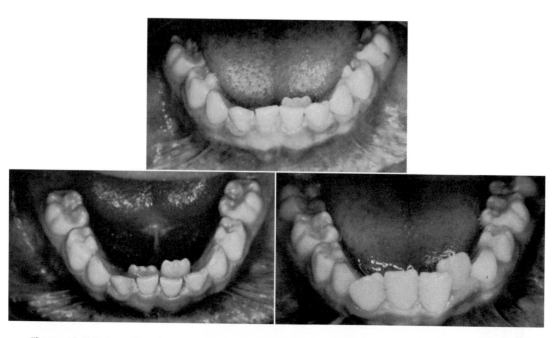

Figure 18-8 Early manifestation of tooth/jaw discrepancy. Although moderate intercanine width increase (2.0 mm) occurred during eruption of 21/12, this was inadequate to permit alignment and positioning of permanent incisors. Case now requires careful analysis involving critical consideration of *1,* existing leeway space, *2,* present state of facial balance, and *3,* clinician's skill in increasing arch length posteriorly with appliances to determine best treatment program. (From Graber TM: *Current orthodontic concepts and techniques,* Philadelphia, 1969, WB Saunders.)

be considered a serious handicap in achieving normal alignment unless there is a favorable interplay with other factors. A greater than average growth response of the dental arches or extremely small permanent teeth are necessary to overcome lack of interdental spacing. Another alternative requires the permanent teeth to assume a greater than normal anterior positioning through orthodontic mechanotherapy, which may compromise their stability (Figure 18-9).

So far, for illustrative purposes, average tooth size has been cited from Black.[53] However, other studies give somewhat different figures, which factor in ethnic variability. Clearly, few patients are an average, so their specific individual measurements must serve for their own case analysis.[56-58,63]

Intercanine Arch Width Changes
A number of clinical studies of dental casts have shown an increase in the intercanine width at the time of eruption of the permanent incisors.[56,57,59-62,64-67] How could this happen? Is this really growth?*

Between the primary and mixed dentitions there is an increase in arch width between the primary canines (Figure 18-10).[59] Yet this increase is the most variable, diagnostically unpredictable change in the mixed dentition. The maxillary arch growth curves for both males and females are illustrated in Figure 18-11. Note that the changes in the curves for intercanine widths

correlate with the timing of the late mixed to early permanent dentition exchange. In the mandibular arch the eruption of the canines and the width change occur earlier (Figure 18-12).

Moorrees and associates[61,63-66] showed sexual dimorphism in the intercanine width in their longitudinal research. The average increase in maxillary intercanine width for males, as measured from canine tips between 2 years and 18 years of age, is almost 6 mm. For females the increase between 2 years and 12 years of age is 4.5 mm (Figure 18-13).

In the mandibular arch (see Figure 18-12), the top pair of curves represents intercanine width changes from 3 years of age to maturity. The solid line shows intercanine changes in males and the broken line shows intercanine width changes in females. Owing to the earlier eruption of the mandibular canines, arch width growth continues practically without pause until about 8½ to 9 years of age in girls and until 10 years of age in boys. After this point the width does not surpass or even reach this level, as seen in the top pair of curves.

It is proper to pause momentarily to ask more precisely what is meant by "growth of the arches." No interstitial bone growth of the apical base occurs. Rather, according to Graber[12,25] and Enlow,[70] appositional growth on selected surfaces produces an increase in the size of these bases while considerable vertical growth of the alveolar process takes place. This occurs in such direction and amount, especially during the transition from the primary to the permanent dentition,

*References 2, 12, 35, 40, 56, 59, 68, 69.

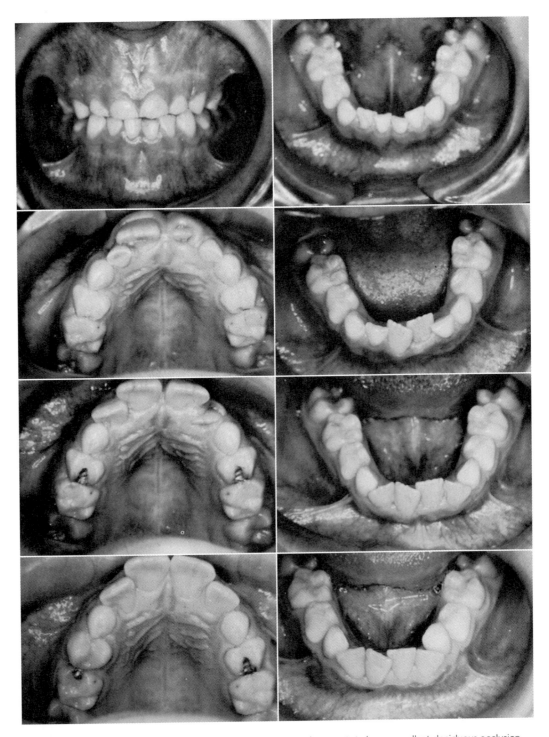

Figure 18-9 Case first seen at age 4 years with what appears to the parents to be an excellent deciduous occlusion. However, to be noted are the very small lower deciduous incisors, which were crowded. Practically no intercanine width increase occurred during the transitional period, and this patient at age 10 years presented a mandibular arch length deficiency of 8.5 mm. It should be observed that the upper permanent incisors have erupted not only well forward of the deciduous predecessors, but have continued this forward displacement throughout the transitional period. (From Graber TM: *Current orthodontic concepts and techniques*, Philadelphia, 1969, WB Saunders.)

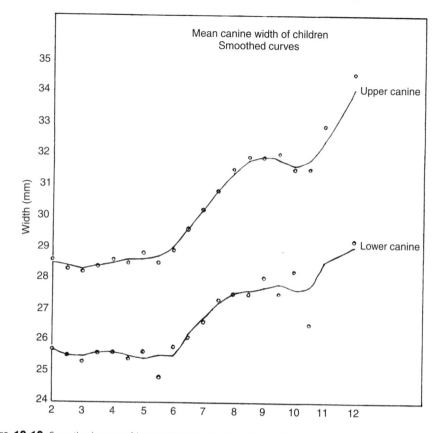

Figure 18-10 Smoothed curve of intercanine growth. (From Graber TM: *Current orthodontic concepts and techniques*, Philadelphia, 1969, WB Saunders.)

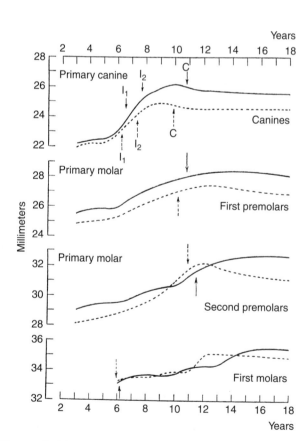

Figure 18-11 Average distances between antimeres in the maxillary dental arch at various ages. *Solid lines,* males; *broken lines,* females. The arrows refer to the mean ages of emergence of the permanent teeth. (From Moorrees CFA: *The dentition of the growing child,* Cambridge, Mass, 1959, Harvard University Press.)

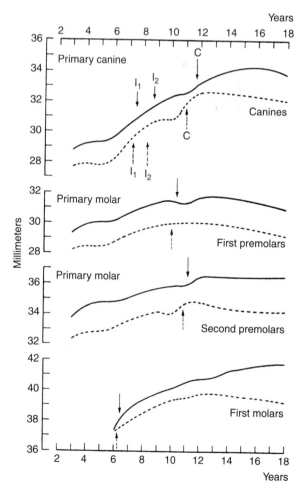

Figure 18-12 Average distances between antimeres in the mandibular dental arch at various ages. *Solid lines,* males; *broken lines,* females. The arrows refer to the mean ages of emergence of the permanent teeth. (From Moorrees CFA: *The dentition of the growing child,* Cambridge, Mass, 1959, Harvard University Press.)

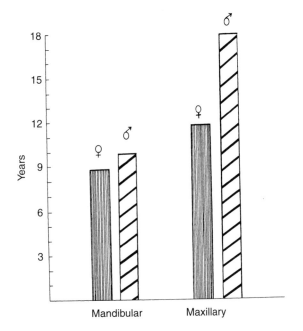

Figure 18-13 Average ages of completion of intercanine growth. (From Graber TM: *Current orthodontic concepts and techniques,* Philadelphia, 1969, WB Saunders.)

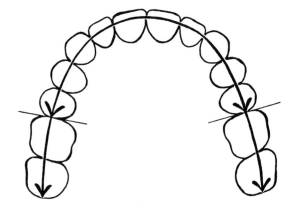

Figure 18-14 Clinical arch length better known simply as *arch length.* (From Graber TM: *Current orthodontic concepts and techniques,* Philadelphia, 1969, WB Saunders.)

as to result in a larger arc. This is especially true anteriorly, allowing the accommodation of the larger, thicker, and more procumbent permanent teeth.

According to Moorrees and others,[54,57,60,63] by 8½ to 9 years of age nearly 100% of the anticipated mandibular intercanine arch width increase in most girls has already occurred. Most boys have undergone approximately 85% of their mandibular intercanine increase by the same age (see Figure 18-13). After 10 years of age there is little mandibular intercanine width change to be expected in either boys or girls. This is in contrast to the pattern of maxillary intercanine dimensional increases already described.

Arch Length Change   Arch length is the distance around the arch from the most distal surface of the last tooth on one side through the region of the interproximal contacts to the most distal surface on the opposite side (Figure 18-14). Of greater clinical importance is the distance around the arch from the mesial surface of one first permanent molar to the counterpart on the other side.

Arch length may, and generally does, change during the growth period. Changes vary considerably between individuals and between the maxillary and mandibular arches. A critical fact that is too often overlooked is that, in most cases, arch length actually *decreases* in the mandibular arch during the growth period (Figure 18-15).[54,57,59-61,63-66,68] The ramifications of this arch length reduction are too often not apparent to the novice.

Labial Positioning of Erupting Incisors
Another factor that may influence arch length is related to changes in the curvature of the anterior segment. The permanent incisors erupt slightly labially and are slightly more procumbent. This increases arch length without compromising intercanine width.[35,36] The maxillary anterior positioning averages 2.2 mm, according to Baume.[68] Again, this is variable depending on tooth size, the interaction between the labial and lingual neuromuscular forces, and overbite. With larger teeth, the maxillary anterior arc might reasonably be slightly greater (Figure 18-16). This adjustment is less of a factor in the mandibular arch.

Variations in the Size Ratio of Primary Teeth and Their Permanent Successors   The fourth factor to consider is the ratio between the size of the primary teeth and the permanent teeth. A relatively smaller permanent tooth size increases the chances of optimal alignment, again, depending on the balance of the other factors just described. In an individual with normal occlusion, the average maxillary incisor liability is 7.6 mm, which is overcome by a combination of various factors, namely, an average interdental spacing of 3.8 mm, an intercanine width increase of 3.0 mm, and anterior tooth positioning of 2.2 mm. The mandibular incisor liability is only 6.0 mm and can be overcome by an average interdental spacing of 2.7 mm, an intercanine width increase of 3.0 mm, and more anterior incisor positioning of 1.3 mm. The deeper the overbite, the greater the challenge of overcoming the mandibular incisor liability. It should be reemphasized that this physiologic and morphologic "give and take" in the mixed dentition is unique for each individual. It requires proper, thorough, and continuing diagnostic evaluation (Figure 18-17).[7,55,71,72]

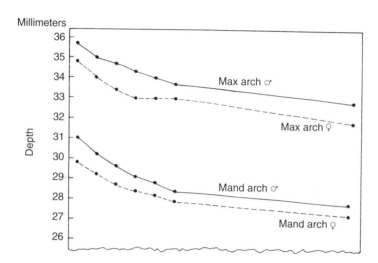

Figure 18-15 Reduction in arch depth. (From DeKock WH: *Am J Orthod* 62:56, 1972.)

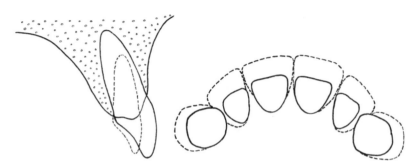

Figure 18-16 Primary and permanent incisor relationships. (From Graber TM: *Current orthodontic concepts and techniques,* Philadelphia, 1969, WB Saunders.)

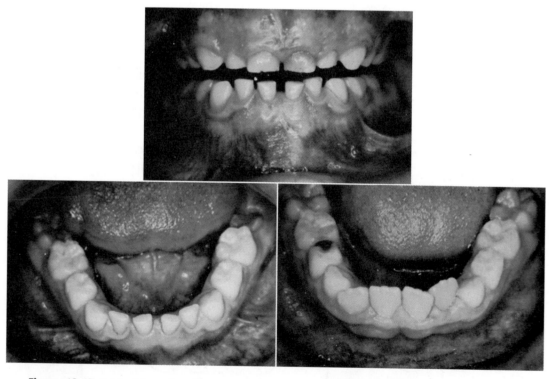

Figure 18-17 Substantial spacing of lower primary incisors, which usually conveys a highly optimistic prognosis regarding alignment of permanent incisors. However, the primary incisors are extremely diminutive and only very modest intercanine arch width increase occurred. The unusually large permanent incisors when fully erupted presented 5.5 mm of crowding. (From Graber TM: *Current orthodontic concepts and techniques,* Philadelphia, 1969, WB Saunders.)

Leeway Space Orthodontics owes much to Nance[9] for his careful observations and tremendous clinical experience. The space differential between the primary and permanent teeth in the posterior segments was termed **leeway space** by Nance[9] and this is still the preferred designation. According to Nance, the combined width of the primary canine and the first and second primary molars on each side in the mandibular arch is, on average, 1.7 mm greater than the permanent canine and the first and second premolars. In the maxillary arch, it averages 0.9 mm greater (Figure 18-18).

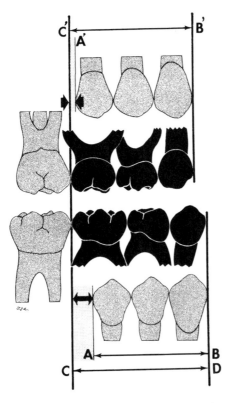

Figure 18-18 Leeway space of Nance. On the average, the combined width of the mandibular primary canine and first and second primary molars is 1.7 mm greater on each side than the permanent canine and first and second premolars. In the maxillary arch the primary canine and first and second primary molars are only slightly wider than the combined width of their permanent successors (0.9 mm). In other words, the distance AC is approximately 2.7 times as great as A'C' on the average (*arrows*). (From Graber TM: *Orthodontics principles and practice*, ed 2, Philadelphia, 1966, WB Saunders.)

It is important to note, however, that the slightly greater space in the mandibular arch is considered *reserved space.* This is because, in many cases, the permanent first molars are in an end-to-end relationship as they erupt into occlusion (Figure 18-19). This relationship changes into a Class I occlusion in 55% of the cases, as the mandibular molars migrate mesially after the loss of the lower second primary molars (see Chapter 5). The other 45% of the cases with **flush terminal plane** end up with a Class II or an end-to-end permanent molar relationship.

Differential mesial migration following the loss of the second primary molars accompanied with differential jaw growth allows for complete cuspal interdigitation in most cases. Thus this reserved space is not to be used for alignment of the lower incisors unless the mixed dentition space analysis indicates the presence of sufficient space for both adjustments. Placing a lower fixed lingual arch to hold this space for incisor alignment prevents the mesial migration of the lower permanent first molars and the proper buccal segment interdigitation. If a diagnostic decision is made to preserve all the available arch length in the lower arch for tooth alignment, the patient will need to wear an extraoral appliance to allow for the molar correction by moving the upper molars distally.

The major emphasis here is that, with normal mandibular development, whatever increase that occurs in the anterior arch segments must be reconciled with the usual reduction in the posterior segments. The net result is a final reduction in the clinical arch length of the mandible in the majority of cases (see Figures 18-15 and 18-20).

ASSESSMENTS TO BE MADE BEFORE A SERIAL EXTRACTION PROCEDURE IS CONTEMPLATED

Intraoral Diagnostic Assessment: What to Watch for Clinically

Serial extraction allows the application of what is known about the total dentofacial morphology and the physiologic ramifications of the growth and develop-

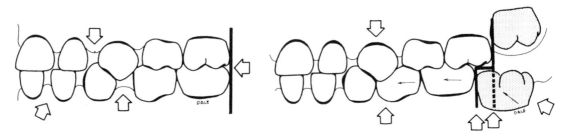

Figure 18-19 Early mesial shift. (From Baume LJ: *J Dent Res* 29:331, 1950.)

mental processes. What a satisfying milieu for clinicians because they use less mechanical procedures to provide a more stable, healthy, gratifying orthodontic result! Literally, less is more! But it makes use of the working "hard drive" of the clinician fortified by a comprehensive and up-to-date batch of mental software with interactive potential.

As explained in previous chapters, the diagnostic clues are obtained from a thorough case history, clinical examination of the patient, photographs, plaster study models, cephalometric radiographs, and panoramic and periapical radiographs. Taken together, these records provide a dynamic working analysis (see Chapters 9 to 13) (Boxes 18-1 and 18-2).

Growth and Development Assessment

Periodic growth assessment records should be made in all patients where growth is still a consideration (i.e., until 14 to 16 years old in girls and until 18 to 19 years old in boys).[12,13,26,27] This is standard of care. Sibling and parental patterns provide significant information on the ultimate status of the dentition, whether there has been orthodontic intervention or not.[7,66,71,73] Every orthodontic patient should benefit from this appraisal, particularly when the patient is in the growing period (i.e., in the mixed dentition). The dynamic effects of growth should not be underestimated, and the morphogenetic pattern evaluation is essential.

BOX 18-1   Potential Genetic Factors to Consider and Evaluate in Clinical Analysis

These factors have been modified from Dale's original suggestions[34,55,71,72]:

1. Maxillary-mandibular dental-alveolar protrusion without interproximal spacing
2. Crowded mandibular incisor teeth (Figure 18-21)
3. Midline displacement of the permanent mandibular incisors, resulting in the premature exfoliation of a primary canine on the crowded side
4. Midline displacement of the permanent mandibular incisors with the lateral incisor on the crowded side blocked out usually to the lingual surface (Figure 18-22 and 18-23)[49]
5. A crescent-shaped area of external root resorption on the mesial aspect of the root of the primary canines caused by the erupting permanent lateral incisors (Figure 18-24)
6. Bilateral mandibular primary canine exfoliation resulting in the lingual uprighting of the permanent incisors, increasing the overjet and allowing a potential lip trap to develop
7. A splaying out of the permanent maxillary or mandibular incisor teeth caused by the crowded malposition of the unerupted permanent canines

8. Gingival recession on one or more of the mandibular incisor teeth (see Figure 18-21)
9. A prominent bulging in the vestibule of the maxillary and mandibular canine teeth as they attempt to erupt (Figure 18-25)[49]
10. A discrepancy in the size of the primary and permanent teeth, reducing the leeway space
11. A discrepancy in the size of the maxillary and mandibular permanent teeth
12. Tooth shape abnormalities, particularly of the mandibular second premolars
13. **Ectopic eruption** of the permanent maxillary first molars resulting in premature exfoliation of the primary second molars, which can be indicative of a lack of developing room in the tuberosity region (Figure 18-26)[12,27,72]
14. "Trapping" of erupting permanent maxillary second and third molars under the distal convexity of the first and second molars—a sign of inadequate space in the alveolar trough
15. "Trapping" or impaction of permanent mandibular second molars, which can be indicative of a critical alveolar trough space shortage

---

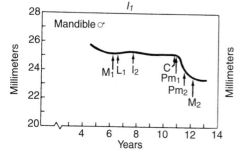

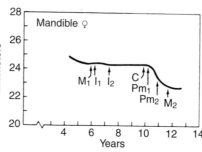

Figure 18-20 Reduction in arch length as a result of the moving forward of posterior teeth. (From Moorrees CFA, Reed RB: *J Dent Res* 44:129, 1965.)

BOX 18-2	Serial Extraction Clues— Environmental Factors[49]

1. Trauma
2. Iatrogenic treatment
3. Transposition of teeth
4. Rotation of teeth
5. Ankylosis of primary teeth (Figure 18-27)[49]
6. Premature loss of primary teeth with subsequent drifting of permanent teeth[49]
7. Prolonged retention of lower second primary molars (Figure 18-28)[49]
8. Interproximal caries, if unrestored
9. Abnormal exfoliation sequence of primary teeth
10. Altered emergence sequence of permanent teeth

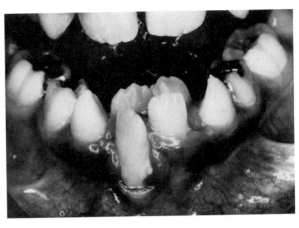

Figure 18-21 Crowding and gingival recession. (From Dale JG: *Dent Clin North Am* 26:565, 1982.)

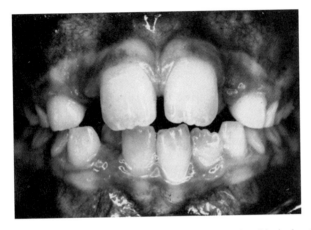

Figure 18-22 One permanent mandibular lateral incisor blocked out lingually with a midline discrepancy. (From Graber TM, Vanarsdall RL: *Orthodontics: current principles and techniques,* ed 3, St Louis, 2000, Mosby.)

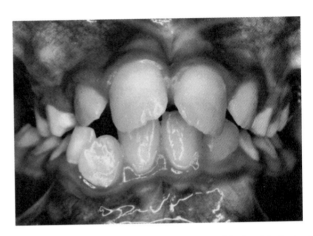

Figure 18-23 One permanent mandibular lateral incisor blocked out labially with a midline discrepancy. (From Dale JG: *Dent Clin North Am* 26:565, 1982.)

Figure 18-24 Root resorption of the primary canine as a result of crowded permanent incisors. (From Graber TM, Vanarsdall RL: *Orthodontics: current principles and techniques,* ed 3, St Louis, 2000, Mosby.)

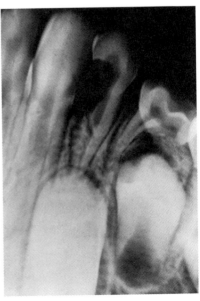

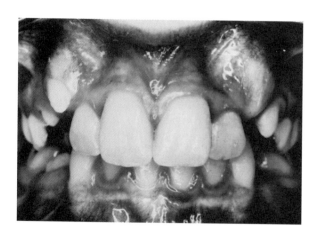

Figure 18-25 Canine bulging in the maxilla. (From Dale JG: *Dent Clin North Am* 26:565, 1982.)

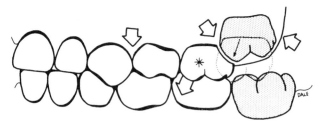

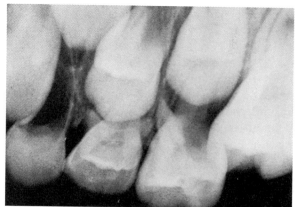

Figure 18-26 Reduction in arch length as a result of ectopic eruption of the permanent maxillary first molars. (From Graber TM, Vanarsdall RL: *Orthodontics: current principles and techniques,* ed 3, St Louis, 2000, Mosby.)

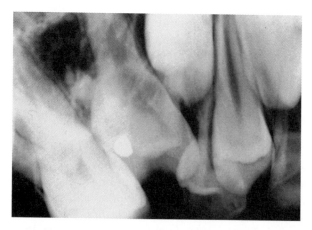

Figure 18-27 Irregularity caused by a suppressed (ankylosed) primary maxillary second molar. (From Graber TM, Vanarsdall RL: *Orthodontics: current principles and techniques,* ed 3, St Louis, 2000, Mosby.)

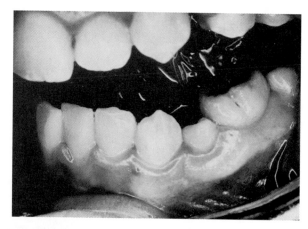

Figure 18-28 Prolonged retention of the mandibular second molar causing crowding of the first premolar. (From Graber TM, Vanarsdall RL: *Orthodontics: current principles and techniques,* ed 2, St Louis, 1994, Mosby.)

Functional Analysis

It has been emphasized that the most successful orthodontic treatment occurs in cases where there is a normal muscular function and a balance of the dynamic components of the stomatognathic system including the teeth, bones, respiration, and the neuromuscular envelope. Class I cases usually have normal muscle balance, and any orthodontic intervention should not disturb such a balance. On the other hand, it is incumbent on the clinician to do an actual functional analysis, even in Class I malocclusions, because neuromuscular aberrations can exist.

Palpation of head and neck muscles is essential. Checking swallowing, respiration, speech, opening and closing and excursive movements of the mandible, and careful palpation of both temporomandibular joints are all basic tools of the diagnostic assessment for all malocclusions. There should be no shortcuts in these evaluations because of the presence of a Class I occlusal relationship.* Existing neuromuscular abnormalities or creating an imbalance between the dentoalveolar structures and the neuromuscular envelope through orthodontic intervention invites relapse, if not outright failure, in the long run, not to mention more potential for iatrogenic changes.

Morphologic Assessment

Mayne[36] has developed a list of morphologic assessment criteria that incorporates some of the developmental and functional aspects discussed previously. The list shows the interrelationship of these components.
1. Tooth mass—present and future
2. Arch form
3. Arch length—present and future
4. Skeletal pattern and denture position
5. Skeletal growth potential
6. Anticipated transitional changes in denture position
7. Orofacial musculature
8. Facial esthetics
9. Oral habits
10. Hereditary assessments of parents and siblings and their application to the patient

The most favorable factors for serial extraction include (1) Class I malocclusion; (2) a favorable morphogenetic pattern—one that does not change; (3) a flush terminal plane or, even better, a mesial step relationship of the second primary molars; (4) minimum overjet; and (5) minimum overbite.[27,55]

SPACE ANALYSIS IN THE MIXED DENTITION

The first step in the guidance of the eruption/serial extraction regimen is to assess the tooth size-arch length relationship in the mixed dentition. The purpose is to determine the presence or absence of any future or existing discrepancy, whether it is crowding or spacing. This topic is described in great detail in Chapter 12. The mixed dentition analysis involves the prediction of the tooth size of the unerupted permanent canines and premolars.

Each patient is unique, and careful measurements must be made from study models and from long-cone periapical radiographs for an accurate determination of the size of the unerupted teeth (see Chapter 12). It is of interest to note in this context that the premolar teeth are usually wider buccolingually than mesiodistally. Therefore if these teeth are rotated in the alveolar process, they appear wider on the radiograph. Care must be taken to determine the anatomy and possible malposition before recording what appears to be the mesiodistal dimensions. An accurate assessment permits diagnostic projections, even if the decision is against serial extraction at that time.

Factors to be Considered in the Space Analysis

As explained in Chapter 12, a number of factors need to be taken into consideration during the space analysis.

The Curve of Spee   A *curve of occlusion* formula is used to determine the additional space required to flatten the **curve of Spee** when required. A flat plastic square is placed on the study model, in contact with the permanent molars and mandibular incisors. The deepest point between the plastic plate and the buccal cusps is measured with a Boley gauge. The depths of the curve on the right and left sides are added and divided by two. An additional 0.5 mm is added to provide the total space required for leveling the curve of Spee (Figure 18-29).[34]

Mandibular Incisors   Tweed[1] observed that the mandibular incisors are often not in a stable relationship to the basal bone after orthodontic therapy, particularly after the use of Class II elastics. Tweed[1] incorporated the anticipated cephalometric changes in the position of the lower incisors in what he termed a **total space analysis.** (In every 1 degree of labial or lingual tipping of the lower incisors there is a 0.8-mm of respective increase or decrease in arch length.) The total space analysis also involves the evaluation of the positions of the permanent second and third molar

---

*References 8, 13, 26, 30, 38, 71, 72, 74.

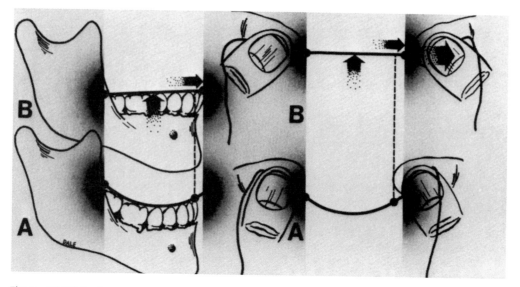

Figure 18-29 Total space analysis. Curve of occlusion. (From Graber TM, Vanarsdall RL: *Orthodontics: current principles and techniques*, ed 3, St Louis, 2000, Mosby.)

teeth. The idea is that there is only so much room in the alveolar trough, and the position of the permanent molars may be a factor affecting the ultimate stability of the orthodontic result.

Soft Tissue Profile   The soft tissue profile is also an important factor to consider in the total space analysis. What actually constitutes an ideal facial balance and harmony is the most contentious aspect of orthodontics. Because patients represent multiracial origins, a unified norm is difficult to determine. Therefore the supreme clinical image involves the interpretation of that individual's *own* data. As one orthodontic wit observed, "We treat only one patient at a time." There is no Procrustean bed of normalcy for all patients.

Serial extraction should be limited essentially to Class I malocclusions with an initial normal sagittal jaw relationship and normal neuromuscular balance. It is the objective of treatment to maintain this balance. All available methods of anchorage control should be used in the final active appliance-finishing phase to maintain the multisystem balance.

It is reiterated that the philosophy is to require as little mechanical intervention as possible using nature's normal stomatognathic balance of the neuromusculature and the maxillary and mandibular bony bases.[18,40-42] Optimal autonomous adjustment without using appliances *first* is a valid goal.

SEQUENCE OF EXTRACTIONS

No single extraction sequence applies to all patients, even when limiting the case selection to Class I malocclusions.

In 1743 Bunon,[75] prompted by nature's own clues, originally conceived the following order of tooth extractions: (1) primary canines, (2) first primary molars, and (3) first premolars. Two and a half centuries later this is still the most satisfactory order in most patients, particularly when the first premolars are erupting ahead of the permanent canines and second premolars. However, individual variations mitigate against adopting this sequence as a hard and fast rule.

The landmark articles on serial extraction by Berger Kjellgren,[2] Rudolph Hotz,[3] John Heath,[10] L.J. Baume,[68] Hayes Nance,[9] and Tod Dewel[4] in the last 50 years discussed the possibility of reversing the order of primary tooth extractions. Removal of the first primary molars before the primary canines is sometimes advocated to promote the earlier eruption of the first premolars. Often this sequence is largely academic, however, because most patients have already lost one or more primary canines by the time they see the orthodontist.[49] In addition, this sequence of extraction is of interest only in the lower arch because the maxillary first premolars usually erupt ahead of the canines.

In general, extraction of the primary canines is preferable.[4,10,11,50,76] The primary objective is to establish the integrity of the upper and lower incisors, preventing lingual crossbite of the maxillary lateral incisors and the resultant mesial migration of the maxillary canines.

Boxes 18-3 to 18-5 include a basic guide for selecting the most suitable extraction sequence, factors to consider during the serial extractions procedure, and representative cases.

Text continued on p. 287

Guide to Selecting Suitable Extraction Sequence

1. Extracting the primary canines only: It produces rapid self-improvement in incisor crowding and alignment, intercepting the development of lingual crossbites of the lateral incisors.
2. Extracting the primary first molars only: This approach produces the earlier eruption of the first premolars but reduces the rapidity and amount of incisor alignment. This is the result of the retention of the primary canines.
3. Extracting both primary canines and first molars: This approach is a compromise between rapid improvement in incisor alignment and the desired early eruption of the first premolars. In some cases this sequence results in the simultaneous eruption of the canines and first premolars, which may cause a reduced distal translation of the permanent canines and possible impaction of the first premolars.
4. Enucleation of first premolar buds: This approach is advocated when the first premolar eruption is behind that of the canines and second premolars. This enucleation permits maximum distal translation of the erupting canines. The danger of **knife-edging** the alveolus at the extraction site (localized collapse of the lingual and buccal walls of the extraction space) mitigates against autonomous adjustment and even later uprighting of teeth contiguous to the extraction site. The surgeon must maintain the buccolingual alveolar dimension by filling the extraction site with bone substitute (freeze-dried bone) following the extractions, if needed. Enucleation is rarely indicated in the maxillary arch.

Factors to Consider During the Serial Extractions Procedure

1. With the proper diagnostic assessment, skilled timing, and careful monitoring, programmed serial extraction procedures are capable of producing extensive amounts of permanent tooth translation. Generally, the earlier the first premolars are removed, the greater the distal eruption of the permanent canines. The obvious question, however, is, "Is it desirable in the total treatment plan to achieve maximum canine distal movement?" This is part of the decisional process that is based on ultimate incisor position and inclination, arch leveling, and anchorage requirements.
2. Another misapplication of the serial extraction procedure is by saving too much arch length early with a holding arch. Too much uprighting of the incisors in the available space can result in too flat a face, caused by the "dishing in" of the anterior segments. On the other hand, occasionally, the lower anterior teeth must be stabilized to prevent excessive lingual tipping. This may be caused by excessive tonicity of the lip musculature (i.e., lip trap). A fixed lower lingual arch from first permanent molar to first permanent molar may be the answer. If prevention of mesial migration of posterior teeth is critical, it may be done by placing a lower lingual arch. However, in the majority of cases, this is not necessary and reduces the autonomous adjustment of the lower anterior teeth.
3. Judicious reproximation disking of primary teeth with no tooth extraction is an occasional option. This decision depends on the careful tooth size-arch length evaluation.
4. Each visit by the patient should be a diagnostic exercise whether extractions are planned at this juncture or not.[6-8,27-29,57] The amount of crowding, the arch length requirements, whether they are symmetric, and the state of the health of the investing tissues are factors that continually impact the occlusal guidance program.
5. On occasion, removal of second premolars or lower second premolars and upper first premolars may be preferred, depending on facial balance, anchorage requirements, size of teeth, and the other factors already stressed.
6. Instead of being a single-decision process, serial extraction is a multidecisional, time-linked process, or a road to success (Figures 18-30 and 18-31).[36] Deciding on the serial extraction avenue is just the first of a series of choices as one fork in the road after another is encountered and the desired avenue is selected. For example, such decisions include whether to remove the primary canines or the primary molars first, when to remove the next pairs of teeth (or maybe only one if there is an asymmetry), and whether to continue on this road or abort the serial extraction program depending on response, growth, development, and patient compliance. To remove or not to remove the first premolars is the question that must be answered; another question that must be answered is whether to place a holding arch because of a critical space problem. Continued vigilance is the name of the game. Annual records such as panoramic radiographs, photographs, and study models are essential, as indicated. This is an exciting and rewarding "game" that is beneficial because it is a win-win situation for both the patient and the orthodontist.
7. The most common unfavorable sequela of the serial extraction procedure is a deepening of the overbite.[6,7,13,55,71] Uprighting of incisors and early loss of posterior teeth may be causative factors. Occasionally, a simple palatal biteplate may correct this problem. But with the now available exotic arch wires, vertical control is efficient and rapid.

8. Paralleling the roots of the teeth contiguous to the extraction sites is usually easy with the autonomous approximation to various degrees before mechanotherapy.

9. Retention demands are significantly less following serial extraction. However, it is better to follow a regular retention regimen for the first 6 months as a safeguard against possible relapse of rotations and to allow settling of the occlusion. An upper Hawley-type retainer and a bonded lower canine-to-canine retainer make an efficient retention regimen.

BOX 18-5

Representative Cases[30,34]

Serial Extraction in Class I Treatment

Group A: Anterior Discrepancy (Crowding)

Step 1 Extraction of the primary canines (Figure 18-32). Typical serial extraction problems are severe crowding of the incisor teeth and an ideal orthognathic facial pattern. Examination of the radiographs often reveals a crescent pattern of resorption on the mesial side of the primary canine roots (see Figure 18-24). This is an indication of a true hereditary tooth-size/jaw-size discrepancy. It signifies that the first premolars are emerging favorably, ahead of the permanent canines. None of the unerupted permanent teeth have reached half of the root length. Because of this the first primary first molars would not be extracted. The primary canines should be extracted to relieve the incisor crowding.

Step 2 Extraction of the primary first molars (Figure 18-33). The incisor crowding has improved, the overbite has increased, and the extraction side is reduced in size. The radiographs reveal that the first premolars have reached half of the root length. It is now time to extract the primary first molars to encourage the eruption of the first premolar teeth.

Step 3 Extraction of the first premolars (Figure 18-34). These teeth are emerging into the oral cavity. Because the permanent canines have developed beyond half of the root length, indicating that they are at a stage of accelerated eruption rate, the orthodontist extracts the premolars.

Step 4 Multibonded treatment (Figure 18-35). The typical result of serial extraction is a relatively deep overbite with a distoaxial inclination of the canines, a mesioaxial inclination of the second premolars, a Class I molar relationship, an improved alignment of the incisors, and residual spaces at the extraction sites.

Step 5 Retention (Figure 18-36). When mechanotherapy is completed, an ideal occlusion should be observed with minimal overjet/overbite relationship of the anterior teeth, parallel canine and premolar roots, ideal arch form, and no spaces. In addition, the dentition should be aligned in harmony with the craniofacial skeleton and soft tissue matrix.

Step 6 Postretention (Figure 18-37). Again, an ideal occlusion with stability should be evident. Initiating the serial extraction procedure with elimination of the primary mandibular canines tends to deepen the overbite. The primary first molars should be extracted when the underlying first premolars have reached half their root length. If this is done, risk of collapse will be minimal. If the mandibular incisors are crowded, the primary canines should be extracted first in preference to the primary first molars. The orthodontist is rarely satisfied with the improved alignment of the incisors when the primary molars are extracted first. Again, the decision is based on the relative position and length of the roots of the first premolars and canines. Figure 18-37 illustrates the occlusion 18 years after treatment. Figure 18-38 illustrates another patient 18 years after treatment.

Group B: Anterior Discrepancy (Alveolodental Protrusion)

Step 1 Extraction of the primary first molars (Figure 18-39). A minor irregularity of the incisor teeth exists. Instead of crowding, the patient has an alveolodental protrusion. The crowns of the first premolars and canines are beyond half of the root length and are erupting faster than the premolars. Because the first premolars have half their root length developed, the primary first molars should be extracted to accelerate eruption of the first premolars. This ensures that the premolars emerge into the oral cavity ahead of the canines. Timing is most important to prevent the formation of a knife-edge ridge (see Figure 18-39).

Step 2 Extraction of the primary canines and first premolars (Figure 18-40). When the first premolars have emerged sufficiently, they are extracted along with whatever primary canines remain. No effort is made to prevent lingual tipping of the incisor teeth because the objective is to reduce the alveolodental protrusion.

Step 3 Multibonded treatment (Figure 18-41). Note how beautifully the dentition is aligning itself. Little mechanical treatment is required.

Step 4 Retention (Figure 18-42). Retention in the mandible is less crucial because minimal irregularity was present before treatment.

From Graber TM, Vanarsdall RL: *Orthodontics: current principles and techniques*, ed 3, St Louis, 2000, Mosby.

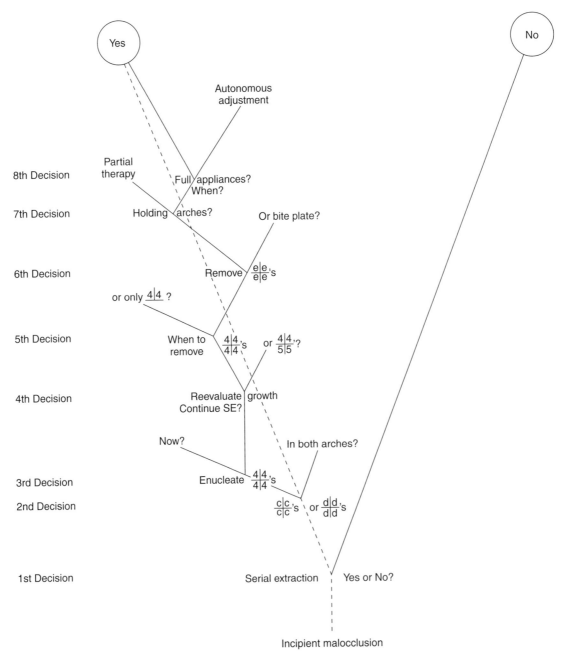

Yes

No

8th Decision — Partial therapy — Autonomous adjustment — Full appliances? When?

7th Decision — Holding arches? — Or bite plate?

6th Decision — Remove $\frac{e|e}{e|e}$'s

or only $4|4$?

5th Decision — When to remove — $\frac{4|4}{4|4}$'s — or $\frac{4|4}{5|5}$'?

4th Decision — Reevaluate growth Continue SE?

Now? — In both arches?

3rd Decision — Enucleate $\frac{4|4}{4|4}$'s

2nd Decision — $\frac{c|c}{c|c}$'s — or $\frac{d|d}{d|d}$'s

1st Decision — Serial extraction — Yes or No?

Incipient malocclusion

Figure 18-30 A more realistic representation of the scope of a serial extraction decision. Rather than a single decision, a series of important decisions are involved. (From Graber TM: *Current orthodontic concepts and techniques,* Philadelphia, 1969, WB Saunders.)

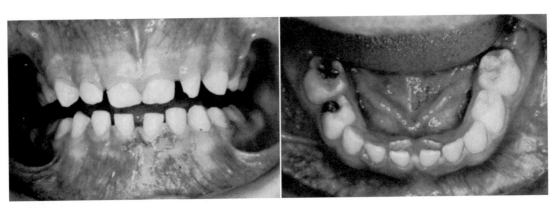

Figure 18-31 Case at age 6 with favorable interdental spacing of lower arch and satisfactory incisor liability, yet the permanent central incisors erupted lingual to deciduous central incisors. The inexperienced clinician might take this ectopic eruption as a diagnostic indication for serial extraction. Such is not true. Case presents favorable measurements throughout offering excellent prognosis. Deciduous central incisors should be extracted. This is not an extraction case, per se, even though extraction of some deciduous teeth may be necessary because of a lack of natural exfoliation. (From Graber TM: *Current orthodontic concepts and techniques,* Philadelphia, 1969, WB Saunders.)

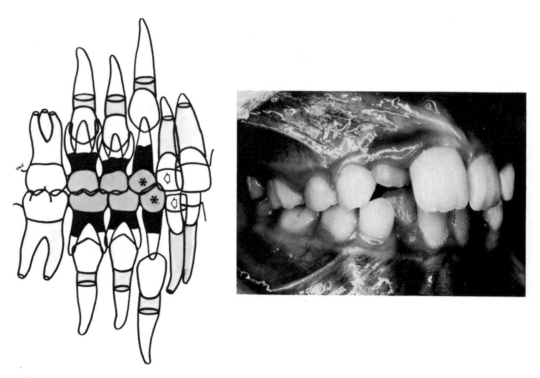

Figure 18-32 Typical serial extraction problem with marked arch length deficiency. (From Graber TM, Vanarsdall RL: *Orthodontics: current principles and techniques,* ed 3, St Louis, 2000, Mosby.)

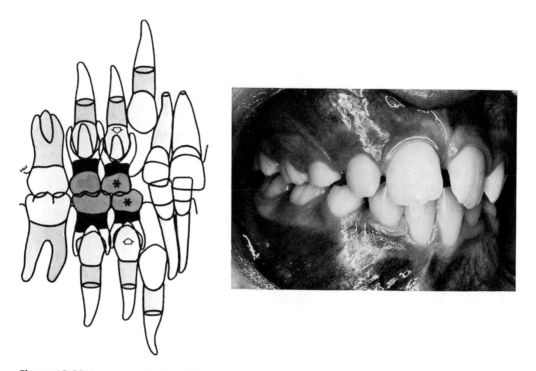

Figure 18-33 Same case as in Figure 18-32 showing improvement following removal of primary canine teeth. (From Graber TM, Vanarsdall RL: *Orthodontics: current principles and techniques,* ed 3, St Louis, 2000, Mosby.)

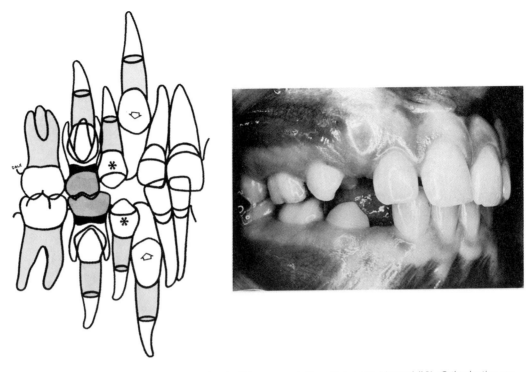

Figure 18-34 First premolars have erupted and will be removed. (From Graber TM, Vanarsdall RL: *Orthodontics: current principles and techniques,* ed 3, St Louis, 2000, Mosby.)

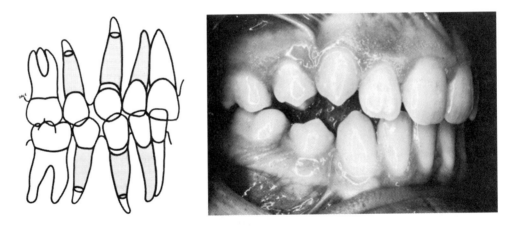

Figure 18-35 Canines erupting after first premolar removal. (From Graber TM, Vanarsdall RL: *Orthodontics: current principles and techniques,* ed 3, St Louis, 2000, Mosby.)

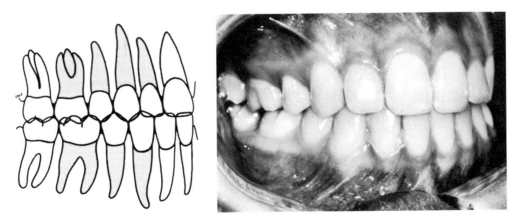

Figure 18-36 Ideal result on appliance removal. (From Graber TM, Vanarsdall RL: *Orthodontics: current principles and techniques,* ed 3, St Louis, 2000, Mosby.)

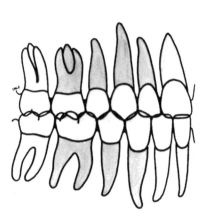 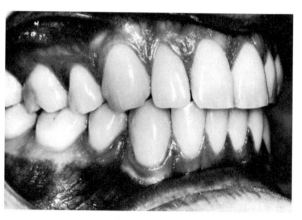

Figure 18-37 Postretention showing a stable result 18 years after treatment. (From Graber TM, Vanarsdall RL: *Orthodontics: current principles and techniques,* ed 3, St Louis, 2000, Mosby.)

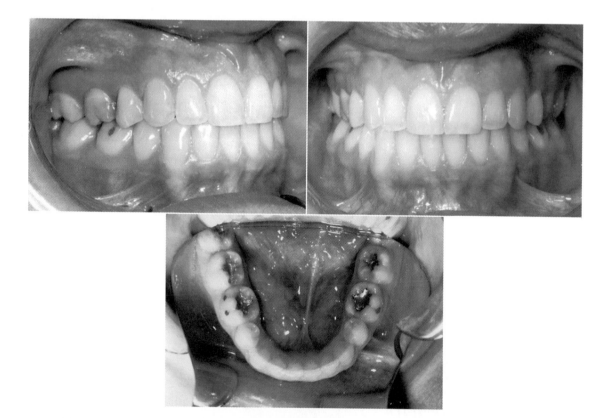

Figure 18-38 Another case 18 years after appliance removal. (From Graber TM, Vanarsdall RL: *Orthodontics: current principles and techniques,* ed 3, St Louis, 2000, Mosby.)

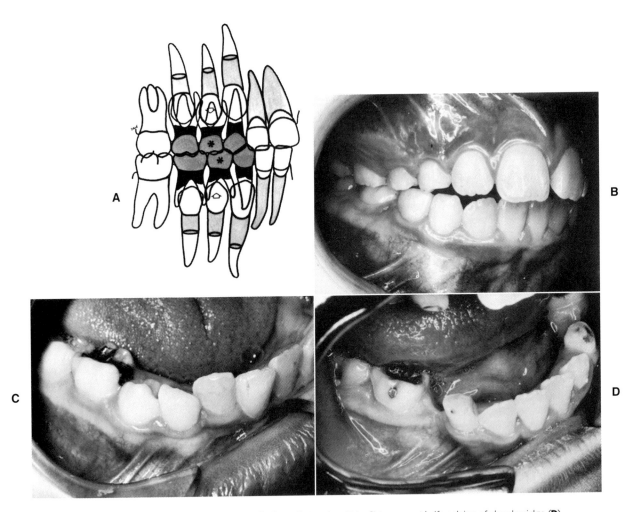

Figure 18-39 Proper timing for extraction of primary first molars (**A** to **C**) to prevent knife edging of alveolar ridge (**D**). (From Graber TM, Vanarsdall RL: *Orthodontics: current principles and techniques,* ed 3, St Louis, 2000, Mosby.)

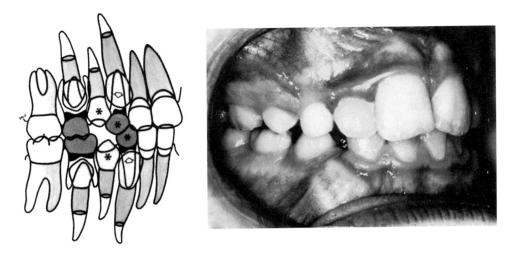

Figure 18-40 Extraction of primary canines and first premolars. (From Graber TM, Vanarsdall RL: *Orthodontics: current principles and techniques,* ed 3, St Louis, 2000, Mosby.)

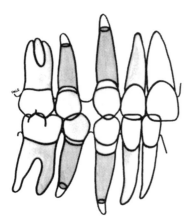

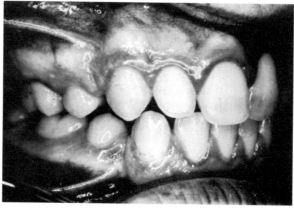

Figure 18-41 Same case as in Figure 18-40 showing excellent autonomous improvement. (From Graber TM, Vanarsdall RL: *Orthodontics: current principles and techniques,* ed 3, St Louis, 2000, Mosby.)

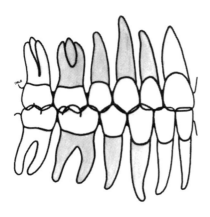

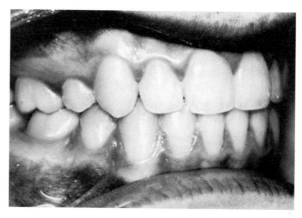

Figure 18-42 Same case as in Figures 18-40 and 18-41. After appliance removal, prospects of long-term stability are excellent. (From Graber TM, Vanarsdall RL: *Orthodontics: current principles and techniques,* ed 3, St Louis, 2000, Mosby.)

SUMMARY

Serial or guided extraction is the removal of certain primary and permanent teeth in a definite sequence. The rationale epitomizes the desire to bring morphologic and biologic concepts together, eventually using fixed appliances when autonomous adjustment does not achieve the optimal therapeutic objectives. To be successful requires a discipline based on comprehensive understanding of orofacial growth and development. Equally important are the fundamental physiologic phenomena of homeostasis and homeorrhesis. A thorough understanding of the components of the stomatognathic system and their dynamic interplay is essential.

A continuing diagnostic exercise is the basis of procedural steps and their timing as the clinician watches the unfolding of that particular patient's pattern and their response to interceptive procedures. The serial extraction program is not irreversible until the decision is made for the removal of permanent teeth. The orthodontist cannot help but be excited by the autonomous adjustment of "Dr. Nature," when the right steps and timing have been employed. Nature is the world's greatest serial extractionist.

A significant number (82%) of patients referred to orthodontists have experienced premature naturally occurring exfoliation of one or more primary canines.[76-78] The early loss of these teeth has strong clinical implications. Unfortunately, many of the naturally occurring exfoliations are unilateral, resulting in significant midline shifts and an associated altered eruptive sequence. To allow the midline shifts to worsen or to allow one primary molar to be lost many months ahead of time (or to be retained too long), when compared with its antimere, serves no useful purpose and can well make the ultimate fixed appliance stage more complicated with consequent iatrogenic potential. The $64.00 question is, "Is this the procedure I would employ for my own child with the same problem?" The question is not, "Is it more efficient for the office from a financial point of view to treat later with comprehensive appliances?"

When limited to Class I malocclusions, the challenges are less and the likelihood of success is greater because the neuromuscular component is not involved etiologically. The effort in these cases should be made to maintain the balance of the tooth component, the osseous component, and the neuromuscular system component of the stomatognathic system.

Concern over growth retardation, resulting from early serial extractions has restricted the wider application of this procedure despite ample long-term evidence to the contrary from excellent studies in Sweden and Switzerland.[2,3] There is no present evidence that either the amount or direction of growth have been modified by guided extraction procedures. Yet attempts to grossly oversimplify the diagnostic discipline by unqualified professionals has given some clinicians cause to pause before taking this biologic highway to ultimate success. The cases shown should assure the hesitant orthodontist that the potential is there if the rules are followed. Likewise, the benefits of serial extraction can be exaggerated by anecdotal cases of minimal or no appliance placement. These are the exceptions. The orthodontist and patient must be prepared for comprehensive detailing and finishing.

REFERENCES

1. Tweed CH: Treatment planning and therapy in the mixed dentition, *Am J Orthod* 49:881-906, 1963.
2. Kjellgren B: Serial extraction as a corrective procedure in dental orthopedic therapy, *Trans Eur Orthodont Soc* 134-160, 1947.
3. Hotz R: Active supervision of the eruption of the teeth by extraction, *Trans Eur Orthodont Soc* 34-47, 1947.
4. Dewel BF: Serial extraction in orthodontics: indications, objections, and treatment procedures, *Int J Orthod* 40:906-926, 1954.
5. Dewel BF: A critical analysis of serial extraction in orthodontic treatment, *Am J Orthod* 40:906, 1959.
6. Dewel BF: Serial extraction: its limitations and contraindications in orthodontic treatment, *Am J Orthod* 45:424, 1967.
7. Dewel BF: Serial extraction: precautions, limitations, and alternatives, *Am J Orthod* 69(1):95-97, 1976.
8. Dewel BF: Serial extraction, second premolars, and diagnostic precautions, *Am J Orthod* 73(5):575-577, 1978.
9. Nance HN: The limitations of orthodontic diagnosis and treatment. I and II, *Am J Orthod* 33:177-223, 253-301, 1947.
10. Heath J: The interception of malocclusion by planned serial extraction, *N Z Dent J* 49:77-88, 1953.
11. Lloyd ZB: Serial extraction as a treatment procedure, *Am J Orthod* 42:728, 1956.
12. Graber TM: *Orthodontics: principles and practices*, ed 3, Philadelphia, 1972, WB Saunders.
13. Mayne WR: Serial extraction. In Graber TM, Swain BF (eds): *Current orthodontic concepts and techniques*, ed 2, Philadelphia, 1969, WB Saunders.
14. Sandstedt K: Einige betrage zur theoriz der zahnregulierung, *Nord Tand Tidskr* 5:236, 1904.
15. Noyes FB: *Textbook of oral histology*, New York, 1912, Lea & Febiger.
16. Oppenheim A: Human tissue response to orthodontic intervention, *Am J Orthod Oral Surg* 28:263, 1942.
17. Weinmann JP, Sicher H: *Bone and bones*, ed 2, St Louis, 1955, Mosby.
18. Ketcham AH: A radiographic study of orthodontic tooth movement: a preliminary report, *J Am Dent Assoc* 42:1577-1598, 1927.
19. Lundström A: *Malocclusion of the teeth regarded as a problem in connection with the apical base*, Stockholm, Sweden, 1923, AB Falcrantz.
20. Lischer BE: *Principles and methods of orthodontics*, Philadelphia, 1912, Lea & Febiger.
21. Angle EH: *Treatment of malocclusion of the teeth*, ed 7, Philadelphia, 1907, SS White Dental Manufacturing.
22. Binder RE: Serial extraction in preventive dentistry, *Clin Prev Dent* 1(4):21-22, 1979.
23. Heath J: Dangers and pitfalls of serial extraction, *Eur Orthod Soc Trans* 37:60, 1961.
24. Graber TM: Extraction in orthodontics, *Colorado Dent J* 43:17, 1966.
25. Graber TM: Serial extraction: a continuous diagnostic and decisional process, *Am J Orthod* 60:541, 1971.
26. Graber TM: Die serie-extraktion—ein kontinuer und entscheidungsvoller prozesz, *Orthodont Kieferorthop* 7:137, 1975.
27. Graber TM: Orthodontic therapy: a continuum of decision making, *Rhodes J Dent* 5:7, 1976.
28. West EE: Pitfalls in serial extractions. In Cook JT (ed): Transactions of the third international orthodontic Congress, pp 282-286, London, 1976.
29. Robertson PB et al: Occurrence and distribution of interdental gingival clefts following orthodontic movement into bicuspid extraction sites, *J Periodontal* 48(4):232-235, 1977.
30. Ono S, Kondo E, Sakamoto M: Serial extraction: clinical advantages and disadvantages, *Shikai Tenbo* 53(5):719-733, 1979.
31. Sharpe W et al: Orthodontic relapse, apical root resorption, and crestal alveolar bone levels, *Am J Orthod Dentofacial Orthop* 91(3):252-258, 1987.
32. Burger H: The danger of unplanned extractions, *J Dent Assoc S Afr* 50(9):436, 1995.
33. Kurol J et al: Hyalinization and root resorption during early orthodontic tooth movement in adolescents, *Angle Orthod* 68(2):161-165, 1998.
34. Dale J: Interceptive guidance of occlusion, with emphasis on diagnosis. In Graber TM, Vanarsdall RL (eds): *Orthodontics: current principles and techniques*, ed 2, St Louis, 1994, Mosby.
35. Mayne WR: *The rationale of serial extraction (audiovisual sequence)*, St Louis, 1965, American Association of Orthodontists.
36. Mayne WR: Serial extraction. In Graber TM, Swain BF (eds): *Current orthodontic concepts and techniques*, Philadelphia, 1969, WB Saunders.
37. Hotz RP: Guidance of eruption versus serial extraction, *Am J Orthod* 58:1, 1970.

38. Carstens NK: Serial extraction, *J Macomb Dent Soc* 13(7):18-19, 1976.
39. Ross SA: Success in serial extraction, *Your Okla Dent Assoc J* 6(2):19-20, 1976.
40. Sebata M, Yamaguchi H: Serial extraction, *Shiyo* 27(12): 2-6, 1979.
41. Drosis C, Markostamos K: Serial extraction for the prevention of orthodontic abnormalities, *Hell Stomatol Chron* 25(5):49-56, 1981.
42. Zietsman ST: Serial extraction in orthodontics, *J Dent Assoc S Afr* 36(4):263-268, 1981.
43. Sfondrini G, Bianchi S, Fraticelli D: Serial extraction, *Riv Ital Stomatol* 50(11):895-901, 1981.
44. Simoes WA: New concept of serial extraction, *J Pedod* 6(2):91-113, 1982.
45. Wolf GR: Case report BC: extraction decisions based on treatment responses, *Angle Orthod* 63(4):251-256, 1993.
46. Luyten C: Guided tooth eruption via serial extraction, *Rev Belge Med Dent* 50(2):67-78, 1995.
47. Vaden JL, Kiser HE: Straight talk about extraction and nonextraction: a differential diagnostic decision, *Am J Orthod Dentofacial Orthop* 109(4):445-452, 1996.
48. Braun S et al: On the management of extraction sites, *Am J Orthod Dentofacial Orthop* 112(6):639-644, 1997.
49. Yoshihara T et al: Effect of serial extraction alone on crowding: relationships between tooth width, arch length, and crowding, *Am J Orthod Dentofacial Orthop* 116(6):691-696, 1999.
50. Greer J: Serial extraction, *J Macomb Dent Soc* 15(6):4-5, 1978.
51. Burlington Orthodontic Research Project: University of Toronto, Faculty of Dentistry, Report #3, 1957.
52. Hurme VO: Assessment of dental age by mean age of tooth emergence, *J Dent Child* 16:11, 1949.
53. Black GV: *Descriptive anatomy of the human teeth*, ed 5, Philadelphia, 1902, SS White Dental Manufacturing.
54. Moorrees CFA: Dental development—a growth study based on tooth eruption as a measure of physiologic age, *Eur Orthod Soc Trans* 40:92, 1964.
55. Dale JG et al: Dr. Jack Dale on serial extraction, *J Clin Orthod* 10(1):44-60, 1976.
56. Baume LJ: Developmental and diagnostic aspects of the primary dentition, *Int Dent J* 9:349, 1959.
57. Moorrees CFA: *The dentition of the growing child: a longitudinal study of dental development between 3 and 18 years of age*, Cambridge, Mass, 1959, Harvard University Press.
58. Bolton WA: The clinical application of a tooth size analysis, *Am J Orthod* 48:504, 1962.
59. Sillman JH: Dimensional changes of the dental arches: longitudinal study from birth to 24 years, *Am J Orthod* 50:824, 1963.
60. Fanning EA, Hunt EE: Linear increments of growth in the roots of permanent mandibular teeth, *J Dent Res* 43(suppl):981, 1964.
61. Moorrees CFA: Normal variation in dental development determined with reference to tooth eruption statistics, *J Dent Res* 44:161, 1965.
62. DeKock WH: Dental arch depth and width studies longitudinally from 12 years of age to adulthood, *Am J Orthod* 62:56, 1972.
63. Moorrees CFA, Chadha JM: Crown diameters of corresponding tooth groups in deciduous and permanent dentition, *J Dent Res* 41:466, 1962.
64. Moorrees CFA, Fanning EA, Gron AM: Consideration of dental development in serial extraction, *Angle Orthod* 33:44, 1963.
65. Moorrees CFA: Changes in dental arch dimensions expressed on the basis of tooth eruption as a measure of biologic age, *J Dent Res* 44:129, 1965.
66. Moorrees CFA, Chadha JM: Available space for the incisors during dental development: a growth study based on physiologic age, *Angle Orthod* 35:12, 1965.
67. Little RM: The effects of eruption guidance and serial extraction on the developing dentition, *Pediatr Dent* 9(1):65-70, 1987.
68. Baume LJ: Physiological tooth migration and its significance for the development of occlusion. Parts 1-4, *J Dent Res* 29:123-132, 331-337, 338-348, 440-447, 1950.
69. Krogman WM: Biological timing and dento-facial complex, *ASDC J Dent Child* 35:377-381, 1968.
70. Enlow DH: *Handbook of craniofacial growth*, ed 2, Philadelphia, 1970, WB Saunders.
71. Dale JG et al: Dr. Jack Dale on serial extraction. 2, *J Clin Orthod* 10(2):116-136, 1976.
72. Dale JG: Dr. Jack Dale on serial extraction. 3, *J Clin Orthod* 10(3):196-217, 1976.
73. Rakoski T, Jonas I, Graber TM: *Orthodontic diagnosis*, Stuttgart, Germany, 1993, Thieme Medical.
74. Banack AR: Controlled serial extraction: a review, *Ont Dent* 55(9):11-12, 1978.
75. Bunon R: *Essay sur les maladies des dents oui l'on propose le moyens se leur procurer une bonne confirmation des la plus tendre enface, et d'eu assurer la conservation pendant tout le cours de la vie*, Paris, 1743.
76. Greer EV: Guidelines for serial extraction, *Your Okla Dent Assoc J* 6(2):19-20, 1976.
77. Little RM: The effects of eruption guidance and serial extraction on the developing dentition, *Pediatr Dent* 9(1):65-70, 1987.
78. Little RM: Serial extraction of first premolars: postretention evaluation of stability and relapse, *Angle Orthod* 60(4):255-262, 1990.

CHAPTER 19

Treatment of Class I Nonextraction Problems, Principles of Appliance Construction, and Retention Appliances

Robert N. Staley and Neil T. Reske

KEY TERMS

finger spring	quad helix appliances	t-loop	Resta clasp
Hawley appliance	fixed W-spring appliance	retromolar rigid endosseous	ball clasp
bonded fixed appliance	modified rapid maxillary	implant	arrow clasp
segmental arch wires	expander appliance	composite resin	C clasp
crossbite elastics	helical spring	Adams clasp	occlusal rests

Patients with Class I malocclusions may need the correction of anterior crossbites, posterior crossbites, incisor diastemas, and tipped teeth at extraction sites, as well as the maintenance of arch length. The diagnosis, treatment planning, and appliances (fixed or removable) used in the treatment and retention of these problems are discussed and illustrated in this chapter.

REMOVABLE APPLIANCES

Principles of Design

A large and effective anchorage system is an important requirement in the design of removable appliances that move teeth. The anchorage unit, which includes those teeth that are not supposed to move as well as the alveolar and palatal tissues, must resist the force directed against the tooth to be moved. These appliances are best kept simple by restricting them to the movement of one or two teeth. For example, Shamy[1] designed a removable appliance to move maxillary first and second molars distally on just one side of the arch in patients with a Class II malocclusion and then constructed a new appliance to retract the molars on the other side of the arch. Therefore whenever several teeth are to be moved substantial distances, it would

be wise to make two or more different appliances to complete the entire treatment.

The anchor teeth are best clasped with Adams clasps.[2] These clasps engage undercut areas on anchor teeth and stabilize them against movement. Clasps are made from stainless steel wires 26 to 28 mil (0.001 inch) in diameter that provide strength and rigidity (Table 19-1).

Finger springs are usually bent from stainless steel wires of 18 to 20 mil in diameter. Springs can be embedded in the acrylic body of an appliance or soldered to a labial bow. Springs move teeth buccolingually or mesiodistally, for the most part.

The acrylic body joins the clasps and finger springs together into one appliance. The acrylic must be closely adapted to the lingual surfaces of clasped teeth to make the clasps effective and the anchor teeth more secure. A spring embedded in the acrylic body has a stable platform from which it can deliver the force required to move a tooth.

In general, removable appliances move a tooth primarily by tipping it as the tooth rotates around its center of resistance and secondarily by translating it bodily a short distance. Finger springs should apply forces that engage the tooth crown as close as physically possible to the center of resistance in the root. Thus the finger

TABLE 19-1	Conversion Table for Orthodontic Wires	
Inches	**Millimeters**	
0.014	0.35	
0.016	0.40	
0.018	0.45	
0.020	0.50	
0.024	0.60	
0.026	0.65	
0.028	0.70	
0.030	0.75	
0.036	0.90	

0.001 inch = 1 mil = 0.0254 mm

spring force should be applied at the level of the gingiva so that bodily movement of the tooth is maximized in proportion to the predominant tipping movement.

When a force of sufficient magnitude is delivered to a healthy tooth by a metal spring in a removable appliance, the tooth will move through the surrounding bone until the force falls below the level sufficient to further move the tooth. The spring then needs to be reactivated.

How much force is required to move a tooth? Crabb and Wilson[3] retracted maxillary canines in 20 patients with finger springs on removable appliances that delivered 30 g in six patients, 40 g in seven patients, and 50 g in seven patients. The canines moved at an equal rate for the three groups, about 1 mm in a month. The 50-g force caused pain in three patients and caused the teeth to tilt distally more so than in the groups with less force. This study indicates that a removable appliance can move a tooth in a biologically sound manner when delivering a force of 30 to 40 g. For example, the lever arm of a maxillary canine is about 10 mm long. The length of the lever is the distance between the point on the crown where a finger spring expresses its force and the center of resistance in the root about which the tooth rotates. A 30-g force from a finger spring produces approximately a 300 g-mm moment as it moves a maxillary canine.

Advantages and Disadvantages

Being able to remove an appliance during treatment allows the patient to keep his or her teeth and gingiva clean and healthy. This same feature can work against treatment success, if the patient chooses not to wear the appliance enough to complete the treatment. Tooth movement is primarily tipping, which may or may not be appropriate for a particular patient.

FIXED APPLIANCES

Principles of Design

Fixed appliances are attached directly to the teeth and include appliances such as lower lingual arches, maxillary expanders, the Begg multiple unit appliance[4] and Angle's multiple unit edgewise appliance.[5,6] The edgewise appliance, with its rectangular tubes and bracket slots, is the most frequently used fixed appliance (see Chapter 14).

The anchorage unit in fixed appliances is less easily defined than in removable appliances. When an initial flexible arch wire is placed in banded and bracketed teeth, all of the teeth move to conform to the shape of the arch wire. In some instances, groups of anchor teeth are tied together to act as an anchor unit. For example, to retract the canines in certain patients with Class II malocclusions, elastics (rubber bands) pit the lower teeth against the upper canines. Another alternative is to use extraoral anchorage from headgear, whether cervical or occipital, to support a group of posterior anchor teeth when canines are retracted.

Because the multiple unit fixed appliances move every tooth that is included in the appliance, care must be taken to correctly fit bands and place brackets in appropriate positions on the teeth. Careless fitting and placement of the appliance create many undesirable tooth movements. In addition, care must be taken in choosing and adjusting the arch wires so that arch form is maintained and the desired tooth movements are obtained (see Chapter 16).

Higher forces are required in the edgewise appliance as compared with removable appliances for two reasons: (1) friction in the tubes and brackets influence the force level and impede tooth movement along an arch wire and (2) the lever arms within the bracket are much shorter in the edgewise appliance than in the removable appliances. Because force delivery must be adjusted according to arch wire size, that is, less force with smaller wires and greater force with larger wires, experience and good judgment are required to successfully use this appliance.

Advantages and Disadvantages

The advantages of the edgewise appliance are its ability to move teeth effectively in all three planes of space, to move teeth bodily, and to torque teeth in the buccolingual plane around an arch. For these reasons, the edgewise appliance, if properly placed and adjusted, can produce the finest and most stable finished occlusion.

Fixed appliances expose patients to enamel decalcification and gingival irritation if oral hygiene is poor. Fixed appliances may cause root resorption, a process that stops when the appliances are removed.

MANAGEMENT OF SPECIFIC CLASS I MALOCCLUSION PROBLEMS

Anterior Crossbites

If maxillary incisors erupt too far lingually, they may be trapped into a crossbite malocclusion. When an anterior crossbite is detected in the mixed dentition, clinicians are concerned that the malocclusion may adversely affect forward maxillary alveolar growth and further complicate the crowding of the maxillary anterior teeth in patients with arch length deficiency problems. For these reasons, anterior crossbites should be corrected as soon as they are discovered.

Variables That Can Influence the Correction of Anterior Crossbites

Anterior Centric Relation to Centric Occlusion Shift

The presence or absence of an anterior shift from centric relation (CR) to centric occlusion (CO) during mandibular closure must be established as part of a diagnosis. Patients with an anterior shift are usually categorized as pseudo Class III and, for the most part, have a Class I molar relationship in CR. In addition to the anterior shift, other signs for pseudo Class III malocclusions include the ability of the patient to make some contact between the incisal edges of the crowns of the maxillary and mandibular incisors in the most retruded mandibular position, maxillary incisors in crossbite may be more lingually inclined than normal, and the mandibular incisors in crossbite may be more labially inclined than normal. When no anterior shift is detected, the probability increases that a true Class III malocclusion is present. Besides the lack of an anterior shift, other signs for a true Class III malocclusion include the inability of the maxillary and mandibular incisors to make incisal contact, maxillary incisors in crossbite may have greater than normal labial inclination, and mandibular incisors may have greater than normal lingual inclination. In addition, the skeletal relationship indicates a mandibular protrusion or maxillary retrusion. The distinction between pseudo and true Class III malocclusions has an important impact on the treatment plan, the prognosis for treatment, and the stability of the correction. Pseudo Class III malocclusions are treated in a relatively short time and, for the most part, successfully retained. True Class III problems are difficult to treat and retain, can involve lengthy treatment when started in younger patients, and may culminate in maxillofacial surgery (see Chapters 21 and 30).

Overbite

The overbite has an impact on the treatment and retention of the teeth involved in crossbite. When an anterior crossbite occurs with a deep anterior overbite, a posterior bite block is needed to allow the lingually positioned maxillary incisors to move anteriorly without occlusal interferences from the lower incisors. When an anterior crossbite is associated with little overbite or an anterior open bite, a posterior bite block is not needed for correction of the crossbite. After the crossbite has been corrected, retention stability depends on the presence of adequate overbite. Thus patients with incisor crossbites associated with little or no overbite are the most difficult to treat and retain. Treatment of anterior crossbites with little overbite is best managed with fixed appliances that can extrude incisors to develop sufficient overbite to retain the teeth in their corrected positions.

Anterior Arch Length

A maxillary incisor in palatal crossbite must have adequate space in the arch into which an appliance can move the tooth out of crossbite. If insufficient arch length is available, an appliance must first create the space needed before trying to move the incisor out of crossbite. In the edgewise-fixed appliance, open coil springs are often used to create sufficient arch length to move the tooth into its proper position. In patients who have significant crowding, premolar extractions and comprehensive orthodontic treatment may be necessary.

Torque of Maxillary Incisor Roots

Many incisors in palatal crossbite have roots that are positioned so far lingually that when their crowns are moved anteriorly out of crossbite, the long axis of the tooth is in a much greater labial inclination than normal. A labially inclined tooth is much more likely to slip back into crossbite following treatment than a tooth with normal inclination. The edgewise-fixed appliance can torque the root labially after the crown has been moved out of crossbite. To accomplish this kind of root movement, a bracket with built-in torque is bonded upside down on the labial surface of the crown. Torquing requires rectangular arch wires of 18×25 mil in a 22×28 mil bracket slot and may take 8 to 12 weeks for completion.

Alignment of Mandibular Teeth

The alignment of mandibular anterior teeth should be delayed until after the upper anterior teeth have been moved out of crossbite. Premature alignment of the lower arch usually complicates treatment of anterior crossbite problems.

Retention

As explained previously, adequate overbite and normal inclination of the long axis of the treated tooth are important for retention stability. After completing treatment, stability can be tested by removing the removable appliance or removing the arch wire from a fixed appliance for a period of 2 to 3 weeks. If the maxillary tooth remains stable, no retainer is needed. However, if the tooth moves lingually, further treatment may be needed and a maxillary retainer should be made to hold the tooth out of crossbite.

A patient who presented with a CR-CO shift may persist habitually with the shift after correction of the crossbite. The habit could persist for a month or more following treatment. These patients should be educated to close into a normal occlusion and to do so purposefully when awake. Eventually the shift will disappear.

Appliances Used to Correct Anterior Crossbites

Removable Appliances The occlusion of a 9-year-old boy with all four of his maxillary incisors in lingual crossbite is illustrated in Figure 19-1. The patient had a CR-CO shift anteriorly. His upper and lower incisors overlapped with about 50% overbite—a favorable condition. His maxillary anterior arch had adequate length to accommodate the incisors in crossbite in their new position. His maxillary incisors were lingually inclined, a finding favorable for simple forward tipping of the teeth.

A removable appliance with a jackscrew and a maxillary posterior bite plate was used to correct the crossbite of the incisors as illustrated in Figure 19-2. Posterior bite blocks were adjusted at the beginning of treatment to provide just enough overbite clearance for the forward movement of the maxillary incisors. Because the screw directed the anterior acrylic segment straight forward, the maxillary central incisors were moved more quickly forward than the lateral incisors. After the central incisors had been moved forward, acrylic was taken away from their lingual surfaces so that acrylic would touch the lingual surfaces of the maxillary lateral incisors (see Figure 19-2). Adjustments of the acrylic were made at each visit until the lateral incisors were out of crossbite.

At the end of treatment, adequate overbite eliminated the need for a retainer. After the crossbite was corrected the patient's occlusion was near normal in CO.

A male patient in the mixed dentition had an upper right central incisor in crossbite (Figure 19-3). The central incisor in crossbite presented with two favorable conditions: an overbite of about 20% and a lingual inclination that is compatible with tipping of the tooth

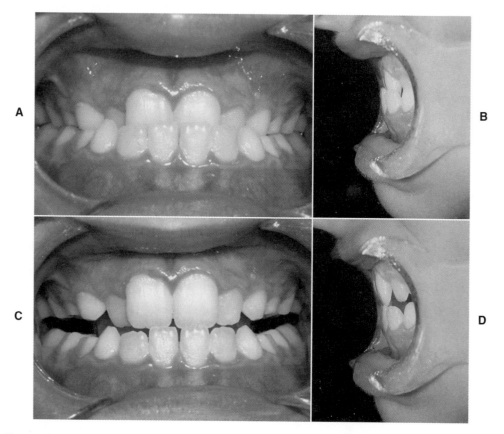

Figure 19-1 A pseudo Class III occlusion with maxillary incisors in crossbite. **A** and **B,** Depiction of centric occlusion. **C** and **D,** Depiction of teeth in centric relation demonstrating the forward shift from centric relation to centric occlusion.

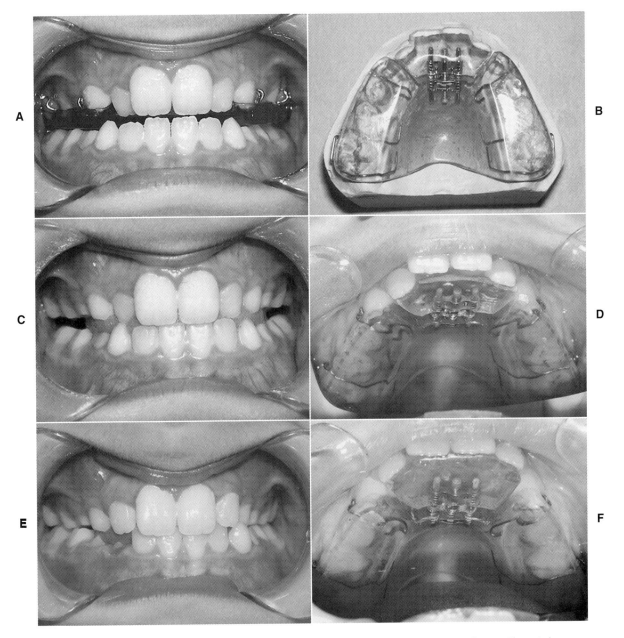

Figure 19-2 The treatment of the incisors in crossbite. **A** and **B,** The removable jackscrew appliance with posterior bite blocks to open the bite. Notice the acrylic touches the lingual of all incisors. **C** and **D,** Appliance in the mouth. Two months later with central incisors almost out of crossbite. Notice the acrylic was relieved from the lingual of the central incisors. Activation of the screw moves lateral incisors labially to align with central incisors. **E,** Occlusion after the crossbites were corrected. **F,** The appliance at the end of treatment.

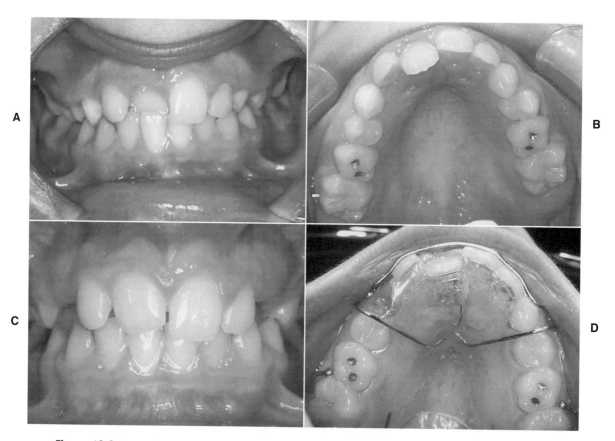

Figure 19-3 A, A right central incisor in crossbite. **B,** The lingually tipped upper right central incisor. Notice that space was available for incisor movement. **C,** The occlusion after treatment. **D,** The removable appliance with a double helical coil spring.

labially. A double helical **finger spring** mounted in a **Hawley appliance** tipped the central incisor forward, out of crossbite (see Figure 19-3).

Fixed Appliances

A 12-year-old male presented with his upper right lateral incisor and upper left central incisor in crossbite (Figure 19-4). His overbite was deep—a favorable condition for retention. He had an anteroposterior shift forward from CR to CO. The gingival recession on his lower left central incisor was severe for his age and perhaps, in part, caused by the crossbite malocclusion (see Figure 19-4). This patient was treated with a combination of fixed and removable appliances shown in Figure 19-4. A fixed appliance was used to align the upper teeth, and a lower acrylic, posterior bite block was used to open the bite so that the lingually positioned incisors could be moved forward. The lower removable bite block was removed as soon as the upper teeth were moved out of crossbite. After the crossbites were corrected, the mandible moved slightly posteriorly as the CR-CO shift disappeared. This allowed for alignment of the lower teeth with a fixed appliance. It must be emphasized that, in the presence of an anterior cross-

bite, the lower anterior teeth should not be aligned before the upper teeth have been brought forward out of crossbite. Aligning the lower teeth first makes correction of the crossbite more difficult. This patient was given upper and lower Hawley retainers.

A young female patient with an upper right lateral incisor in crossbite is shown in Figure 19-5. She had several less favorable conditions when she presented for treatment: (1) the overbite was minimal, (2) the tooth in crossbite was rotated, and (3) the arch length was slightly deficient. A fixed appliance was chosen to align the teeth, to provide space for the right lateral incisor, and to rotate the lateral incisor and bring it out of crossbite. The fixed appliance also helped develop adequate overbite by extruding the tooth after it was brought forward out of crossbite. This patient was given upper and lower Hawley retainers after treatment. A gingival fibrotomy would help stabilize the upper right lateral incisor.

An adolescent male patient who had two upper lateral incisors in crossbite is shown in Figure 19-6. This patient had several conditions that made the correction of his crossbites difficult: (1) minimal overbite, (2) inadequate arch length for the upper lateral incisors,

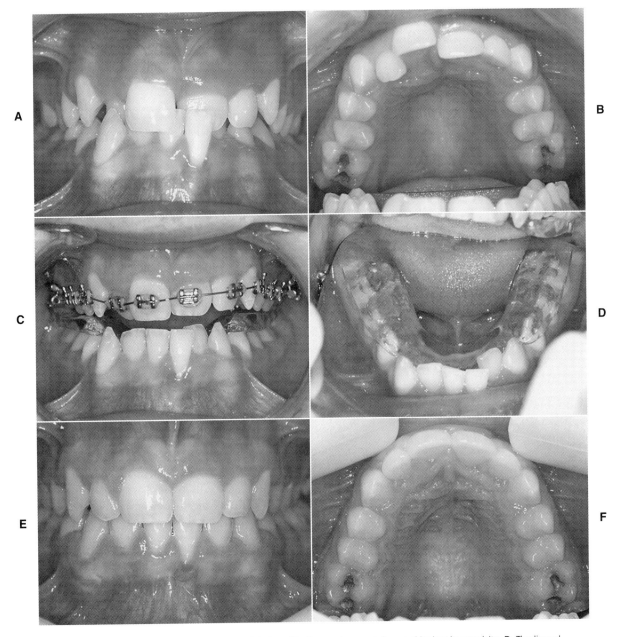

Figure 19-4 **A,** A patient with his upper right lateral incisor and upper left central incisor in crossbite. **B,** The lingual inclination of the teeth in crossbite—a favorable condition. **C** and **D,** A fixed appliance in the upper arch and a removable acrylic posterior bite block in the lower arch that opened the bite enough to easily move the teeth forward out of crossbite. **E** and **F,** The occlusion and upper arch after removal of the appliances.

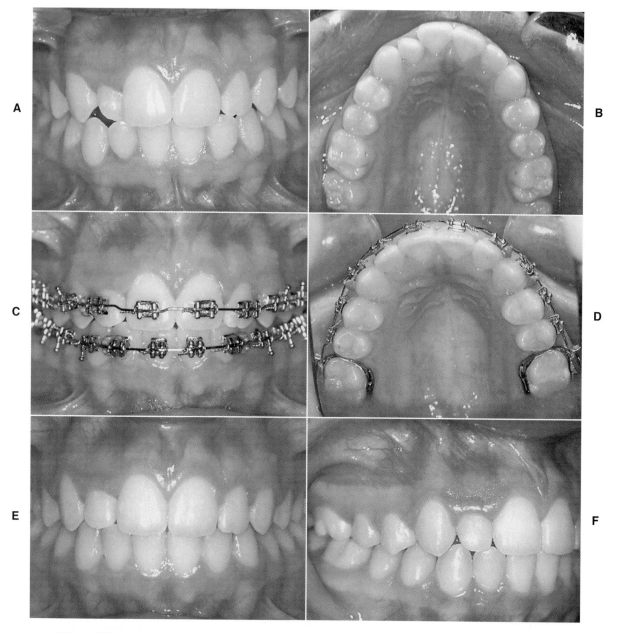

Figure 19-5 A female patient with an upper right lateral incisor in crossbite. **A** and **B,** She had minimal overbite, the tooth in crossbite was rotated, and arch space was slightly deficient. **C** and **D,** The fixed appliance used to correct the crossbite. **E** and **F,** The final treatment result.

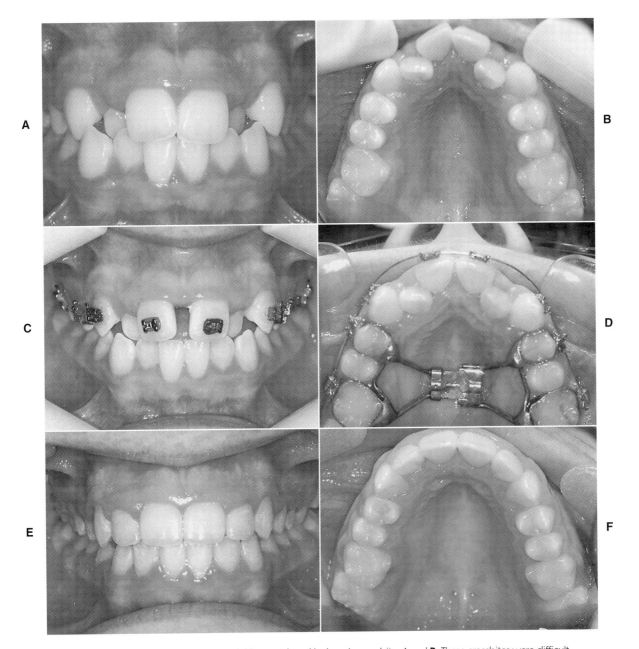

Figure 19-6 An adolescent male with his upper lateral incisors in crossbite. **A** and **B,** These crossbites were difficult to treat because arch length was deficient, overbite was minimal, and the lateral incisors had to be moved bodily out of crossbite. **C** and **D,** The treatment of these crossbites involved rapid maxillary expansion and a fixed appliance. **E** and **F,** Achieving the finished occlusion required comprehensive orthodontic treatment with fixed appliances in both arches and rectangular upper arch wires to move (torque) the lateral incisor roots labially.

and (3) lateral incisors that had both crowns and roots positioned lingually to the alveolar ridge, thus requiring bodily movement for correction. Treatment was started with a rapid maxillary expander to widen the maxillary arch about 5 mm and a fixed appliance with coil springs to create arch length for the lateral incisors (see Figure 19-6). After the lateral incisors were brought out of crossbite, the roots of these teeth were torqued labially with rectangular arch wires.

TREATMENT OF POSTERIOR CROSSBITES

Posterior crossbites usually involve the lingual displacement of a maxillary tooth and the buccal displacement of an occluding mandibular tooth. The buccal displacement of a maxillary tooth and lingual displacement of an occluding mandibular tooth creates a less common posterior crossbite called a *scissors bite.*

Scissors bites occur most often in the first premolars of patients with Class II Division 1 malocclusion. When all the teeth are in scissors bite, the condition usually results from a retrusive (retrognathic) mandible and is called the *Brodie syndrome*. The reverse relationship may also be observed in severe Class III malocclusions in which all the teeth in a small maxillary arch are entirely lingual to the mandibular teeth. When the term *posterior crossbite* is used hereafter, it refers to the lingual displacement of upper teeth and buccal displacement of lower teeth.

The number of teeth involved in a posterior crossbite can vary from one upper and one lower tooth to all the posterior teeth on one or both sides of both arches. The number of teeth involved in crossbite is a guide to the severity of the problem with fewer involved teeth usually associated with less severity. Posterior crossbites, as observed in CO, fall into two categories: unilateral and bilateral.

Variables That Can Influence the Correction of Posterior Crossbites

Buccolingual Inclination of Teeth The buccolingual inclinations of the upper and lower posterior teeth involved in crossbite provide valuable information. If an upper molar in crossbite is abnormally inclined lingually, this position is advantageous because correction of the crossbite usually improves the inclination by tipping the molar buccally. On the other hand, if the upper molar in crossbite is abnormally inclined buccally, the cause is probably the result of a narrowness of the entire upper arch in relation to the width of the lower arch. In such instances, widening of the entire upper arch with a rapid maxillary expander appliance is desirable, as opposed to further tipping of the upper molars buccally.

The abnormal buccal inclination of a lower molar in crossbite is a favorable sign because the molar can be moved to a more normal lingual inclination as part of the treatment. When the lower molar in crossbite has abnormal lingual inclination, the cause is probably related to a discrepancy between the widths of the upper and lower arches. In these cases, movement of the lower molars buccally toward more normal inclination worsens the crossbite and reveals the true width discrepancy between the arches.

Lateral Shift During Mandibular Closure
Most patients who have a unilateral posterior crossbite shift their mandibles toward the side with the crossbite when closing into CO. The lateral functional shift means that the crossbite is, in actuality, bilateral and therefore readily treatable with an appliance that moves both sides of the upper arch buccally. Usually,

in CO, the lateral functional shift has deviated the lower dental midline toward the side with the crossbite. When a functional shift is not easily detected, the patient should be asked to open his or her mouth widely. If the lower dental midline shifts on opening toward the patient's facial midline or lines up at full opening with the upper dental midline, then a functional shift is present. A diagnostic occlusal splint worn 1 to 2 weeks can verify the presence or absence of a functional shift. Diagnostic splints help detect lateral functional shifts in patients whose muscles of mastication have been programmed to close the mandible into the deviated position.

If a thorough examination rules out the presence of a functional shift, the crossbite is caused by a skeletal asymmetry. When the maxilla is expanded by an appliance that bilaterally widens the upper arch in skeletally based unilateral posterior crossbites, the noncrossbite side of the upper arch moves laterally into a buccal crossbite (scissors bite) as the crossbite side is corrected. These patients can benefit from unilateral mechanics such as unilateral cross-elastics or unilateral expansion aided by orthognathic surgery.

Estimate of Expansion Needed In bilateral posterior crossbites and unilateral posterior crossbites with functional shifts involving permanent first molars and other posterior teeth, an estimate of the amount of expansion needed for a Class I molar relationship can be obtained by (1) subtracting the width between the buccal grooves of the mandibular first molars from the width between the mesiobuccal cusp tips of the maxillary first molars and (2) adding to this difference 2 or 3 mm for overcorrection as a protection against return of the crossbite after treatment. The measurements are described and norms are listed in Chapters 10 and 11. The difference between the intermolar widths is positive and is on the order of 1.5 mm for individuals who have no posterior crossbite.

If the needed expansion of the upper arch is 4 mm or less and the upper molars are inclined lingually, a number of fixed and removable appliances such as the quad helix, W-spring fixed or removable appliances, transpalatal arch, and arch wires in the edgewise fixed appliance can be used to expand the upper arch. Expansion of the upper arch between 5 and 12 mm is best accomplished by fixed, maxillary, midpalatal expanders with jackscrews.[7,8] A patient needing expansion greater than 12 mm may require a combination of the use of a jackscrew and surgical orthodontic treatment.

Age of Patient Bilateral posterior crossbites and unilateral posterior crossbites with a lateral shift are best treated in children and young adolescents. It is thought that the prolonged lateral shifting of the mandible in patients with a unilateral crossbite may predispose them to temporomandibular joint dysfunction.[9] Unilateral posterior crossbites with a lateral shift can be corrected in the primary, mixed, or permanent dentitions with a stress on early detection and treatment.

Posterior crossbites can be corrected in adolescents with good success; however, older adolescents and adults are often resistant to standard jackscrew expansion because the more ossified midpalatal suture of adults is more difficult to separate.[7] Furthermore, the resistance of bony tissue and other soft tissues increases the tendency for relapse. Surgically assisted jackscrew expansion is often employed in the treatment of posterior crossbites in adults.[10]

Adults with significant bilateral posterior crossbites who have no shift between CR and CO are sometimes left in crossbite as an acceptable compromise. This compromise is supported by the fact that posterior crossbites corrected primarily by tipping of the upper and lower molars in adults are often unstable, resulting in a return of the crossbite.

Vertical Changes During the treatment of posterior crossbites, anterior overbite usually decreases because the lingual cusps of the corrected upper posterior teeth occlude with the occlusal surfaces of the lower posterior teeth for the first time. This opening of the bite is, for the most part, temporary, and as the teeth settle into their new occlusal relationships, the anterior overbite returns to its pretreatment condition.[7] The tendency for opening the bite must be handled carefully in patients who have a posterior crossbite combined with an anterior open bite (see Chapter 23).

Appliances to Treat Posterior Crossbites

Slow and Rapid Expansion The removable expanders and the simpler fixed expanders work best with a slow approach to expansion. Essentially, the posterior teeth are being tipped buccally. The goal for the rate of activation of the appliance with slow expansion is 1 mm each month. For removable appliances, secure clasping of the anchor teeth and cooperation in wearing the appliance by the patient are essential for a successful treatment.

A more rapid approach is taken with the fixed jackscrew appliances. The recommended rates for expansion in children and young adolescents are 3 mm the first week and 1.75 mm each week thereafter.[11] In older adolescents the recommended rates for expansion are 2.2 mm during the first week, 1.75 mm the second week, and 1.0 mm each week thereafter. Some suggest a much slower approach to expansion with fixed jackscrew expanders, essentially similar to the 1-mm/month speed recommended for removable and simpler expanders.

Removable Appliances A Hawley-type appliance with a jackscrew can be used in the treatment of posterior crossbites of smaller magnitude in children and young adolescents (Figure 19-7). Posterior tooth crowns with adequate undercut areas to provide a secure retentiveness for Adams clasps and cooperation of the patient are needed for a successful treatment. A slow rate of expansion is recommended. A Hawley retainer can be used after the upper arch is widened.

A young female patient in the mixed dentition stage presented with a unilateral posterior crossbite involving her right primary canines and molars and permanent first molars (see Figure 19-7). The difference between her upper and lower intermolar widths was −5.1 mm, indicating that she needed about 7.1 mm of expansion across her upper permanent first molars. Her upper intermolar width was within 1 SD of the female norm, whereas her lower intermolar width was 3 SD wider than the mean. Because her incisors were not fully erupted, she had an anterior open bite. Her crossbite was corrected with a split-plate Hawley appliance with a jackscrew (see Figure 19-7). The jackscrew was opened slowly. The appliance was retained with Adams clasps on her upper permanent first molars and ball clasps between her upper primary molars. Secure retention and cooperative wear of the appliance were important for the successful treatment of the posterior crossbite illustrated in Figure 19-7.

A W-spring appliance can also be used to correct posterior crossbites in children and young adolescents. Again, the appliance cannot work without Adams clasp retention of the teeth and a cooperative patient. A slow rate of expansion is best suited for removable appliances. Treatment is followed with a Hawley retainer.

Fixed Appliances A simple fixed appliance useful in the correction of unilateral crossbites consists of two bands fitted on upper and lower teeth in crossbite. Latex elastics are worn between the button on the lingual surface of the upper tooth and the attachment on the buccal surface of the lower tooth to correct the crossbite. Bonded attachments or bands can be used. This appliance is most effective when the upper tooth is inclined lingually and the lower tooth is inclined buccally. The vertical force from the elastics may extrude the teeth, causing an opening of the bite.

An adolescent female patient presented with her upper left second premolar in crossbite (Figure 19-8). The premolar was displaced lingually as seen in the occlusal view (see Figure 19-8, *A*). Her lower arch was well aligned. The crossbite was corrected using a **bonded fixed appliance, segmental arch wires,** and **crossbite elastics** (see Figure 19-8). The corrected occlusion shown in Figure 19-8 illustrates the improved position of her upper left second premolar.

Fixed appliances that expand the maxilla bilaterally include the banded W-spring, quad helix, transpalatal

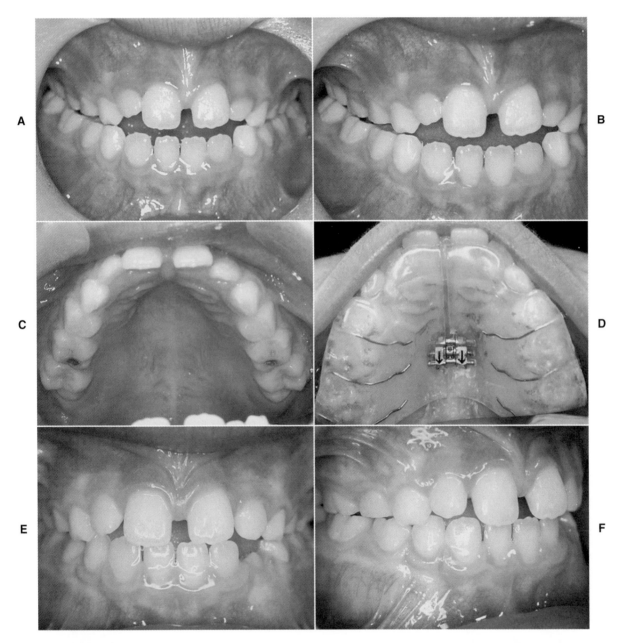

Figure 19-7 **A** and **B,** A female patient in the mixed dentition with a right unilateral posterior crossbite. **C,** An occlusal view of the upper arch before treatment. Her anterior open bite is probably related to partially erupted incisors. **D,** The crossbite was corrected with a removable Hawley split plate with a jackscrew. **E** and **F,** Her treated occlusion.

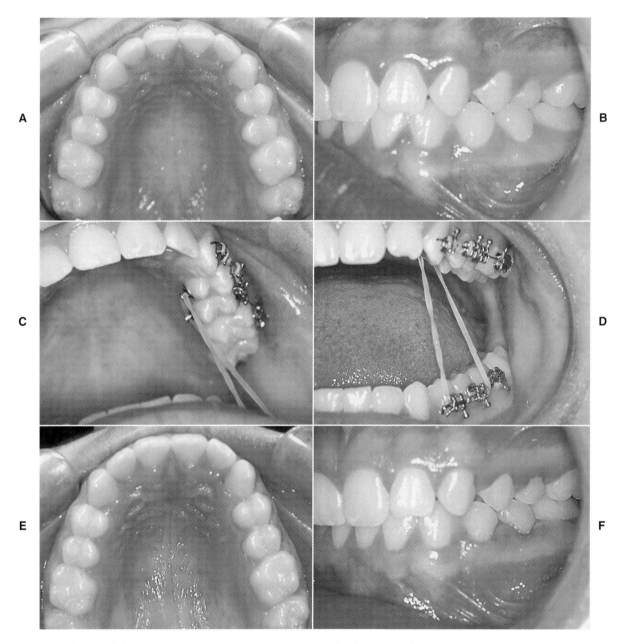

Figure 19-8 **A** and **B,** An adolescent female patient presented with an upper left second premolar in crossbite. The occlusal view of the upper arch shows the lingual malposition of this tooth **(A)**. **C** and **D,** The crossbite of the upper left second premolar was corrected with two segmental arch wires and crossbite elastics. **E** and **F,** The corrected occlusion. The upper occlusal view **(E)** shows the improved position of the upper left second premolar.

arch, and modified rapid maxillary expander. These appliances are used to correct crossbites of moderate magnitude. Fixed appliances such as these require little cooperation by the patient. Slow expansion is best with these appliances. For reactivation, the W-spring and **quad helix appliances** are removed from the banded teeth, are widened, and are recemented on the teeth to complete the expansion.

A female patient in the mixed dentition presented with a unilateral posterior crossbite involving her right

primary second molars and first permanent molars (Figure 19-9). The difference between her upper and lower intermolar widths was −3.9 mm, indicating that she needed about 5.9 mm of expansion across her upper permanent first molars. Her upper intermolar width was 2 SD narrower than the female norm, whereas her lower intermolar width was within 1 SD of the norm. During closure into CO, her mandible shifted to the right, causing the lower dental midline to be deviated toward the side of the crossbite (see Figure

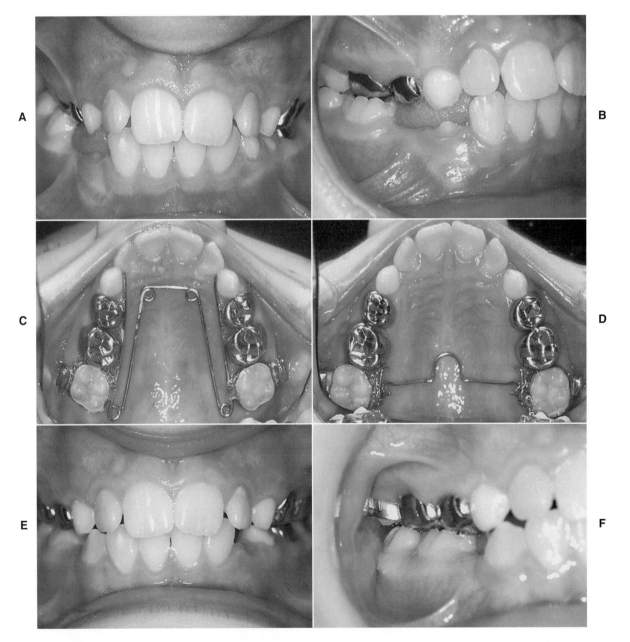

Figure 19-9 **A** and **B,** A female patient in the mixed dentition presented with a unilateral posterior crossbite on the right side. She had a functional shift during closure into centric occlusion toward the crossbite side as evidenced by the deviation of her lower dental midline to the right **(A). C,** A quad helix appliance corrected the unilateral posterior crossbite **(D** and **E).** The dental midlines were closer in the corrected occlusion, demonstrating that the functional shift was eliminated during treatment **(D). F,** The expansion of the maxillary arch was retained with a removable transpalatal arch.

19-9, *A*). Upon opening her mouth, the lower dental midline moved leftward toward the upper dental midline, providing evidence of a lateral functional shift. She had, in fact, a bilateral posterior narrowing of the maxilla masking as a unilateral crossbite because of the functional shift. A quad helix appliance was used to correct the posterior crossbite (see Figure 19-9).

After treatment her lower dental midline was nearer to the upper midline, demonstrating the elimination of the functional shift (see Figure 19-9, *E*). The expansion of the maxilla was retained with a fixed, removable transpalatal arch (see Figure 19-9, *C*).

A female patient in the mixed dentition presented with a unilateral posterior crossbite on the right side involving her right primary canines and molars (Figure 19-10). Her lower dental midline was positioned toward the side of the crossbite, but there was no evidence of a mandibular shift rightward on closure (see Figure 19-10). Her permanent first molars on the right side were not in crossbite. The bands of the **fixed W-spring appliance** were cemented on the upper primary second molars (see Figure 19-10, *D*). The objective of treatment was to reposition the upper right primary canine and molars buccally so that the

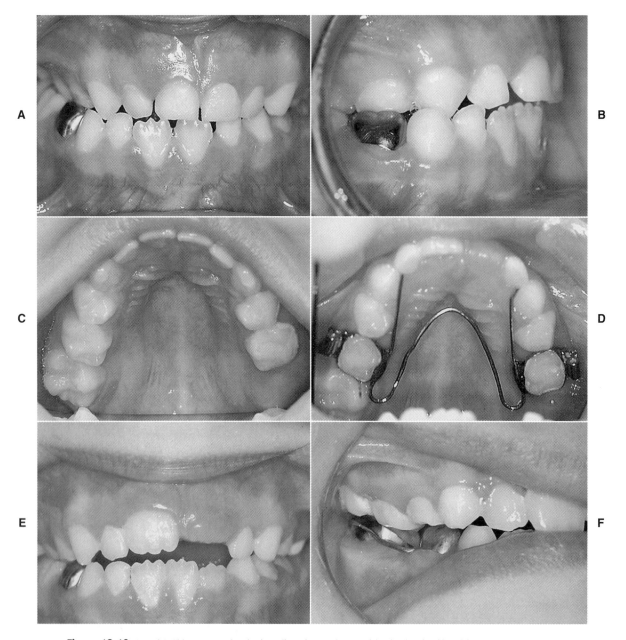

Figure 19-10 A and **B,** This young patient had a unilateral posterior crossbite that involved her right primary canines and molars. **C,** An occlusal view of the upper arch before treatment. A noticeable discrepancy is seen between her upper and lower dental midlines **(A). D,** The crossbite was corrected with a fixed W-spring appliance. **E,** Her treated occlusion at the time of appliance removal in the early mixed dentition. **F.** About 1½ years after treatment the crossbite correction was stable.

upper right permanent canine and premolars would not be influenced to erupt into crossbite positions. The treated result is shown in Figure 19-10, *E*. The lower dental midline after treatment was still deviated to the right of the upper dental midline. The expanded upper arch was retained with the W-spring appliance for 1 year. This patient had a Class II permanent molar relationship on the right side and will, therefore, need full orthodontic treatment at an older age. The right side is shown about 1½ years after treatment in Figure 19-10, *F*. The crossbite correction was stable, and a band and loop retainer was placed in the lower arch to hold arch length after the loss of a lower right primary second molar.

Patients in the mixed dentition who need more than 5 mm of expansion are recommended to use a **modified rapid maxillary expander appliance** to correct the posterior crossbite. A young male patient in the mixed dentition presented with a unilateral posterior crossbite involving his right primary canines and molars and permanent first molars (Figure 19-11). The difference between his upper and lower intermolar widths was −4.4 mm, indicating that he needed about 6.4 mm of expansion across his upper permanent first molars.

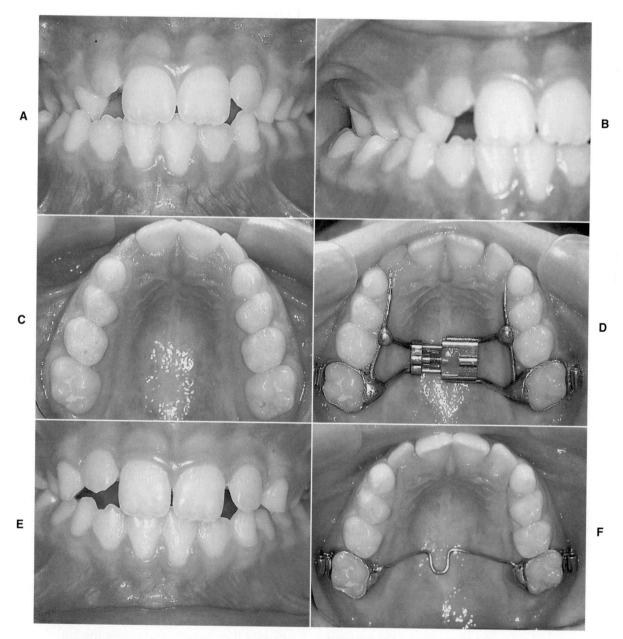

Figure 19-11 A and **B,** This young male patient had a unilateral posterior crossbite involving his right primary canines and molars and permanent first molars. **C,** An occlusal view of the upper arch. The discrepancy between his dental midlines (**A**) was caused by a functional shift toward the crossbite side. **D,** A modified rapid maxillary expander was used to correct this posterior crossbite. **E,** The patient's treated occlusion. **F,** The expansion was retained with a soldered transpalatal arch.

His upper intermolar width was 3 SD narrower than the male norm, whereas his lower intermolar width was within 1 SD of the norm. His right permanent first molars were Class II, an additional problem that must be addressed after the crossbite problem is treated (see Figure 19-11). The patient had a functional CR-CO shift of the mandible to the right side, as can be observed in the discrepancy between the upper and lower dental midlines (see Figure 19-11, A). The modified rapid maxillary expander used in his treatment is shown in Figure 19-11, D. The occlusion after maxillary expansion is shown in Figure 19-11, E and F. His occlusion on the right side improved to an end-to-end molar relation because the expansion of his upper arch eliminated the functional shift. The upper and lower dental midlines are closer together after maxillary expansion—another sign that the functional shift was eliminated. The expander was kept in place for 3 months after activation was stopped, and after that a soldered transpalatal arch was cemented to the permanent first molars to retain the expansion (see Figure 19-11, F).

ORTHODONTIC TREATMENT OF MESIALLY TIPPED MOLARS RELATED TO EXTRACTION AND PREMATURE LOSS OF A TOOTH OR IMPACTION

When a patient loses a permanent tooth or several permanent teeth because of caries or trauma, the surrounding permanent teeth gradually move toward the space that the lost tooth had occupied. For example, if a lower right first molar is extracted, the lower right second and third molars eventually drift and tip mesially and the lower right canine and premolars drift and tip distally. In time, the lower incisors and teeth on the left side of the arch may move toward the right side of the arch. To prevent this shifting and tipping of teeth after a permanent tooth is lost, the patient has two options to consider: prosthetic replacement of the extracted tooth and orthodontic movement of teeth adjacent to the extraction site to close the space. Prosthetic replacement or orthodontic treatment should be pursued promptly after the extraction to avoid the shifting of teeth and the resorption of the alveolar ridge at the extraction site. Both changes complicate orthodontic treatment.

In the mixed dentition the premature loss of a primary second molar can quickly lead to the mesial tipping of the adjacent permanent first molar. In turn, the mesial drifting and tipping of the permanent first molar can easily lead to the impaction of the adjacent unerupted second premolar located mesial to the molar. Impaction of the unerupted second premolar

can be prevented by prompt placement of a maxillary or mandibular holding arch or other space-maintaining appliances (see Chapter 17).

If the loss of a tooth or teeth is not promptly addressed with appropriate measures, orthodontic treatment will probably be required to correct the resulting malpositions of the teeth in conjunction with prosthetic treatment.

Variables That Can Influence the Uprighting of a Molar Tipped into an Extraction Site

Extraction Timing If a young patient loses a first molar while the second molar is still unerupted, the second molar may erupt forward in the arch and eventually take a position either near or in contact with the second premolar. The angulation of this second molar may or may not be desirable, and the opposing upper molar may have supererupted into the area occupied by the lost molar.

If the first molar is lost after the second molar has erupted fully, the second molar will usually tip forward into the extraction site of the first molar. Later, the third molar will erupt and probably tip forward as it makes contact with the tipped second molar. When an adult with good occlusion loses a first molar, the second molar may remain in a reasonably good position because the good interdigitation of the opposing teeth helps keep the molar from tipping mesially. This is especially true for maxillary second molars situated behind first molar extraction sites. However, in most adults who lose first molars, the second molars tip forward to varying degrees depending on the time elapsed since the first molar was lost.

Periodontal Condition Patients have difficulty cleaning the partially submerged mesial surface of the tipped molar. Plaque accumulates on the mesial surface of the tooth and eventually produces periodontal disease including loss of alveolar bone that can threaten the longevity of the molar. Uprighting the molar helps stop the periodontal disease process on its mesial surface.

Vertical Dimension The position of teeth in the opposite arch occluding with the tipped molar should be carefully observed. Sometimes the teeth in the opposing arch have overerupted into the area of the tipped tooth, and sometimes teeth are no longer present to occlude with the tipped molar. Repositioning the tipped molar in a distal direction extrudes it occlusally and opens the bite. An already overerupted opposing tooth exaggerates the opening of the bite. An overerupted tooth in the opposing arch can be intruded by an orthodontic appliance, or its crown can be shortened by occlusal equilibration to control bite opening. The absence of opposing teeth can allow the tipped molar to extrude too far occlusally when it is repositioned. In these circumstances the choice of appliance and occlusal equilibration can help control the vertical position of the repositioned molar. Because the distal movement and uprighting of a molar usually creates an open bite, the use of occlusal equilibration to close the bite after uprighting must be discussed with the patient before starting treatment to obtain an informed consent for this procedure.

Number of Missing Teeth

The number of teeth missing mesial to the tipped molar must be considered because fixed appliances cannot effectively control the movement of a tipped second or third molar that is isolated at the distal end of an edentulous ridge with only a first premolar or canine available forward of the molar. When the patient is missing several teeth, removable appliances can be used to better upright a molar because removable appliances derive their anchorage from both the teeth and the alveolar ridge.

Position of Third Molar

When a tipped lower second molar to be repositioned distally for a prosthetic appliance is in close contact with a lower third molar, the lower third molar is often extracted at the beginning of treatment to make room for the repositioning of the second molar. This approach to treatment is appropriate when the opposing upper third molar is absent or impacted.

Resorbed Alveolar Ridge

When adolescents and adults lose a permanent tooth, the alveolar ridge at the extraction site resorbs. The resorbed ridge is short and narrow. Some resorbed ridges may have an hourglass appearance from the occlusal view. Molars cannot be easily moved through an hourglass ridge, and if they are forced to do so, the molar roots may partially resorb. A first molar space can be more easily closed mechanically by retracting the premolars into the narrower hourglass ridge. However, this movement is not desirable for most patients. The resorption of an alveolar ridge can be exacerbated when the buccal alveolar plate of bone is removed with the extracted tooth. Moving teeth into resorbed ridges can result in a compromised periodontal attachment. Therefore when a lower second molar is tipped mesially into the extraction site of a first molar and the alveolar ridge has resorbed to an hourglass shape, the most common orthodontic treatment involves tipping the second molar distally to an upright position to prepare for a prosthetic replacement. An hourglass ridge

may also prevent the placement of a single tooth implant replacement without bone grafting or distraction osteogenesis.

Impacted Mandibular Second Molars   In some patients the mandibular second molar is partially erupted and tipped forward with its mesial surface locked beneath the distal surface of the first molar. If an impacted third molar lies behind and over the distal surface of the impacted second molar, it must be extracted to make room in the alveolus for uprighting the second molar. Because impacted second molars are usually only partially erupted, bonding a rectangular tube on the exposed buccal surface is easier than fitting a band on the tooth. Sometimes a tube or bracket must be bonded to a small part of the occlusal surface that is exposed to the oral cavity.

These tipped molars must be moved distally and occlusally so that the molar occludes at a normal axial angulation with the upper teeth. In adolescent patients the opposing upper molars are usually present but not overerupted. However, in adult patients the opposing upper molars are likely to be overerupted—a situation that limits how far the tipped molar can extrude as it tips backward (see Chapter 28). Thus the primary difficulty encountered is that the uprighted molar moves upward too much and opens the bite. The choice of appliances can help with this problem, but, more important, adult patients must be told that the occlusal surfaces of the crowns of both the upper and lower molars at the site of the uprighting may need to be mechanically reduced to reestablish a healthy overbite.

Appliances to Upright Molars

Removable Appliances   A removable appliance with an uprighting **helical spring** made from 21×25 mil stainless steel wire can be used to move a molar distally and upright it to a more normal angulation.[1] These appliances are most useful when larger edentulous regions isolate the tipped tooth from other teeth. The removable appliance has limited control over the vertical, buccolingual, and mesiodistal movements of the molar. Keeping the spring at the gingival margin as close as possible to the center of resistance of the tooth is important for the best control of tooth movement. Secure anchorage of the appliance on the clasped teeth is important for the effective delivery of force to upright the molar.

A young male in the mixed dentition prematurely lost his upper left second primary molar (Figure 19-12). A removable appliance with Adams clasps and a 21×25 mil rectangular helical uprighting spring was placed in the maxillary arch to regain arch length (see Figure 19-12).

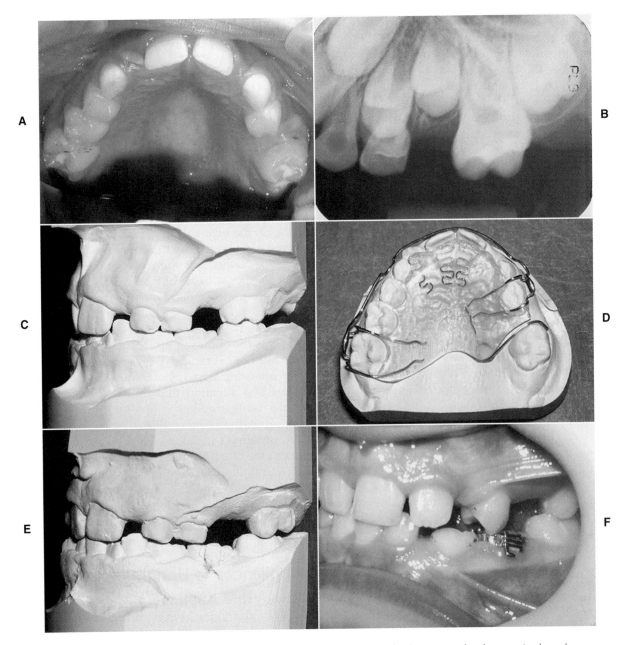

Figure 19-12 **A** to **C,** This patient in the mixed dentition lost his upper left primary second molar prematurely, and his upper left permanent first molar slipped mesially. **D,** A removable appliance was made to regain arch length. **E** and **F,** The occlusion after the space for the unerupted second premolar is regained.

Fixed Appliances A coil spring placed on a flexible arch wire tied into an edgewise fixed appliance is a mechanically simple device that is most effective in moving a second molar distally and tipping it into a more normal angulation. This appliance will allow the second molar to extrude and open the bite, depending on the flexibility of the arch wire. The continued leveling of the arch with larger arch wires may intrude the uprighted molar sufficiently to avoid occlusal equilibration.

A **t-loop** placed in a rectangular stainless steel arch wire 18 × 25 mil in size in a 22 × 28 mil edgewise fixed appliance is an excellent appliance for uprighting and distalizing a lower second molar.[12] As stated previously, the arch wire can, if properly made, assist in controlling the extrusion of the uprighted molar. The t-loop must be made so that it does not injure the surrounding soft tissues. The t-loop can tip the crown distally and bring the roots mesially by rotating the tooth around the buccal tube. The rectangular wire of the t-loop can also control buccolingual inclination of the uprighted tooth.

An adult female patient presented with an impacted lower left permanent second molar (Figure 19-13). She

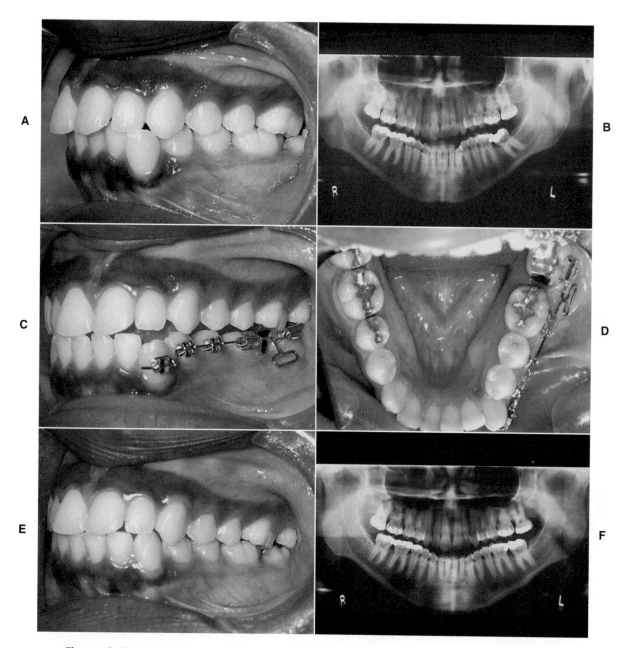

Figure 19-13 A, An adult woman presented with an impacted lower left permanent second molar. **B,** The panorex revealed a periodontal defect mesial to the impacted molar. **C** and **D,** A t-loop rectangular segmental arch wire uprighted and distalized the impacted molar. **E,** The lower left premolars and first molar were retracted to make room for the lower left canine. **F,** A panorex taken after treatment was completed.

had no third molar distal to the impacted molar—an advantage. Her overbite was about 20%—a favorable finding. Her lower left canine was buccally displaced out of the arch—a complication. A t-loop 18 × 25 mil rectangular segmental wire uprighted and distalized the lower molar (see Figure 19-13). After placing a full lower arch wire with stops mesial to the lower right first molar and lower left second molar, the lower left first molar and premolars were retracted to make room in the arch for the lower left canine. Intentional depression of the uprighted molar kept the bite from opening too much.

A helical spring appliance can be used to upright and extrude a tipped lower second molar. The spring is made of an 18 × 25 mil stainless steel arch wire that hooks onto an 18 × 25 mil arch wire in a 22 × 28 mil fixed edgewise appliance to activate the spring. Because the spring is separate from the arch wire, the uprighted molar is free to extrude. Extrusion of a molar is sometimes needed to bring it up to the occlusal plane, but, in most cases, deliberate extrusion of a tipped molar is avoided. The helical spring has little control over buccolingual movement of the uprighted molar and tends to incline the crown lin-

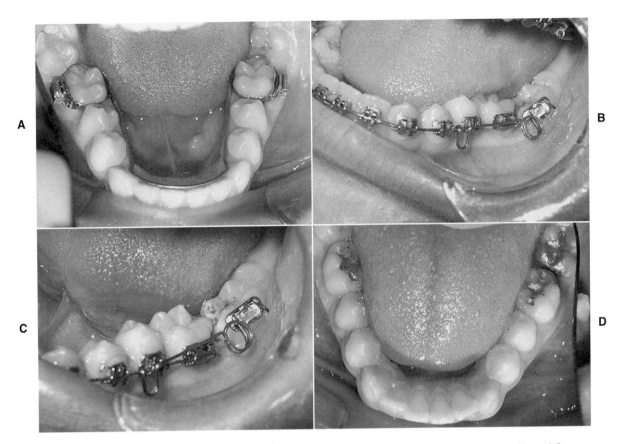

Figure 19-14 A, A male patient who had worn a lower lingual holding arch presented with an impacted lower left permanent second molar. **B** and **C,** A helical uprighting spring anchored on a full lower arch wire was used to upright the impacted molar. **D,** The uprighted molar was carious and required immediate restoration.

gually as it extrudes the tooth. Replacing the helical spring with a continuous arch wire after the molar has uprighted can help control the unwanted side effects of the spring.

An adolescent male who had been wearing a soldered lower lingual arch presented with an impacted lower left permanent second molar (Figure 19-14). The impacted molar was uprighted with a helical coil spring anchored on a full lower arch wire that extended from first molar to first molar. The impacted molar was carious and required an immediate restoration after the uprighting (see Figure 19-14).

Appliances to Upright a Molar and Close an Extraction Site If the extraction of a molar is quickly followed by orthodontic treatment, a fixed edgewise appliance can be used to protract the second or third molar into the extraction site. This necessitates comprehensive orthodontic treatment involving bodily tooth movement. Protraction headgear or interarch elastics may be used as additional sources of anchorage to accomplish such a treatment. The mesial movement of the molar is best accomplished with a large rectangular stainless steel wire of 18 × 25 mil dimensions in the 22 × 28 mil edge-

wise appliance that helps the molar move forward bodily as opposed to tipping. Lingual buttons on the molar and premolars with plastic chains stretched between the buttons keep the molar from rotating while using force delivery systems such as elastics or springs on the buccal surfaces.

A young woman presented with a badly carious lower left permanent second molar (Figure 19-15). Her partially erupted lower left third molar was protracted to replace the extracted lower second molar (see Figure 19-15, C and D). The protracted third molar opened the bite (see Figure 19-15, E). After occlusal equilibration, the bite closed (see Figure 19-15, F).

Distraction osteogenesis techniques are being developed to widen resorbed alveolar ridges so that a molar can be moved mesially with a fixed appliance to close an edentulous space.

A fixed appliance using a **retromolar rigid endosseous implant** anchor can effectively protract molars through an edentulous alveolar ridge (see Chapter 28).[13,14] The surgically placed implant becomes ankylosed in the bone and acts as a secure anchor against which forces can be delivered to protract a molar or molars without displacing either other teeth or

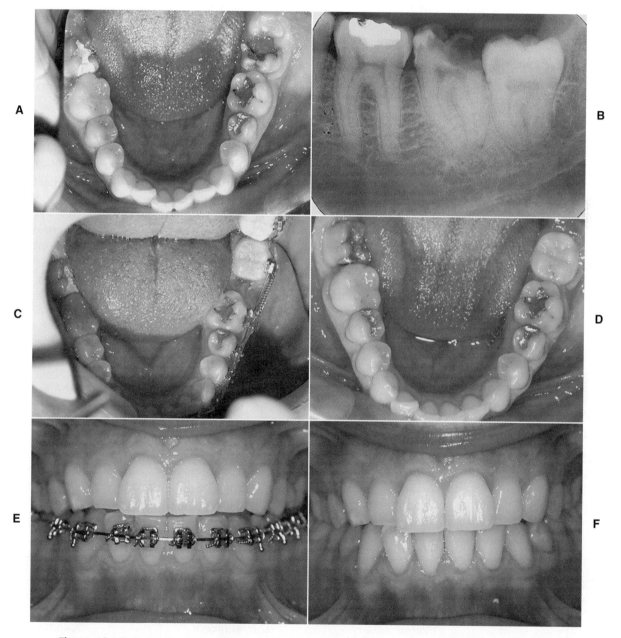

Figure 19-15 **A,** A young woman presented with a lower left permanent second molar that required extraction. **B,** A periapical radiograph illustrates the carious condition of her lower left second molar. **C** and **D,** Her partially erupted third molar was protracted shortly after the carious second molar was extracted using a coil spring. All teeth mesial to the extraction site were continuously tied to enhance the ancorage while protracting the third molar. **E,** The protraction opened the bite, and, **F,** occlusal equilibration was used to close the bite.

the dental midline toward the molar extraction site. Molars can be moved with this appliance even through hourglass-shaped ridges; however, some root resorption and periodontal attachment problems may still be encountered. This appliance can eliminate the need for a fixed prosthesis in an area of the arch in which a fixed prosthesis may not function well or have a limited longevity.

MANAGEMENT OF INCISOR DIASTEMAS IN THE PERMANENT DENTITION

Patients seek treatment for diastema and spacing problems primarily for esthetic reasons. Orthodontic treatment can be an important part of the correction of these diastemas.[15] Diastemas between permanent maxillary incisors occur for several reasons in persons with Class I occlusion: (1) the incisors have normal size and the dental arch is large, (2) the incisors are small and the dental arch is normal, (3) the incisors are small and the dental arch is large, (4) the incisors are positioned labially to the mandibular incisors with overjet larger than normal, (5) one or more incisors are severely rotated, and (6) a midline frenum is abnormally attached to soft and bony tissues at the site of the diastema. Diastemas also occur when one or more incisors are congenitally missing or extracted. This discussion does not address the topic of missing and extracted teeth.

Variables That Can Influence the Treatment of Diastemas

Size of Teeth   To evaluate the cause of a diastema, measurements of the mesiodistal widths of the anterior teeth can be taken. The widths of the anterior teeth of European-American persons with normal occlusion

are given in Table 19-2.[16] If arch size is thought to contribute to the cause, arch widths can be measured and compared with the norms found in Chapter 9.

The four incisors have harmonious dimensions in persons with normal occlusions. In the maxilla, central incisor crowns have larger vertical and mesiodistal dimensions than lateral incisors. Upper central incisors are stable teeth with regard to size, whereas lateral incisors are prone to greater variation in size.[17] Mesiodistal widths may demonstrate that all four incisors are too small or that the central incisors have normal size and the lateral incisors are smaller than normal.

Treatment Considerations with Regard to Tooth Size   Knowledge of tooth size and interrelations in tooth size is important when deciding the appropriate treatment plan. If all the maxillary incisors are too small, the objective of orthodontic treatment would be to position the teeth so that appropriate crown widths can be established with **composite resin** build ups or crowns on all four incisors. If only the lateral incisors are small, the central incisors would be moved together orthodontically to properly position the lateral incisors before restoring crown size.

The interarch relationships between the mesiodistal widths of the maxillary and mandibular anterior teeth can contribute to the presence of a diastema. Bolton[18] established a ratio between the mesiodistal widths of the maxillary and mandibular teeth in excellent occlusion. When the combined widths of the mandibular anterior teeth are too large for the combined widths of the maxillary anterior teeth, a well-aligned lower arch is matched to an upper arch with spacing between the incisors. In these patients maxillary spacing can be reduced by removing some of the interproximal enamel from the mandibular anterior teeth. However, mandibular anterior crown width reduction is limited

TABLE 19-2	Mesiodistal Widths of Anterior Teeth in European-American Persons with Normal Occlusion[16] (Mean ± 1 SD in mm)								
	Central Incisor			*Lateral Incisor*			*Canine*		
	Mean	Min	Max	Mean	Min	Max	Mean	Min	Max
Maxillary Arch									
Males (n=37)	8.8 ± 0.6	7.7	9.9	6.9 ± 0.5	5.8	8.8	8.1 ± 0.5	6.6	9.0
Females (n=33)	8.7 ± 0.6	7.5	10.6	6.7 ± 0.5	5.2	7.8	7.7 ± 0.3	7.0	8.5
Mandibular Arch									
Males (n=37)	5.6 ± 0.4	4.8	7.3	6.0 ± 0.4	5.1	6.9	7.0 ± 0.4	6.0	7.9
Females (n=33)	5.4 ± 0.4	4.5	6.3	5.9 ± 0.4	5.2	7.0	6.6 ± 0.4	5.8	7.5

SD, Standard deviation.

to a small amount, and most mandibular incisors have too little enamel thickness for any significant, that is, effective reduction. The treatment of interarch tooth width discrepancies with enamel reduction require the use of orthodontic fixed appliances in both arches.

Some patients with a diastema between their maxillary central incisors can best be treated by composite resin recontouring of the central incisors without any orthodontic treatment. It must be emphasized that orthodontic treatment always carries with it the potential for posttreatment tooth movement, therefore limiting the treatment of a midline diastema to composite resin esthetic recontouring produces a more stable result with respect to tooth position.

Mandibular Arch Alignment
Maxillary diastema management is affected by the alignment of the mandibular teeth. If the mandibular teeth are well aligned with no spacing between them, the maxillary diastema can be treated without the need for an appliance in the lower arch. However, if spacing exists between the mandibular teeth, this spacing should be closed as part of the management of the maxillary diastema. After the lower arch spaces are closed, the maxillary incisors can be retracted to contact the mandibular anterior teeth. The retraction of the maxillary incisors will reduce and sometimes eliminate the diastema problem in the upper arch.

Labially Positioned Maxillary Incisors
In a Class I molar and canine occlusion, the maxillary incisors are sometimes labially inclined with diastemas between them. This condition can be caused by a thumbsucking habit. If the habit is active at the time of the orthodontic examination, it should be addressed as part of the treatment. When excessive overjet is present, retraction of the maxillary incisors is necessary, and may, in itself, close the diastemas. If diastemas persist following incisor retraction, treatment is directed toward proper spacing of the teeth before their esthetic enlargement.

Rotated Incisors
In some patients incisor diastemas are created when one or more incisors are rotated 90 degrees from their appropriate positions in the arch. Correction of such diastemas requires orthodontic movement of the rotated teeth. Rotation of the teeth into proper position may eliminate the diastemas. The retention of rotated incisors is important, and includes supracrestal fibrotomy around the tooth and fixed retainers.[19,20]

Maxillary Labial Frenum
A midline diastema between the maxillary central incisors can be associated with an abnormal maxillary labial frenum. A normal frenum inserts into the attached gingiva superior to the central incisors. The characteristics that are associated with an abnormal frenum include the following: (1) the frenum attaches into the soft tissues between the central incisors or into the palatal soft tissues lingual to the incisors, (2) the frenum is wider than usual at its insertion site, and (3) when the upper lip and frenum are stretched, the tissue between the central incisors moves and is blanched.[21]

A frenectomy greatly increases the long-term stability of the closure of a midline diastema when the frenum has an abnormal insertion.[21] Before the frenectomy, most clinicians advise that the diastema be orthodontically closed so that scar tissue does not impede closure of the diastema (Figure 19-16). The frenectomy alone, without orthodontic treatment, is unlikely to result in complete closure of the diastema. The frenectomy is best performed by a periodontist.

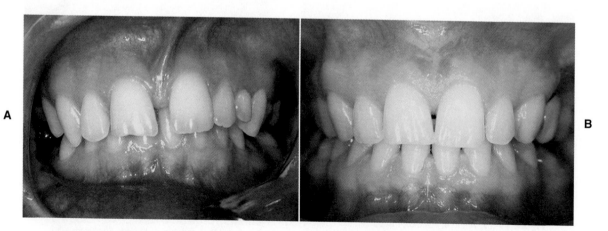

Figure 19-16 **A,** A patient is shown with a large frenum that is attached between the maxillary central incisors at the site of a diastema. **B,** After the diastema was closed with orthodontic treatment, a surgical frenectomy was performed to ensure stability of the orthodontic closure.

Appliances to Close Diastemas

Removable Appliances The treatment of a female patient in the mixed dentition with a diastema between her maxillary central incisors is illustrated in Figure 19-17, *A* and *B*. A removable appliance with finger springs was used to close the diastema (see Figure 19-17, *C* and *D*). Wire loops embedded in the acrylic body of the appliance were used to control tongue thrusting (see Figure 19-17). The closure of the diastema created arch length for an erupting upper right lateral incisor. The lower den-

tal midline had shifted to the right in response to the unilateral loss of the lower right primary canine (see Figure 19-17, *E*). This patient needs additional treatment.

Fixed Appliances An adult female presented with diastemas in the anterior regions of her maxillary and mandibular arches (Figure 19-18, *A* to *C*). A fixed appliance was used to first close the lower arch spaces and then to close the upper arch spaces (see Figure 19-18, *D*). Treatment eliminated the diastemas. She was retained with Hawley appliances and a bonded

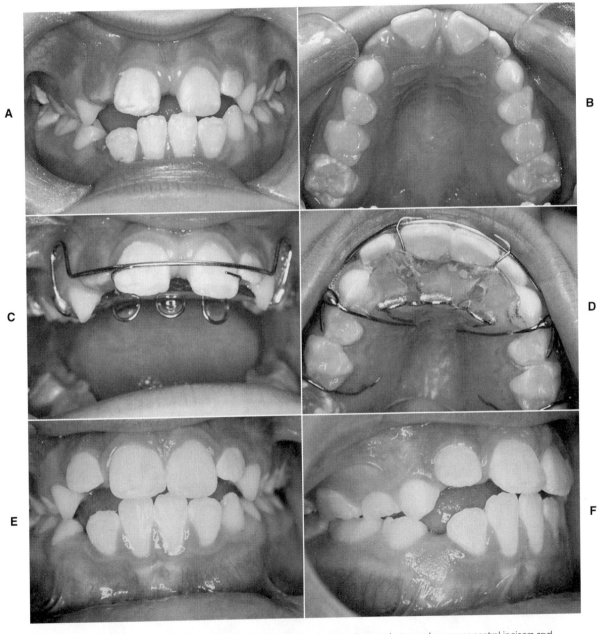

Figure 19-17 **A** and **B,** A female mixed dentition patient had a large diastema between her upper central incisors and an upper right lateral incisor that needed additional arch length to erupt. **C** and **D,** A removable Hawley appliance with finger springs was used to close the diastema. Loops were placed in the palatal acrylic of the appliance to discourage tongue thrusting by the patient **(C** and **D). E,** Her upper and lower dental midlines were not coincident after treatment because the unilateral loss of a mandibular right primary canine resulted in a rightward shifting of the mandibular incisors. **F,** The erupting upper right lateral incisor had adequate room to erupt after the diastema was closed.

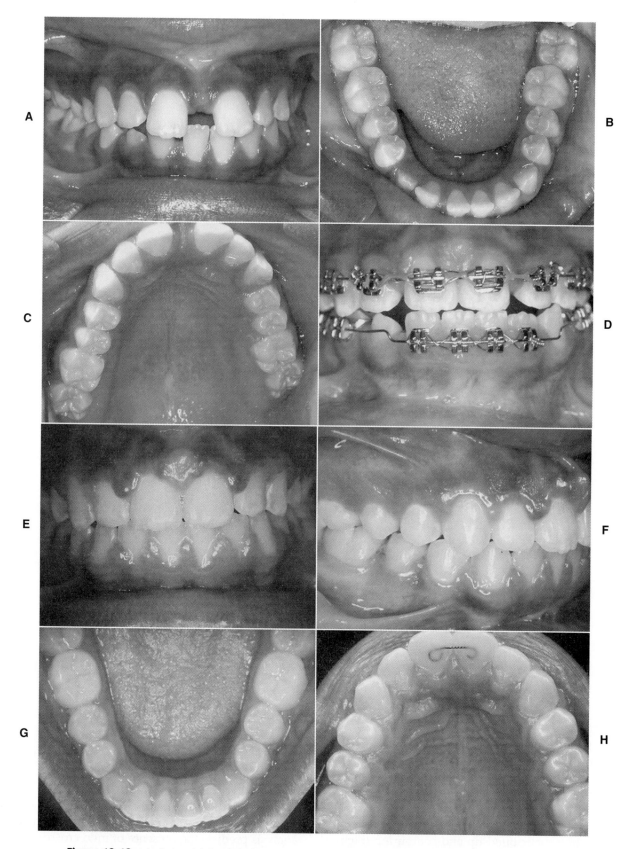

Figure 19-18 A to **C,** An adult female is shown with diastemas in the anterior parts of her maxillary and mandibular arches. **D,** A fixed appliance was used to close spaces in both arches. **E** to **G,** The posttreatment results. **H,** A bonded wire was placed between her upper central incisors as a permanent retainer.

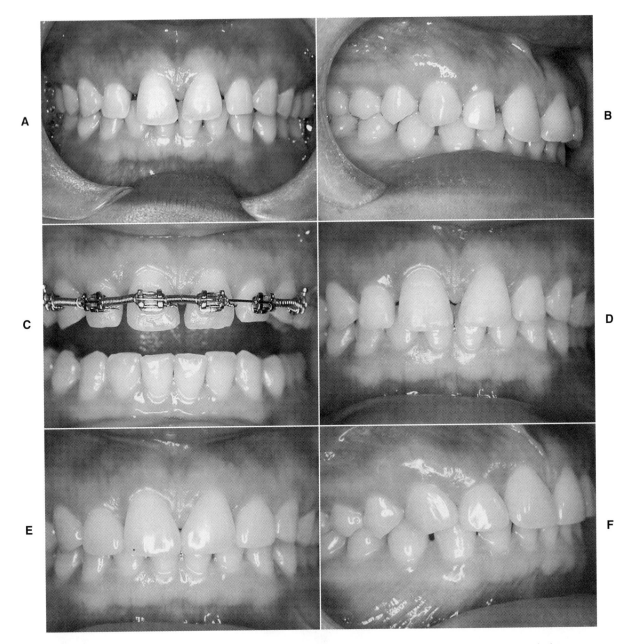

Figure 19-19 **A** and **B,** An adult female is shown with diastemas between her upper incisors. **C** and **D,** Her incisors were spaced evenly with a fixed appliance for composite resin build-up and contouring. **E** and **F,** The finished result with composite resin build-ups.

fixed retainer between her upper central incisors (see Figure 19-18, *G*).

An adult female with diastemas between her maxillary incisors is shown in Figure 19-19, *A* and *B*. An upper arch fixed appliance was used to evenly space and position the incisors (Figure 19-19, *C* and *D*) for composite resin esthetic build-up and contouring (Figure 19-19, *E* and *F*). The small size of her maxillary incisors was the primary etiologic factor (see Figure 19-19). She was retained with a maxillary Hawley appliance.

Maintenance of Arch Length and Width

In the mixed dentition a need may arise for a space maintainer when a primary canine or molar is lost prematurely or when a mixed dentition arch length analysis predicts the presence of mild crowding in the mandibular arch. In the latter case, the space maintainer is used after arch length is regained or the incisors are aligned.

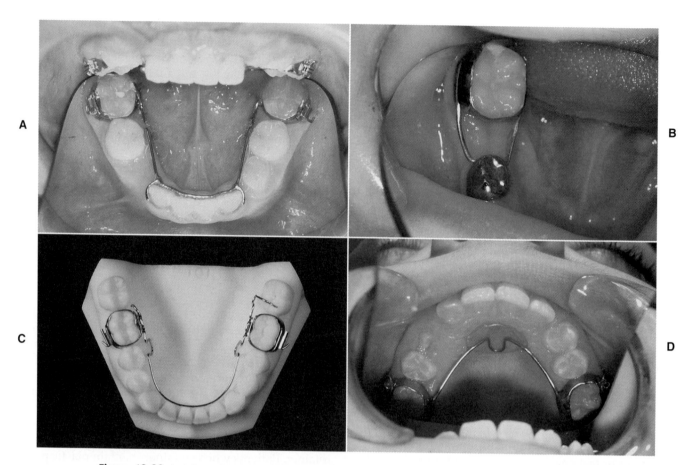

Figure 19-20 A, A lower lingual holding arch (LLHA) with soldered wires to keep the lower incisors from shifting. **B,** A band and loop space retainer. **C,** A removable LLHA with an optional spring to upright the lower left second molar. **D,** A Nance palatal holding arch.

Appliances

Lower Lingual Holding Arch This appliance comes in fixed and fixed-removable versions. The fixed holding arch is most commonly used to maintain arch width and arch length. A wire with adjustment loops is soldered to bands cemented on the first permanent molars. The wire should rest on the cingula of the mandibular incisors. Adjustment loops allow clinicians to shorten, lengthen, raise, or lower the wire into passive contact with the incisor cingula.

If mandibular incisors have drifted off center because one of the mandibular primary canines exfoliated prematurely, an appliance can be used to correct the deviation of the teeth. Midline deviations are usually corrected with a fixed appliance and retained with a fixed lower lingual holding arch (Figure 19-20, A).

If a primary second molar is prematurely lost, a band and loop retainer will hold the arch length for an unerupted second premolar (see Figure 19-20, B).

Fixed removable lower lingual arches such as the Wilson arch (Rocky Mountain Orthodontics, Inc., Denver) can be used to maintain arch dimensions but are primarily useful in the expansion of arch length and width. They can also be used to upright mesially tipped molars, rotate molars and torque molar crowns either buccally or lingually (see Figure 19-20, C). The fitting and adjustment of these wires require skills that are detailed in a manual written by the inventor. Essentially, the arch wire must first be adjusted to fit passively into the vertical tubes on the bands and on the cingula of the incisors. Then adjustments in the wire are made to move the teeth.

Palatal Arches The Nance holding arch can be used to maintain maxillary arch length. The arch consists of a wire embedded in an acrylic button on the anterior palate and soldered to bands on the maxillary first permanent molars (see Figure 19-20, D).

Transpalatal arches consist of a wire passing over the palatal vault and soldered to the first permanent molars (see Figure 19-11, F). The purposes of these arches are to maintain arch width and molar position after buccal expansion of the maxillary arch and to keep the molars from tipping buccally in response to forces from an occipital pull facebow headgear.

Fixed, removable transpalatal arches are used to maintain, expand, or constrict intermolar width, to rotate upright mesially tipped molars, and to torque maxillary molars (see Figure 19-9). The fitting and adjustment of these arches require skills similar to those described for the fixed, removable lower lingual arches.

Other Appliances Other arch length maintenance appliances include those used to hold space for an incisor that was lost because of trauma. These appliances are removable or fixed prosthodontic devices that give patients an important esthetic service. The band and loop appliance is most helpful in saving arch length when a primary molar is lost prematurely.

Retention Principles and Appliances

When orthodontic appliances are removed at the end of treatment, a clinician must decide whether or not to place a retainer to hold the teeth in their new positions. Studies on posttreatment changes have shown that, over time, some movement of the treated teeth is common to many patients.[22-28]

Patients who desire no posttreatment changes in their occlusion must be willing to wear a retainer daily at least part-time for an indefinite period. This is not an unreasonable request, considering that failure to wear the retainer regularly may bring the patient back to the clinician for retreatment at a later time. The recommendation to wear a retainer is based on the concern that the factors that caused the malocclusion may continue to unfavorably impact the alignment and occlusion of the teeth following treatment.

Patients who have a single maxillary incisor in crossbite and adequate overbite probably do not need to have a retainer after the tooth has been moved out of crossbite. On the other hand, patients who have anterior crossbite problems associated with little or no overbite are in need of a retainer following treatment because the treated tooth can easily drop back into a crossbite position.

Circumferential supracrestal gingival fibrotomy[29] is a helpful procedure in retaining rotated teeth. However, a retainer is still needed to hold the teeth during the several months required for healing and reorientation of the gingival fibers. There are two types of retainers available to clinicians: removable and fixed.

Removable Hawley Retainers

Advantages and Disadvantages Removable Hawley retainers[30] have many advantages that make them the preferred retainer for most patients. Hawley retainers allow a patient to sustain a program of good oral hygiene. They also allow for the settling of the teeth into full occlusal contact after the removal of orthodontic appliances.[31] Well-made retainers can hold the teeth in good occlusion and alignment for many years. Hawley retainers are excellent for long-term retention and a wise course for many patients who receive the benefits of orthodontic treatment. Several disadvantages come to mind such as wires passing over the occlusal surfaces that interfere with occlusion and prevent the settling of the teeth and the dependence on the patient to wear and clean the retainer as directed.

Types of Hawley Retainers Several different types of Hawley retainers are shown in Figure 19-21. Each type is made in response to the specific needs of patients. The parts of a Hawley retainer are described later in this chapter.

Wear Time In general, Hawley retainers should be worn full-time, except when eating and brushing, for at least 6 months after removal of the tooth-moving appliance. Thereafter, night wear should be continued at least through the period of active growth. For many patients, wear should continue at night indefinitely to minimize posttreatment changes. For long-term wear, removal of the retainer for most of the day is beneficial to the oral soft tissues in contact with the retainer. Patients whose retainers contain plastic pontic teeth that require daytime wear for esthetic reasons should remove the retainers at night to give oral tissues a rest.

Components of the Hawley Retainer A typical Hawley retainer has four major components: (1) clasps that hold the retainer on the teeth, (2) occlusal rests that keep the mandibular retainer in place, (3) a labial bow wire to hold the teeth in place in conjunction with (4) an acrylic body that supports the lingual surfaces of the teeth and holds the clasps and labial bow in place.

Clasps and Occlusal Rests A number of different clasps are used to anchor a Hawley retainer to the teeth. The **Adams clasp**[2] is an excellent clasp when spaces are available through which to pass the mesial and distal wires of the clasp over the occlusal surface of the clasped tooth without interfering with the occlusion (Figures 19-21, *A* and *B*, and 19-22, *A*). If a patient presented with a deep overbite problem, an anterior bite plate on an upper Hawley would help retain the overbite correction and provide interocclusal clearance for the Adams clasp. The Adams clasp grips the anchor tooth securely by engaging the undercuts on the mesiobuccal and distobuccal surfaces of the tooth. This clasp has the best retentive properties. The drawback of this clasp in retainers is that it will not allow settling of the clasped tooth. The clasp is formed from

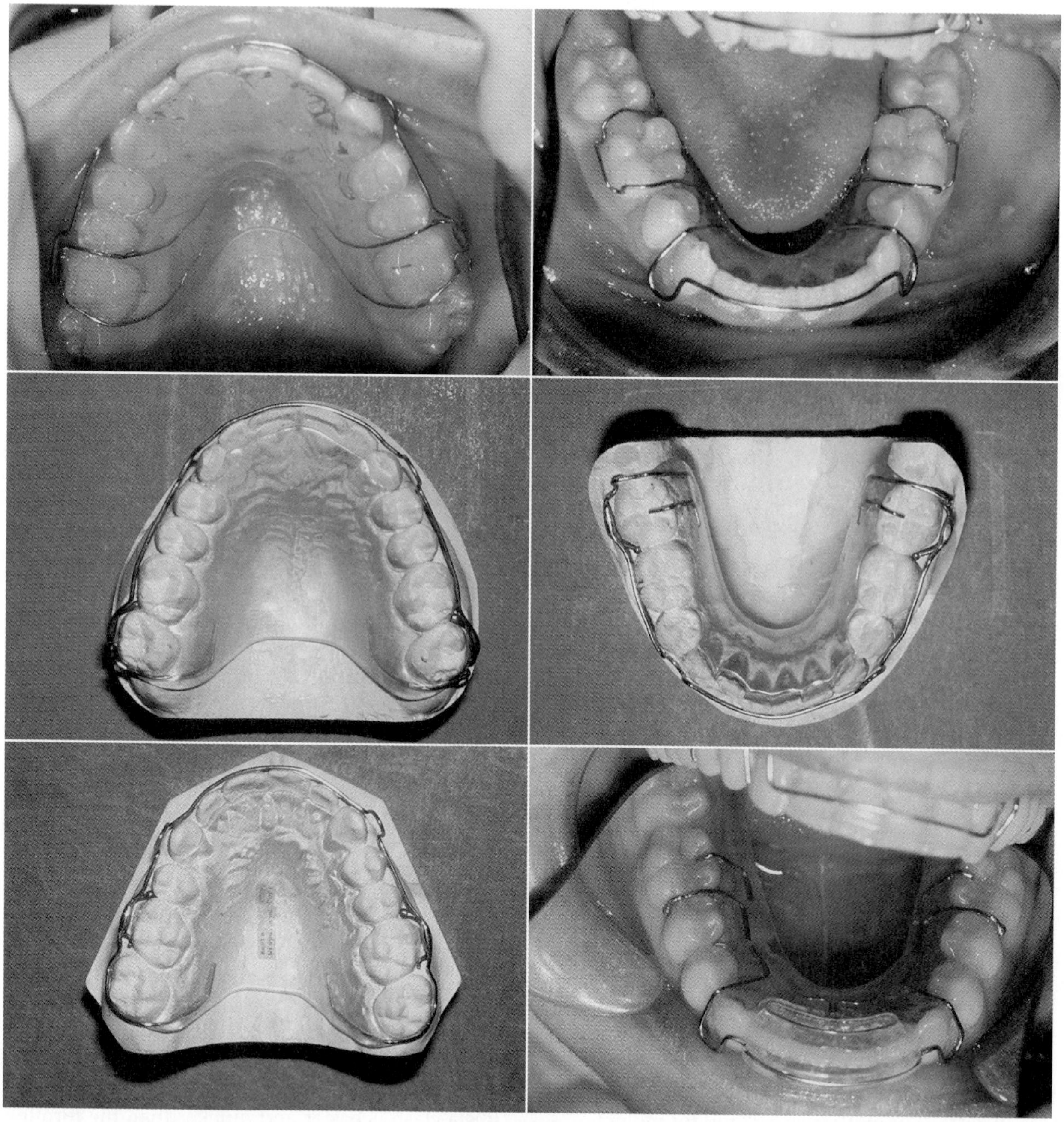

Figure 19-21 Types of Hawley retainers. **A,** An upper retainer with Adams clasps soldered to a labial bow. **B,** A lower retainer with Adams clasps and a separate labial bow. **C,** An upper retainer with a wraparound labial bow soldered to Resta clasps on the second molars. **D,** A lower retainer with a wraparound labial bow soldered to Resta clasps on the second molars that have occlusal rests. **E,** An upper retainer with a wraparound labial bow soldered to modified Resta clasps on the first molars. **F,** A lower spring retainer to securely maintain the position of the lower incisors with ball clasps and occlusal rests to hold the appliance.

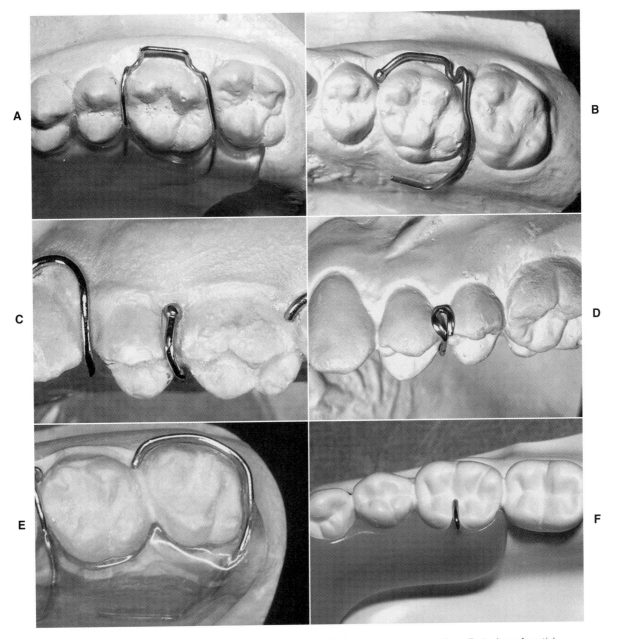

Figure 19-22 A, An Adams clasp. **B,** A Resta clasp. **C,** A ball clasp. **D,** An arrow clasp. **E,** A circumferential clasp. **F,** An occlusal rest.

cylindrical (round) stainless steel wires having diameters of 26 mil for premolars and 28 mil for molars.

The **Resta clasp**[32,33] is a modified version of the Adams clasp. It uses the arrowhead retentive point from the Adams clasp and the ball from a ball clasp to engage two undercut areas on the buccal surface of the anchor tooth. The clasp wire passes over the occlusal surface of the clasped tooth either on its mesial or on its distal side (see Figures 19-21, *C* and *D*, and 19-22, *B*). The clasp is useful when interocclusal clearance or space is available on only the mesial or distal side of the tooth to be clasped. Although not as retentive as an Adams clasp, the Resta clasp has the

ability to perform well in retainers. The making of a Resta clasp is easier and quicker than the forming of an Adams clasp. The Resta clasp can be modified to be part of a wraparound retainer design. The Resta clasp is formed from preformed stainless steel ball clasp wires having diameters of 28 mil for premolars and 30 or 32 mil for molars.

The **ball clasp** is a simple clasp that can be used in retainers to engage undercuts on two adjacent teeth (see Figures 19-21, *F,* and 19-22, *C*). Its simplicity is an advantage. On the other hand, it has the same disadvantages of the Adams clasp in that the wire passes over the occlusal surfaces and can only be used when sufficient interocclusal space is available. The clasp can also be used in mixed dentition patients between primary molars that have no available retentive surfaces for an Adams clasp or a Resta clasp.

The **arrow clasp** is similar in its function to a ball clasp (see Figure 19-22, *D*). The arrow part of the clasp is preformed by manufacturers and is placed between adjacent teeth to engage undercuts on each tooth. Retentiveness of the clasp is similar to the ball clasp because it engages the same undercuts. It is easier for a patient to grasp the larger arrowhead clasp than the smaller ball clasp when removing the retainer from the mouth.

Figure 19-22, *E*, illustrates the circumferential clasp, or **C clasp,** which can be used on any tooth but is most useful on the most distal teeth in the upper arch where it can pass over the distal surface of the molar and engage the undercut on the mesiobuccal surface of the tooth. The clasp in such circumstances does not interfere with the occlusion. The clasp is not highly retentive because it engages only one undercut area on the clasped tooth. Because of its length, the clasp can be easily distorted by a patient when the retainer is inserted or removed. A variation of this clasp is incorporated into many wraparound labial bow wire designs.

Occlusal rests are an essential part of a mandibular Hawley retainer, especially when clasps that cross over the occlusal surface are not included in the retainer (see Figures 19-21, *D*, and 19-22, *F*). Without occlusal rests, the acrylic body drops downward onto and irritates the alveolar soft tissues and loses proper contact with the teeth. Rests are usually made from 32-mil round stainless steel wires.

Labial Bow

The labial bow of a Hawley retainer holds the teeth in place from the labial and buccal tooth surfaces and keeps the teeth in contact with the acrylic body located on the palatal or lingual surfaces (see Figure 19-22). The typical labial bow passes through the occlusion between the canines and first premolars when space is available. In many patients the maxillary labial bow wire cannot easily pass through the occlusion distal to the canine. Therefore the labial bow is usually soldered to clasps on the molars. In the mandibular arch the labial bow is often able to pass through the teeth without interfering with the occlusion. In some patients in whom we wish to avoid any interference with occlusion and the settling of teeth, the labial bow of the upper Hawley is incorporated into the wraparound design (see Figure 19-21, *E*). The labial wire must be intimately adapted to the incisors to prevent rotational relapses of these teeth. The labial bow contains two loops buccal to the canines that allow adjustment in the anteroposterior position of the wire adapted to the incisors. Adjustment of the loops permits the clinician to fit the

wire snugly but not too tightly against the labial surfaces of the incisors. The labial bow wire is commonly formed from 28- or 30-mil diameter round stainless steel wires. A flat preformed labial bow wire is also available for use in removable retainer construction.

Acrylic Body The acrylic body of the Hawley retainer can be constructed from liquid and powdered methyl methacrylate, light-cured acrylic resins, or thermoplastic materials that are formed on special machines that heat the plastic and force it with pressurized air on the cast. For all three materials the wires are fixed into position on the cast before processing the acrylic. The acrylic body must be trimmed so that it leaves a 1½- to 2-mm band of acrylic touching the lingual surfaces of the teeth. In the incisor-canine region of the upper arch the acrylic covers the cingula of the anterior teeth to better hold them in the retainer. The posterior border of the acrylic body should be extended forward from the second molars in the upper arch so that it does not cause the patient to gag. The acrylic body of the upper retainer needs to be uniform and approximately 2 mm thick. In the lower arch the acrylic body should not extend to the floor of the mouth or irritate the tongue. Any undercuts on the lingual surfaces of the alveolar ridges should be waxed out on the dental cast so that the acrylic does not engage them. The lower retainer needs proper thickness to provide for adequate strength but should not encroach on the space of the tongue. It should be uniformly 2 to 2½ mm thick. The acrylic should be polished and smooth on the surfaces that touch the tongue but left unpolished on the surfaces adjacent to the palate and alveolar ridges. When using the liquid and powdered methyl methacrylate, porosity within the body can be reduced by using a high-quality, fine-grained, acrylic resin and by processing the newly made unpolymerized acrylic in a pressure pot.

Transparent Plastic Invisible Retainers Other commonly used removable retainers include clear plastic retainers constructed from thermoplastic materials on vacuum or air pressurized machines (Figure 19-23, *A*). These retainers are easily and quickly constructed when compared with Hawley retainers. The invisible retainers that cover all the teeth do not allow for the settling of the teeth into better occlusal contact and, because of this, can maintain a slight anterior open bite.[31] Some clinicians use full-coverage invisible retainers as temporary appliances until permanent Hawley retainers can be fabricated.

The Essix retainer[34] (Raintree Essix, Inc., New Orleans) is an example of the invisible retainer that only incorporates the six anterior teeth of each arch (see Figure 19-23, *B*). These appliances allow for the settling of the posterior teeth into better occlusion and, if worn according to instructions, can serve as good retainers.[35]

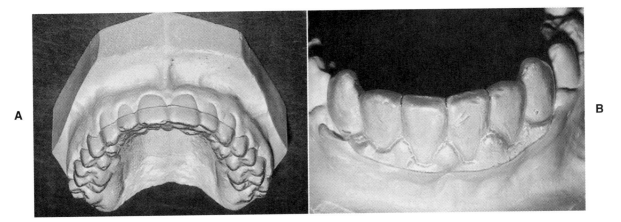

Figure 19-23 A, An invisible retainer that covers the palate, the lingual and occlusal surfaces and part of the labial-buccal surfaces of the teeth. **B,** A modified invisible retainer that covers the lower six anterior teeth.

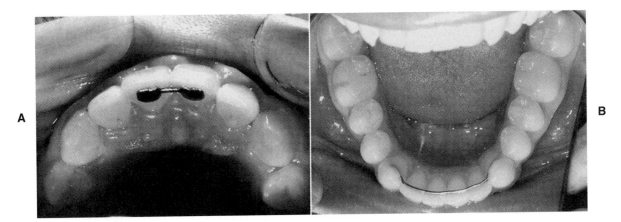

Figure 19-24 Fixed retainers in the upper arch to retain a closed diastema **(A)** and in the lower arch to maintain anterior arch dimensions and tooth alignment **(B).**

Fixed Retainers The most common type of fixed retainer is a wire formed to fit the lingual surfaces of the lower incisors and bonded to the lower canines (Figure 19-24). The wire must be placed far enough incisally to hold the form of the dental arch. In addition to the canines, one or more incisors can also be bonded to the wire for maximum retention. Lingual fixed retainers in the mandibular arch do not interfere with occlusion. However, sufficient overjet is required for the placement of fixed bonded wires on the lingual surfaces of upper incisors so that the fixed retainer does not interfere with the occluding lower anterior teeth.

In the upper arch, bonded wire fixed retainers are often used to retain closed diastemas between the upper central incisors (see Figures 19-18, *G,* and 19-24, *A*). These retainers are also used to retain upper central incisors that were severely rotated or malaligned before treatment.

Other fixed retainers include lower lingual holding arches and transpalatal arches that retain arch widths (see Figures 19-9, *D,* 19-11, *F,* and 19-20, *D*).

Advantages and Disadvantages The advantages of fixed retainers are that they are effective and do not rely on patient compliance. The major disadvantage is that the retainer interferes with flossing and oral hygiene maintenance. Patients should agree to periodic cleaning of the teeth and retainer by a dental hygienist as a necessary component of the care of fixed retainers. The lower fixed retainer from canine to canine should not be placed in patients who readily collect dental calculus. The clinician should periodically see patients with fixed retainers to monitor their performance and hygiene practices. Fixed retainers can loosen when a bond fails. The patient should seek treatment for replacement or recementing of the retainer.

SUMMARY

This chapter discussed a number of different Class I malocclusions that may be encountered by clinicians. The objective of this chapter is to give an overview of the treatment of the problems addressed. To successfully treat patients with these malocclusions, the clinician must have a thorough understanding of the diagnostic and treatment planning criteria discussed in other chapters. In addition, the clinician must have acquired the skills needed to successfully design and manipulate the appliances used in treatment and retention.

REFERENCES

1. Shamy FE: Retraction of maxillary bicuspids and molars with a removable appliance, *N Z Orthod J* 1:17-24, 1972.

2. Adams CP: *The design, construction, and use of removable orthodontic appliances,* ed 5, Bristol, Great Britain, 1984, John Wright & Sons.

3. Crabb JJ, Wilson HJ: The relation between orthodontic spring force and space closure, *Dent Pract Dent Rec* 22:233-240, 1972.

4. Begg PR: *Begg orthodontic theory and technique,* Philadelphia, 1965, WB Saunders.

5. Angle EH: The latest and best in orthodontic mechanism, *Dental Cosmos* 70:1143-1158, 1928.

6. Angle EH: The latest and best in orthodontic mechanism, *Dental Cosmos* 71:164-174, 260-270, 409-421, 1929.

7. Bishara SE, Staley RN: Maxillary expansion: clinical implications, *Am J Orthod Dentofacial Orthop* 91(1):3-14, 1987.

8. Krebs A: Midpalatal suture expansion studied by the implant method over a seven year period, *Eur Orthod Soc Rep* 40:131-142, 1964.

9. Ingervall B, Mohlin B, Thilander B: Prevalence of symptoms of functional disturbances of the masticatory system in Swedish men, *J Oral Rehabil* 7:185-197, 1980.

10. Epker BN, Fish LC: *Dentofacial deformities: integrated orthodontic and surgical correction,* St Louis, 1996, Mosby.

11. Zimring JF, Isaacson RJ: Forces produced by rapid maxillary expansion (III) forces present during retention, *Angle Orthod* 35:178-186, 1965.

12. Hoenigl KD et al: The centered T-loop: a new way of preactivation, *Am J Orthod Dentofacial Orthop* 108:149-153, 1995.

13. Roberts WE, Marshall KJ, Mozsary PG: Rigid endosseous implant utilized as anchorage to protract molars and close an atrophic extraction site, *Angle Orthod* 60:135-152, 1990.

14. Roberts WE, Nelson CL, Goodacre CJ: Rigid implant anchorage to close a mandibular first molar extraction site: a viable alternative to a fixed partial denture (FPD) or a single tooth replacement (STR) implant, *J Clin Orthod* 28:693-704, 1994.

15. Bishara SE: Management of diastemas in orthodontics, *Am J Orthod* 61:55-63, 1972.

16. Staley RN: Unpublished data taken from Iowa Facial Growth Study Projects, 1985.

17. Dahlberg AA: Concepts of occlusion in physical anthropology and comparative anatomy, *J Am Dent Assoc* 46:530-535, 1945.

18. Bolton WA: Disharmony in tooth size and its relation to the analysis and treatment of malocclusion, *Angle Orthod* 28:113-130, 1958.

19. Edwards JG: A study of the periodontium during orthodontic rotation of teeth, *Am J Orthod* 54:441-459, 1968.

20. Edwards JG: A surgical procedure to eliminate rotational relapse, *Am J Orthod* 57:35-46, 1970.

21. Edwards JG: The diastema, the frenum, the frenectomy: a clinical study, *Am J Orthod* 71:489-508, 1977.

22. Swanson WD, Riedel RA, D'Anna JA: Postretention study: incidence and stability of rotated teeth in humans, *Angle Orthod* 45(3):198-203, 1975.

23. Little RM, Wallen TR, Riedel RA: Stability and relapse of mandibular anterior alignment: first premolar extraction cases treated by traditional edgewise orthodontics, *Am J Orthod* 80(4):349-365, 1981.

24. Sadowsky C, Sakols EI: Long-term assessment of orthodontic relapse, *Am J Orthod* 82:456-463, 1982.

25. Uhde MD, Sadowsky C, BeGole EA: Long-term stability of dental relationships after orthodontic treatment, *Angle Orthod* 53(3):240-252, 1983.

26. Puneky PJ, Sadowsky C, BeGole EA: Tooth morphology and lower incisor alignment many years after orthodontic therapy, *Am J Orthod* 86(4):299-305, 1984.

27. Shields TE, Little RM, Chapko MK: Stability and relapse of mandibular anterior alignment: a cephalometric appraisal of first-premolar-extraction cases treated by traditional edgewise orthodontics, *Am J Orthod* 87(1):27-38, 1985.

28. Harris EF et al: Effects of patient age on postorthodontic stability in Class II, division 1 malocclusions, *Am J Orthod Dentofacial Orthop* 105:25-34, 1994.

29. Edwards JG: A long-term prospective evaluation of the circumferential supracrestal fiberotomy in alleviating orthodontic relapse, *Am J Orthod* 93:380-387, 1988.

30. Hawley CA: A removable retainer, *Int J Orthod Oral Surg* 2:291-298, 1919.

31. Sauget E et al: Comparison of occlusal contacts with use of Hawley and clear overlay retainers, *Angle Orthod* 67:223-230, 1997.

32. Staley RN, Reske NT: A one-arm wrought wire clasp that engages two buccal surface undercuts, *Quintessence Dent Technol* 11:123-127, 1987.

33. Staley RN, Reske NT: A new clasp for orthodontic retainers: the Resta clasp, *Oral Health* 79:19-22, 1989.

34. Sheridan JJ, LeDoux W, McMinn R: Essix retainers: fabrication and supervision for permanent retention, *J Clin Orthod* 27:37-45, 1993.

35. Lindauer SJ, Shoff RC: Comparison of Essix and Hawley retainers, *J Clin Orthod* 32:95-97, 1998.

CHAPTER 20

Treatment of Class II Malocclusions

Peter Spalding

KEY TERMS

overjet
protrusion
ectopic molar eruption
interarch tooth size
  discrepancy
retrusion
dental compensation
skeletal discrepancy
mesiolingual rotation
nasolabial angle
lip incompetence
mandibular plane
mandibular body
mandibular rami
posterior face height
lower anterior face height
anterior overbite
gummy smile
clockwise rotation
midface protrusion
facial skeletal convexity
Norman Kingsley
retract
Calvin Case

Edward Angle
Class II elastics
facial orthopedic treatment
dental camouflage
protract
growth modification
orthognathic surgery
extraoral orthopedic force
anteroposterior maxillary
  excess
occipital or cervical
  attachment
facebow
J-hook headgear
outer bow
inner bow
center of resistance
extrusion
combination headgear
orthodontic force magnitude
orthodontic force duration
intermittent force
continuous force

force direction or vector
pubertal growth spurt
derotation
bodily movement
tipping movement
fundamental growth pattern
overcorrection
retrospective studies
prospective
tooth-borne appliance
intrusion
activator
functional corrector
  (or functional regulator)
condylar cartilage
bionator
twin block appliances
Herbst appliance
"working" or "construction"
  bite registration
mandibular growth potential
differential eruption
rotation of the occlusal plane

maxillary posterior anchorage
mandibular anterior
  anchorage
transpalatal arch
Nance holding arch
osseointegrated attachment
nickel-titanium
titanium molybdenum
miniscrews
onplants
rigid internal fixation
intraoral ramus osteotomy
sagittal split
vertical "L" or "C" osteotomy
vertical ramus osteotomy
interarch compatibility
Le Fort I maxillary
  osteotomies
root divergence
interdental osteotomy
root parallelism
Peer Assessment Rating (PAR)
  Index

REVIEW AND HISTORY OF CLASS II MALOCCLUSION

Malocclusions in human populations and attempts to treat these conditions have been evident since early civilization. The description or classification of a con-dition is an essential prerequisite to determining the prevalence or severity of that condition in human populations. Although numerous attempts were made throughout the nineteenth century to classify malocclusions, it was not until the end of that century that a widely accepted classification became important to the

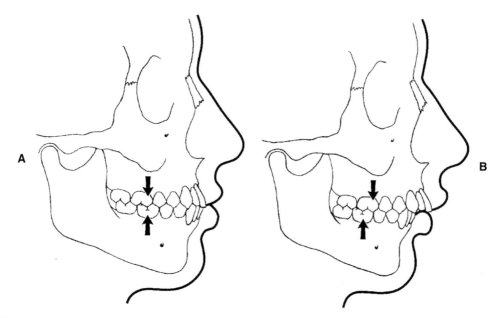

Figure 20-1 **A,** The anteroposterior occlusal relationship of the first permanent molars that was defined by Edward Angle as the mesiobuccal cusp of the maxillary first molar occluding with the buccal groove of the mandibular first molar. This occlusal relationship characterizes both normal occlusion and Class I malocclusion. **B,** Class II malocclusion, or distal occlusion, is characterized by anteroposterior relation of the mandibular first molars distal to normal occlusion or Class I malocclusion.

dental profession. Orthodontic problems before this time had been viewed with less importance in the face of such widespread need for restorative treatment to manage the ravages of dental and periodontal disease. After the vast improvements in dental restorative techniques during the nineteenth century, it no longer seemed frivolous to consider the functional and cosmetic positions of the teeth that were being salvaged.

In 1899 Edward Angle's background in prosthodontics with his keen interest in dental occlusion led the American dentist to publish a paper entitled *The Classification of Malocclusion.* It became a part of the fifth edition of his orthodontic textbook in which he described three classes of malocclusion, based on the anteroposterior occlusal relationship of the first permanent molars. The neutrooclusion, or Class I malocclusion, relationship was characterized by the mesiobuccal cusps of the maxillary molars occluding with the buccal grooves of the mandibular molars (Figure 20-1, *A*). The second class of malocclusion (Class II malocclusion, or distal occlusion) was used to describe the condition in which the mandibular first molars occluded distal to the normal relationship with the maxillary first molars (see Figure 20-1, *B*). Angle further differentiated the Class II malocclusions into Division 1 in which the maxillary incisors are protruding, and Division 2 in which the maxillary incisors are retruding. Finally, he described a subdivision for each of these divisions in which the distal occlusion is unilateral with the opposite side exhibiting the normal relationship (see Chapter 8).

Angle's classification provided the first orderly means of characterizing malocclusions, and its universal acceptance by the dental profession was a testament to its practical simplicity. This acceptance permitted epidemiologic assessment of malocclusion for the first time. In spite of Angle's important contribution, it became clear during the early part of the twentieth century that this classification system was inadequate to characterize the variety of manifestations of malocclusion presented by skeletal and dental discrepancies in all three planes of space. Nevertheless, the use of Angle's basic classification has survived the century. His definition of *distal occlusion,* termed *distoclusion* by Benno Lischer in 1912, was adopted as one descriptor of malocclusion and was also used to establish an international system of orthodontic classification in the early 1970s by the World Health Organization and the Federation Dentaire International.[1] This malocclusion descriptor continues to be incorporated in epidemiologic surveys of malocclusion to this day.

PREVALENCE OF CLASS II MALOCCLUSION IN THE POPULATION

American Epidemiologic Studies

Based on several thousand cases he examined, Angle,[2] himself, suggested in his textbook that an estimated 27% of malocclusions could be classified as Class II malocclusions. Since that time numerous efforts have been made to determine the prevalence of Class II malocclusions in the population. Although a number of attempts have been made to estimate malocclusion prevalence in the United States, the first national epidemiologic study of malocclusion was a part of the National Health and Nutrition Examination Survey (NHANES I) conducted in the 1960s by the Public Health Service of the U.S. Department of Health, Education, and Welfare.[3,4] This study examined a cross section of approximately 23 million U.S. children between the ages of 6 and 17 years. For nearly 30 years its data were the only reliable information dentists had regarding the prevalence of malocclusion in the United States. Fortunately, a second federal epidemiologic survey (NHANES III) designed to represent 150 million U.S. citizens was completed in 1991. It expanded the breadth of the previous sample, including adults (ages 18 to 50) and the racial subcategory of Mexican Americans to the previously designated non-Hispanic whites and blacks (see Chapter 8).[5]

Although the malocclusions revealed by both of these studies were derived from limited dental occlusal characteristics and there were minor differences in their results, they do conclude that Class II malocclusion is common, representing about 20% of our U.S. population. The prevalence appears to decrease with age, affecting about 25% to 30% of children in the mixed dentition, 20% to 25% of children in the early permanent dentition, and 15% to 20% of the adult population. The data do not support clear gender difference and possible racial or ethnic differences in the United States.

Smaller local or regional U.S. epidemiologic studies of malocclusion indicate that Class II malocclusion occurs twice as often in whites as it does in blacks.[6-9] Although the more comprehensive NHANES I survey supported this racial difference, the NHANES III survey seemed to indicate the opposite was true. The only data regarding Latinos (Mexican Americans) were obtained from the second survey in which the overall prevalence of Class II malocclusions is similar to that of blacks but in which the more severe expression of this malocclusion is rarer in the Latino group. It is noteworthy that the few attempts to assess malocclusion in Native American populations have shown a much smaller prevalence (5% to 10%) of Class II malocclusions in these groups.[10,11]

International Epidemiologic Studies

Surveys conducted outside the United States, although usually not as extensive as the NHANES studies, still provide some appreciation for the world-wide variations in the prevalence of Class II malocclusion. The most abundant epidemiologic data have been produced in northern Europe, particularly Scandinavia

and the British Isles, owing in large part to the well-developed, socialized health care systems in these regions. Surveys conducted in Finland, Sweden, and Denmark demonstrate a prevalence of distal molar occlusion comparable to the U.S. population.[12-14] British surveys have revealed similar prevalence for their population.[15,16] Although more limited data are available for continental Europe, Dutch and French surveys show that the prevalence of Class II malocclusion is no different than for Scandinavia and the British Isles.[17,18]

The prevalence of Class II malocclusion in the "caucasoid" populations of northern Africa appears to be similar to that of Europe.[19-21] However, sub-Saharan populations that are primarily black Africans demonstrate a dramatically decreased prevalence of Class II malocclusion, usually between 1% and 10%.[22-27]

In the Arab populations native to the Middle East, the prevalence of Class II malocclusion appears to be about 10% to 15%, intermediate between the European "caucasoid" populations and the black populations of sub-Saharan Africa.[28,29] Although little malocclusion prevalence data are available for central Asia, surveys from east and southeast Asia demonstrate a Class II malocclusion prevalence somewhat similar to that of the Middle East and lower than that of European and North American populations.[30-33]

The native homogeneous populations of the South Pacific have a low Class II malocclusion prevalence of about 0% to 5% unless there is a mixture of heritage with Asian or European populations.[34-37] This phenomenon is clearly evident on the continent of Australia where the majority population, primarily of European origin, has a Class II malocclusion prevalence similar to that of Europeans,[38,39] whereas the native Aboriginal population has less than 1% prevalence.[40]

Class II malocclusion prevalence in Latin America appears to be about 10% to 15% (comparable to that of the Middle East and Asia).[41-44] However, a survey demonstrated a much higher prevalence of Class II malocclusion that was similar to North American and European populations in an ethnically diverse area of southern Brazil.[45]

It is striking how few individuals have a Class II malocclusion in more isolated populations of Amerindian origin. Prevalence in these homogeneous ethnic groups ranges from 0% to 5%.[38,46-49] The Native Americans of the continental United States and southern Canada seem to have a somewhat increased prevalence of Class II malocclusion (10% to 15%) relative to more isolated Amerindian populations in the Western Hemisphere. This increased prevalence, however, appears to decrease with greater indigenous heritage.[10,50]

Further data are necessary to make conclusive statements regarding world-wide differences in the prevalence of Class II malocclusions. However, the international epidemiologic studies conducted to date suggest that there seems to be over 20% prevalence of Class II malocclusions in North America, Europe, and North Africa. In Latin America (including Mexico and South America), the Middle East, and Asia there appears to be a lower prevalence of 10% to 15%. Black populations of sub-Saharan Africa have an even lower prevalence of about 1% to 10%. Homogeneous Amerindian, Pacific islanders, and other indigenous groups have the lowest prevalence of Class II malocclusion of all (0% to 5%).

TYPES OF CLASS II MALOCCLUSIONS

General Characteristics

During the twentieth century Angle's original description of Class II malocclusion was expanded by others to include premolar and canine occlusal relationships. This became necessary because the limitation of only describing the molar relationship did not provide a more complete characterization of anteroposterior occlusal discrepancies. It was possible to find individuals with a Class I molar relationship and a Class II canine relationship with excessive **overjet** caused by spacing and **protrusion** of the maxillary teeth. It also was possible to find a Class II molar relationship associated with a Class I canine relationship and normal overjet caused by crowding or loss of maxillary teeth mesial to the first molars. It became clear that Angle's original simplified approach was inadequate to describe the diversity of Class II malocclusion arising from both dental and skeletal origin. The introduction of standardized cephalometric radiographs and their widespread use in clinical orthodontics in the second half of the twentieth century permitted further appreciation of the dental and skeletal features that may be associated with individuals who have Class II malocclusions.

Dental Class II Malocclusions

Although most Class II malocclusions are caused by an underlying skeletal discrepancy or deformity, it is possible to have a normal skeletal jaw relationship associated with a dental Class II malocclusion. In these conditions the maxillary molars have moved forward more than normal during dental development, whereas the mandibular molars have remained in a more posterior position relative to the maxillary molars. The causes of these dental Class II malocclusions can be subdivided into two groups: (1) maxillary dental protrusion and (2) mesial drift of the maxillary first permanent molars.

Maxillary Dental Protrusion Maxillary dental protrusion may be confused with anteroposterior maxillary excess or midface protrusion. Although both conditions are characterized by facial convexity, maxillary dental protrusion is not a skeletal problem but a dentoalveolar one that is limited to the maxillary dental arch. The facial appearance of anteroposterior maxillary excess is a protrusion of the entire midface, whereas maxillary dental protrusion only affects the lips. Excessive overjet is a reliable feature of this dental malocclusion, and there may be generalized maxillary spacing associated with the protruded maxillary incisors. The mandible and mandibular dentition are in a normal anteroposterior position.

The cephalometric presentation of maxillary dental protrusion shows a normal anteroposterior and vertical skeletal relationship characterized by a normal ANB, SNA, and SNB angle; A-B difference projected on the occlusal plane; true horizontal anteroposterior position of A and B relative to Nasion perpendicular; and normal linear measures of the maxilla and mandible. The mandibular incisors also will be in a normal anteroposterior position relative to the NB line, mandibular plane, and Frankfort horizontal. The departure from normal values will be the maxillary incisors, which will be in a protrusive position relative to lines NA, SN, and Frankfort horizontal.

Mesial Drift of the Maxillary First Permanent Molars Normal eruption of permanent teeth is dependent on the normal position and integrity of the primary teeth. Congenital absence or loss of the primary teeth before normal exfoliation may disturb the normal eruption of permanent teeth. This is particularly the case with the premature loss of posterior primary teeth. Mesial and occlusal drift of the permanent first molars occurs if there is loss of mesial proximal contact with the second primary molars from congenital absence, extraction, dental caries or ankylosis. The mesial drift is more pronounced if the lack of proximal contact occurs in the maxilla or if the loss occurs before clinical emergence of the first permanent molar.[51] **Ectopic molar eruption,** in which the eruption of the first permanent molar causes premature root resorption of the adjacent primary second molar, also occurs more frequently in the maxillary arch.[52]

In both of these situations, if left untreated, the maxillary first permanent molar assumes a more mesial position, resulting in a Class II permanent molar relationship if the mandibular arch is unaffected (Figure 20-2). This dental Class II relationship may be unilateral or bilateral and, if there is no incisor protrusion, results in a normal overjet with crowding of the maxillary arch caused by the loss of space in the arch perimeter.

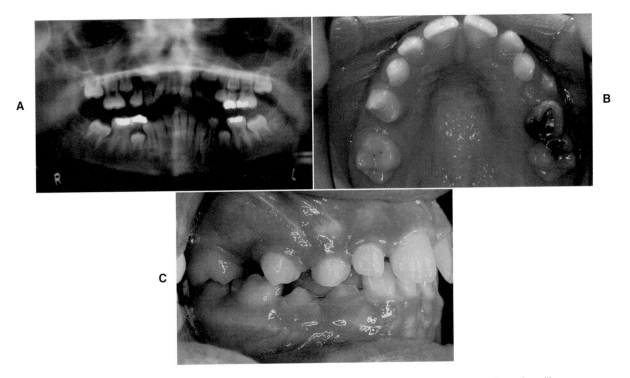

Figure 20-2 A and **B,** Mesial drift of the maxillary right first permanent molar following premature loss of maxillary right second primary molar. **C,** This usually results in a Class II permanent molar relationship.

For normal occlusion of the permanent teeth, the size of the maxillary teeth must be proportional to the size of the mandibular teeth. An **interarch tooth size discrepancy** caused from smaller or absent maxillary permanent teeth results in a maxillary tooth size deficiency. In an individual with a normal skeletal relationship and normal overjet, this problem usually is exhibited as maxillary spacing. However, it also is possible for the maxillary permanent molars to drift forward into a Class II relationship and for the interdental spacing to be minimal.

With the exception of the third molars, the most common permanent teeth to be small or congenitally absent are the mandibular second premolars followed by the maxillary lateral incisors and maxillary second premolars.[53,54] In a normal skeletal relationship with a mandibular arch unaffected by congenital absence or small teeth, the congenital absence of the maxillary second premolars almost always results in the mesial drift of the maxillary first permanent molars into a Class II relationship. This is especially the case if there has been early loss or extraction of the maxillary second primary molars.[55] Congenital absence of the maxillary permanent lateral incisors can result in mesial migration of the canines, but substantial mesial drift of the posterior maxillary teeth does not occur unless selective early extraction of the maxillary primary teeth is undertaken.

It is unusual to have a generalized maxillary tooth size deficiency in which all of the maxillary teeth are small in proportion to the mandibular teeth. It is common, however, to have individual teeth that are deficient in size, with the most frequently affected being the maxillary second premolars and lateral incisors. If the lateral incisors are small, the maxillary deficiency in tooth size usually is characterized by spacing of incisors. If the second premolars are small, their proximity to the first permanent molars often results in a Class II molar relationship.

Even if the maxillary and mandibular teeth are proportional in size, it is possible to have displaced or impacted teeth as a result of maxillary crowding or dental eruption problems. Because the maxillary canines and second premolars are the last teeth to erupt anterior to the molars, their displacement out of the arch or impaction is common and is often caused by inadequate space in the dental arch. If this occurs and the mandibular arch is unaffected by abnormal eruption or displaced posterior teeth, it may result in the mesial drift of the maxillary molars into a Class II relationship.

Skeletal Class II Malocclusions

Although orthodontists historically have appreciated the relationship between facial morphology and maloc-

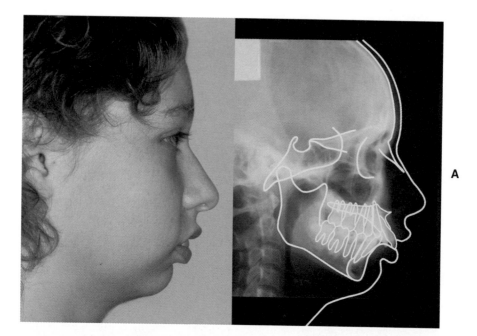

A

Figure 20-3 **A,** A patient with mandibular deficiency characterized by both a small mandibular ramus and body. There is decreased posterior face height. In this case the deficiency is great enough to cause eversion or redundancy of the lower lip with its position lingual to the maxillary incisors, preventing resting lip apposition.

Continued

clusion, cephalometrics provided a more comprehensive awareness of the underlying skeletal features that affect the occlusion. Angle's original dental classification was extended by the next generation of orthodontists to describe anteroposterior skeletal discrepancies or disproportions of the maxilla and mandible. Skeletal discrepancies associated with Class II malocclusions have been termed *skeletal Class II relationships.* This term indicates that the Class II malocclusion is one resulting from an anteroposterior disproportion in size or discrepancy in position of the jaws rather than malposition of the teeth relative to the jaws (**retrusion** of mandibular teeth or protrusion of maxillary teeth or both).

These skeletal Class II relationships often are associated with Class II dental malocclusions. Typically, some natural **dental compensation** is observed in the presence of the **skeletal discrepancy.** This compensation tends to make the dental discrepancy less severe than the skeletal discrepancy and is exhibited most often as protrusive mandibular incisors and less frequently as retrusive maxillary incisors. Another typical compensation is a maxillary dental arch that is more narrow or constricted than normal because it is in occlusion with a narrower part of the mandibular dental arch. This transverse dental compensation is characterized further by **mesiolingual rotation** of the maxillary first molars.

Skeletal Class II malocclusions can be subdivided conveniently into those comprised of either mandibular deficiency or maxillary excess.

Mandibular Deficiency Caused by Size or Position

A skeletal Class II relationship resulting from a mandible that is small or retruded relative to the maxilla is termed a *mandibular deficiency.* Regardless of whether the mandibular deficiency is an absolute deficiency (because of size) or a relative deficiency (because of position), the resulting anteroposterior dental relationship is usually Class II. The patient with this condition typically presents with a facial appearance characterized by a normal **nasolabial angle,** relative protrusion of the maxillary anterior teeth and a relative deficiency of the chin caused by the small size or retruded position of the mandible (Figure 20-3, *A*). The lower lip tends to be more everted or redundant, resulting in a pronounced labiomental fold. This is the result of the lingual contact of the maxillary incisors with the lower lip, which prevents it from being supported by the mandibular incisors. If the deficiency is great enough, the lower lip will be positioned lingually to the maxillary incisors at rest (everted lower lip), resulting in **lip incompetence** (i.e., an absence of upper and lower lip apposition) (see Figure 20-3, *A*). The consequence of this resting lip position is further protrusion of the maxillary incisors. This lip posture also prevents the lower lip from providing adequate vertical support for the maxillary incisors, promoting overeruption of these incisors.

One manifestation of mandibular deficiency in cephalometric analysis is exhibited as a downward and backward rotation of the mandible caused by the

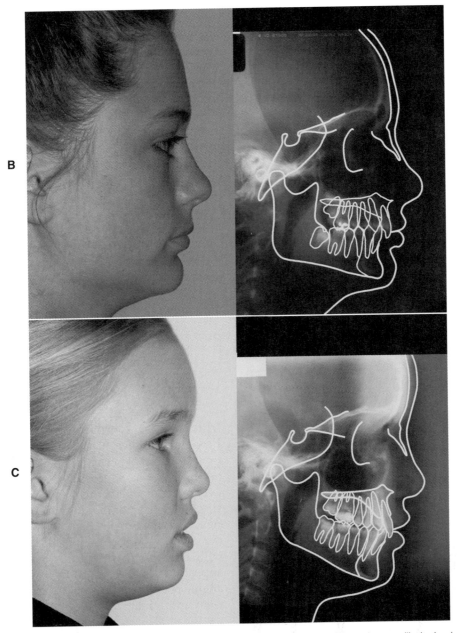

Figure 20-3, cont'd B, A patient with mandibular deficiency limited primarily to the mandibular body with a normal-sized ramus. This usually results in a normal posterior face height with a decreased anterior face height and a flat mandibular plane. **C,** A patient with mandibular deficiency characterized by retrusion of a normal sized mandible. The cranial base angle is increased, resulting in a more posterior position of the mandible.

small size of the ramus and body of the mandible (see Figure 20-3, *A*). This relationship often results in a decreased posterior facial height, a steeper **mandibular plane** angle, an increased ANB angle, a normal SNA angle with a decreased SNB angle, an increased angle of convexity, and an increased overjet. There is an increased A-B difference depicted as a greater positive value by the WITS analysis. Another distinguishing cephalometric measurement is a normal position of point A but a posterior position of point B relative to Nasion perpendicular.

Excessive overjet is the feature that was used by Angle to distinguish his classification of Class II Division 1. The overjet may become more severe if the anteroposterior discrepancy between the maxillary and mandibular teeth is great enough to cause the lower lip to be positioned lingual to the maxillary incisors, further protruding them (see Figure 20-3, *A*). Excessive overjet prevents occlusion between the maxillary and mandibular incisors which may result in overeruption, causing an excessive anterior overbite. It is common in a severe mandibular deficiency to have dental compensation for the skeletal disproportion displayed cephalometrically as protruded mandibular incisors (increased angulation of mandibular incisors relative to mandibular plane or N-B line and a decreased angulation relative to the occlusal plane or Frankfort horizontal).

Another variation of mandibular deficiency is one in which the decreased size is localized more to the **mandibular body** with **mandibular rami** of normal or increased length (see Figure 20-3, *B*). This usually appears cephalometrically as normal or increased **posterior face height** and a flatter mandibular plane. Linear assessment of mandibular length as measured from Ar to Gn or Pog may appear normal because of an excessive bony chin projection. This chin projection may be great enough to mask the facial appearance of the mandibular deficiency, but it may still leave a lack of support for the lower lip. These individuals typically have a short **lower anterior face height,** often resulting in both the upper and lower lips having a more everted position at rest. This type of mandibular deficiency is often associated with a deep **anterior overbite** with the maxillary incisors lingually inclined, decreasing overjet and further masking the anteroposterior dental discrepancy (see Figure 20-3, *B*). The lingual inclination of the maxillary incisors and reduced overjet are the features that distinguish Angle's Class II Division 2 classification. Although there is a prevailing empirical belief that there are distinguishing skeletal and facial differences between individuals with Division 1 and Division 2 Class II malocclusions, there is support that no such distinction exists.[56-58]

Individuals with mandibular deficiency resulting from retrusion of a normal-sized mandible share cephalometric features of other types of mandibular deficiency with respect to points A and B relative to Sella and the occlusal plane (see Figure 20-3, *C*). The cranial base angle, defined by points Nasion, Sella, and Basion, often is more obtuse with the glenoid fossa in a relatively posterior position. The distinguishing characteristics will be the normal size of the mandibular ramus and body, usually resulting in normal mandibular linear anteroposterior length and a normal lower face height in spite of the anteroposterior discrepancy between the maxilla and mandible.

Maxillary Excess Maxillary excess frequently may be the underlying skeletal cause of a Class II malocclusion. Maxillary excess may present as overdevelopment in the vertical or anteroposterior dimension or both. In the case of vertical maxillary excess, the excess may be more localized to the posterior area, associated with the maxillary posterior teeth being in an inferior position with a normal vertical position of the incisors (Figure 20-4, *A*). This condition is usually associated with an anterior open bite but with a normal vertical display of the maxillary incisors relative to the upper lip both in repose and upon smiling. Vertical maxillary excess also may present as overall excess with the anterior as well as the posterior maxillary teeth located inferiorly (see Figure 20-4, *B*). In this condition there will be no anterior open bite, but there will be an excessive vertical display of the maxillary incisors relative to the upper lip in repose as well as a **gummy smile** (excessive exposure of the gingiva upon smiling). In either of these two presentations of vertical maxillary excess, the mandible is rotated downward and posteriorly (the term **clockwise rotation** often is used), resulting in the Class II skeletal relationship.

With vertical maxillary excess the mandible may be of normal size but in a retrusive position because of the inferior position of the maxilla. The facial presentation of an individual with this skeletal deformity may not appear different from the mandibular deficiency when viewed by the untrained eye. However, the facial appearance often includes a narrow nose with a prominent dorsum and narrow alar bases. There is usually an increased lower anterior face height with a normal or obtuse nasolabial angle. As with the mandibular deficiency, there will be a relative chin retrusion and relative maxillary incisor protrusion because of the anteroposterior jaw discrepancy. Lip incompetence, or lack of lip apposition at rest, is even more common with maxillary vertical excess than with mandibular deficiency because the increased vertical height of the lower face causes the lips to be apart vertically, adding to the anteroposterior lip separation caused by the mandibular retrusion (see Figure 20-4).

Cephalometrically, the vertical maxillary excess is typified by an increased anterior face height and steeper mandibular plane angle. Just as with mandibular deficiency, vertical maxillary excess is usually characterized by an increased ANB angle, a normal SNA angle with a decreased SNB angle, an increased angle of convexity, and an increased overjet. Although there is usually an increased distance between points A and B as projected on the occlusal plane (WITS), this difference may be minimized by the steepness of the occlusal plane. When projected on a true horizontal line, the anteroposterior skeletal discrepancy becomes more readily apparent. Just as with the mandibular deficiency, A point appears in a normal anteroposterior position and B point appears in a posterior position relative to Nasion perpendicular. The anteroposterior discrepancy usually results in dental compensation with mandibular incisor protrusion similar to the mandibular deficient condition. However, anteroposterior mandibular length may appear normal relative to anteroposterior maxillary length. The most distinguishing cephalometric features of the vertical maxillary excess are in the vertical plane and

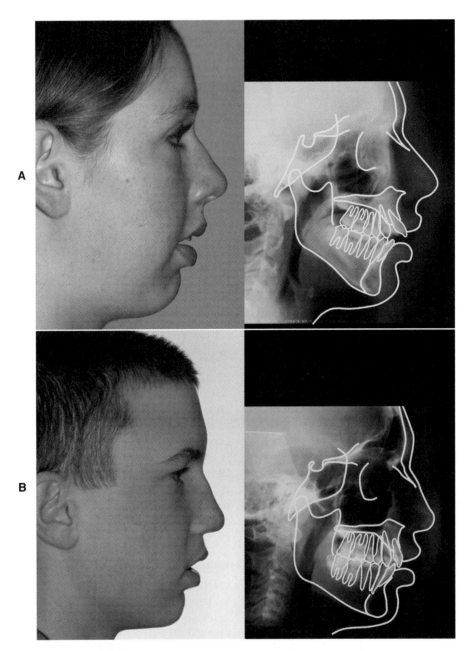

Figure 20-4 A, A patient with posterior vertical maxillary excess. Although there is increased anterior face height, steep mandibular plane, and incompetent lips, there is normal vertical display of maxillary incisors in repose and while smiling. This is typically associated with an anterior open bite. **B,** A patient with overall vertical maxillary excess. The increased anterior face height, steep mandibular plane, and incompetent lips are features in common with posterior vertical maxillary excess. However, the additional vertical excess in the anterior part of the maxilla results in excessive vertical display of maxillary incisors in repose and while smiling. An anterior open bite usually is not a feature of this condition.

include an increased lower anterior face height, steeper mandibular plane angle, and more inferior position of maxillary molars relative to the palatal plane. If the vertical excess includes the anterior part of the maxilla, the maxillary incisors will also be in a more inferior position relative to the palatal plane (see Figure 20-4, *B*).

It is possible, although less common, to have maxillary excess in the anteroposterior dimension or **midface**

protrusion. The facial appearance of this deformity can be easily confused with maxillary dental protrusion. Although both conditions exhibit **facial skeletal convexity** with a normal anteroposterior position of the mandible, maxillary anteroposterior excess is characterized by a protrusion of the entire midface, including the nose and infraorbital area as well as the upper lip (Figure 20-5, *A*). Cephalometric features of anteroposterior maxillary excess, as with all skeletal Class II rela-

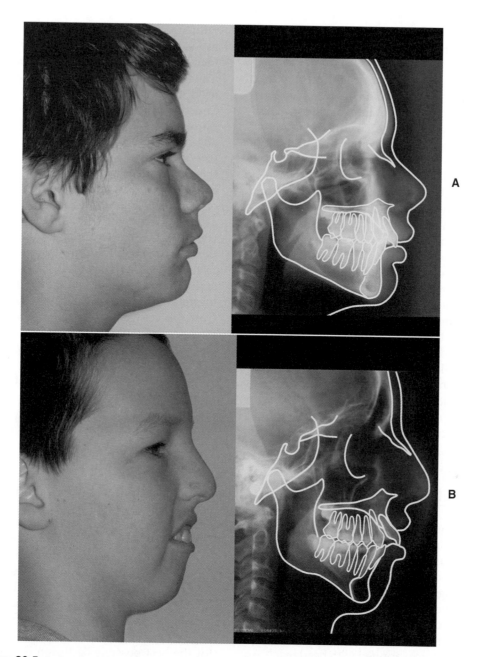

Figure 20-5 A, A patient with anteroposterior maxillary excess. This is characterized by midface protrusion with a normal size and position of the mandible. **B,** A patient with a combination of mandibular deficiency and vertical maxillary excess.

tionships, typically include an increased ANB angle and A-B difference projected on occlusal plane (WITS analysis) and true horizontal line, as well as increased facial convexity. In addition, however, SNA angle usually is increased. In contrast to mandibular deficiency, SNB angle is normal, A point is anterior, and B point is normal relative to Nasion perpendicular. Anteroposterior maxillary length is increased and anteroposterior mandibular length usually is normal. As with the other types of skeletal Class II relationships, there usually is anteroposterior dental compensation in the form of mandibular incisor protrusion and transverse dental

compensation in the form of maxillary constriction. The excessive overjet usually is associated with overeruption of the mandibular incisors and excessive overbite. If the midface protrusion is severe, the lower lip may play a similar role as with the severe mandibular deficiency with its position lingual to the maxillary incisors encouraging their protrusion and overeruption. It is important for the clinician to remember that in the numeric interpretation of the cephalometric measurements, a steep cant of the anterior cranial base or an anterior displacement of Nasion can influence the magnitude of these angles. Therefore such anatomic variations should be taken into consideration during cephalometric interpretations.

Combination of Mandibular Deficiency and Maxillary Excess

It is common to have a combination of mandibular deficiency and maxillary excess, each of which would add to the severity of the anteroposterior skeletal problem (see Figure 20-5, *B*). It is not possible to differentiate all the skeletal features that contribute to the Class II anteroposterior discrepancy without a thorough evaluation of facial form and cephalometric analyses. Historically, there has been a focus on the mandible as the problem, largely as a result of Angle's century-old classification scheme that was based on the assumption that the position of the maxillary first molar, relative to the maxilla, is a biologic constant. However, appreciation of maxillary skeletal deformities, particularly aided with the advent of cephalometric analyses, has significantly improved in the latter part of the twentieth century. It is now understood that vertical or anteroposterior excess of the maxilla may be as frequently at fault as mandibular deficiency in causing skeletal Class II relationships. In fact, it is likely that most patients with skeletal Class II problems have a combination of mandibular deficiency and maxillary excess.

HISTORY OF CLASS II MALOCCLUSION TREATMENT

Orthodontic treatment of Class II malocclusion at the latter part of the nineteenth century was limited primarily to retraction of maxillary anterior teeth to decrease excessive overjet. In 1880 an American dentist, **Norman Kingsley,** published a description of treatment techniques for addressing protrusion. The primary technique of the time was to extract the maxillary first premolars and **retract** the maxillary anterior teeth with extraoral forces applied with headgear.[59] An American orthodontist, **Calvin Case,** continued to refine these methods and those of tooth extraction.[60] In the early twentieth century, however, extraction of teeth fell into disfavor under the dominating influence of **Edward Angle.** Angle championed the belief that teeth should not be extracted in the course of treatment but should be maintained by any means possible. This led him to depend on expansion of crowded dental arches in addition to intraoral elastic traction from the maxillary anterior to the mandibular posterior teeth, later termed **Class II elastics,** for the correction of Class II malocclusions.

Orthodontics in the early part of the twentieth century was characterized by an almost universal belief that forces applied to a growing face could alter the morphologic outcome. There was optimism about the influence orthodontic treatment could have on skeletal growth. In the United States the principal appliance for **facial orthopedic treatment** was headgear, whereas the functional appliance was the appliance predominantly used in Europe. Although functional appliances continued being used in Europe throughout the twentieth century, the use of headgears in the United States was all but abandoned by the 1920s. The elimination of the use of extraoral force by orthodontists was primarily the result of the dominating influence of Angle, who believed that intraoral appliances, specifically Class II elastics, were just as effective as extraoral force in achieving favorable Class II skeletal correction. He was confident that this technique resulted in skeletal as well as dental correction of the anteroposterior problem. In fact, he was convinced that Class II elastics produced a stimulation of mandibular growth as well as a restraint on the continued growth of the maxilla. It was largely from this conviction by Angle, as well as the improved patient compliance with Class II elastics caused by the ease of wear and lack of visibility, that orthodontists discontinued the use of extraoral force in the 1920s. Angle's influence on the orthodontic profession in the United States was profound, and it would be nearly half of a century before extractions and extraoral force would return to become a well-accepted part of clinical practice.

After the 1920s there was a decline in the enthusiasm by U.S. orthodontists for the possibilities of altering facial morphology with orthopedic forces. It reached its lowest level in the 1950s. This change largely was the result of the persuasive influence of one of Angle's orthodontic students and successors, Alan Brodie, who believed that the growing face could not be significantly altered from its genetically predetermined form. With this prevailing attitude, orthodontists felt their only option in treating malocclusions caused by skeletal discrepancies was dental camouflage or moving the teeth within their respective jaws for the best possible occlusion in spite of the skeletal discrepancy. This led to a renewed acceptance of extractions as necessary in orthodontic treatment because orthodontic dental compensation, or **dental camouflage,** almost invariably required removal of teeth. In the case of a Class II skeletal problem, this usually obligated the orthodontist to extract maxillary premolars to provide room for retraction of the maxillary incisors to reduce overjet. It became more common to extract mandibular premolars to provide sufficient room in the mandibular arch to **protract** the mandibular molars into a normal Class I relationship. Two pivotal events completed the reintroduction of extractions in U.S. orthodontic practices—the death of Edward Angle and the influence of one of his orthodontic students, Charles Tweed. Tweed[61] had been discouraged by the prevalence of relapse in many of his treated patients, so he decided to oppose conventional wisdom and retreat a group of these cases with extractions. His findings that the results were more stable had an enormous impact on orthodontists in the 1940s. This led to a renewed enthusiasm for treatment of Class II malocclusions with extractions.

At about this same time the standardized lateral cephalostat, an invention that had received limited attention since its creation in 1931, began to be used to evaluate growth and treatment influence on facial form and occlusion. At first, longitudinal cephalometric evaluations seemed to confirm the prevailing belief of the time that significant skeletal changes were not possible with facial orthopedic treatment. This was the case because intraoral forces using Class II elastics was the only treatment being used for Class II correction because of Angle's enduring influence and the clinical tradition of the previous half century. It required the innovation of the American orthodontist, Silas Kloehn,[62] to reintroduce extraoral force in the form of the cervical headgear for treatment of skeletal Class II relationships. Just as longitudinal lateral cephalometric films were used as evidence to refute the assumption that Class II elastics produced a skeletal correction, it was somewhat of a paradox that Kloehn used this same radiographic technique to demonstrate that extraoral force produced positive skeletal changes as well as dentoalveolar changes in the correction of skeletal Class II problems.[62] Kloehn's reintroduction was followed by continued development of extraoral force during the next two decades as the favored orthopedic means for treating skeletal Class II relationships in the United States. It took more than half a century for the pendulum to swing back in favor of extraoral dentofacial orthopedic treatment.

Meanwhile, European orthodontics took a different path than American orthodontics during the first half of the twentieth century. European treatment emphasized removable rather than fixed appliances, and the confidence in the skeletal effects of facial orthopedic treatment endured throughout the century. A number of factors affected this circumstance. Communication across the Atlantic was limited within the orthodontic profession, and the disruption of the two World Wars further isolated the European and American orthodontists from each other. The scarcity of precious metals and the development of social welfare systems may have been important additional factors in the European reliance on removable appliances.[63]

It was not until the 1960s that the separate paths followed by American and European orthodontists began to converge. Professional and personal associations between orthodontists across the Atlantic flourished, bringing functional appliances to the United States and fixed appliances and headgears to Europe. Since that time there have been vast improvements in

the interaction, collaboration, and cooperation of orthodontists worldwide through continuing education, international meetings, collaborative research, and publications. This has led to a much less provincial and a more interactive and productive specialty, providing a climate more receptive to diverse orthodontic treatment approaches.

In addition to growth modification, orthognathic surgical techniques have been an important adjunct in the treatment of skeletal Class II malocclusions. These techniques originally were developed in Europe and were further advanced in the United States during the 1960s and 1970s. Surgical methods that permit treatment of the skeletal problem at the actual source of the problem, correcting the specific jaw discrepancy or disproportion, are now available.

CURRENT TREATMENT APPROACHES TO DENTAL CLASS II MALOCCLUSIONS

The most common Class II malocclusion is one that is caused by an underlying Class II skeletal discrepancy. The Class II malocclusion that is present in an individual with a normal skeletal jaw relationship is less frequent and caused by forward movement during dental development of the maxillary molars relative to the mandibular molars. This less common condition may be unilateral or bilateral in presentation. There are two alternatives for treatment of the dental Class II malocclusion: a nonextraction approach involving distal movement of the maxillary teeth and the extraction approach involving unilateral or bilateral dental extractions.

Extraction vs. Nonextraction Treatment

If the Class II dental relationship is the result of mesial drift of maxillary permanent molars caused by premature loss or small maxillary primary molars, it may be possible to move the maxillary permanent molars distally to achieve a normal Class I relationship and regain space for the other permanent maxillary teeth. Successful distal movement of the molars depends on the severity of the mesial drift. If the molars are tipped forward, their crowns can be moved distally using either extraoral force applied to the molars with a headgear or an intraoral spring force applied with a removable or fixed appliance (see Chapters 13 and 19). If the roots as well as the crowns of the molars are forward, often caused by loss of second primary molars before eruption of the permanent molars, it is a much more difficult challenge for the clinician. This circumstance requires distal bodily molar movement that usually is possible only with full-time headgear wear. Appliances that generate an intraoral distal force to the molars must be dependent on anterior anchorage to prevent anterior movement of the maxillary anterior teeth as a side effect. Usually the magnitude and duration of force necessary to bodily move the molars distally overwhelm the anterior anchorage and result in unacceptable protraction of maxillary incisors.

A more practical approach to treatment of the dental malocclusion, characterized by maxillary molars with their roots and crowns mesially positioned in a Class II relationship, is to accept the molar relationship and obtain space for the remaining maxillary teeth by extracting maxillary first or second premolars.

Unilateral vs. Bilateral Class II

It is possible that the factors causing a Class II dental relationship may occur only on one side of the arch, resulting in a unilateral Class II problem. If this is associated with dental midlines that are coincident with the facial midline, extraction of a maxillary premolar on the affected side, unless one is already missing, may be indicated to provide adequate space for the remaining teeth. The unilateral Class II problem may be associated with a maxillary midline deviation toward the affected side caused by the loss or displacement of a premolar or canine on that side. Treatment may require extraction of a maxillary premolar on the unaffected side to center the maxillary midline with the face. If inadequate overjet is present, mandibular extractions may be necessary as well.

CURRENT TREATMENT APPROACHES TO SKELETAL CLASS II MALOCCLUSIONS

It is important for the clinician to be competent in differentiating between dental orthodontic problems caused by malpositioned teeth on well-proportioned jaws and skeletal orthodontic problems caused by a disproportion in the size or position of the jaws. Although it is most appropriate for the orthodontist to treat skeletal problems, the general dentist should have a good understanding of the different treatment alternatives. Essentially, there are three alternatives for treating any skeletal problem: **growth modification,** dental camouflage, and **orthognathic surgery.** In the growing child, all three may be possible, whereas in the adult, only the latter two are options.

Growth Modification for Class II Skeletal Problems

The goal of growth modification is to alter the unacceptable skeletal relationships by modifying the patient's remaining facial growth to favorably change the size or position of the jaws. Certainly, it would be ideal to successfully treat all Class II skeletal problems with growth modification because it would preclude the need for dental extractions or surgery. Unfortunately, the patient may be unwilling to wear an orthopedic appliance, have too little favorable facial growth remaining, or the skeletal problem may be too severe for the orthodontist to treat to an acceptable outcome. It is with these potential limitations in mind that the orthodontist must select the best treatment alternative. Basically, three types of orthodontic appliances are used for growth modification of Class II skeletal problems: extraoral force appliances, functional appliances, and interarch elastic traction.

Extraoral Force (Headgear) Appliances

Mode of Action and Goals of Treatment with Headgears A headgear intended for use in growth modification is designed to deliver an adequate **extraoral orthopedic force** to compress the maxillary sutures, modifying the pattern of bone apposition at these sites. Although posterior and superior extraoral orthopedic forces primarily are intended to inhibit anterior and inferior development of the maxilla, they also inhibit mesial and occlusal eruption of the maxillary posterior teeth. The goal of treatment is for this restriction of maxillary growth to occur while the mandible continues to grow forward an adequate amount to "catch up" with the maxilla. The forces need to be of sufficient magnitude, applied in an appropriate direction, and delivered for an adequate length of time during a period of active mandibular growth for there to be a positive treatment prognosis.

Although the headgear can be an effective appliance in the treatment of a variety of Class II problems, the most ideal indication for the use of extraoral force in the correction of skeletal Class II malocclusions is with **anteroposterior maxillary excess.** Because the headgear is intended to restrict anterior and inferior maxillary growth while growth in other areas progresses, the maxillary anteroposterior excess (maxillary protrusion) would seem to be the most suitable skeletal problem for treatment in this manner. Another optimum indication for treatment with headgear accompanying the maxillary excess would be normal mandibular skeletal and dental morphology because the extraoral force would minimally influence these features. Finally, the ideal circumstance for use of headgear must be one where there is continued active mandibular growth, primarily displacing the mandible in a forward, rather than downward direction.

Types of Headgears *Headgear* is a common term for an appliance that is used for delivering a posteriorly directed extraoral force to the maxilla. Each headgear consists of a metal device attached extraorally to an **occipital or cervical attachment** and intraorally to an appliance fixed to the teeth. There are essentially two types of headgear available for delivering extraoral force to the maxilla: the **facebow** and the **J-hook headgear.**

The first and most common type of headgear is the facebow, which is a large-gauge wire framework consisting of an **outer bow** for the extraoral attachment soldered to an **inner bow** that attaches intraorally in tubes attached to the maxillary first permanent molar bands (Figure 20-6). This is the more versatile of the two types of headgear because it can be used with either a maxillary fixed or removable appliance. The fixed appliance can be as simple as banded maxillary first permanent molars alone or can include banding or bonding of the remaining dentition. A removable appliance may be a possible alternative as long as there is sufficient acrylic bulk to prevent displacement

of the tubes that serve as the intraoral attachment. Because the intraoral point of attachment usually is localized to the bands on the maxillary first permanent molars, it usually is the molar **center of resistance** that is considered when determining the direction or vector of force. If the facebow is attached to a removable appliance, the center of resistance is more forward between the anterior and posterior maxillary teeth.

The second type of headgear, commonly referred to as a *J-hook headgear,* is two separate, curved, large-gauge wires that are formed on their ends into small hooks, both of which attach directly to the anterior part of the maxillary arch wire (Figure 20-7). This type of headgear is more commonly used for retraction of canines or incisors rather than orthopedic purposes. The J-hook headgear is limited to use only with a maxillary fixed appliance with a continuous arch wire. It is preferable if all the maxillary teeth are incorporated in the fixed appliance, but a minimum requirement is

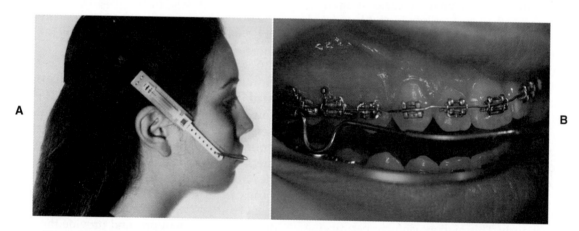

Figure 20-6 A, The occipital extraoral attachment dissipates the force on the cranium. **B,** The intraoral attachment for the facebow is a tube that is an integral part of the bracket welded to each of the maxillary first molar bands. The facebow can be placed with a complete fixed appliance or simply with bands on the maxillary first molars.

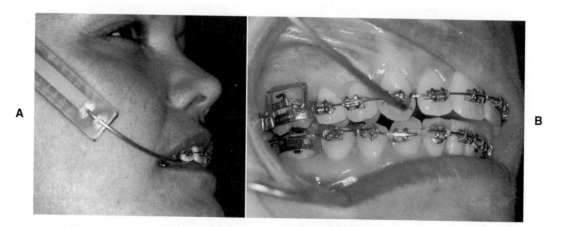

Figure 20-7 A, The intraoral attachment for the J-hook headgear is directly to the maxillary arch wire, usually placed mesial to the maxillary canines. This anterior location permits the J-hook wires to emerge from the mouth without impinging the lip commissures. **B,** A J-hook headgear for orthopedic purposes only should be placed with a complete fixed appliance in the maxillary arch.

inclusion of the maxillary first molars and incisors. The intraoral point of attachment is directly to the maxillary arch wire, which usually is attached to all of the maxillary teeth. As a result, the center of resistance has to be considered to be similar to the circumstance with the facebow attached to a removable appliance (i.e., with the midpoint between the most anterior and posterior maxillary teeth).

There are two basic types of extraoral attachments that provide anchorage for the headgear. The first is the cervical attachment or neck strap (Figure 20-8, *A*). Because the point of attachment is usually below the occlusal plane, the extraoral force is directed inferiorly as well as posteriorly. This force vector may help anteroposterior correction but may amplify vertical maxillary excess problems. With the facebow the cervical attachment creates an extrusive and distal force to the maxillary molars, whereas this same attachment to a J-hook promotes **extrusion** and retraction of the maxillary incisors. These extrusive effects are usually counterproductive to treatment of Class II skeletal problems because they also result in the backward rotation of the mandible. Therefore the cervical strap should only be considered for individuals with flat mandibular and occlusal planes (closer to true horizontal) in which an increase in facial vertical dimension is desired. This extrusive force is minimized if, in some cases, the attachment on the neck delivers a horizontal force vector that is directed through the center of resistance of the maxillary molars.

The second type of extraoral anchorage for a headgear is the occipital attachment or headcap (see Figure 20-6, *B*). With the point of attachment well above the occlusal plane, the extraoral force is directed superiorly and posteriorly. This high attachment permits the creation of a force vector that contributes to correction of not only anteroposterior maxillary excess, but also to vertical maxillary excess. The higher angle of the force vector created results in a distal and intrusive force to the maxillary molars. When the occipital attachment is used with a J-hook, the force vector is further forward so that it tends to have an intrusive force to the maxillary incisors and may have an indirect extrusive force to the maxillary molars as a result of tipping the occlusal plane.

It is possible to use a combination of the cervical and occipital attachments, termed **combination headgear,** to distribute the external force over more surfaces and to provide a convenient means of modifying the direction of the force vector (see Figure 20-8, *B*). If the forces are equal for each attachment, the resulting force vector is usually above the occlusal plane but inferior to the vector created with the occipital attachment alone. The advantage of a combination headgear is the ease with which the force vector can be modified and the improved comfort afforded by the increased force distribution. The disadvantage is that it increases the number of parts that the patient has to wear, manage, and possibly lose. Thus cooperation becomes more challenging.

Selection of Magnitude, Duration, Direction, and Timing of Extraoral Force
The **orthodontic force magnitude** used to move a tooth usually varies between 15 and 400 g depending on the size of the tooth or, more specifically, the periodontal ligament surface area and the type of tooth movement.[64] Low orthodontic force magnitude, as light as 10 to 15 g (less than half of an ounce) per anterior tooth, may create the most efficient tooth movement, cause the least morbidity for the teeth and periodontium, and provide the least discomfort for the patient.[65] Even the tooth movements that

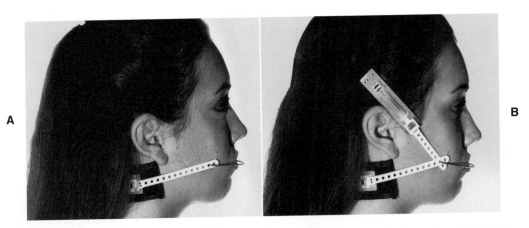

Figure 20-8 Alternative extraoral attachments. **A,** Cervical attachment. **B,** Combination (cervical and occipital) attachment. The extraoral force vector is the most inferior with the cervical attachment and the most superior with the occipital attachment. The combination attachment creates a force vector between the ones created by either attachment alone. An increase in the occipital force or decrease in the cervical force raises the force vector angle. An increase in the cervical force or decrease in the occipital force lowers the force vector angle.

require the greatest force usually do not exceed 150 g per tooth.[64] A force beyond 300 g per anterior tooth appears to surpass the threshold for tooth movement.[66] Light orthodontic forces, however, are not effective for facial orthopedic purposes to modify skeletal growth. Extraoral force must be of much greater magnitude, in the range of 400 to 600 g (1 to 1½ pounds) per side for a total of 800 to 1200 g (2 to 3 pounds), to maximize the potential for skeletal change and to minimize dental change.[63]

The **orthodontic force duration** that most effectively moves teeth is continuous in nature.[67] Much effort has been made in the development of orthodontic materials that apply a force that decays as slowly as possible over time. This has an added practical benefit to the orthodontist in that the patient does not need to be appointed as often for reapplication of the optimum force. In contrast to orthodontic tooth movement, intermittent forces of 12 to 16 hours' duration appear to be effective for facial orthopedic changes.[68] One should not infer that sutures respond best to **intermittent force.** In fact, it makes biologic sense that a **continuous force** affects them more. Because the headgear is tooth-borne, however, an intermittent force minimizes tooth movement while still providing for skeletal change. In fact, if the headgear is worn more than about 16 hr/day at force levels below approximately 400 g or 1 pound, less skeletal effect and more tooth movement will occur.[69] An intermittent heavy force also is less damaging to the teeth and periodontium than a continuous heavy force.[70] The intermittent use of the headgear is another practical benefit to treatment of skeletal problems because few children are willing to wear a headgear full time.

Extraoral orthopedic force must be applied in the appropriate direction to have a maximum skeletal effect. The **force direction or vector** can be altered by a variety of means. The extraoral attachment, as mentioned previously, can be cervical or occipital to establish a low or high angle of force vector, respectively. If a combination extraoral attachment is being used, the force magnitude can be increased to the occipital attachment or decreased to the cervical attachment to raise the force vector angle superiorly. Finally, the outer bow of the facebow can be shortened or raised or both vertically to produce a more superior force vector (Figure 20-9). Although a superior and posterior force through the center of resistance appears to be the most appropriate direction to affect the maxillary sutures, some modification of the angle of this force vector may be necessary in specific situations. As mentioned previously, extraoral orthopedic force with a cervical attachment may have a force vector that is below the center of resistance of the maxillary molars that results in distal movement of the molar crowns as well as extrusion of the molars. Although the distal movement is in the direction favoring the overall Class II correction, the extrusion is not because it opens the bite by rotating the mandible downward and backward. Fortunately, the typical occipital headgear force on the maxillary molars is an intrusive as well as a distal one, minimizing their natural eruption anteriorly and inferiorly. Exceptional headgear wear can even intrude maxillary first molars and move them distally. Either of these possible tooth movements from the orthopedic force applied will be beneficial because they are in the direction of the overall Class II correction.

A final consideration for extraoral orthopedic force is the timing of force application. It is a basic principle of facial orthopedic treatment that the greatest amount of skeletal improvement can be obtained while wearing the appliance during the most active period of

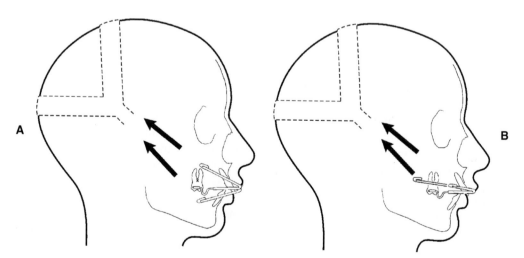

Figure 20-9 Change in extraoral force vector with changes in height and length of outer bow. **A,** Change in height of outer bow. **B,** Change in length of outer bow. Raising or shortening the outer bow moves the force vector superiorly, whereas lowering or lengthening the outer bow moves the force vector inferiorly.

facial growth.[71,72] Because the most active period of all is early in life, before eruption of the permanent teeth, one may think that this would be the most ideal time. Although dramatic skeletal growth modification can be achieved quickly in young children, the renewed expression of the original growth pattern following treatment may negate part of the corrections with no permanent long-term effect on the original skeletal growth pattern.[63,73] The second most active period of facial growth is during the **pubertal growth spurt** in early adolescence when skeletal changes achieved with Class II treatment are much more resistant to relapse, probably because of the minimal maxillary growth and residual mandibular growth that often remains at this stage of growth. Unfortunately, the facial pubertal growth spurt does not occur in all patients and is not accurately predictable regarding its timing, magnitude, direction, or duration. Another risk of starting treatment during the pubertal growth spurt is that its occurrence coincides with the physically and emotionally labile period of adolescence, which often limits the patient compliance for headgear wear. It is for these reasons that orthodontists may choose to have the patient begin headgear wear while still in the mixed dentition. It is fortunate that permanent teeth other than the maxillary first molars are not required for the support of the appliance. One final note on optimum timing of extraoral force is the recognition that increased release of growth hormone and other endocrine factors that promote growth occurs more during the evening and night than during the day[74] and is associated with sleep onset.[75] A similar nocturnal phenomenon has been documented for dental eruption with the most active eruption occurring in the late evening until 1 AM.[76] There also is evidence that skeletal growth follows a similar circadian pattern.[77] Because evening and nighttime usually is the only time one can reliably expect an adolescent to wear a headgear, these nocturnal phenomena are fortuitous biologic benefits for these patients.

Although there is an improved understanding of the magnitude, duration, direction, and timing of force application that is most effective in achieving skeletal changes, there are some practical limitations in orthodontic clinical practice. The maxillary teeth provide the only current means for applying orthopedic forces to the maxillary sutures. Because the intraoral part of the appliance is tooth-borne, it is unrealistic to assume that one can direct forces to the maxillary sutures without these forces affecting the position of the teeth. In spite of using heavy, intermittent forces, it is inevitable that significant tooth movement will occur.

Another limitation that is all too familiar to orthodontists is the dependence on patient compliance to wear and care for the headgear for successful treatment progress. Headgears, by definition, are remov-

able appliances and can be effective only when they are worn. Finally, an important limitation is the dependence on an adequate amount and direction of mandibular growth on successful treatment. It has become clear that one cannot necessarily be assured of this even though the timing of treatment coincides with the pubertal growth spurt.[78]

In summary, the most effective extraoral force application for skeletal Class II treatment is with a facebow attached to an occipital attachment using a heavy force (400 to 600 g per side) applied for 12 to 16 hours daily (evening and night). The force vector should be directed superiorly and posteriorly through or above the center of resistance for the maxillary molars. Finally, the treatment must occur during active growth (see Chapter 7).

Clinical Procedures for Use of Headgears

Preparation of Dentition for Headgears If the headgear being used is one that is attached intraorally to the maxillary first permanent molars, usually the only preparation of the dentition is fitting and cementing bands with headgear tubes on these molars. It is common to have some degree of mesiolingual rotation of the maxillary first molars if the occlusion of these teeth with the mandibular first molars is a Class II relationship. Occasionally, this rotation is severe, making the insertion of the inner bow impossible. In this situation a short period of orthodontic treatment, usually with an active transpalatal arch to rotate the maxillary first molars to permit facebow insertion, is required before delivering the headgear. Other than this exception, no other preparation of the dentition usually is necessary.

When the headgear is attached intraorally to a removable acrylic splint or functional appliance, the headgear tubes are incorporated directly into the acrylic, occlusal to the maxillary premolars (Figure 20-10). This attachment location approximates the force vector through the center of resistance for the maxilla. Under these circumstances, no special preparation of the dentition is necessary, although accurate impressions and a bite registration are necessary to fabricate the acrylic portion of the appliance.

The J-hook headgear can be delivered only after bonding of the maxillary incisors as well as banding of the maxillary molars. It is recommended that complete banding and bonding of all the maxillary teeth are considered to provide for a more stable appliance, avoiding distortion or breakage. Delivery of the J-hook headgear requires much more preparation of the teeth than the facebow. An arch wire of adequate stiffness to support orthopedic forces, such as 0.017-inch × by 0.025-inch stainless steel in 0.018-inch slot or 0.018-inch × 0.025-inch stainless steel in 0.022-inch slot, is recommended. For this reason, a period of time often

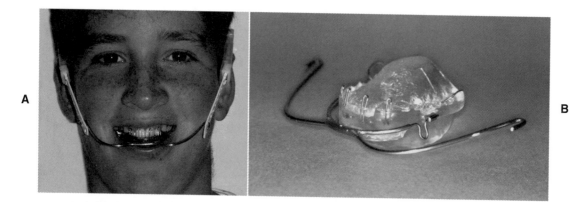

Figure 20-10 **A,** Combination of facebow with a removable functional appliance. **B,** The headgear tubes are placed in the acrylic occlusal to the maxillary premolars. This more anterior placement requires a facebow with a shorter inner bow.

lasting a number of months is necessary to align and level the teeth attached to the arch wire to permit placement of the stiffer wire before headgear delivery.

Fabrication and Delivery of Headgears The facebow must be selected and adjusted to permit adequate clearance of the inner bow away from the maxillary teeth and positioned to rest comfortably between the lips at rest. Expansion of the inner bow usually is necessary to help facilitate correction of the constricted maxillary arch that is typical of a Class II malocclusion. The outer bow is adjusted to conform to the cheeks. The selection of the occipital or cervical attachment, in combination with the length and height of the outer bow dictates the final force direction. A release mechanism is recommended to prevent the facebow or J-hook wires from springing back and injuring the patient's eyes or face if it is pulled away from the face while still connected to the attachment. Final adjustments, modifying the force magnitude or direction, should be accomplished with the patient in an upright sitting or standing position.

When the clinician is satisfied with the final adjustments, it is best to demonstrate placement and removal of the headgear to the patient with one of the parents present. This permits both the child and parent to understand how to manipulate the appliance in a safe and efficient manner because it usually is necessary for the child to have some assistance during the first week of wear. The dentist demonstrates how to carefully insert and remove the facebow without applying vertical forces with the distal ends of the inner bow in the headgear tubes that promote loosening of the molar bands. In a similar manner the J-hook wires have to be inserted and removed without applying a force to the arch wire that can deform it or debond brackets. The patient is shown how to safely connect and disconnect the headgear attachment to the facebow with an explanation and demonstration of

the safety release mechanism. The child is then allowed to place and remove the appliance until the parent and child are confident with the process. There must be assurance that the headgear components are being properly positioned so that improper wear is avoided. Finally, instruction is given for safe use and avoidance of wear during most sports and other physical activity where the child may be vulnerable to blows to the face. The optimum wear of 12 to 16 hours per day is best achieved by consistent wear by the child while in the home, which usually includes evenings and while sleeping.

Management of Treatment with Headgears There needs to be a period of adaptation by the child to wearing the headgear. The patient should be warned that some soreness is to be expected during the first week or two of wear while the teeth and supporting bone adapt to the force. The discomfort would be intolerable if the child were to wear the appliance with the expected orthopedic force and duration from the outset. To prevent this discomfort and permit easier acclimation to the appliance, one of two strategies can be employed. Either the initial duration or the magnitude of force can be minimized and gradually increased until the optimum levels are reached within the first 2 weeks.

The next scheduled office visit by the patient should not occur later than 2 weeks after delivery of the headgear to verify that the patient is managing well with the appliance and that adequate oral hygiene is being maintained. It is especially important during this initial period of acclimation that the patient and parent are encouraged to contact the dentist if there are any difficulties that prevent the planned headgear wear. The second appointment after initial delivery should be no later than 1 month to confirm that the patient is continuing to do well. More frequent office visits during this time provide the dentist with more opportunities to monitor compliance as well as to reinforce the patient when compliance is good. There are a number of indicators that assist the dentist in assessing headgear wear compliance. The most reliable ones include the ease with which the patient can place and remove the appliance and the mobility of the maxillary first molars when a facebow is used. After the first few months of wear, there will be other indicators, including signs of wear on the extraoral attachment components and calculus on the facebow. Ultimately, anteroposterior improvement in the occlusion, including less severe Class II buccal occlusion and decreased overjet, is the most desirable indication of good headgear wear. Once the dentist is confident that the patient has acclimated well to the appliance and is wearing it consistently, time between office visits to monitor progress can be increased to a 6- to 8-week interval.

At each appointment it is important for patients to bring their headgear in for inspection and possible adjustment. Usually the force magnitude decreases after initial placement of the headgear because the occipital or cervical attachment fabric stretches and conforms to the patient's head or neck after initial wear. This may require increasing the force as well as adjusting the facebow to reestablish the appropriate force magnitude and direction. At each appointment it is necessary to adjust the inner bow to achieve the desired **derotation** and expansion of the maxillary molars. After a number of months of wear, there is some dental movement that will require facebow adjustments. If the maxillary first molar crowns are tipping posteriorly, it will be necessary to raise and possibly shorten the outer bow to direct the force vector above the center of resistance of the molars to prevent further distal tipping of the molar crowns. If there is any distal displacement of the molars, it is desirable for it to be **bodily movement** as opposed to **tipping movement.** If the maxillary first molars move distally in the arch, it will also be necessary to open the vertical adjustment loops to lengthen the inner bow. This maintains the clearance from the facial surfaces of the maxillary incisors and prevents a lingually directed force from inadvertently being applied to the incisors.

The decision to discontinue orthopedic treatment with headgear must be made only after carefully considering the type of skeletal problem and the potential for remaining growth. Although facial orthopedic treatment may successfully modify skeletal growth expression, it will have a negligible effect on the **fundamental growth pattern** of the patient.[79] For this reason, it is possible for the growth pattern to continue to express itself after orthopedic treatment is discontinued, causing the skeletal discrepancy to return.[80] In the case of mandibular deficiency in the growing child, the mandible is likely to grow less after orthopedic treatment and stop growing sooner than a normal

mandible. If the normal maxilla continues growing downward and forward, the original jaw discrepancy may reoccur. If the original cause of the skeletal Class II problem is excessive maxillary growth, continued growth after successful orthopedic treatment may result in the maxilla growing more and for a longer time than a normal maxilla, either of which may result in a return of the original jaw discrepancy.

This phenomenon of the patient's fundamental growth pattern reexpressing itself following cessation of orthopedic treatment must be considered when determining the endpoint for headgear wear. Two treatment recommendations that can minimize this problem are the inclusion of **overcorrection** and the continuance of some degree of orthopedic treatment until maxillary growth is complete. The patient must continue to wear headgear for the same daily duration until sufficient overcorrection is achieved, usually 1 to 2 mm beyond ideal buccal occlusion with no overjet. When adequate overcorrection is present, it is advisable to discontinue the headgear wear incrementally while monitoring the occlusion. In some cases of maxillary excess continued growth after initial orthopedic treatment may require the nightly use of headgear until completion of adolescent growth.

Effects of Treatment with Headgears

Skeletal effects of headgears The objective of orthopedic treatment with the headgear is to compress the maxillary sutures, altering the growth and apposition of bone at these sutures. The result is to suppress or restrict normal downward and forward maxillary growth while the mandible continues to grow normally. The intention is for the mandible to "catch up" with the maxilla, correcting the anteroposterior skeletal discrepancy. Obviously, restriction of maxillary growth with effective headgear wear provides an insignificant treatment benefit unless there is also adequate mandibular growth in a forward direction occurring during treatment. Clinical benefits were demonstrated with the reintroduction of headgear in the 1940s,[62] and it was clearly shown, by means of early cephalometric studies, that redirection of maxillary growth could be accomplished with headgear use.[81] Numerous clinical studies have confirmed this effect on the maxilla.[82-103] Animal models also have been used to demonstrate that an extraoral force directed against the maxilla restricts forward growth and alters the pattern of bone apposition at the maxillary sutures.[104-112] The growth response of the maxilla to orthopedic force is much more predictable than the growth response of the mandible.[113]

It is possible that the effect of extraoral force with a headgear is not limited to the maxilla.[114] There are some clinical **retrospective studies** that suggest that headgear treatment may cause a small increase in mandibular growth, although there is debate whether this amount is of clinical significance.[99,115,116] Recently, there is supporting evidence from a **prospective** randomized controlled clinical trial that indicates enhanced mandibular growth from headgear treatment.[117] However, this is not supported by other recent prospective randomized controlled trials.[78,103]

Dental effects of headgears Although skeletal change without dental movement is usually desired when using the headgear for orthopedic purposes, it is not possible for a **tooth-borne appliance** to selectively alter skeletal relationships without dental change.[99] The typical response from effective headgear wear is to prevent the maxillary first molars from erupting downward and forward, indirectly enhancing the forward direction of mandibular growth. Extrusion of the maxillary molars by a distal force that is directed more inferiorly can result in more downward and backward rotation of the mandible, which limits the forward expression of mandibular growth. With most skeletal Class II problems it is more desirable to have the intrusive effect on the maxillary molars to maximize the anteroposterior skeletal correction. In the minority of cases in which vertical mandibular growth expression is also desired to increase lower face height, some maxillary molar extrusion may be acceptable because the skeletal mandibular growth pattern tends to be expressed more forward with or without treatment.[118] Although minimal dental change is expected in the mandibular arch or in the anterior maxillary arch as a direct result of headgear wear,[117] there is some evidence that the mandibular incisors may become slightly more protrusive.[103] No appreciable movement of the maxillary incisors occurs from the use of a headgear in the absence of an arch wire connecting them to the first molars. If there is a continuous arch wire present, any distal movement of the maxillary molar crowns may also result in slight lingual movement of the incisor crowns. In the absence of an arch wire, it is possible to have **intrusion** and lingual tipping of the maxillary incisors if the facebow being used is a Cervera facebow, which has a metal plate incorporated in the anterior part of the inner bow. A similar intrusive and distal force can be applied to all the erupted maxillary teeth if a standard facebow is attached directly to a maxillary acrylic splint or a functional appliance (see Figure 20-10).

Functional Appliances

Norman Kingsley,[59] an early influential American orthodontist, has been credited with the development of the first appliance to position the mandible forward as early as 1879. However, most consider Pierre Robin[119] to have developed the earliest removable functional appliance, the monobloc, in France in 1902.

Only 3 years later at the International Dental Congress in Berlin, Emil Herbst[120] introduced a fixed pin and tube appliance to posture the mandible forward. The most popular functional appliance, the **activator,** was independently developed by Viggo Andresen[121] in Denmark in 1908 and later modified in Norway by his colleague, Karl Häupl.[122] A more recent innovation in functional appliance design, the **functional corrector (or functional regulator),** was developed by Rolf Fränkel[123] in Germany and was introduced in 1966. This appliance was unique in that it was principally tissue-borne, mostly supported in the vestibule rather than supported by the teeth. Countless modifications of these removable functional appliances followed their introduction. The individuals who made the modifications usually renamed the appliance, more often than not, with their own name. All of these appliances postured the mandible downward and forward with the intent that the muscle and soft tissue pressure attempting to reposition the jaw back to its original position would modify jaw growth to correct the Class II skeletal problem. Needless to say, the success of these appliances was dependent on excellent patient compliance because of their removable nature.

Indications for and Goals of Treatment with Functional Appliances Class II functional appliances are designed to position the mandible downward and forward to stimulate or accelerate mandibular growth. Theoretically, the distraction of the mandibular condyles out of the glenoid fossae reduces the pressure on the actively growing **condylar cartilage** and alters the muscle tension on the condyles, increasing the amount of endochondral growth more than would normally occur.[72] Although a functional appliance is primarily intended to enhance the downward and forward growth of the mandible, it usually is designed to inhibit mesial and occlusal eruption of the maxillary posterior teeth and encourage mesial eruption of the mandibular posterior teeth. Just as with the headgear, the appliance needs to be worn an adequate length of time during a period of active mandibular growth to have a positive prognosis. Although the functional appliance, like the headgear, can be an effective appliance in the treatment of a variety of Class II problems, the ideal indication for the use of the appliance in the correction of skeletal Class II malocclusions is a mandibular deficiency. Another ideal circumstance for treatment with a functional appliance, in addition to the mandibular deficiency and normal maxillary development, is a normal or mildly decreased face height because, theoretically, most of these appliances encourage mandibular posterior dental eruption. An additional optimal indication for functional appliances is slightly protrusive maxillary incisors and slightly retrusive mandibular incisors because the expected dental effect of these appliances includes some maxillary incisor retraction and mandibular incisor protraction. Finally, as with headgear therapy, the ideal patient must have active mandibular growth, primarily in a forward direction. It is important to note that although the indications for use of functional appliances and headgears may slightly differ, comparisons of their treatment effects indicate similar outcomes.

Types of Functional Appliances

Functional appliance is a common term for a variety of appliances, most of which are designed to correct skeletal Class II relationships by positioning the mandible downward and forward to theoretically enhance mandibular growth. All functional appliances are intraoral devices, and nearly all of them are tooth-borne or supported by the teeth. With a few exceptions, these appliances are removable, consisting primarily of acrylic with wire components for retention and support. Although there is an extensive diversity of different functional appliances, they can be divided conveniently into three types: removable tooth-borne, removable tissue-borne, and fixed tooth-borne.

The most common functional appliances are the removable tooth-borne appliances, including the activator, **bionator,** and **twin block appliances.** To achieve the desired skeletal and dental effects, these appliances depend on the stretch of the soft tissues caused by the mandible being positioned downward and forward as well as by the muscle activity generated by the mandible attempting to return to its original position.

The activator consists of a large acrylic splint with a large lingual flange to maintain the mandible downward and forward (Figure 20-11, *A*). The original appliance was retained loosely by means of a maxillary labial bow with a transpalatal wire for support. This loose retention was intended because it was thought that the patient continually would be functioning, or using, muscle activity to actively hold the appliance in position, accentuating the treatment effects. These characteristics gave rise to the terms *functional appliance* and *activator.* Facets are cut into the acrylic to guide eruption of the posterior teeth to assist in correcting the Class II occlusion. The maxillary posterior teeth are encouraged to erupt distally, occlusally, and buccally, whereas the mandibular posterior teeth are guided mesially and occlusally.

Another type of activator resulted from modifications by Egil Harvold[123a] of Denmark and Donald Woodside[124] of Canada, including an increased mandibular opening for improved retention and increased soft tissue stretch. In addition, posterior facets were replaced with interocclusal acrylic to prevent eruption of the maxillary posterior teeth and to leave space for unhindered eruption of the mandibu-

lar posterior teeth as well as acrylic capping over the mandibular incisal edges to minimize protraction of these teeth during treatment. The maxillary wire crossing the palate was replaced with palatal acrylic. Springs were embedded in the acrylic to displace the appliance forward, forcing the patient to actively "function" to maintain the appliance in place. Other modifications have been made that do not depart from this basic design, including eliminating displacing springs, replacing the maxillary labial bow with labial torquing springs, adding molar clasps, adding lip or cheek pads to remove lip or cheek pressure from the teeth, and adding active components such as expansion screws for transverse or anteroposterior activation or springs for tipping of teeth. These various modifications have provided ample opportunity to rename or discover a new appliance multiple times.

The bionator was developed in Germany by Wilhelm Balters[125] in the early 1950s to increase patient comfort and facilitate daytime wear to increase the functional use of the appliance. Balters[125] accomplished this by drastically reducing the acrylic bulk of the activator (see Figure 20-11, *B*).[126] There is a much smaller mandibular lingual flange, minimal interocclusal acrylic, a transpalatal wire in place of palatal acrylic, and a modified labial bow with buccal extensions that minimize cheek pressure on the teeth. The bionator can incorporate either posterior facets or interocclusal acrylic to prevent or selectively guide eruption. As with the activator, active components such as expansion screws, which make the appliance more versatile but decrease its sturdiness, can be added to the bionator.

The twin block appliance was introduced by a Scottish orthodontist, William Clark,[127] in 1977 as a two-piece or split activator using separate maxillary and mandibular appliances with occlusal acrylic portions that serve as inclined guide planes and bite blocks to determine the extent that the mandible is postured downward and forward (see Figure 20-11, *C*). Although this appliance provides for more range of mandibular movement and is adjusted and modified more easily than other functional appliances, it has a greater tendency to protract mandibular incisors. The twin block appliance also can have active components incorporated similar to the other removable tooth-borne functional appliances.

The second main type of functional appliance is the removable tissue-borne one that is represented by only one appliance (see Figure 20-11, *D*). Named the *functional corrector or functional regulator* by its German developer, Rolf Fränkel,[128] this appliance was created in an attempt to minimize unwanted tooth movement and to recontour the facial soft tissue adjacent to the teeth as well as posture the mandible downward and forward. A mandibular lingual acrylic flange positions

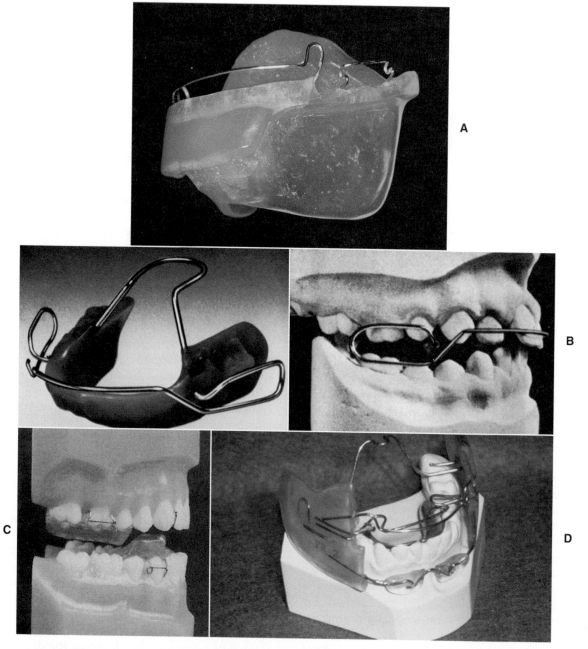

Figure 20-11 Types of removable functional appliances. **A,** Andresen's activator appliance is intended to fit loosely in the mouth, requiring the patient to "function" with their muscles to "actively" maintain the appliance in position, giving rise to the terms *functional appliance* and *activator*. The more contemporary version pictured has an increased vertical opening, posterior interocclusal acrylic to prevent eruption of maxillary posterior teeth and to promote eruption of mandibular posterior teeth, and large lingual flanges. **B,** Balter's bionator appliance, a "trimmed down" activator that has considerably less acrylic bulk, increasing patient comfort and facilitating daytime wear. However, this reduction in bulk decreases the appliance durability. **C,** Clark's twin block appliance, which modifies the activator by splitting it into a maxillary and mandibular portion. The height of the bite blocks determines the extent of vertical opening, and the inclination of the guide planes determines the extent of forward mandibular positioning. **D,** Fränkel's removable "functional regulator" appliance that is primarily tissue-borne, being largely supported in the vestibular areas by acrylic buccal shields and mandibular labial lip pads. (**B** From Graber TM, Vanarsdall RL: *Orthodontics: current principles and techniques,* ed 3, St Louis, 2000, Mosby. **C** From Graber TM, Vanarsdall RL: *Orthodontics: current principles and techniques,* ed 2, St Louis, 1994, Mosby.)

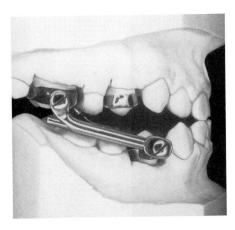

Figure 20-12 Herbst's fixed pin and tube appliance for maintaining the mandible in a forward position. This is the only fixed functional appliance being used in contemporary orthodontic treatment. (From McNamara JA, Brudon WL: *Orthodontic and orthopedic treatment in the mixed dentition,* Ann Arbor, Mich, 1994, Needham Press.)

the mandible forward, whereas mandibular labial acrylic lip pads and large acrylic buccal shields hold the lip and cheek pressure away from the teeth and provide soft tissue support for the appliance. These acrylic components are held together with a wire framework that includes a labial bow and transpalatal wire. Although the appliance is largely supported in the vestibular areas by means of the acrylic components, there still is some contact with the dentition, including wire rests occlusal to the maxillary molars to minimize their eruption, wires lingual to the mandibular incisors, and the labial bow. This appliance has a greater influence on arch expansion than the more traditional functional appliances without active expansion screws.

The fixed tooth-borne appliance is the third type of functional appliance, which also is represented by only one appliance. In 1905 Emil Herbst introduced a fixed appliance in Germany that maintained the mandible in a forward position while permitting the teeth to occlude. The appliance was not widely used and was largely forgotten after the mid 1930s.[129] After 2 years of clinical research, Hans Pancherz[130] reintroduced the appliance in Germany in 1979. It has gained increased popularity worldwide since that time. The **Herbst appliance** consists of a rigid maxillary and mandibular framework that is usually made of acrylic and bonded as a splint to each arch or soldered to thick bands or stainless steel crowns and cemented in place (Figure 20-12). The mandible is maintained in a forward position by means of a metal rod and tube telescopic mechanism that is attached bilaterally from the maxillary first molars to the mandibular first premolars. An American orthodontist, James Jasper,[131] has replaced the rigid telescopic mechanism with a flexible plastic covered open coil spring that can be attached directly to auxiliary wires with a complete or partial fixed appliance in place.

Selection of Functional Appliance Features and Timing of Treatment

Although functional appliances can be divided into the preceding three types for ease of description, it is important to appreciate the extent of diversity represented by the appliances used in clinical practice worldwide. Inexperienced clinicians can find the selection of the appropriate functional appliance to be a daunting task. An accurate, comprehensive diagnosis of the orthodontic problems and an adequate knowledge of the function of the available appliance features aid in the selection of the appropriate appliance. When a functional appliance is indicated in the treatment of a skeletal Class II problem, the best strategy for choosing the appropriate appliance is to select the features that address the specific problems presented by the patient. This means ignoring the part of the preprinted laboratory prescriptions that requests a choice of a named appliance and designing a custom appliance by requesting specific features or components.[132] William Proffit,[63] a renowned American orthodontic educator, characterizes this as the *component approach* to treatment with functional appliances.

As a general guideline, more simplified and bulky functional appliances like the activator are durable and less prone to deformation or breakage. The more complex appliances with more active components may be more versatile but usually at the expense of durability. The functional regulator has few active components yet is fragile because of the minimal bulk of acrylic and the abundant use of wires to hold parts of the appliance together. Its decreased durability is offset by the fact that it seems to work better as a daytime appliance because of the improved ability to speak with it in place. It also provides the possibility of generalized transverse expansion from the buccal shields, although active transverse screws can be incorporated in activators or bionators to achieve a similar effect.[133-135] The twin block appliance provides for greater range of mandibular movement and is easily modified for increasing the vertical or anterior positioning of the mandible. However, the direct pressure against the mandibular incisors to maintain the mandible in its forward position results in increased protraction of these teeth. The Herbst appliance has the advantage of full-time wear, but it is less durable and mandibular incisor protraction usually is more common than with the other appliances.[136]

If the lower face is vertically deficient with a longer ramus and flat mandibular plane, posterior eruption can be encouraged, particularly in the mandible, to more effectively correct the Class II occlusion. If the lower face is vertically excessive with a short ramus and a steep mandibular plane, posterior bite blocks or headgear tubes for intrusive extraoral force to the maxilla can be included to minimize posterior dental eruption, thereby encouraging more anterior and less vertical mandibular growth direction.

The same principles of facial growth modification regarding the appropriate timing of treatment with headgears apply to functional appliances as well. As mentioned previously, the greatest treatment effectiveness can be obtained during the most active period of facial growth. The original growth pattern continues its expression following orthopedic treatment until adolescent growth ends. For this reason and to take advantage of improved compliance, it usually is prudent to begin treatment with functional appliances during the mixed dentition. In as much as wear compliance remains an important factor with functional appliances and headgear, it is fortuitous that the greatest magnitude of daily growth and dental eruption occurs in the late evening and night.[74-77]

The same factors relevant to the decision to discontinue treatment with a headgear apply to the functional appliance. Both the type of skeletal problem and the potential for remaining growth are important considerations. It is typical for the fundamental growth pattern to continue to express itself after headgear use when appreciable growth remains. In the case of mandibular deficiency or maxillary excess, it is prudent to continue orthopedic treatment until complete cessation of maxillary growth. As is the case for headgear, it is recommended to achieve some overcorrection and to discontinue appliance wear in an incremental fashion while monitoring the occlusion. It sometimes is necessary, particularly when maxillary excess is the underlying problem, to continue appliance wear at night until completion of adolescent growth.

Clinical Procedures for Use of Functional Appliances

Preparation of Dentition for Functional Appliances
Facial growth modification can only take place if the orthopedic treatment occurs early enough in adolescence to take advantage of active mandibular growth. This stage of physical development usually occurs during the mixed dentition, particularly in females who are more physically precocious. The functional appliance as well as the headgear can be used during the mixed dentition. However, the position and relationship of the incisors must be acceptable to place most functional appliances.

Functional appliances and overjet If a functional appliance is being planned, it is necessary to have sufficient overjet to permit adequate forward positioning of the mandible. Although most individuals with a Class II occlusion have ample overjet for this purpose, it is not possible if the maxillary incisors are inclined lingually, as is the case with the Class II Division 2 malocclusion, or if the mandibular incisors are inclined labially. Adequate overjet can also be precluded from irregular or crowded incisors with either lingual displacement of

one or more maxillary incisors or labial displacement of one or more mandibular incisors. If any of these circumstances is present, it is necessary to complete a preliminary phase of orthodontic treatment to create the necessary overjet. This may require protraction and alignment of maxillary incisors or retraction of mandibular incisors. Because the mandibular incisors are often in a protrusive position as a result of natural dental compensation for the skeletal discrepancy and some additional protrusion can be expected from functional appliance wear, it may be necessary to retract the mandibular incisors before starting treatment with a functional appliance. It should be kept in mind that adequate space must be present in the mandibular arch to permit retraction of the mandibular incisors. Otherwise there will be a risk of impaction or displacement of the unerupted canines or premolars. Following this preliminary orthodontic treatment, the teeth should be retained for 2 to 3 months to minimize relapse and prevent excessive incisor movement during the functional appliance phase of treatment.

If adequate overjet is present to permit the desired forward position of the mandible, accurate impressions and a **"working" or "construction" bite registration** are required. The maxillary and mandibular impressions must be accurate in regard to the teeth and all the areas where the parts of the appliance will contact the soft tissue. If a deep mandibular lingual flange is desired, special effort must be made to extend impression material in this area. If lip pads or buccal shields are planned, in the case of the functional regulator, the clinician must be careful to avoid excessive extension of impression material in these areas that will overly displace the soft tissue. Once acceptable impressions are obtained, they should be poured in stone as soon as possible to provide the most accurate and stable representative casts. If use of a nonbonded Herbst appliance is being planned, bands or steel crowns must be transferred to the impressions before pouring the casts. Box 20-1 lists a number of factors that must be considered before procuring the construction bite registration.

A number of techniques are available for obtaining the construction bite registration. It is possible to simply practice with the patient to consistently be guided to the desired anterior and vertical position in the softened wax. It is often helpful to provide an interincisal guide of the desired thickness, such as a dowel or tongue blade(s) with carved notches representing the desired position for the maxillary and mandibular incisal edges (Figure 20-13). It is important that the final construction bite not only represent the planned anterior and vertical position of the mandible, but also the transverse position. If stone models have been fabricated before the appointment for procuring the construction bite, it is convenient to mount the models in a plasterless, or Galetti, articulator to affirm that the

BOX 20-1

Factors to Consider before Construction Bite Registration

1. It is critical that the interocclusal wax be easily warmed to a softness that permits indentations of all the posterior teeth on either side of the bite registration, yet be easily chilled to adequate hardness at room temperature to be stable until the appliance can be fabricated.

2. The wax should not extend anteriorly to cover the incisors, preventing reliable observation of the mandibular position by means of the interincisal relationship. It also should not extend posteriorly into the retromolar area that may exaggerate the vertical opening in this area.

3. The extent of downward and forward mandibular positioning must be predetermined on the basis of patient tolerance and appliance design. Usually 4 to 6 mm of forward positioning is sufficient to avoid frequent remaking of the appliance for additional advancement and yet is tolerated well by the patient.

4. The amount of downward positioning is dependent on the interocclusal space required for wire and acrylic components of the appliance and, in some cases, the treatment objectives. If only adequate space for wires connecting lingual and labial portions of the appliance is necessary, 3 to 4 mm of posterior opening are sufficient. If interocclusal stops or facets are needed to guide posterior eruption, usually 4 to 5 mm of opening are required. On the other hand, an additional 1 to 2 mm may be necessary to extend the patient beyond their resting vertical dimension if posterior eruption is to be restricted.

5. In most cases the mandible should be advanced symmetrically so that the original relationship between the maxillary and mandibular midlines is maintained in the construction bite. The only exception is when a mandibular skeletal asymmetry is present where the more deficient side is advanced further forward.

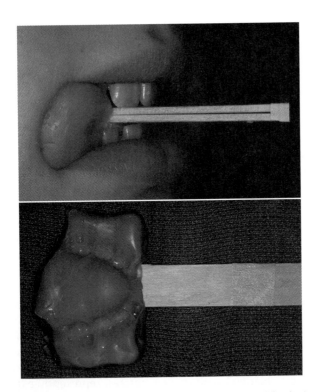

Figure 20-13 It is helpful to have an interincisal guide while obtaining the functional appliance construction wax bite, such as tongue blades with notches on the surface, to easily establish the predetermined mandibular position downward and forward. The construction wax bite should clear the incisors and retromolar areas. Incisor clearance permits visualization of the incisors when the patient closes into the wax to avoid errors in achieving the predetermined mandibular position. Clearance from the retromolar area helps avoid excessive vertical opening in this area.

wax bite accurately represents the desired mandibular position.

Fabrication and Delivery of Functional Appliances
Once accurate stone models are created from the impressions and an acceptable construction bite is obtained, a laboratory prescription needs to be completed with specific instructions for the planned design of the functional appliance. If there is any doubt about the accuracy of the construction bite, it can be easily checked by mounting the models in a plasterless articulator. Although it usually is acceptable to send the models unmounted to the laboratory, it is important to exercise care in wrapping the construction bite to avoid its distortion during transport, preventing improper fit of the finished appliance. Mounting of the casts in a simple nonadjustable articulator with the fresh construction bite and sending the articulated models to the laboratory as a unit provides some assurance that this will not occur.

Upon receipt of the finished appliance from the laboratory, the casts should be seated in the appliance to check the fit. This should occur well in advance of the first scheduled patient appointment so that any errors in fabrication can be rectified. At the delivery appointment, care must be taken to ensure that the appliance fits well without soft tissue impingement. Once the fit is confirmed, the patient needs to be guided in the insertion and removal of the appliance until the child and the parent are confident with the process. If the appliance is removable, instruction should be given regarding proper storage when it is not being worn. Optimal wear of removable functional appliances is similar to that recommended for headgear (usually 12 to 16 hours per day, during evenings and sleep) for comparable reasons. Although continuous wear may have a greater skeletal effect, it is likely to do so at the expense of increased unwanted dental movement in the direction of the skeletal correction, including maxillary incisor retraction and mandibular incisor protraction.[136,137] There is a minority of functional appliances that are intended to be worn full-time, including the functional regulator and the fixed Herbst appliance.

Management of Treatment with Functional Appliances Initial wear of a functional appliance requires a period of adaptation by the child in much the same manner as the headgear. The patient should be warned of some mild generalized soreness during the first few weeks but needs to distinguish this generalized soreness from localized soft tissue sore spots caused by appliance impingement or overextension. Localized tissue sore spots need to be addressed immediately. The initial general discomfort can be minimized by gradually increasing the duration of wear from 1 to 8 hr/day over the first week so that it can be worn all night by the start of the second week. If there is difficulty wearing the appliance all night, extra daytime wear is required until complete nighttime wear is routine. During the second week, the patient can add the final 3 to 5 daytime hours to the full nighttime wear.

The next scheduled office visit should be no later than 2 weeks after delivery of the functional appliance. It is important for the patient or parent to contact the clinician immediately if there are any reasons that prevent the recommended wear. It is prudent to have more frequent office visits during this adaptation period to monitor and reinforce compliance. The most obvious indicator of good wear compliance is the ease with which the patient inserts and removes the appliance. Other indicators that will be more obvious after a few months of wear are habitual anterior posturing of the mandible without the appliance in place, referred to by some as the *pterygoid effect*, and formation of calculus on the appliance. Anteroposterior improvement in occlusion and decrease of overjet are the most desirable indicators. Once the clinician is convinced that the patient is consistently wearing the functional appliance, appointments can be spaced 6 to 8 weeks apart.

It is important for the patient to bring the appliance to each appointment for inspection and possible adjustment. Common adjustments include removing interocclusal acrylic to permit selective eruption of teeth and adjustment of the labial bow or other wire elements to prevent unwanted dental movement or encourage desired dental movement. In the case of the functional

regulator, there needs to be periodic adjustment of the buccal shields laterally to continue arch expansion. If there are active expansion screws in the appliance, these are normally activated by the patient at 2-week intervals. However, overactivation prevents proper seating of the appliance and must be avoided. Many functional appliances are not designed with an expansion component. In these circumstances there is the assumption that transverse correction of the maxillary arch will either precede or follow appliance use, if needed.

Reactivation of the appliance After 6 to 9 months of compliant wear, enough positive change in the occlusion may take place to warrant additional advancement of the mandible. This requires a new construction wax bite and adjustment or replacement of the appliance, depending on the type being used. An activator can be sectioned to separate the upper and lower portions and rejoined with acrylic to hold the mandible in the new position. The functional regulator also can have the lower lip pads and lingual flange advanced and rejoined with acrylic. It is difficult to accomplish these modifications without compromising the fit of the appliance, thus it usually is prudent to remake the appliance when additional mandibular advancement is required. Although attempts have been made to create an activator split between its upper and lower parts with a prefabricated anteroposterior expansion screw to advance the lower portion, the stability and durability of the appliance are compromised significantly. The twin block appliance was designed as a means of avoiding this dilemma by creating separate upper and lower halves that could be modified easily to periodically advance the mandible. It is an even easier task with the Herbst appliance, in which additional washers can be threaded on to the rod to supplement the length of the tube and maintain the mandible in a more advanced position.

If 6 to 9 months have passed with minimal favorable response, one or more of three possibilities exist: (1) poor compliance, (2) unfavorable skeletal growth, or (3) inappropriate design of appliance. New records will be needed in this situation to evaluate the changes and to make the treatment plan more productive.

Effects of Treatment with Functional Appliances The theoretic primary effect of functional appliances for skeletal Class II relationships is to stimulate mandibular growth to the extent that its final anteroposterior length is greater than it would have been if no treatment had occurred. The intention is to accelerate the growth of the deficient mandible to the extent that it will reach a normal size relative to the normal growing maxilla. It is clear that substantial **mandibular growth potential** is expected and that this growth can be directed in a forward direction during treatment. Although acceleration of mandibular growth has been demonstrated in animal studies,[138,139] the long-term benefit in terms of achieving a greater absolute growth has not been confirmed by clinical studies.[78]

Although functional appliances have been used throughout the century in Europe and in the last 40 years in the United States, it was not until the late 1960s that scientific data were available to evaluate the empiric rationalization for their clinical effectiveness. This early data consisted of animal experiments demonstrating histologic and radiographic evidence of increased growth of the condylar cartilage when the mandible was held in a forward position. Breitner's early monkey studies[140,141] and Alexandre Petrovic and coworkers' initial findings[142,143] using rats as models were complemented by later primate[139,144-156] and rat[72,138,157-159] studies conducted by a number of independent investigators. Petrovic suggested that the unique characteristics of the condylar cartilage, including the cell division of the prechondroblasts (as opposed to the chondroblasts in epiphyseal cartilage of the long bones or cartilage in the synchondroses of the cranial base) make this cartilage more responsive to orthopedic devices. The animal studies of the 1960s and 1970s created enormous enthusiasm in the professional community and played an important role in the rapid acceptance and use of functional appliances in the United States that had been largely ignored up until that time.

The controversy There were two important considerations that were left unanswered. First, would the increases in overall mandibular length achieved with orthopedic devices placed in growing rats and monkeys also occur in growing children? Second, was the quantitative increase in condylar growth demonstrated at a cellular level enough of an increase to make a relevant clinical difference in a human? In response to these issues, various investigators in the 1970s and 1980s conducted retrospective clinical studies. This was occurring at the same time that many clinicians were embracing functional appliances as the answer for mandibular deficient patients. A number of these retrospective studies demonstrated some average modest increases in mandibular growth (2 to 4 mm/yr) during treatment with functional appliances.[130,136,138,160-170] Other investigators, however, did not consider the effect of functional appliances on quantitative lengthening of the mandible to be clinically significant.[86,162,171-189] In addition, it became clear that there was much greater variability in the mandibular growth response of humans to functional appliances than in the animal models.[102] Also, the variability of growth potential and response to orthopedic treatment was much greater for the mandible than for the maxilla.[113]

The enthusiasm for functional appliances in the United States during the 1980s considerably moderated in the 1990s in light of the less impressive results of the retrospective clinical studies complemented by clinical experiences. Although a modest mean increase in mandibular growth may occur for a group of patients being treated with functional appliances, the increase is not predictable because of the great variability in patient response.[102] In addition, there still is uncertainty whether discernible mandibular growth acceleration is merely temporal and does not result in an absolute final gain in mandibular length.[78] In other words, it is possible that the ultimate length of the mandible may not be altered appreciably in spite of accelerated growth during treatment. There still has not been a clear demonstration that the observed treatment effects represent true growth stimulation beyond the limits of human growth variation. In spite of the continued controversy around the reliability of gains in mandibular length from functional appliance treatment, there are other effects that contribute to the correction of Class II malocclusions.

Skeletal effects of functional appliances Although Class II functional appliances are designed to stimulate mandibular growth, there is evidence of other skeletal effects from their use. There is a superior and posterior force delivered by these appliances to the maxilla. This headgearlike effect is caused by the stretched facial muscles and soft tissues attempting to return the postured mandible back to its more posterior and superior position. Because the maxillary part of the appliance contacts the maxillary arch, the forces from the muscles and soft tissues are transmitted through the appliance to the maxillary teeth and maxilla. There is some evidence that this effect restricts maxillary growth in a manner not unlike the effect of headgear.[86,174,175,180,190-194] Well-planned retrospective clinical studies comparing the skeletal response between headgear and functional appliance treatment have found few differences in treatment outcome between the two methods.[98,99,165] There is some speculation that downward and forward remodeling of the glenoid fossa might account for some of the skeletal correction with functional appliances.[195]

Dental effects of functional appliances There are clear differences in the effects that headgear and functional appliance treatment have, respectively, on the dentition. Although headgear has negligible effects on teeth other than the maxillary posterior teeth, functional appliances typically cause some retrusion of maxillary incisors.[86,172,175,177] This is caused by a lingual force transmitted from the labial bow or torquing springs against these teeth when the mandible attempts to reposition back to its normal position. This same natural repositioning attempt by the mandible causes protrusion of mandibular incisors caused by a labial force transmitted from the portion of the appliance lingual to these teeth.[161,171,175,180] The clinician partially controls the extent to which these movements occur.

Labial bows can be positioned labially away from the maxillary incisors and remain in contact more with the soft tissue to minimize the lingual tipping of these teeth. The labial tipping of mandibular incisors can be minimized by depending more on lingual acrylic flanges that are not in contact with the dentition to position the mandible forward. In the case of the activator or bionator, the addition of acrylic coverage overlapping the facial surfaces of the incisal edges of the mandibular incisors can also help.[183]

Functional appliances, unlike headgears, also have a direct effect on mandibular posterior and anterior dentition. It is common with contemporary activators and other functional appliances to promote the eruption of mandibular posterior teeth while inhibiting the eruption of maxillary posterior teeth often referred to as **differential eruption.** This encourages differential posterior eruption that tends to correct the Class II occlusion while rotating the occlusal plane up in the posterior and down in the anterior.[172,177] It also is a common feature to have anterior interocclusal acrylic to inhibit eruption of maxillary and mandibular anterior teeth to decrease excessive anterior overbite. The promotion of posterior dental eruption to gain Class II correction or decrease anterior overbite is not prudent where there is greater potential for vertical or downward, as opposed to forward, mandibular growth potential. This would be the case with an increased lower face height accompanied by a shorter ramus and steeper mandibular plane. Permitting posterior differential eruption in such a situation would be self-defeating because posterior eruption would tend to steepen the mandible further with the growth being expressed vertically instead of anteriorly. Functional appliances have an additional effect on the mandibular dentition that is not influenced by headgear. There is invariably some protraction of mandibular incisors in response to the force of the mandible contacting the appliance lingual to these teeth as it attempts to reposition itself back to its natural, posterior, and superior positions.

Combined Growth Modification Treatment

Headgears or functional appliances can be used effectively to treat skeletal Class II problems. Although headgears are intended for restriction of maxillary growth and functional appliances for stimulation of mandibular growth, the skeletal changes from the two treatment methods are surprisingly similar. Although headgears restrict maxillary growth, they work best when the mandible grows well. In the same manner, functional appliances may stimulate some mandibular growth acceleration, but the headgearlike effect is probably necessary for successful treatment. It seems reasonable that a combined appliance approach to orthopedic treatment using extraoral force in combination with a functional appliance may provide greater cumulative skeletal growth effects than use of either appliance alone. The integration of the two methods was developed in the late 1960s in Europe.[176]

This combined approach utilizes an occipital attachment connected to a facebow inserted into headgear tubes that are incorporated into the interocclusal acrylic in the premolar area.[196,197] Because the tubes are more anterior than their usual location attached to the first molar bands, it is necessary to have a much shorter inner bow to fit appropriately with the lips and maxillary incisors (see Figure 20-10). It also is possible to use a J-hook headgear attached to wire hooks incorporated in the acrylic.[198] The high-pull headgear can benefit the treatment by improving the functional appliance retention and directly applying extraoral force through the center of resistance of the maxilla. The functional appliance can complement the headgear benefits by encouraging mandibular growth while controlling posterior and anterior dental eruption.[197,199]

It is not practical to use this combined approach with a removable functional appliance lacking adequate acrylic bulk like the functional regulator or most bionators. The lack of acrylic bulk prevents these appliances from providing adequate rigidity to withstand the extraoral force without deforming or damaging the appliance. It also is recommended to use torquing springs on the maxillary incisors as opposed to a labial bow to help minimize the retraction of these teeth. The combined approach often is reserved for more severe skeletal Class II problems, particularly if maxillary vertical excess is a prominent feature.

Interarch Traction

Indications for and Goals of Treatment with Interarch Traction   Interarch traction from the anterior part of the maxillary arch to the posterior part of the mandibular arch, commonly referred to as *Class II elastics,* is intended to deliver an anterior force to the mandibular teeth and a posterior force to the maxillary teeth. This results primarily in protraction of mandibular teeth and, to a lesser extent, retraction of maxillary teeth. Although these dental movements usually are desirable with Class II elastics, there are other simultaneous dental movements that clinicians usually attempt to limit as much as possible. Because of the vertical vector of force that accompanies the use of Class II elastics, some extrusion of mandibular posterior and maxillary anterior teeth is to be expected (Figure 20-14). This results in **rotation of the occlusal plane** up posteriorly and down anteriorly. In addition, because of a slight force in the transverse dimension, there is some tendency for mandibular molars to tip buccally.

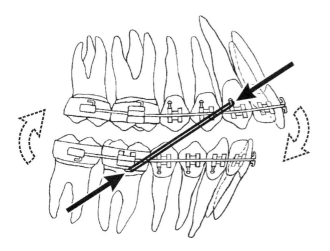

Figure 20-14 The vertical effect of Class II elastics causes extrusion of mandibular posterior teeth and maxillary anterior teeth. This results in rotation of the occlusal plane up in the posterior and down in the anterior.

The most appropriate indication for the use of Class II elastics is where anterior movement of the mandibular teeth is desired and rotation of the occlusal plane with extrusion of mandibular molars and maxillary incisors is not detrimental to the treatment outcome. The most ideal circumstance for treatment with Class II elastics is a dental Class II malocclusion in the presence of a normal skeletal jaw relationship. Although most skeletal Class II problems are characterized by protrusive mandibular incisors caused by dental compensation, it is more favorable to initially have retrusive mandibular incisors when using Class II elastics. Other optimum indications include protrusive and slightly intrusive maxillary incisors and slight constriction of the mandibular molars. A final favorable indication would include at least some minimal mandibular growth potential with flat occlusal and mandibular planes where an increase in lower face height is desired. If space were present in the dental arches, it would be preferable for the space to be mesial to the mandibular molars and distal to the maxillary molars.

Types of Class II Interarch Traction *Class II elastics* is the term used to describe intraoral traction between points of attachment buccal to the mandibular posterior and labial to maxillary anterior teeth. More specifically, it refers to any interarch elastic that has its mandibular point of attachment more distal than its maxillary attachment. The more distance there is between the attachments, the more horizontal and less vertical the force vector. There are only two types of traction—one fabricated from latex or synthetic rubber and the other fabricated from a metal alloy.

The first and most common type of traction is elastics fabricated from latex rubber. Natural latex rubber bands have been used in orthodontics since the mid-

nineteenth century when the vulcanization process made the material much more stable. Orthodontists have taken advantage of the increased elastic range of latex rubber with its ability to be stretched over a great distance without breaking or dramatically changing force. Further twentieth century improvements in the quality of latex elastics have reduced dramatically the intraoral deterioration of the material. Even with the introduction of synthetic rubbers after World War II, latex rubber elastics continue to be the favored material for Class II elastics. Nevertheless, recent concerns regarding allergic sensitivity to latex has resulted in the proliferation of synthetic rubber elastic alternatives. It is likely that this health concern will reduce the use of latex rubber in the future.

The second type of interarch traction is one fabricated from stainless steel in the form of a large spring. In contrast to the rubber elastics that are placed and removed by the patient, these springs are designed to be ligated directly to the orthodontic appliance and only removed by the clinician. This form of interarch traction has not been widely accepted because of problems with breakage caused by fatigue, oral hygiene, and comfort for the patient. Usually this type has been used only as a last resort after continued poor compliance with latex elastics.

Clinical Procedures for Use of Class II Interarch Traction

Preparation of Dentition for Class II Interarch Traction The use of Class II elastics should be limited to the permanent dentition with a complete fixed orthodontic appliance and continuous arch wires in place. Headgears and functional appliances usually are indicated for use during the mixed dentition. This is primarily to take full advantage of the growth acceleration that often begins before the complete eruption of the permanent teeth. Because the effects of Class II elastics are limited to dental movement with no appreciable influence on the skeletal relationship, their use before eruption of the premolars and canines would be contraindicated in most cases. There is a second important reason for not using interarch traction with only partial eruption of the permanent teeth. The vertical forces associated with Class II elastics tend to extrude the maxillary incisors and the mandibular molars. If the fixed appliance is only in place on the first molars and incisors, there is a much greater extrusive effect because of the absence of adjacent teeth that can serve to reinforce anchorage or resistance to the unwanted extrusive tooth movement.

Preparation of the teeth for the use of Class II elastics involves alignment and leveling of the dental arches. It requires the placement of initial flexible arch wires that provide light and continuous forces fol-

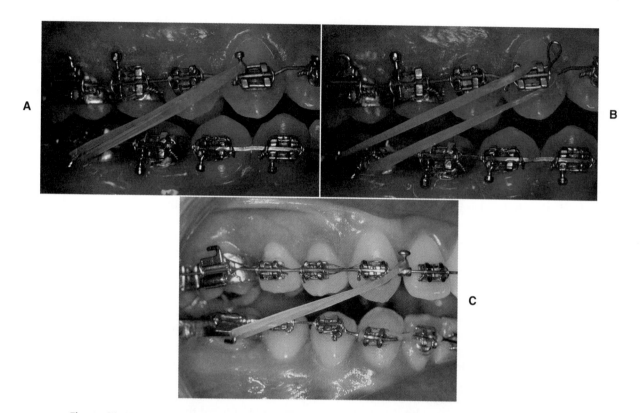

Figure 20-15 Alternative hooks to use as attachments for Class II elastics. **A,** A hook that is integral to the bracket. **B,** Kobayashi hook, a 0.012-gauge ligature wire welded to form a loop and ligated to the bracket. **C,** A hook that is fabricated to be crimped directly onto the arch wire.

lowed by progressively stiffer wires in a sequential manner until continuous rectangular steel wires can be placed without generating excessive forces. Both alignment and leveling are necessary for the teeth to slide along the arch wire. The mandibular teeth need to slide forward and the maxillary teeth need to slide back in response to the horizontal force from the Class II elastics. If alignment or leveling is inadequate, the bracket will more readily bind with the arch wire and prevent horizontal movement of the teeth along the wire. Therefore, before the placement of the interarch elastics, rectangular steel arch wires are recommended to provide adequate stiffness and reduced friction.[63] If the plan is to have the dental movement limited to one arch more than the other, a large rectangular steel arch wire that fully engages the bracket slot should be placed on the arch where minimal dental change is desired. In most Class II malocclusions, the least change usually is indicated in the mandibular arch.

Fabrication Force and Delivery of Class II Interarch Traction Interarch elastics are manufactured in a large selection of sizes, varying in the cross section of the elastic filament as well as in length. Varying these two characteristics determines the magnitude of the force being delivered for a given amount of extension or stretch of the elastic. The manufacturers classify the elastics by stipulating two measurements: the diameter (inches or millimeters) of the circle created by a passive elastic and the force (ounces or grams) created by the stretching of the elastic a specific length (the average distance between the mandibular first molar and the maxillary canine). In this manner, both the cross section and the length of the elastic filament can be varied to provide the clinician with the appropriate force when the elastic is stretched a certain distance.

The magnitude of force required depends on the clinical situation. If single teeth are to be moved (maxillary canine distally or mandibular molar mesially), selection of an elastic that delivers about 100 g (3 to 4 oz) per side is appropriate. If groups of teeth or entire arches are expected to move, approximately 300 g per side is indicated. These force levels can be measured with a force gauge to ensure accuracy.

Class II elastics usually are placed with the maxillary canines as the maxillary points of attachment and the mandibular first molars as the mandibular points of attachment. Interarch elastics can be placed on hooks that are integral or ligated to the brackets, or they can be welded, soldered, or crimped directly to the arch wire (Figure 20-15). If it is desired to have individual or groups of teeth moved along the arch wire, it is necessary to have the point of attachment directly on the brackets of these teeth. If the entire dental arch is to be moved, the point of attachment to the arch wire is an option. The horizontal component of force can be accentuated and the vertical component deemphasized by making the mandibular second molars as the mandibular point of attachment and the maxillary incisors as the maxillary point of attachment. If these attachment points are placed closer to each other, the horizontal force becomes more limited and the vertical force becomes more substantial.

Once the clinician has selected the proper size of elastic and provided accessible hooks for attachment, it is important to demonstrate placement and removal of the elastics with the patient and parent. It usually is easiest to attach the elastic first to the least accessible point of attachment, which is the mandibular attachment. The hooks need to be extending laterally to the extent that they are readily accessible, yet not positioned so far as to irritate the buccal mucosa. The patient is then encouraged to place and remove the elastics until he or she is confident with the process. The optimum wear is 24 hr/day because continuous forces move teeth more efficiently. The only time they should be removed is while eating, cleaning the teeth, or wearing a mouthguard. Elastics have been shown to deteriorate in the intraoral environment.[200] Therefore the patient should be supplied with an ample quantity of elastics so that they can be replaced at least 2 or 3 times per day.

Management of Treatment with Class II Interarch Traction A period of acclimation with progressive increase in the duration of wear is usually unnecessary with interarch elastics because of the light forces being applied. Nevertheless, the patient should expect some mild soreness during the first week of wear. The next scheduled appointment need not be for less than 3 to 4 weeks unless the patient has difficulties with elastic management, in which case the appointment should be as soon as possible. The first recall appointment provides the opportunity to monitor compliance and determine whether progress is taking place. If no appreciable change is evident after 4 to 6 weeks, the duration of wear or the magnitude of force that was selected is inadequate. Although extensive use of headgear or functional appliances for 6 or more months is often indicated for skeletal Class II problems, the use of Class II elastics for correction of dental Class II problems is usually limited to 3 to 6 months of wear. Use of these elastics for longer than this period of time usually results in excessive extrusion of maxillary incisors and mandibular molars. This can result in a poor cosmetic appearance with excessive vertical display of incisors, a gummy smile, and increased lower face height with a steeper mandibular plane.

Effects of Treatment with Class II Interarch Traction There was a period of time during the first half of the twentieth century, due in large part to the influence of Edward Angle, when it was assumed that Class II elastics had an orthopedic effect. With the advent of cephalometric analysis of treatment response in the 1940s, it became readily apparent that the improvement in Class II malocclusions with Class II elastics was the result of dental movement with negligible skeletal effects. There is some recent evidence demonstrating that Class II elastics placed for 14 hours daily in growing rats can have a stimulating effect on mandibular condylar cartilage growth at the microscopic level.[113] The authors of this study believe that this stimulating effect can result in clinically relevant lengthening of the mandible if treatment is initiated during the beginning of the pubertal growth spurt.[201,202] This view is not supported, however, by numerous clinical studies that demonstrate that the effects of Class II elastics are limited to the dentition.[203]

The dental response to Class II elastics is characterized by substantial protraction or mesial movement of the mandibular teeth and, to a much lesser extent, retraction or distal movement of the maxillary teeth. Because the mandibular incisors may already have a protrusive position caused by dental compensation, further protraction of these teeth may be contraindicated. There also is a vertical component to the force vector produced from Class II elastics, causing some extrusion of mandibular molars and maxillary incisors that accompanies the anteroposterior changes. If substantial extrusion of these teeth is permitted to take place, the occlusal plane becomes steeper, rotating up in the posterior and down in the anterior. Although this will decrease the anterior overbite, a benefit in many Class II malocclusions, it will do so while rotating the mandible open if growth of the mandibular rami does not keep up with the amount of molar extrusion. If this occurs, the anterior face height and the steepness of the mandibular plane will increase, which is undesirable if the original face height is normal or long. As explained previously, the extrusion of maxillary incisors from Class II elastic wear can result in excessive vertical display of these teeth relative to the upper lip, creating a poor cosmetic appearance characterized by a gummy smile.

Class II elastics can also be used with sliding jigs to apply a distal force to the maxillary molars. However, extrusion of mandibular molars from the reactive force limits this method to patients who can tolerate increased lower face height and have some vertical growth of the mandibular ramus remaining.

Dental Camouflage of Class II Skeletal Problems

The goal of dental camouflage is to disguise the unacceptable skeletal relationship by orthodontically repositioning the teeth in the jaws so there is an acceptable dental occlusion and esthetic facial appearance. The primary dental movement needed is retraction of maxillary teeth and protraction of mandibular teeth to eliminate overjet and correct buccal occlusion. Individuals who already have extensive natural dental compensation present before treatment with the mandibular incisors in a protrusive position are poor candidates for dental camouflage because dental camouflage is aimed at creating or accentuating dental compensation for the skeletal discrepancy (Figure 20-16).

Appropriate patients for dental camouflage treatment should be limited to older adolescents or adults who no longer have adequate facial growth potential to make it worthwhile to attempt or continue growth modification. This type of treatment also should be considered only when the skeletal Class II problems are mild to moderate in severity. In these individuals, dental camouflage may be the only reasonable treatment alternative to combined surgical orthodontic approach. More severe skeletal problems cannot be treated effec-

tively with Class II mechanics because the achievement of an acceptable occlusion may require so much retraction of maxillary incisors that it results in an unesthetic facial appearance. This appearance includes a more retrusive upper lip, giving greater projection to the nose, an increased nasolabial angle, and a smile characterized by lingually inclined maxillary incisors. Candidates for dental camouflage treatment should also have no more than minimal dental crowding and, ideally, extra space in the dental arches. This is desirable so that there is adequate space to move teeth the necessary distance to correct the anteroposterior discrepancy. For this reason, dental camouflage almost always requires extraction of teeth (unless teeth are already missing) in one or both dental arches. A final criterion for selecting dental camouflage is that it results in normal vertical facial proportions. It is difficult to increase the vertical facial dimension and decrease the anterior overbite when extracting teeth in an individual with a short face and a deep bite that is

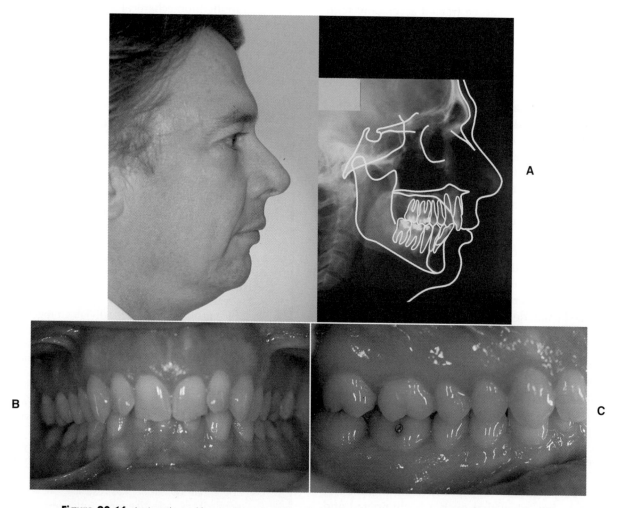

Figure 20-16 A, A patient with extensive natural Class II dental compensation typically characterized by retrusive maxillary incisors and protrusive mandibular incisors. **B** and **C,** This may result in minimal overjet in spite of Class II posterior dental occlusion.

often associated with mandibular deficiency and a flat mandibular plane. In an individual with a long face associated with maxillary excess and a steep mandibular plane with or without mandibular deficiency, it is difficult to achieve adequate anteroposterior occlusal correction without extruding mandibular molars and worsening the vertical problem.

Usually the most optimal treatment for a moderate to severe skeletal Class II malocclusion in a patient with minimal remaining facial growth potential is to directly address the source of the problem with orthognathic surgery. If there is a skeletal discrepancy or deformity, surgical repositioning of the bony structures at fault permits the most ideal functional occlusion and esthetic facial balance. Therefore orthodontic treatment combined with orthognathic surgery is particularly appropriate for severe skeletal problems in patients with minimal growth potential. Unfortunately, not all individuals with a skeletal Class II problem are willing or able to undergo the necessary surgery. Although there are limits to the extent that dental camouflage can be used, there are many mild to moderate skeletal Class II problems that can be treated acceptably with dental camouflage.

The types of dental camouflage for Class II skeletal problems can be divided conveniently according to whether or not the treatment requires extraction of teeth.

Dental Camouflage without Extractions
It is a rare case where a skeletal Class II relationship can be treated successfully using dental camouflage without extractions. It is necessary that the skeletal problem be mild enough with a Class II posterior occlusion of less than a half unit and a mild, excessive overjet. It also is necessary for adequate space to be present in the dental arches. Space is required in the maxillary arch to retract the incisors and eliminate overjet, and it is required in the mandibular arch to be able to protract the mandibular teeth into a normal posterior occlusion. The presence of such excess interdental space in both arches is uncommon and is evident in the case of generalized small dentition. The only other possibility is where the maxillary molars can be moved posteriorly enough to provide the necessary space to retract maxillary incisors and treat to a normal buccal occlusion. Distal bodily movement of maxillary molars is a formidable challenge with traditional orthodontic biomechanical methods. On the other hand, recent development of absolute intraoral anchorage attachments, to be described later, may make this option a more realistic one.

The goals of nonextraction treatment are to retract the maxillary dentition and protract the mandibular dentition to the extent that overjet is eliminated and normal posterior occlusion is achieved. As explained earlier, sufficient space must be present or orthodontically created in the arches to permit acceptable dental camouflage treatment with this approach. If inadequate space is present, unacceptable compromises are the inevitable results of treatment. Occlusal goals achieved at the expense of overly retracted and extruded maxillary incisors result in compromised facial esthetics. If the occlusal goals require excessive protraction of mandibular teeth, the stability of the final mandibular incisor positions is compromised.

Types of Appliances. Treatment by means of dental camouflage must be undertaken with a complete fixed orthodontic appliance in place. Orthodontic treatment of this nature normally requires significant bodily repositioning of teeth to achieve a stable treatment result. It is impossible to control root movement to the extent necessary to bodily move teeth with removable appliances.

If sufficient space is present in the dental arches, it is possible to design treatment to retract maxillary teeth and protract mandibular teeth to achieve a normal occlusion and overjet in spite of an underlying mild skeletal Class II problem being present. The appropriate orthodontic biomechanical approach is to provide for maximum **maxillary posterior anchorage** and maximum **mandibular anterior anchorage** (Boxes 20-2 and 20-3). This is necessary to minimize mesial movement

---

> ### BOX 20-2   Reinforcing Maxillary Posterior Anchorage
>
> 1. Posteriorly directed extraoral force, either with a facebow delivering force directly to the maxillary first molars or a J-hook headgear delivering force directly to the anterior teeth being retracted (see Figure 20-7)
> 2. Lingual arch fixed to the maxillary first molars, either with a **transpalatal arch** or **Nance holding arch** (Figure 20-17)
> 3. A removable palatal retainer
> 4. Multiple maxillary posterior teeth joined together as a combined resistance unit while retracting only one anterior tooth at a time
> 5. Segmented arch mechanics for retraction of anterior teeth to avoid friction from retracting teeth along the arch wire
> 6. Maxillary posterior teeth positioned with mesial root tip to encourage their bodily movement against the anterior retractive force
> 7. Distal crown tipping of the retracting maxillary anterior teeth followed by their uprighting to minimize strain on posterior anchorage
> 8. Use of the mandibular arch as resistance while providing maxillary retractive force with Class II elastics
> 9. **Osseointegrated attachment** in the palate that serves as absolute intraoral anchorage (Figure 20-18)

of maxillary molars while maxillary premolars, canines, and incisors are retracted and to minimize distal movement of mandibular incisors while mandibular molars, premolars, and canines are protracted.

When adequate generalized spacing in the arches is not present, it may be difficult but possible to move maxillary posterior teeth distally to create sufficient space to retract maxillary teeth. This requires bodily distal movement of maxillary molars—a difficult challenge with current orthodontic techniques. Traditionally, the only possible method was full-time use of extraoral force with a facebow attached to the first molars. Successful distal molar movement requires full-time headgear wear, and appreciable movement is possible only if the second molars are not present. If patient compliance is inadequate, the only other option is to place an orthodontic appliance that delivers an intraoral distal force to the maxillary molars. Unfortunately, intraoral forces always have a reciprocal reactive force affecting the other teeth that is usually counterproductive to the orthodontic treatment. If the intraoral distal force to the maxillary molars is generated by a spring, the reactive force is an equal mesial force to the maxillary anterior teeth, moving them in the opposite direction desired (Figure 20-19, A).

In the 1980s and 1990s a number of new appliances were introduced by individuals who contend that they have overcome these biomechanical problems and can effectively distalize the maxillary molars. These appliances have been designed to deliver a continuous reciprocal force of 100 to 300 g generated with reciprocal repelling magnets,[205] **nickel-titanium** open coil springs,[206] nickel-titanium arch wires deflected to form active loops,[207] or **titanium molybdenum** helical

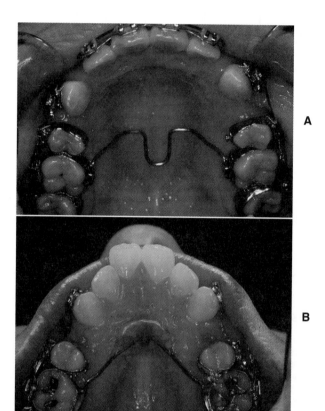

A

B

Figure 20-17 **A,** The transpalatal arch extends across the palatal vault but is clear of the soft tissue. **B,** The Nance holding arch extends more anteriorly on the palate, incorporating a palatal acrylic pad that directly conforms to the anterior palatal mucosa. The wires for these appliances are typically made of 0.036- to 0.040-inch stainless steel wire. These appliances, which serve to join the two maxillary posterior quadrants together, help stabilize these teeth, preventing their mesiolingual rotation and minimizing their anterior movement while retracting the anterior teeth.

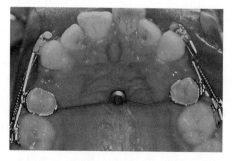

Figure 20-18 Absolute intraoral orthodontic anchorage with the use of an osseointegrated titanium implant to prevent reciprocal forces from acting upon teeth. When using an osseointegrated titanium implant or a miniscrew, the implant or the miniscrew must be placed anteriorly in the palate. The osseointegrated titanium onplant can be located more posteriorly because the increased thickness of palatal bone is not needed for the onplant. (From Wehrbein H, Feifel H, Diedrich P: *Am J Orthod Dentofacial Orthop* 116:678-686, 1999.)

BOX 20-3	**Reinforcing Mandibular Anterior Anchorage**

1. Anteriorly directed extraoral force with elastics extending from mandibular posterior teeth to attachment on facemask
2. Lingual arch fixed to mandibular canines
3. Multiple mandibular anterior teeth joined together as a combined resistance unit while protracting only one posterior tooth at a time
4. Segmented arch mechanics for protraction of posterior teeth to avoid friction from protracting teeth along arch wire
5. Incorporation of lingual root torque to mandibular incisors and distal root tip to mandibular canines to encourage their bodily movement against the posterior protractive force
6. Mesial crown tipping of the protracting posterior teeth followed by their uprighting to minimize strain on anterior anchorage
7. Use of maxillary arch as resistance while providing mandibular protractive force with Class II elastics
8. Osseointegrated attachments distal to mandibular molars that serve as absolute intraoral anchorage[204]

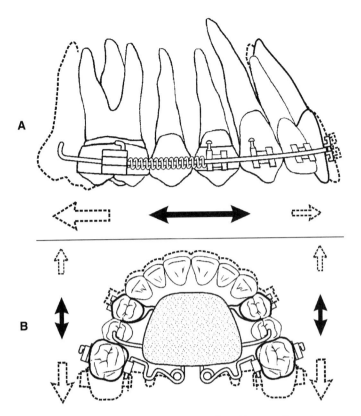

Figure 20-19 A, An open coil spring placed in an appliance to move molars distally creates a counteracting anterior force that moves the anterior teeth mesially. The addition of palatal acrylic, like a Nance holding arch, attached to the teeth anterior to the molars helps dissipate the reciprocal anterior force, minimizing the movement of the anterior teeth forward. **B,** The use of helical springs directly attached to the palatal acrylic pad is an alternative method to move molars distally. Again, the acrylic pad serves to decrease the extent of reciprocal anterior tooth movement (reaction) from the force created by the activated springs.

springs (see Figure 20-19, B).[208,209] In the absence of the erupted maxillary second molars, sufficient distal crown movement of the maxillary first molars is achieved in 3 to 7 months. Primarily tipping, not bodily, movement of the molars characterizes this movement. The springs also generate a reciprocal anterior force that can potentially protract the teeth anterior to the first molars, moving these teeth in the opposite direction of the planned retraction. The teeth anterior to the first molars and the anterior palate are used to resist this undesirable anterior force and minimize protraction of the anterior teeth and worsening the overjet. A modified Nance holding arch fixed to multiple teeth anterior to the maxillary first molars is typically used for this purpose (see Figure 20-19, B). In spite of these anterior anchorage measures, there is still some protraction of the maxillary anterior teeth that invariably accompanies the distal movement of the maxillary molar crowns.[207] When the protracted teeth are later retracted to close the space, some or all of the distal movement of the molars is sacrificed because of poste-

rior anchorage loss. This anchorage loss primarily results from the ease with which the distally tipped molars tip back forward into an upright position.[210]

To achieve distal bodily movement of the maxillary molars, the distal tipping of molars accomplished with these appliances must be followed by a posterior and superior force to move the molar roots distally as well. Two possibilities for delivering this force are full-time use of high-pull headgear[206] or use of a Herbst appliance.[208] The headgear option has the disadvantage of its dependence on patient compliance, whereas the Herbst option has the disadvantage of mandibular dental protraction as a side effect. Nevertheless, a few millimeters of distal bodily movement of molars may be achievable under optimal conditions. If this is not sufficient to correct the Class II occlusion, the remaining correction of the buccal occlusion and overjet requires some mandibular dental protraction. If no space is present in the mandibular arch and the mandibular incisors should not be moved to a more protrusive, potentially unstable position, no further anteroposterior occlusal correction is possible. On the other hand, if there is mandibular space or retrusive incisors, additional correction can be achieved with mandibular protraction.

It continues to be a challenge to find an effective means of achieving bodily distal movement of maxillary molars in spite of the recent appliance innovations. The primary reason for this is the inability to contrive an absolute method of anchorage to either distalize the first molars or to prevent mesial movement of teeth anterior to the first molars. All of the traditional orthodontic intraoral anchorage techniques are tooth-borne, so some anchorage loss is inevitable. However, there is some promise that osseointegrated attachments may provide the absolute intraoral anchorage that has been unavailable to date. Titanium implants,[211,212] **miniscrews,**[213] and **onplants**[214] are being developed as temporary osseointegrated attachments to be placed, which can serve as absolute anchorage to prevent reactive anterior orthodontic forces (see Figure 20-18).

Clinical Procedures If adequate space is present already in both dental arches to permit anteroposterior correction of the occlusion, a comprehensive fixed orthodontic appliance can be placed at the outset of treatment. Alignment and leveling must be completed with gradual increases in arch wire size until rectangular steel wires of at least 0.017-inch × 0.025-inch dimension in a 0.022-inch × 0.028-inch slot are in place for space closure. If space has to be created with distal movement of maxillary molars, a partial fixed orthodontic appliance may be placed, bypassing the canines and premolars and limited to the maxillary arch. This appliance is adequate if extraoral force is the principal means of creating space by moving the maxillary molars distally. If this space is created with an intra-oral force, a partial fixed appliance must be reinforced to partially dissipate the reactive anterior force against the incisors (see Figure 20-19, *B*). Once the space has been gained, the remainder of the fixed appliance is placed and alignment and leveling are completed before space closure.

Successful space closure is achieved if the maxillary teeth can be retracted and the mandibular teeth can be protracted sufficiently to correct the buccal occlusion and reduce overjet. As previously explained, the clinician must take great care in maximizing maxillary posterior anchorage and mandibular anterior anchorage to achieve this result. If Class II elastics are being used and space is already closed in the mandibular arch, a full dimension rectangular steel arch wire should be placed in this arch to minimize excessive protraction of the mandibular incisors.

In summary, few cases can be successfully treated with dental camouflage without extraction. The severity of the Class II malocclusion must be mild in a patient with no mandibular growth potential. In addition, adequate spacing must be available in the dental arches to permit correction to a normal molar relationship. Typically, the severity of the occlusal problem and the lack of spacing force the clinician to resort to dental extractions to permit successful treatment with dental camouflage.

Dental Camouflage with Extractions

It is usually necessary to extract maxillary first premolars when treating a Class II malocclusion with dental camouflage to gain sufficient space to retract maxillary canines and incisors. Adequate space is available only if there is no excessive protrusion of maxillary incisors. Furthermore, if there is no appreciable crowding or protrusion of the mandibular incisors, no mandibular extractions are necessary. The treatment goal in this instance is to maintain the molars in a Class II relationship but achieve complete reduction of the overjet. A more challenging approach is to extract maxillary second molars and retract all of the remaining maxillary teeth to achieve a normal molar relationship and overjet. The limits of moving maxillary molars distally have been previously discussed. An additional limitation of this approach is the unpredictability of the formation and eruption of the maxillary third molars. Successful treatment should include orthodontic movement of the maxillary third molars to serve as replacements for the extracted maxillary second molars. Unfortunately, the chance that the third molars may not form or properly erupt presents a substantial risk that this treatment will be compromised. Even if the challenging retraction of all of the maxillary teeth is successful, this additional risk of not having well-formed third molars to substitute for the extracted second molars may compromise the treatment outcome.

Another approach to dental camouflage with extraction is to extract mandibular first or second premolars as well as maxillary premolars. The treatment goal in this instance is to use the extraction space to move the mandibular posterior teeth forward into a normal molar relationship. If there is preexisting crowding or protrusion of the mandibular incisors, mandibular extractions are essential.

Types of Appliances Once the space is available from extractions, a springlike force (elastic, closing loop, closed coil spring) is applied across the space to close it. The response of the teeth to this intraarch force is for the posterior teeth to move mesially and the anterior teeth to move distally. The biomechanical challenge for the orthodontist is to close the space with retraction or distal movement of maxillary incisors and minimal protraction or mesial movement of maxillary posterior teeth. A number of technical approaches are available to accomplish this treatment (see Box 20-2).

If the patient is willing to wear it, a headgear can be of enormous benefit to minimize mesial movement of maxillary molars while retracting the maxillary anterior teeth. The extraoral force can be applied either directly to the maxillary molars with the facebow or directly to the anterior teeth with the J-hook headgear. With the facebow, the intention is to use the extraoral force posteriorly against the maxillary molars to counteract the intraarch elastic or spring force that is serving to close the space. In this way, the molars are anchored more effectively so that most of the space closure will be from retraction of the anterior teeth, decreasing overjet without compromising the posterior occlusion. A disadvantage of this technique is that the patient must wear the headgear as much as possible to provide adequate anchorage and achieve an optimal outcome. Another disadvantage is that the intraarch force is continuous and the extraoral force is intermittent. Thus it is realistic to assume that some mesial molar movement will occur unless the headgear is worn nearly full-time or the elastics are worn only when the headgear is on, which provides an intermittent force.

The J-hook headgear applies the extraoral force directly to the anterior teeth to retract them distally to close the space. Because the extraoral force closes the space without the need for an intraarch force, there is no counteracting force pulling the molars forward so posterior anchorage is unnecessary. Just as with the facebow, a disadvantage is the dependence on patient compliance to wear the headgear enough for tooth movement to occur. Another disadvantage is that the force to retract the anterior teeth is intermittent, which is not as optimal for tooth movement. In addition, it is more difficult to control the level of force to keep it light enough to effectively retract the incisors.

Because extraoral force often is not an option if the patient is unwilling to wear the headgear, alternative treatment approaches become necessary. Without extraoral force, some other means of improving the anchorage of the maxillary molars must be contrived. One method of supplementing the posterior anchorage is to join as many posterior teeth together as possible while minimizing the number of anterior teeth to be retracted. This permits the intraoral elastic or spring force to act on a few anterior teeth at a given time while dissipating the reactive force over multiple posterior teeth. This can be accomplished by ligating the maxillary second molars, first molars, and second premolars together.

Another means of supplementing posterior anchorage is the use of a fixed lingual arch such as a transpalatal arch or a Nance holding arch. A transpalatal arch is a large-gauge wire that traverses the palate to rigidly connect the lingual aspect of both maxillary first molars. If the other posterior teeth are ligated together, the transpalatal arch joins both sides of the arch together, creating one multirooted dental unit of six teeth to counteract the intraarch force (see Figure 20-17, A). A Nance holding arch is an alternative type of fixed lingual arch soldered to the maxillary molars, with the anterior part embedded in an acrylic pad that conforms to the anterior aspect of the palate (see Figure 20-17, B). With this in place, the protractive force acting on the maxillary molars during space closure is partially dissipated against the palate by means of the acrylic pad.

A possibility to reinforce maxillary posterior anchorage is a removable palatal retainer that can use the resistance of the palate, similar to a Nance holding arch, to hold the maxillary molars posteriorly during space closure.

Another strategy to minimize the anterior movement of the maxillary molars is to decrease the magnitude of intraarch force required to retract the anterior teeth while closing the space. One way is to reduce the number of anterior teeth to the two maxillary canines for initial retraction. This effectively pits the six posterior teeth against the two canines, improving the posterior anchorage. Once the canines have been retracted, they can be joined to the posterior teeth to create an eight-tooth unit that can then be pitted against the four maxillary incisors to obtain maximum retraction of these teeth. The disadvantage of this technique is the extended treatment time required.

A final technique to maximize retraction of maxillary incisors with minimal protraction of maxillary molars is to use the mandibular teeth for anchorage. Class II elastics, extending from the maxillary anterior teeth to the mandibular posterior teeth, can provide the retractive force. The posterior reactive force is dissipated among all of the mandibular teeth, avoiding any mesial movement by the maxillary posterior teeth. The disadvantage of this technique is that the vertical and anteroposterior forces from the Class II elastics tend to extrude the mandibular molars and maxillary incisors as well as protract the mandibular teeth. These may not be desirable tooth movements, especially with patients who already have protrusive mandibular teeth or excessive inferior position of the maxillary incisors.

Clinical Procedures   Dental camouflage with extractions may involve only removal of the maxillary first premolars or may include removal of mandibular first or second premolars. In either case it is prudent to place a comprehensive fixed orthodontic appliance to provide adequate control of both dental arches during treatment. In the same manner as dental camouflage without extractions, it is necessary to bond and band all of the teeth and level and align the dentition in each arch. As explained previously, this requires a gradual increase in arch wire size and stiffness to a minimum of 0.017-inch × 0.025-inch or 0.018-inch × 0.022-inch stainless steel arch wires in a 0.022-inch × 0.028-inch slot to prepare for space closure.

The appropriate time to extract teeth to provide space for dental camouflage treatment can depend on the presence or absence of dental crowding or protrusion. If some of the extraction space is required to eliminate crowding or reduce protrusion of the incisors, extractions should take place at the onset of treatment. If no appreciable crowding or protrusion of teeth is present, the clinician has the option of waiting until leveling and alignment are complete before having the premolars extracted. This latter possibility provides the advantage of having fresh extraction sites present at the start of space closure. Older extraction sites may have more resorbed alveolar bone with constricted facial and lingual cortical plates that inhibit effective space closure. New extraction sites not only preclude this possibility, but also are characterized by highly active osseous turnover, offering an ideal environment for efficient space closure.

Once leveling and aligning of the arches with extractions have been completed, retraction of maxillary anterior teeth to eliminate excessive overjet can begin. As with dental camouflage without extractions, the same anchorage principles apply, namely maximum maxillary posterior anchorage and mandibular anterior anchorage, to achieve a successful treatment outcome. The desired final anteroposterior position of the incisors also is an important consideration when planning anchorage before space closure. The planned final incisor position and the extent of the Class II occlusal discrepancy define the amount the extraction spaces are closed by incisor retraction versus molar protraction.

Most cases of mild to moderate skeletal Class II problems that can be treated effectively with dental camouflage require extractions. The severity of the Class II malocclusion must be minimal enough to permit sufficient retraction of the maxillary anterior teeth to eliminate overjet, following the extraction of maxillary first premolars. No extractions in the mandibular arch should be necessary if there is no substantial crowding or protrusion of the mandibular teeth. However, if either of these is present, mandibular premolar extractions are necessary to eliminate the crowding or to retract the mandibular incisors while providing space for protraction of mandibular molars—a difficult task to accomplish (i.e., to achieve a Class I occlusion) without headgear wear cooperation and favorable mandibular growth.

GROWTH MODIFICATION: ONGOING CONTROVERSY

Although little argument remains that skeletal growth modification of the maxilla and mandible may be possible with the use of orthopedic forces, controversy continues regarding the precise nature of the skeletal change as well as the optimal timing and the type of appliances that produce the best treatment outcome. Numerous well-designed retrospective clinical studies have been undertaken to examine these factors, comparing outcome in the treated population vs. the untreated controls. Keeling and coworkers[117] have published an excellent summary of these clinical studies.

These retrospective studies generally support the effectiveness of the use of headgear or functional appliances on improving anteroposterior apical base and occlusal changes. There is not agreement, however, on the nature or mechanism of these changes. It appears that headgear inhibits downward and forward maxillary displacement, but functional appliances seem to demonstrate a similar effect. In spite of animal studies that demonstrate histologic increase in mandibular growth, these studies generally refute the contention that either of these appliances can enhance mandibular growth to produce a mandibular position that is significantly more anterior than untreated controls.[215] Headgear and functional appliances demonstrate dental effects that include decreasing the mesial movement of maxillary molars. Retraction of maxillary anterior teeth and protraction of mandibular anterior teeth occur more frequently with functional appliances.

There also is not agreement on the timing of skeletal Class II orthopedic treatment for the best treatment outcome.[216-219] There is considerable support by orthodontists for starting facial orthopedic treatment during the mixed dentition to take advantage of active mandibular growth during this time. This approach requires two phases of orthodontic treatment. The first phase includes a removable or limited fixed appliance intended to achieve growth modification and skeletal correction. The second phase begins after eruption of the permanent teeth with the placement of a complete fixed appliance to finish the orthodontic treatment. Retrospective clinical studies have not always supported this two-phase approach as a necessity for successful treatment outcome.[220,221]

Potential disadvantages presented by retrospective studies often include biased samples, inadequate sample size, inadequate matching of control sample, and other inherent problems.[222] There has been a recent attempt in the United States to shed new light on these issues with the support by the National Institute of Health for three prospective randomized clinical trials. All three of these investigations were prospectively designed to compare treatment outcome from early orthopedic treatment with headgear or functional appliances with untreated controls. Although the complete results following definitive orthodontic treatment with a complete fixed appliance and following adolescent growth will not be available for some time to come, their present findings are worth summarizing.

The first of these trials, conducted at the University of Florida, included the comparison of children randomly assigned to one of three groups: control, bionator, and headgear (cervical or high-pull) with an anterior biteplane.[117] The results demonstrated that the use of the headgear or the bionator did not significantly affect maxillary growth but both appeared to enhance mandibular growth with this effect remaining stable 1 year following treatment. The dental changes that occurred with the treatment, namely retraction of maxillary teeth and protraction of mandibular teeth, did not appear to be stable following removal of the appliances.

The second prospective randomized clinical trial has been taking place at the University of North Carolina where a somewhat smaller sample of children was assigned randomly to one of three groups: control, bionator, and combination headgear.[78] The findings following initial treatment with the orthopedic appliances revealed a maxillary inhibitory effect with the headgear group and a mandibular-enhancing effect with the bionator group on average. However, the investigators were struck by the considerable variation in response and by the lack of major difference in treatment outcome among all three groups following definitive fixed orthodontic treatment.

The third prospective clinical trial is being undertaken at the University of Pennsylvania. It has the smallest sample of children. Children from this sample are randomly assigned to two treatment groups with no control group.[103] The two treatments used were either functional regulator or combination headgear. The investigators found that the functional regulator promoted a more anterior mandibular position, whereas the headgear appeared to have more of a maxillary inhibitory effect. Retraction of maxillary incisors and protraction of mandibular incisors characterized the dental movement with the functional regulator, whereas the headgear appeared to promote protraction of both maxillary and mandibular incisors.

It is apparent that the preliminary results of these recent prospective randomized clinical studies have not provided clear answers to the controversy regarding the efficacy and effects of current methods of facial orthopedic growth modification. Although there is growing support for simplifying treatment of skeletal problems to one phase in the permanent dentition, there is still widespread support for an early orthopedic phase in the mixed dentition, followed by a final fixed phase. It is hoped that all three of these studies ultimately will provide a clearer picture of the true impact of the various appliances on growth modification. Future studies may identify which treatment is most efficacious in individual patients. Treatment response appears to be influenced strongly by the variability of skeletal growth pattern in addition to patient compliance, clinician expertise, appliance type, and other possible unknown factors. Until such time as these factors can be more clearly identified and understood, a variety of appliances will be used in the growing child to attempt treatment of Class II skeletal problems.

Surgical Correction of Class II Skeletal Discrepancy in Adult

There are many skeletal Class II problems in individuals with little or no remaining growth potential that cannot be treated properly with orthodontic treatment alone. This can be the case if at least one of two features is present with the malocclusion. The first is that the skeletal disharmony is so severe that the extent of dental movement (maxillary retraction or mandibular protraction) necessary to eliminate the overjet is either too great to permit a stable treatment outcome or too great to permit an esthetic facial result. The second feature that precludes acceptable dental camouflage treatment is the presence of crowding or protrusion of incisors that is severe enough to require all of the lower extraction space to correct these problems, leaving no additional space to retract maxillary teeth or protract mandibular teeth.

In preparation for orthognathic surgery, it is necessary to remove any dental compensations present and to place the teeth in a favorable position with their supporting bone. In contrast to dental camouflage treatment that seeks to create dental compensation (retrusive maxillary teeth and protrusive mandibular teeth) for the skeletal Class II problem, orthodontic preparation for surgery often requires the removal of

natural dental compensations. This usually means that the planned movement of the teeth before surgery must be in the opposite direction, typified by maxillary protraction and mandibular retraction, from the movement with dental camouflage treatment. For this reason it is important to avoid extensive dental camouflage treatment for challenging skeletal Class II problems. If there is a failure to reach an acceptable orthodontic treatment outcome, additional extensive treatment aimed at moving the teeth in the opposite direction will be required if orthognathic surgery is later contemplated. Therefore inordinate treatment protraction, causing increased patient unhappiness and morbidity such as root resorption, can be avoided by careful treatment planning. If a successful orthodontic treatment outcome with dental camouflage cannot be predicted with assurance, orthodontic treatment with orthognathic surgery is the treatment of choice for skeletal Class II problems.

Originally developed in Europe, orthognathic surgical techniques were further advanced in the United States during the 1960s and 1970s. By the 1980s it was possible to reposition the jaws or dentoalveolar segments in all three planes of space. The adoption of **rigid internal fixation** during the 1980s provided further progress in the management and stability of orthognathic surgical treatment. At the end of the twentieth century, facial skeletal problems can be treated directly at the source of the malocclusion with surgical correction of the specific jaw discrepancy or disproportion at fault. In terms of Class II skeletal malocclusions, the surgical treatment options are at least as abundant as the underlying causes of the problems. These options can be divided conveniently into five categories: mandibular advancement, mandibular total subapical advancement, maxillary impaction, anterior maxillary subapical setback, or a combined surgery including both the maxilla and mandible.

Mandibular Advancement: Indications and Treatment In patients with skeletal Class II malocclusions in which neither growth modification nor dental camouflage offer an acceptable treatment, surgical advancement of the mandible is often necessary in combination with orthodontic treatment. A mandibular advancement is indicated in most skeletal Class II cases where mandibular deficiency is present (Figure 20-20). If the lower face height is short with an excessive anterior overbite, these vertical problems and the anteroposterior discrepancy can be effectively treated with rotation of the mandible downward anteriorly as it is advanced. This provides an effective and stable means of increasing the deficient lower face height and eliminating the excessive anterior overbite.

Although a number of techniques for surgically advancing the mandible were introduced in the first half of the twentieth century, there was little acceptance due to the morbidity and instability associated with these methods. These concerns were mitigated with the development of an **intraoral ramus osteotomy** that has become known as the **sagittal split** (Figure 20-21). Originally developed by the Austrian surgeon, Richard Trauner, and the Swiss surgeon, Hugo Obwegeser,[223] in 1957 and introduced to American surgeons in the 1960s, most surgeons now prefer this method for advancing the mandible. The technique commonly used today is based on modifications by the American surgeons Ervin Hunsuck[224] and

Bruce Epker.[225] Because the distal, tooth-bearing segment of the osteotomy is the part advanced and rotated downward, there is no significant lengthening of the pterygomasseteric musculature that would produce an unstable outcome. When extreme mandibular advancements of greater than 10 to 15 mm are necessary, a **vertical "L" or "C" osteotomy** often is preferred.[226,227] This surgical technique combines the sagittal split with a **vertical ramus osteotomy** that requires an extraoral approach.

The orthodontic treatment necessary to prepare a patient for a mandibular advancement includes align-

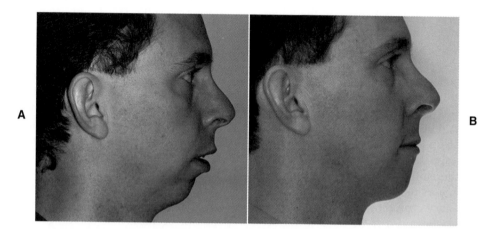

Figure 20-20 A, A surgical mandibular advancement is indicated where the mandibular deficiency is severe enough and mandibular growth potential is minimum enough to preclude acceptable treatment with dental camouflage or growth modification. **B,** The skeletal problem can be directly addressed with the surgical procedure, providing an improved functional and cosmetic treatment outcome. An augmentation genioplasty could be included with the mandibular advancement for this patient to further enhance the cosmetic outcome.

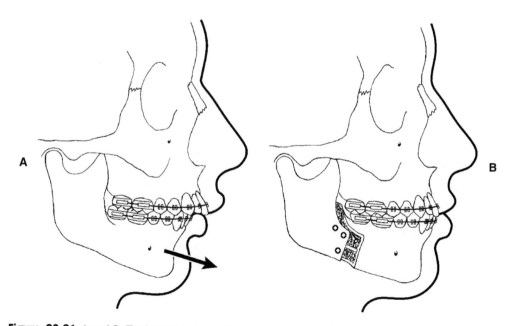

Figure 20-21 A and **B,** The intraoral sagittal split ramus osteotomy is the most popular technique for surgical mandibular advancement.

ment of the teeth and establishing the final vertical and anteroposterior incisor positions and **interarch compatibility.** Normally, some maxillary expansion is necessary to accommodate the advanced mandible. If significant expansion is required and the midpalatal sutures are no longer patent enough to allow orthopedic expansion, surgically assisted expansion may be necessary. Usually orthodontic leveling of the maxillary and mandibular arches is completed before surgery, but in cases with a short lower face and severe curve of Spee, leveling of the mandibular arch may be performed postsurgically. In these cases extrusion of the mandibular posterior teeth to level the arch is more simply and efficiently accomplished after surgery. Postsurgical leveling also permits a more effective increase in the lower face height and stable decrease in excessive anterior overbite. Intrusion of incisors with segmental mechanics is rarely needed in these cases. If required, it should be completed before surgery. Another approach for these cases is to accomplish posterior molar extrusion before surgery by using an anterior bite plate and posterior vertical elastics, eliminating the need for a prolonged period of postsurgical orthodontic treatment.

A final consideration for orthodontic preparation for surgery is whether to extract in the mandibular arch. Maxillary premolars may need to be extracted if there is severe maxillary crowding or incisor protrusion or if Class III elastics need to be used to retract and upright the mandibular incisors. In some cases the extent of crowding or protrusion of the maxillary incisors is usually not severe enough to require additional space in the arch. In addition, the need for an expanded maxillary arch to prevent posterior crossbite after mandibular advancement may preclude maxillary extractions. In contrast, extraction of mandibular premolars is often necessary to prepare the mandibular arch for the surgery. Extra space is required within the arch to alleviate the typical crowding and protrusion (natural dental compensation for the skeletal Class II problem) of the mandibular incisors to permit adequate mandibular advancement. When extraction of premolars will be performed in the lower arch only, the molar occlusion postsurgically will be Class III. Proper posterior interdigitation in some of these cases may be difficult to accomplish.

Presurgical orthodontic treatment is completed when full-dimension rectangular steel arch wires are in place to facilitate stabilization at surgery. Upon removal of the surgical splint following surgery, postsurgical orthodontic treatment includes the placement of light working arch wires and interarch elastics improve occlusal interdigitation.

Mandibular Total Subapical Advancement: Indications and Treatment
A less common mandibular surgical technique for correction of

selected cases of mandibular deficiency is the total subapical osteotomy used to advance the mandibular dentoalveolus. Although a mandibular anterior subapical advancement was described in the European literature as early as 1936,[228] it was a 1959 publication in English by the Austrian surgeon, Heinrich Köle,[229] describing various types of segmental osteotomies, that influenced American surgeons to begin performing this surgery. Since the mid 1970s, a method for removing the inferior alveolar neurovascular bundle from the canal has permitted this surgery to be accomplished safely and effectively.[230,231] This procedure is indicated where there is only slightly short or normal lower face height and slightly excessive or normal anterior overbite. This is important because significant surgical rotation of the mandibular dentoalveolar segment with the subapical technique to increase lower face height and decrease overbite usually is not stable. Two other prerequisites for this surgical procedure are the presence of an exceptionally prominent chin (prominent relative to the dentoalveolar segment but normal relative to the face) and the presence of sufficient vertical bone height between the mandibular teeth and the inferior mandibular border for the osteotomy to be safely accomplished. The goal of this surgery is to advance the entire dentoalveolar segment along the mandibular corpus, correcting the anteroposterior occlusal discrepancy and eliminating excessive overjet without significantly changing face height or overbite. The procedure provides better support for the lower lip, decreasing the acute labiomental fold and the relative excessive prominence of the chin for a more esthetically pleasing face.

Maxillary Impaction: Indications and Treatment
The type of orthognathic surgery indicated for vertical maxillary excess is maxillary impaction.[232] Although superior surgical movement of the maxilla was first reported by Schuchardt in 1959,[233] it was Heinrich Köle's publication[229] in that same year that encouraged more widespread development of maxillary surgical techniques in the United States. Contributions by Hugo Obwegeser[234] and the American surgeons, William Bell and Barnet Levy[235,236] at the end of the 1960s persuaded surgeons that **Le Fort I maxillary osteotomies** could be performed safely and successfully. Maxillary surgical impaction may include either a total maxillary osteotomy if the excess is anterior as well as posterior (Figure 20-22, A and B)[232] or bilateral posterior segmental maxillary osteotomies if the excess is more in the posterior (see Figure 20-22, C and D).[237] Bone is removed at the osteotomy site to permit superior repositioning of the maxilla. As the maxilla moves up, the mandible rotates upward and forward around the condylar axis, correcting the anteroposterior occlusal discrepancy. The vertical prob-

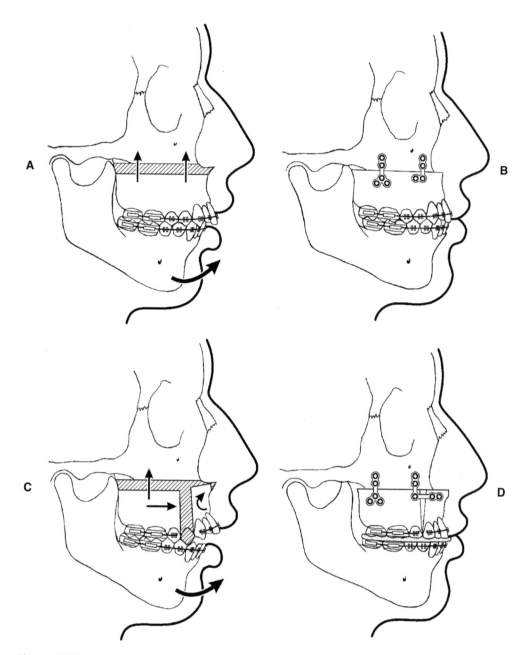

Figure 20-22 A surgical maxillary impaction permits the mandible to rotate upward and forward to help correct a skeletal Class II problem. This surgical procedure also can improve the vertical display of maxillary incisors as well as the associated long anterior face height and incompetent lips. **A** and **B,** A total maxillary osteotomy is indicated when there is no expansion necessary and the vertical maxillary excess is both anterior and posterior. **C** and **D,** A segmental maxillary osteotomy is indicated when the excess is more posterior. This procedure often requires extraction of maxillary first premolars to provide adequate space for the presurgical alignment and the interdental osteotomies at the time of surgery. This results in the maxillary posterior segments being brought forward during surgery into a Class II occlusion of the posterior teeth. It is prudent to use an interocclusal splint ligated to the segmented maxillary arch to enhance the stability of the surgical outcome.

lems associated with vertical maxillary excess, including excessive lower face height, incompetent lips, anterior open bite, or excessive vertical display of the maxillary incisors, can be treated effectively in the older teenager or adult with maxillary impaction. If the maxilla is too narrow to provide interarch compatibility, the maxillary osteotomy needs to be in two or three segments to permit expansion of the maxilla. If there is a vertical discrepancy between the anterior and posterior occlusal plane, the osteotomy needs to be in three segments to permit greater impaction of the two posterior segments than the anterior segment. Finally, four segments may be necessary in a severely constricted maxilla with a midline separation of the anterior segment to allow for adequate intercanine expansion.

Orthodontic preparation for maxillary impaction includes many of the same goals as presurgical orthodontic treatment for mandibular advancement. These include dental alignment and establishment of incisor position and interarch compatibility. However, an important difference is the need to complete leveling of the mandibular arch before surgery. Another difference is that the maxillary arch should not be presurgically leveled with a continuous arch wire if there is a significant vertical discrepancy between the anterior and posterior occlusal plane. In this case presurgical leveling should occur in separate segments to prepare for a three- or four-segment maxillary osteotomy.

The decision whether or not to extract teeth in preparation for maxillary impaction depends on the amount of crowding and anterior protrusion of the incisors. If either of these is severe enough, extractions are necessary to provide space for alignment or retraction. An additional consideration is the amount of space for the interdental osteotomies if a segmental maxillary surgery is planned. There must be adequate space at the osteotomy sites between the roots to permit the vertical bone cuts without risking root damage or periodontal defects to the adjacent teeth. Although an interdental space of 3 to 4 mm is critical between the roots, some surgeons prefer some space between the crowns as well.

Presurgical orthodontic preparation is complete after the placement of full-dimension rectangular steel arch wires. If the maxillary surgery is to include multiple segments, segmented maxillary arch wires need to be placed with adequate **root divergence** at the planned **interdental osteotomy** sites. Following surgery where the maxillary arch is leveled, orthodontic treatment is resumed at the time of splint removal. Postsurgical orthodontic treatment includes light continuous arch wires and light vertical elastics. The maxillary arch wire often needs to be a flexible (nickel-titanium) full-dimension wire to maintain anterior torque while achieving **root parallelism** at the interdental osteotomy sites.

Anterior Maxillary Subapical Setback: Indications and Treatment

In rare situations in which the skeletal Class II malocclusion is caused by a maxillary excess limited to the anteroposterior dimension with no associated maxillary vertical or transverse skeletal problems and a normal size and position of the mandible, an anterior maxillary subapical setback may be indicated. Midface protrusion is characteristic of this condition and must be distinguished from protrusion of the maxillary teeth alone, which may be treated effectively with orthodontic treatment without surgery. Another necessary feature for successful treatment with this surgical procedure is the absence of significant crowding or dental protrusion of the maxillary and mandibular incisors. The treatment goal is to use the maxillary first premolar space for surgical retraction of the maxillary anterior teeth, maintaining the Class II molar relationship and achieving a Class I canine relationship while reducing overjet.

The anterior maxillary subapical osteotomy was the first maxillary orthognathic surgical technique introduced in the United States. Although a method was described in the European literature in 1921,[238] it was Heinrich Köle's publication,[229] together with other reports in the American literature,[239,240] that influenced American surgeons to use this technique in the 1960s. At that time, this was the favored method for treating a variety of skeletal Class II problems until mandibular and total maxillary osteotomies became available options for American surgeons. Significant esthetic and functional compromises were common with this procedure because it did not directly address vertical and transverse discrepancies that are so common with skeletal Class II problems. Although infrequently used today, there are limited cases of midface protrusion that may benefit from a surgical setback of the anterior maxilla.[241] The surgical technique may be either one described by Wassmund[242] or one described by Wunderer[243] and includes extraction of the maxillary first premolars followed by vertical interdental osteotomies in this area and removal of vertical bone segments. Additional osteotomies are performed to mobilize the anterior maxilla to permit the posterior movement of the anterior maxilla to correct excessive overjet.

Orthodontic preparation for this surgery includes leveling and aligning the dental arches as well as achieving root divergence of the maxillary canines and second premolars adjacent to the interdental osteotomy sites. If the maxillary anterior teeth are vertically extruded relative to the other maxillary teeth, it is necessary to level the anterior segment separately from the two maxillary posterior segments so that intrusion of the maxillary anterior teeth can be accomplished at the time of surgery. If there is inadequate maxillary intercanine width and orthodontic expansion is not possible because of periodontal limitation, it is necessary to include an additional interdental osteotomy between the maxillary central incisors to permit surgical expansion of the anterior maxilla.

Presurgical orthodontic treatment includes leveling and aligning both arches with continuous arch wires and is completed with placement of full-dimension stainless steel wires. Root divergence of the maxillary canines and second premolars must be achieved to permit adequate space to complete the interdental osteotomies, and a sufficient amount of bone must be removed to permit complete surgical retraction of the anterior teeth. If the maxillary anterior teeth need to be surgically intruded as well as retracted, the maxillary anterior teeth should be leveled as a separate segment before surgery. Following surgery, orthodontic treatment is resumed with placement of continuous flexible arch wires and light interarch elastics. Similar to the postsurgical orthodontic treatment that follows total maxillary segmental impaction, placement of a maxillary full-dimension nickel-titanium arch wire is recommended to maintain anterior torque while completing root parallelism in the osteotomy sites.

Combined Surgical Approaches: Indications and Treatment

Although many skeletal Class II problems in individuals with minimal growth potential can be treated effectively with one of the surgical approaches mentioned previously, it is not uncommon to require a combination of maxillary and mandibular surgeries to adequately address the malocclusion.[244] This is the case where there is a significant maxillary deformity (vertical or anteroposterior excess or transverse deficiency) combined with a mandibular deficiency. The forward projection of the mandible resulting from its rotation after maxillary impaction may be inadequate to provide normal occlusion and facial balance. In this situation, a mandibular advancement is required in addition to the maxillary impaction to complete the anteroposterior correction. Even if there is no maxillary excess, surgery to the maxilla in the form of expansion may be necessary to complement a mandibular advancement. This can occur when the maxilla is so constricted relative to the advanced mandible that dental expansion alone is inadequate to achieve a stable buccal overjet.

Treatment Outcome

In the last half of the twentieth century, there has been extensive international development, particularly in Europe, of socialized health care systems. Proper management of these systems requires accurate information not only about the nature and prevalence of health problems, but also about the quality of alternative treatments for these problems. This has resulted in an emphasis on developing more specific quantitative criteria to describe and assess the severity of malocclusions and the quality of treatment outcome. None of the assessment systems proposed to date have been accepted universally, but the **Peer Assessment Rating (PAR) Index,** developed in 1987 by a group of British orthodontists at the University of Manchester, is recognized as the most reliable and valid method available at this time.[245,246] There has been increased pressure on the dental profession in the United States during the last decade of the twentieth century to adopt more precise means of quantifying the need for treatment and its quality. The PAR Index is being used in clinical studies as an outcome measure for evaluating the efficacy of alternative treatments for Class II malocclusions.[78,247-249] It is possible that the PAR Index, or a modification of it, will be used in the future by practicing clinicians as a means of evaluating the need for, progress of, and outcome of the care they provide.[250-253] There is also the potential for third-party payers to assign orthodontic benefits and evaluate treatment efficacy based on the PAR Index.[254,255]

SUMMARY

The prevalence of Class II dental malocclusions is high, ranging from 15% to 20% of the population in most regions of the world. This common malocclusion is associated most often with an anteroposterior skeletal jaw discrepancy, associated with mandibular deficiency or maxillary excess. Although less common, a Class II dental malocclusion may be present in association with a normal skeletal jaw relationship.

Three alternatives for treating skeletal Class II malocclusions are growth modification, dental camouflage, and orthognathic surgery. Until the last three decades of the twentieth century, only the first two alternatives were possible. Growth modification of skeletal Class II problems has been undertaken with principally two types of appliances: headgears and functional appliances. During the first two decades of the century, headgears were initially used in the United States and then generally abandoned until their reintroduction in the 1950s. In Europe functional appliances were almost exclusively used throughout this entire period. In the 1960s the increased association of orthodontists across the Atlantic resulted in the acceptance of both appliances as treatment alternatives. Dental camouflage is another alternative that has been used for correction of skeletal Class II malocclusions in patients in whom minimal facial growth remains. Class II interarch elastics, usually with selected dental extractions, have been used throughout the century to provide the dental camouflage for these skeletal problems. With the introduction of reliable and safe orthognathic surgical techniques, another alternative for correction of skeletal Class II malocclusions in the absence of growth became possible.

Early in the new millennium, the U.S. Human Genome Project will provide us with the complete genetic sequence for the entire human genome.[256] This information will furnish the basis for a revolution in the understanding of the purpose, interaction, and chemistry of individual genes.[257] It is expected that with the concomitant advances in molecular and cellular biology, genetic engineering to prevent or modify many skeletal and dental malocclusions may be possible during the twenty-first century. A much better understanding of the role of epigenetic or environmental factors on facial morphology and dental malocclusion will also be necessary for complete management of these problems.

For the present, there continues to be a controversy regarding the nature of facial growth modification, its optimal timing, and the efficacy of the various appliances used. There also appears to be an unpredictable, broad, and poorly understood variability in the response of individuals to similar treatment. Skeletal Class II problems in children are not necessarily predictable in terms of their developmental extent of severity or their response to treatment. Skeletal Class II problems in patients with minimal facial growth remaining require complex, sophisticated orthodontic treatment whether or not orthognathic surgery is performed. For these reasons it seems prudent for dental clinicians who are not orthodontists but yet are trained in the use of a fixed appliance to limit their treatment of Class II problems to those that are strictly dental in nature. These dental Class II problems include those associated with children who have a normal skeletal pattern or with adults who have a normal skeletal jaw relationship. Reliable identification of such cases requires the development of extensive diagnostic skills.

REFERENCES

1. Baume LJ, Maréchaux SC: Uniform methods for the epidemiologic assessment of malocclusion, *Am J Orthod* 66:121-129, 1974.
2. Angle EH: *Treatment of malocclusion of the teeth,* ed 7, Philadelphia, 1907, S.S. White Dental Manufacturing.
3. Kelly JE, Sanchez M, Van Kirk LE: *An assessment of the occlusion of the teeth of children ages 6-11 years,* DHEW Pub No (HRA) 74-1612, Washington, DC, 1973, National Center for Health Statistics.
4. Kelly JE, Harvey CR: *An assessment of the teeth of youths 12-17 years,* DHEW Pub No (HRA) 77-1644, Washington, DC, 1977, National Center for Health Statistics.
5. Brunelle JA, Bhat M, Lipton JA: Prevalence and distribution of selected occlusal characteristics in the U.S. population, 1988-1991, *J Dent Res* 75:706-713, 1996.
6. Emrich RE, Brodie AG, Blayney JR: Prevalence of Class 1, Class 2, and Class 3 malocclusions (Angle) in an urban population: an epidemiological study, *J Dent Res* 44:947-953, 1965.
7. Horowitz HS, Doyle J: Occlusal relations in children born and reared in an optimally fluoridated community, *Angle Orthod* 40:104-111, 1970.
8. Infante PF: Malocclusion in the deciduous dentition in white, black, and Apache Indian children, *Angle Orthod* 45:213-218, 1975.
9. Trottman A, Elsbach HG: Comparison of malocclusion in preschool black and white children, *Am J Orthod Dentofacial Orthop* 110:69-72, 1996.
10. Grewe JM et al: Prevalence of malocclusion in Chippewa Indian children, *J Dent Res* 47:302-305, 1968.
11. Wood BF: Malocclusion in the modern Alaskan Eskimo, *Am J Orthod* 60:344-354, 1971.
12. Laine T, Hausen H: Occlusal anomalies in Finnish students related to age, sex, absent permanent teeth and orthodontic treatment, *Eur J Orthod* 5:125-131, 1983.
13. Thilander B, Myrberg N: The prevalence of malocclusion in Swedish schoolchildren, *Scand J Dent Res* 81:12-21, 1973.
14. Helm S: Orthodontic treatment priorities in the Danish Child Dental Health Services, *Community Dent Oral Epidemiol* 10:260-263, 1982.
15. Goose DH, Thompson DG, Winter FC: Malocclusion in school children of the West Midlands, *Br Dent J* 102:174-178, 1957.
16. Lavelle CL: A study of multiracial malocclusions, *Community Dent Oral Epidemiol* 4:38-41, 1976.
17. Burgersdijk R et al: Malocclusion and orthodontic treatment need of 15-74-year-old Dutch adults, *Community Dent Oral Epidemiol* 19:64-67, 1991.
18. Tschill P, Bacon W, Sonko A: Malocclusion in the deciduous dentition of Caucasian children, *Eur J Orthod* 19:361-367, 1997.
19. Gardiner JH: An orthodontic survey of Libyan schoolchildren, *Br J Orthod* 9:59-61, 1982.
20. El-Mangoury NH, Mostafa YA: Epidemiologic panorama of malocclusion, *Angle Orthod* 60:207-214, 1990.
21. Maatouk F et al: Dental manifestations of inbreeding, *J Clin Pediatr Dent* 19:305-306, 1995.
22. Houpt MI, Adu-Aryee S, Graninger RM: Dental survey in the Brong Ahafo region of Ghana, *Arch Oral Biol* 12:1337-1341, 1967.
23. Diagne F et al: Prevalence of malocclusion in Senegal, *Community Dent Oral Epidemiol* 21:325-326, 1993.
24. Kerosuo H et al: Occlusion among a group of Tanzanian urban schoolchildren, *Community Dent Oral Epidemiol* 16:306-309, 1988.
25. Ng'ang'a PM et al: The prevalence of malocclusion in 13- to 15-year-old children in Nairobi, Kenya, *Acta Odontol Scand* 54:126-130, 1996.
26. Isiekwe MC: Malocclusion in Lagos, Nigeria, *Community Dent Oral Epidemiol* 11:59-62, 1983.
27. Hirschowitz AS, Rashid SA, Cleaton-Jones PE: Dental caries, gingival health and malocclusion in 12-year-old urban Black schoolchildren from Soweto, Johannesburg, *Community Dent Oral Epidemiol* 9:87-90, 1981.
28. al-Emran S, Wisth PJ, Boe OE: Prevalence of malocclusion and need for orthodontic treatment in Saudi Arabia, *Community Dent Oral Epidemiol* 18:253-255, 1990.
29. Steigman S, Kawar M, Zilberman Y: Prevalence and severity of malocclusion in Israel Arab urban children aged 13 to 15 years of age, *Am J Orthod* 84:337-343, 1983.
30. Tang EL: Occlusal features of Chinese adults in Hong Kong, *Aust Orthod J* 13:159-163, 1994.
31. Menezes DM, Shaw JG, Anderson RJ: The dental condition of 10-12 year old children in Rangoon and Wolverhampton, *Arch Oral Biol* 17:1187-1195, 1972.

32. Woon KC, Thong YL, Abdul-Kadir R: Permanent dentition occlusion in Chinese, Indian and Malay groups in Malaysia, *Aust Orthod J* 11:45-48, 1989.

33. Schull WL, Neel JV: *The effects of inbreeding on Japanese children,* New York, 1965, Harper & Row.

34. Baume LV: The pattern of dental disease in French Polynesia, *Int Dent J* 23:579-584, 1973.

35. Lombardi AV, Bailit HL: Malocclusion in the Kwaio, a Melanesian group on Malaita, Solomon Islands, *Am J Phys Anthropol* 36:283-293, 1972.

36. Barmes DE: Dental and nutritional surveys of primitive peoples in the Pacific Islands, *Aust Dent J* 12:442-454, 1967.

37. Sutton PR: Dental health survey of Gilbert and Ellice islanders, *Aust Dent J* 11:405-409, 1966.

38. Howell S, Morel G: Orthodontic treatment needs in Westmead Hospital Dental Clinical School, *Aust Dent J* 38:367-372, 1993.

39. Tod MA, Taverne AA: Prevalence of malocclusion traits in an Australian adult population, *Aust Orthod J* 15:16-22, 1997.

40. Homan BT, Davies GN: An oral health survey of Aborigines and Torres Strait Islanders in far North Queensland, *Aust Dent J* 18:75-87, 1973.

41. de-Muniz BR: Epidemiology of malocclusion in Argentine children, *Community Dent Oral Epidemiol* 14:221-224, 1986.

42. Palomino H: The Aymara of western Bolivia: III. Occlusion, pathology, and characteristics of the dentition, *J Dent Res* 57:459-467, 1978.

43. D'Escrivan de Saturno L: Characteristics of the occlusion of 3630 schoolchildren in the metropolitan area of Caracas, *Acta Odontol Venez* 18:237-263, 1980.

44. Sanchez-Perez TL, Saenz LP, Alfaro P: Occlusion distribution in a 7- to 14-year old student population, *Rev ADM* 48:52-55, 1991.

45. da-Silva-Filho OG, de-Freitas SF, Cavassen A: Prevalence of normal occlusion and malocclusion in Bauru (Sao Paulo) students. 2. Influence of socioeconomic level, *Rev Odontol Univ Sao Paulo* 4:189-196, 1990.

46. Moorrees CFA: *The Aleut dentition,* Cambridge, Mass, 1957, Harvard University Press.

47. Newman GV: The Eskimo's dentofacial complex, *U.S. Armed Forces Med J* 3:1653-1662, 1952.

48. Niswander JD: Further studies on the Xavante Indians. VII. The oral status of the Xavantes of Simoes Lopes, *Am J Hum Genet* 19:543-553, 1967.

49. Kuftinec MM: Oral health in Guatemalan rural populations, *J Dent Res* 50:559-564, 1971.

50. Harrison RL, Davis DW: Dental malocclusion in native children of British Columbia, Canada, *Community Dent Oral Epidemiol* 24:217-221, 1996.

51. Owen DG: The incidence and nature of space closure following the premature extraction of deciduous teeth: a literature survey, *Am J Orthod* 59:37-49, 1971.

52. Young DH: Ectopic eruption of the first permanent molar, *J Dent Child* 24:153-162, 1957.

53. Rose JS: A survey of congenitally missing teeth, excluding third molars, in 6000 orthodontic patients, *Dent Pract Dent Rec* 17:107-113, 1966.

54. Maklin M, Dummett CO, Weinberg R: A study of oligodontia in a sample of New Orleans children, *J Dent Child* 46:478-482, 1979.

55. Joondeph DR, McNeill RW: Congenitally absent second premolars: an interceptive approach, *Am J Orthod* 59:50-66, 1971.

56. Hitchcock HP: The cephalometric distinction of class II, division 2 malocclusion, *Am J Orthod* 69:447-454, 1976.

57. Pancherz H, Zieber K, Hoyer B: Cephalometric characteristics of Class II division 1 and Class II division 2 malocclusions: a comparative study in children, *Angle Orthod* 67:111-120, 1997.

58. Ruf S, Pancherz H: Class II division 2 malocclusion: genetics or environment? A case report of monozygotic twins, *Angle Orthod* 69:321-324, 1999.

59. Kingsley NW: *Treatise on oral deformities as a branch of mechanical surgery,* New York, 1880, Appleton & Lange.

60. Case C: *Dental orthopedia and cleft palate,* New York, 1921, Les L Bruder.

61. Tweed CH: Indications for the extraction of teeth in orthodontic procedure, *Angle Orthod* 30:405-428, 1944.

62. Kloehn S: Guiding alveolar growth and eruption of the teeth to reduce treatment time and produce a more balanced denture and face, *Angle Orthod* 17:10-33, 1947.

63. Proffit WR et al: *Contemporary orthodontics,* ed 2, St Louis, 1993, Mosby.

64. Gianelly AA, Goldman HM: *Biological basis of orthodontics,* Philadelphia, 1971, Lea & Febiger.

65. Iwasaki LR et al: Human tooth movement in response to continuous stress of low magnitude, *Am J Orthod Dentofacial Orthop* 117:175-183, 2000.

66. Hixon EH et al: Optimal force, differential force, and anchorage, *Am J Orthod* 55:437-457, 1969.

67. Daskalogiannakis J, McLachlan KR: Canine retraction with rare earth magnets: an investigation into the validity of the constant force hypothesis, *Am J Orthod Dentofacial Orthop* 109:489-495, 1996.

68. Graber TM, Chung DDB, Aoba JT: Dentofacial orthopedics versus orthodontics, *J Am Dent Assoc* 75:1145-1166, 1967.

69. Armstrong MM: Controlling the magnitude, direction, and duration of extraoral force, *Am J Orthod* 59:217-243, 1971.

70. Reitan K: Some factors determining the evaluation of forces in orthodontics, *Am J Orthod* 43:32-45, 1957.

71. McNamara JA, Bookstein FL, Shaughnessy TG: Skeletal and dental adaptations following functional regulator therapy, *Am J Orthod* 88:91-110, 1985.

72. Petrovic A, Stutzmann JJ, Oudet C: Control process in the postnatal growth of the condylar cartilage. In McNamara JA (ed): *Determinants of mandibular form and growth,* Monograph 4, Ann Arbor, Mich, 1975, Center for Human Growth and Development, The University of Michigan.

73. Graber TM: Extraoral force: facts and fallacies, *Am J Orthod* 41:490-505, 1955.

74. Jorgensen JO et al: Evening versus morning injections of growth hormone (GH) in GH-deficient patients: effects on 24-hour patterns of circulating hormones and metabolites, *J Clin Endocrinol Metab* 70:207-214, 1990.

75. Born J, Muth S, Fehm HL: The significance of sleep onset and slow wave sleep for nocturnal release of growth hormone (GH) and cortisol, *Psychoneuroendocrinology* 13:233-243, 1988.

76. Risinger RK, Proffit WR: Continuous overnight observation of human premolar eruption, *Arch Oral Biol* 41:779-789, 1996.

77. Stevenson S et al: Is longitudinal bone growth influenced by diurnal variation in the mitotic activity of chondrocytes of the growth plates? *J Orthop Res* 8:132-135, 1990.

78. Tulloch JFC, Phillips C, Proffit WR: Benefit of early Class II treatment: progress report of a two-phase randomized clinical trial, *Am J Orthod Dentofacial Orthop* 113:62-72, 1998.

79. Brodie AG: On the growth pattern of the human head from the third month to the eighth year of life, *Am J Anat* 68:209-262, 1941.

80. Horowitz S, Hixon E: Physiologic recovery following orthodontic treatment, *Am J Orthod* 55:1-4, 1969.

81. Wieslander L: The effects of orthodontic treatment on the concurrent development of the craniofacial complex, *Am J Orthod* 49:15-27, 1963.

82. Poulton DR: Changes in Class II malocclusions with and without occipital headgear therapy, *Angle Orthod* 29:234-250, 1959.

83. Ricketts RM: The influence of orthodontic treatment in facial growth and development, *Angle Orthod* 30:103-133, 1960.

84. Poulton DR: A three-year survey of Class II malocclusions with and without headgear therapy, *Angle Orthod* 34:181-193, 1964.

85. Creekmore TD: Inhibition or stimulation of the vertical growth of facial complex: its significance to treatment, *Angle Orthod* 37:285-297, 1967.

86. Jakobsson SO: Cephalometric evaluation of treatment effect on Class II, Division 1 malocclusions, *Am J Orthod* 53:446-457, 1967.

87. Ringenberg QM, Butts WC: A controlled cephalometric evaluation of single-arch cervical traction therapy, *Am J Orthod* 57:179-185, 1970.

88. Barton JJ: High-pull headgear vs. cervical traction: a cephalometric comparison, *Am J Orthod* 62:517-529, 1972.

89. Wieslander L: The effect of force on craniofacial development, *Am J Orthod* 65:531-538, 1974.

90. Wieslander L, Buck DL: Physiologic recovery after cervical traction therapy, *Am J Orthod* 66:294-301, 1974.

91. Cross JJ: Facial growth: before, during and following orthodontic treatment, *Am J Orthod* 71:68-78, 1977.

92. Melsen B: Effects of cervical anchorage during and after treatment: an implant study, *Am J Orthod* 73:526-540, 1978.

93. Baumrind S et al: Mandibular plane changes during maxillary retraction. Part 1, *Am J Orthod* 74:32-40, 1978.

94. Mills CM, Holman RG, Graber TM: Heavy intermittent cervical traction in Class II treatment: a longitudinal cephalometric assessment, *Am J Orthod* 74:361-379, 1978.

95. Baumrind S et al: Mandibular plane changes during maxillary retraction. Part 2, *Am J Orthod* 74:603-620, 1978.

96. Brown P: A cephalometric evaluation of high-pull molar headgear and facebow neck strap therapy, *Am J Orthod* 74:621-632, 1978.

97. Baumrind S et al: Distal displacement of the maxilla and upper first molar, *Am J Orthod* 75:630-640, 1979.

98. Baumrind S et al: Changes in facial dimensions associated with the use of forces to retract the maxilla, *Am J Orthod* 80:17-30, 1981.

99. Baumrind S et al: Quantitative analysis of the orthodontic and orthopedic effects of maxillary retraction, *Am J Orthod* 84:384-398, 1983.

100. Howard RD: Skeletal changes with extraoral traction, *Eur J Orthod* 4:197-202, 1982.

101. Firouz M, Zernik J, Nanda R: Dental and orthopedic effects of high-pull headgear in treatment of Class II, division 1 malocclusion, *Am J Orthod Dentofacial Orthop* 102:197-205, 1992.

102. Tulloch JF et al: The effect of early intervention on skeletal pattern in Class II malocclusion: a randomized clinical trial, *Am J Orthod Dentofacial Orthop* 111:391-400, 1997.

103. Ghafari J et al: Headgear versus function regulator in the early treatment of Class II, division 1 malocclusion: a randomized clinical trial, *Am J Orthod Dentofacial Orthop* 113:51-61, 1998.

104. Sproule WR: Dentofacial changes produced by extraoral cervical traction to the maxilla of the Macaca mulatta: a histologic and serial cephalometric study, *Am J Orthod* 56:532-533, 1969.

105. Fredrick DL: *Dentofacial changes produced by extraoral high-pull traction to the maxilla of the Macaca mulatta: a histologic and serial cephalometric study,* thesis, Seattle, 1969, University of Washington.

106. Droschl H: The effect of heavy orthopaedic forces on the maxilla of the growing Siamiri sciureus (squirrel monkey), *Am J Orthod* 63:449-461, 1973.

107. Thompson RW: Extraoral high-pull forces with rigid palatal expansion in the Macaca mulatta, *Am J Orthod* 66:302-317, 1974.

108. Elder JR, Tuenge RH: Cephalometric and histologic changes produced by extra-oral high pull traction to the maxilla of Macaca mulatta, *Am J Orthod* 66:599-617, 1974.

109. Meldrum RJ: Alterations in the upper facial growth of Macaca mulatta resulting from high-pull headgear, *Am J Orthod* 67:393-411, 1975.

110. Yamamoto J: Effects of extraoral forces in the dentofacial complex of the Macaca irus, *Nippon Kyosei Shika Gakkai Zasshi* 34:173-197, 1975.

111. Triftshauser R, Walters RD: Cervical retraction of the maxilla in the Macaca mulatta monkey, *Angle Orthod* 46:37-46, 1976.

112. Brandt HC, Shapiro PA, Kokich VG: Experimental and postexperimental effects of posteriorly directed extraoral traction in adult Macaca fascicularis, *Am J Orthod* 75:301-317, 1979.

113. Petrovic AG, Stutzmann JJ: Research methodology and findings in applied craniofacial growth studies. In Graber TM et al (eds): *Dentofacial orthopedics with functional appliances,* ed 2, St Louis, 1997, Mosby.

114. John JP: Change in form and size in the mandible in the orthopedically treated Macaca iris (an experimental study), *Trans Eur Orthod Soc* 161-173, 1968.

115. Baumrind S, Korn EL: Patterns of change in mandibular and facial shape associated with the use of forces to retract the maxilla, *Am J Orthod* 80:31-47, 1981.

116. Ben-Bassat Y, Baumrind S, Korn EL: Mandibular molar displacement secondary to the use of forces to retract the maxilla, *Am J Orthod* 89:1-12, 1986.

117. Keeling SD et al: Anteroposterior skeletal and dental changes after early Class II treatment with bionators and headgear, *Am J Orthod Dentofacial Orthop* 113:40-50, 1998.

118. Björk A: Prediction of mandibular growth rotation, *Am J Orthod* 55:585-599, 1969.

119. Robin P: Observation sur un novel appareil de redressement, *Rev Stomatol* 9:561-590, 1902.

120. Herbst E: Dreissigjährige erfahrungen mit dem retentions-scharnier, *Zahnärztl Rundschau* 43:1515-1524, 1563-1568, 1611-1616, 1934.

121. Andresen V: Beitrag zur retention, *Z Zahnaertzl Orthop* 3:121, 1910.

122. Andresen V, Häupl K: *Funktionskieferorthopädie: die grundlagen des "norwegischen systems,"* ed 2, Leipzig, 1939, H. Meusser.

123. Fränkel R: The theoretical concept underlying treatment with function correctors, *Trans Eur Orthod Soc* 233-250, 1966.

123a. Evald H, Harvold EP: The effect of activators on maxillary-mandibular growth and relationships, *Am J Orthod* 52:857, 1966.

124. Woodside DG: The activator. In Graber TM, Neumann B (eds): *Removable orthodontic appliances,* Philadelphia, 1977, WB Saunders.

125. Balters W: Ergebnis der gesteuerten selbstheilung von kieferorthopädischen anomalien, *Dtsch Zahnaerztl* 15:241, 1960.

126. Rakosi T: The bionator: a modified activator. In Graber TM et al (eds): *Dentofacial orthopedics with functional appliances,* ed 2, St Louis, 1997, Mosby.

127. Clark WJ: The twin block traction technique, *Eur J Orthod* 4:129-138, 1982.

128. Fränkel R: The treatment of Class II Division 1 malocclusion with functional correctors, *Am J Orthod* 55:265-275, 1969.

129. Pancherz H: The modern Herbst appliance. In Graber TM et al (eds): *Dentofacial orthopedics with functional appliances,* ed 2, St Louis, 1997, Mosby.

130. Pancherz H: Treatment of Class II malocclusion by jumping the bite with the Herbst appliance, *Am J Orthod* 76:423-442, 1979.

131. Jasper JJ, McNamara JA: The correction of interarch malocclusions using a fixed force module, *Am J Orthod Dentofacial Orthop* 108:641-650, 1995.

132. Orton HS: *Functional appliances in orthodontic treatment: an atlas of clinical prescription and laboratory construction,* London, 1990, Quintessence Publishing.

133. Skeiller V: Expansion of the midpalatal suture by removable plates, analysed by the implant method, *Trans Eur Orthod Soc* 143, 1964.

134. McDougall PD, McNamara JA, Dierkes JM: Arch width development in Class II patients treated with the Fränkel appliance, *Am J Orthod* 82:10-22, 1982.

135. Briedon CM, Pangrazio-Kulbersh V, Kulbersh R: Maxillary skeletal and dental change with Fränkel appliance therapy: an implant study, *Angle Orthod* 54:226-232, 1984.

136. McNamara JA, Howe RP, Dischinger TG: A comparison of the Herbst and Fränkel appliances in the treatment of Class II malocclusion, *Am J Orthod Dentofacial Orthop* 98:134-144, 1990.

137. Pancherz H: The mechanism of Class II correction and Herbst appliance treatment: a cephalometric investigation, *Am J Orthod* 83:104-113, 1982.

138. Petrovic AG: Experimental and cybernetic approaches to the mechanism of action of functional appliances on mandibular growth. In McNamara JA, Ribbens KA (eds): *Malocclusion and the periodontium,* Monograph 15, Ann Arbor, Mich, 1984, Center for Human Growth and Development, The University of Michigan.

139. McNamara JA, Bryan FA: Long-term mandibular adaptations to protrusive function in the rhesus monkey (Macaca mulatta), *Am J Orthod Dentofacial Orthop* 92:98-108, 1987.

140. Breitner C: Experimental change of the mesio-distal relations of the upper and lower dental arches, *Angle Orthod* 3:67-76, 1933.

141. Breitner C: Bone changes resulting from experimental orthodontic treatment, *Am J Orthod* 26:521-527, 1940.

142. Charlier JP, Petrovic A: Recherches sur la mandibule de rat en culture d'organes: le cartilage condylien a-t-il un potentiel de croissance indépendant? *Orthod Fr* 38:165-175, 1967.

143. Charlier JP, Petrovic A, Hermann-Stutzmann J: Effects of mandibular hyperpropulsion on the prechondroblastic zone of young rat condyle, *Am J Orthod* 55:71-74, 1969.

144. Derichsweiler H: Experimentelle tieruntersuchungen über veränderungen des kiefergelenkes bei bisslage-veränderung, *Fortschr Kieferorthop* 19:30-44, 1958.

145. Vogel G, Pignanelli M: Indagini istochimiche sull' Articolazione T.M. del Macacus rhesus in corso di trattamento gnato-orthopedico, *Pass Int Stomatol Prat* 9:46-50, 1958.

146. Baume LJ, Derichsweiler H: Is the condylar growth center responsive to orthodontic therapy? *Oral Surg* 14:347-362, 1961.

147. Joho JP: Changes in form and size of the mandible in the orthopaedically treated Macacus Irus (an experimental study), *Rep Congr Eur Orthod Soc* 44:161-173, 1968.

148. Stöckli P, Willert HG: Tissue reactions in the temporomandibular joint resulting from anterior displacement of the mandible in the monkey, *Am J Orthod* 60:142-155, 1971.

149. Elgoyhen JC et al: Craniofacial adaptation to protrusive function in young rhesus monkeys, *Am J Orthod* 62:469-480, 1972.

150. McNamara JA: *Neuromuscular and skeletal adaptations to altered orofacial function,* Monograph 1, Ann Arbor, Mich, 1972, Center for Human Growth and Development, The University of Michigan.

151. McNamara JA: Neuromuscular and skeletal adaptations to altered function in the orofacial region, *Am J Orthod* 64:578-606, 1973.

152. McNamara JA: Functional adaptability of the temporomandibular joint, *Dent Clin North Am* 19:457-471, 1975.

153. McNamara JA, Connelly TG, McBride MC: Histological studies of temporomandibular joint adaptations. In McNamara JA (ed): *Determinants of mandibular form and growth*, Monograph 4, Craniofacial Growth Series, Ann Arbor, Mich, 1975, Center for Human Growth and Development, University of Michigan.

154. McNamara JA, Carlson DS: Quantitative analysis of temporomandibular joint adaptations to protrusive function, *Am J Orthod* 76:593-611, 1979.

155. McNamara JA: Functional determinants of craniofacial size and shape, *Eur J Orthod* 2:131-159, 1980.

156. Woodside DG et al: Primate experiments in malocclusion and bone induction, *Am J Orthod* 83:460-468, 1983.

157. Petrovic A: Mechanisms and regulation of mandibular condylar growth, *Acta Morphol Neerl Scand* 10:25-34, 1972.

158. Petrovic A, Stutzmann J: Further investigations into the functioning of the "comparator" of the servosystem in the control of the condylar cartilage growth rate and the lengthening of the jaw. In McNamara (ed): *The biology of occlusal development*, Monograph 7, Ann Arbor, Mich, 1977, Center for Human Growth and Development, The University of Michigan.

159. Petrovic A, Stutzmann JJ, Gasson N: The final length of the mandible: is it genetically determined? In Carlson DS (ed): *Craniofacial biology*, Monograph 10, Ann Arbor, Mich, 1981, Center for Human Growth and Development, The University of Michigan.

160. Marschner JF, Harris JE: Mandibular growth and Class II treatment, *Angle Orthod* 36:89-93, 1966.

161. Parkhouse RC: A cephalometric appraisal of cases of Angle's Class II, Division I malocclusion treated by the Andresen appliance, *Dent Pract Dent Rec* 19:425-433, 1969.

162. Woodside DG et al: Some effects of activator treatment on the growth rate of the mandible and the position of the midface. In Cook JT (ed): *Transactions of the third international orthodontic congress*, St Louis, 1975, Mosby.

163. Pancherz H: The effect of continuous bite-jumping on the dentofacial complex: a follow-up study after Herbst appliance treatment of Class II malocclusion, *Eur J Orthod* 3:49-60, 1981.

164. Luder HU: Effects of activator treatment: evidence for the occurrence of two different types of reaction, *Eur J Orthod* 3:205-222, 1981.

165. Righellis EG: Treatment effects of Fränkel, activator and extraoral traction appliances, *Angle Orthod* 53:107-121, 1983.

166. Wieslander L: Intensive treatment of severe Class II malocclusions with a headgear-Herbst appliance in the early mixed dentition, *Am J Orthod* 86:1-13, 1984.

167. McNamara JA, Bookstein FL, Shaughnessy TG: Skeletal and dental relationships following functional regulator therapy on Class II patients, *Am J Orthod* 88:91-110, 1985.

168. Remmer KR et al: Cephalometric changes associated with treatment using the activator, the Fränkel appliance, and the fixed appliance, *Am J Orthod* 88:363-372, 1985.

169. DeVincenzo JP, Huffer R, Winn M: A study in human subjects using a new device designed to mimic the protrusive functional appliances used previously in monkeys, *Am J Orthod Dentofacial Orthop* 91:213-224, 1987.

170. Jakobsson SO, Paulin G: The influence of activator treatment on skeletal growth in Angle Class II: 1 cases: a roentgenocephalometric study, *Eur J Orthod* 12:174-184, 1990.

171. Björk A: The principle of the Andresen method of orthodontic treatment: a discussion based on cephalometric x-ray analysis of treated cases, *Am J Orthod* 37:437-458, 1951.

172. Softley J: Cephalometric changes in seven "post normal" cases treated by the Andresen method, *Dent Record* 73:485-494, 1953.

173. Björk A: Variability and age changes in overjet and overbite: report from a follow-up study of individuals from 12 to 20 years of age, *Am J Orthod* 39:779-801, 1953.

174. Meach CL: A cephalometric comparison of bony profile changes in Class II, division 1 patients treated with extraoral force and functional jaw orthopedics, *Am J Orthod* 52:353-370, 1966.

175. Trayfoot J, Richardson A: Angle Class II Division 1 malocclusions treated by the Andresen method: an analysis of 17 cases, *Br Dent J* 124:516-519, 1968.

176. Hasund A: The use of activators in a system employing fixed appliances, *Rep Congr Eur Orthod Soc* 329-341, 1969.

177. Harvold EP, Vargervik K: Morphogenetic response to activator treatment, *Am J Orthod* 60:478-490, 1971.

178. Stöckli PW, Dietrich UC: Sensation and morphogenesis: experimental and clinical findings following functional forward displacement of the mandible, *Trans Eur Orthod Soc* 435-442, 1973.

179. Woodside DG: Some effects of activator treatment on the mandible and the midface, *Trans Eur Orthod Soc* 443-447, 1973.

180. Dietrich UC: Aktivator: mandibuläre reaktion, *Schweiz Monatsschr Zahnheilkd* 83:1093-1104, 1973.

181. Wieslander L, Lagerström L: The effect of activator treatment on class II malocclusions, *Am J Orthod* 75:20-26, 1979.

182. Forsberg CM, Odenrick L: Skeletal and soft tissue response to activator treatment, *Eur J Orthod* 3:247-253, 1981.

183. Calvert FJ: An assessment of Andresen therapy on class II division 1 malocclusion, *Br J Orthod* 9:149-153, 1982.

184. Creekmore TD, Radney LJ: Fränkel appliance therapy: orthopedic or orthodontic? *Am J Orthod* 83:89-108, 1983.

185. Gianelly AA et al: Mandibular growth, condyle position, and Fränkel appliance therapy, *Angle Orthod* 53:131-142, 1983.

186. Janson I: Skeletal and dentoalveolar changes in patients treated with a bionator during prepubertal and pubertal growth. In McNamara JA, Ribbens KA, Howe RP (eds): *Clinical alteration of the growing face*, Monograph 14, Craniofacial Growth Series, Ann Arbor, Mich, 1983, Center for Human Growth and Development, University of Michigan.

187. Mills JRE: Clinical control of craniofacial growth: a skeptic view point. In McNamara JA, Ribbens KA, Howe RP (eds): *Clinical alteration of the growing face*, Monograph 14, Craniofacial Growth Series, Ann Arbor, Mich, 1983, Center for Human Growth and Development, University of Michigan.

188. Looi LK, Mills JR: The effect of two contrasting forms of orthodontic treatment on the facial profile, *Am J Orthod* 89:507-517, 1986.

189. Nelson C, Harkness M, Herbisson P: Mandibular changes during functional appliance treatment, *Am J Orthod Dentofacial Orthop* 104:153-161, 1993.

190. Moss JP: Cephalometric changes during functional appliance therapy, *Trans Eur Orthod Soc* 327-341, 1962.

191. Reference deleted in proofs.

192. Freunthaller P: Cephalometric observations in Class II, Division I malocclusions treated with the activator, *Angle Orthod* 37:18-25, 1967.

193. Hotz R: Application and appliance manipulation of functional forces, *Am J Orthod* 58:459-478, 1970.

194. Ahlgren J, Laurin C: Late results of activator-treatment: a cephalometric study, *Br J Orthod* 3:181-187, 1976.

195. Woodside DG, Metaxas A, Altuna G: The influence of functional appliance therapy on glenoid fossa remodeling, *Am J Orthod Dentofacial Orthop* 92:181-198, 1987.

196. Teuscher UM: A growth-related concept for skeletal Class II treatment, *Am J Orthod* 74:258-275, 1978.

197. Stöckli PW, Teuscher UM: Combined activator headgear orthopedics. In Graber TM, Swain BF (eds): *Orthodontics: current principles and techniques*, St Louis, 1985, Mosby.

198. Bass NM: Dento-facial orthopaedics in the correction of the class II malocclusion, *Br J Orthod* 9:3-31, 1982.

199. Lagerström LO et al: Dental and skeletal contributions to occlusal correction in patients treated with the high-pull headgear-activator combination, *Am J Orthod Dentofacial Orthop* 97:495-504, 1990.

200. Andreasen GF, Bishara SE: Comparison of alastik chains and elastics involved with intra-arch molar to molar forces, *Angle Orthod* 40:151-158, 1970.

201. Petrovic AG, Stutzmann JJ: Timing aspects of orthodontic treatment, *Bull Orthod Soc Yugoslav* 26:25-36, 1993.

202. Petrovic AG: Auxologic categorization and chronologic specification for the choice of appropriate orthodontic treatment, *Am J Orthod Dentofacial Orthop* 105:192-205, 1994.

203. Hanes RA: Bony profile changes resulting from cervical traction compared with those resulting from intermaxillary elastics, *Am J Orthod* 45:353-364, 1959.

204. Roberts WE, Nelson CL, Goodacre CJ: Rigid implant anchorage to close a mandibular first molar extraction site, *J Clin Orthod* 18:693-704, 1994.

205. Gianelly AA, Vaitas AS, Thomas WM: The use of magnets to move molars distally, *Am J Orthod Dentofacial Orthop* 96:161-167, 1989.

206. Gianelly AA, Bednar J, Dietz VS: Japanese Ni-Ti coils used to move molars distally, *Am J Orthod Dentofacial Orthop* 99:564-566, 1991.

207. Gianelly AA: Distal movement of the maxillary molars, *Am J Orthod Dentofacial Orthop* 114:66-72, 1998.

208. Hilgers JJ: The pendulum appliance for Class II non-compliance therapy, *J Clin Orthod* 26:706-714, 1992.

209. Keleş A, Sayinsu K: A new approach in maxillary molar distalization: intraoral bodily molar distalizer, *Am J Orthod Dentofacial Orthop* 117:39-48, 2000.

210. Andreasen G, Naessig C: Experimental findings on mesial relapse of maxillary first molars, *Angle Orthod* 38:51-55, 1968.

211. Odham J et al: Osseointegrated titanium implants: a new approach in orthodontic treatment, *Eur J Orthod* 10:98-105, 1988.

212. Wehrbein H, Feifel H, Diedrich P: Palatal implant anchorage reinforcement of posterior teeth: a prospective study, *Am J Orthod Dentofacial Orthop* 116: 678-686, 1999.

213. Costa A, Raffaini M, Melsen B: Miniscrews as orthodontic anchorage: a preliminary report, *Int J Adult Orthod Orthognath Surg* 13:201-209, 1998.

214. Block MS, Hoffman DR: A new device for absolute anchorage for orthodontics, *Am J Orthod Dentofacial Orthop* 107:251-258, 1995.

215. Johnston LE: Growth and the Class II patient: rendering unto Caesar, *Semin Orthod* 4:59-62, 1998.

216. Bishara SE, Justus R, Graber TM: Proceedings of the workshop discussions on early treatment, *Am J Orthod Dentofacial Orthop* 113:5-6, 1998.

217. Yang EY, Kiyak HA: Orthodontic treatment timing: a survey of orthodontists, *Am J Orthod Dentofacial Orthop* 113:96-103, 1998.

218. Bowman SJ: One-stage versus two-stage treatment: are two really necessary? *Am J Orthod Dentofacial Orthop* 113:111-116, 1998.

219. Vig PS, Vig KD: Decision analysis to optimize the outcomes for Class II Division 1 orthodontic treatment, *Semin Orthod* 1:139-148, 1995.

220. Livieratos FA, Johnston LE: A comparison of one-stage and two-stage nonextraction alternatives in matched Class II samples, *Am J Orthod Dentofacial Orthop* 108:118-131, 1995.

221. McKnight MM, Daniels CP, Johnston LE: A retrospective study of two-stage treatment outcomes assessed with two modified PAR indices, *Angle Orthod* 68:521-526, 1998.

222. Tulloch JFC, Medland W, Tuncay OC: Methods used to evaluate growth modification in Class II malocclusion, *Am J Orthod Dentofacial Orthop* 98:340-347, 1990.

223. Trauner R, Obwegeser H: The surgical correction of mandibular prognathism and retrognathia with consideration of genioplasty, *Oral Surg* 10:787-792, 1957.

224. Hunsuck EE: A modified intra-oral sagittal splitting technique for correction of mandibular prognathism, *J Oral Surg* 26:249-252, 1968.

225. Epker BN: Modifications in the sagittal osteotomy of the mandible, *J Oral Surg* 35:157-159, 1977.

226. Caldwell JB, Hayward JR, Lister RL: Correction of mandibular retrognathia by vertical L-osteotomy: a new technique, *J Oral Surg* 26:259-264, 1968.

227. Hayes P: Correction of retrognathia by modified "C" osteotomy of the ramus and sagittal osteotomy of the mandibular body, *J Oral Surg* 31:682-686, 1973.

228. Hofer O: Die vertikale osteotomies sur verlangerung des einseitig verkurzten aufsteigenden unterkieferastes, *Z Stomatol* 34:826-829, 1936.

229. Köle H: Surgical operations on the alveolar ridge to correct occlusal abnormalities, *Oral Surg* 12:277-288, 1959.

230. MacIntosh RB: Total mandibular alveolar osteotomy, *J Max Fac Surg* 2:210-218, 1974.

231. Frost DE, Fonseca RJ, Koutnik AW: Total subapical osteotomy: a modification of the surgical technique, *Int J Adult Orthod Orthognath Surg* 2:119-128, 1986.

232. Bell WH: LeForte I osteotomy for correction of maxillary deformities, *J Oral Surg* 33:412-426, 1975.

233. Schuchardt K: Experiences with the surgical treatment of deformities of the jaws: prognathia, micrognathia, and open bite. In Wallace AG (ed): *Second Congress of International Society of Plastic Surgeons*, London, 1959, E & S Livingstone.

234. Obwegeser H: Surgical correction of small or retrodisplaced maxillae, *Plast Reconstr Surg* 43:351-365, 1969.

235. Bell WH: Revascularization and bone healing after anterior maxillary osteotomy: a study using rhesus monkeys, *J Oral Surg* 27:249-255, 1969.

236. Bell WH, Levy BM: Revascularization and bone healing after posterior maxillary oseotomy, *J Oral Surg* 29:313-320, 1971.

237. Bell WH: Correction of skeletal type anterior open bite, *J Oral Surg* 29:706-714, 1971.

238. Cohn-Stock G: Die chirurgische immediatre-gulierung der Kiefer, speziell die chirvrgische Behandlung der Prognathie, *Vjschr Zahnheilk Berlin* 37:320, 1921.

239. Murphey PJ, Walker RV: Correction of maxillary protrusion by ostectomy and orthodontic therapy, *J Oral Surg* 21:275-290, 1963.

240. Mohnac AM: Maxillary osteotomy in the management of occlusal deformities, *J Oral Surg* 24:305-317, 1966.

241. Bell WH: Correction of maxillary excess by anterior maxillary osteotomy, *Oral Surg* 43:323-332, 1977.

242. Wassmund J: *Lehrbuch der praktischen chirurgie des Mundes und der Kierfer*, vol 1, Leipzig, 1935, Meusser.

243. Wunderer S: Erfahrungen mit der operativen Behandlung hochgradiger prognathien, *Dtsch Zahn-Mund Kieferheilk* 39:451, 1963.

244. Turvey TA: Simultaneous mobilization of the maxilla and mandible: surgical technique and results, *J Oral Maxillofac Surg* 40:96-99, 1982.

245. Richmond S et al: The development of the PAR Index (peer assessment rating): reliability and validity, *Eur J Orthod* 14:125-139, 1992.

246. Buchanan IB et al: A comparison of the reliability and validity of the PAR index and Summer's occlusal index, *Eur J Orthod* 15:27-31, 1993.

247. Otuyemi OD, Jones SP: Long-term evaluation of treated class II division 1 malocclusions utilizing the PAR index, *Br J Orthod* 22:171-178, 1995.

248. O'Brien KD et al: The effectiveness of Class II, division 1 treatment, *Am J Orthod Dentofacial Orthop* 107:329-334, 1995.

249. McGorray SP et al: Evaluation of orthodontists' perception of treatment need and the peer assessment rating (PAR) index, *Angle Orthod* 69:325-333, 1999.

250. Burden DJ et al: Predictors of outcome among patients with class II division 1 malocclusion treated with fixed appliances in the permanent dentition, *Am J Orthod Dentofacial Orthop* 116:452-459, 1999.

251. Richmond S et al: The PAR index (Peer Assessment Rating): methods to determine outcome of orthodontic treatment in terms of improvement and standards, *Eur J Orthod* 14:180-187, 1992.

252. Richmond S et al: Calibration of dentists in the use of occlusal indices, *Community Dent Oral Epidemiol* 23:173-176, 1995.

253. DeGuzman L et al: The validation of the Peer Assessment Rating index for malocclusion severity and treatment difficulty, *Am J Orthod Dentofacial Orthop* 107:172-176, 1995.

254. Turbill EA, Richmond S, Wright JL: Assessment of General Dental Services orthodontic standards: the Dental Practice Board's gradings compared to PAR and IOTN, *Br J Orthod* 23:211-220, 1996.

255. Turbill EA, Richmond S, Wright JL: A critical assessment of orthodontic standards in England and Wales (1990-1991) in relation to changes in prior approval, *Br J Orthod* 23:221-228, 1996.

256. Collins FS et al: New goals for the U. S. Human Genome Project: 1998-2003, *Science* 282:682-689, 1998.

257. Burley SK et al: Structural genomics: beyond the human genome project, *Nat Genet* 23:151-157, 1999.

CHAPTER 21

Treatment of Class III Malocclusion in the Primary and Mixed Dentitions

Peter Ngan

KEY TERMS

Class III malocclusion	etiology	growth prediction
frequency	diagnosis	

Angle first published his classification of malocclusion in 1899[1] based solely on the dental arch relationship using study casts. According to Angle, Class I occlusion occurred when the mesiobuccal cusp of the upper first permanent molar occluded on the buccal groove of the lower first molar. **Class III malocclusion** occurred when the lower teeth occluded mesial to their normal relationship the width of one premolar or even more in extreme cases. Jaw discrepancies were also described by Goddard[2], Dewey[3], Hellman[4], and Moore.[5] Individual Class III cases were characterized as having a retruded maxilla or a prognathic mandible and, in some cases, by a combination of the two.

With the advent of cephalometric radiography in 1931, it was possible to discern the underlying skeletal pattern of the Class III malocclusion.[6] Tweed[7] divided Class III malocclusions into two categories; pseudo Class III malocclusions with normally shaped mandibles and underdeveloped maxillae and skeletal Class III malocclusions with large mandibles. Moyers[8] further classified Class III malocclusion according to the cause of the problem: osseous, muscular, or dental in origin. For patients with neuromuscular or "functional" malocclusions, Moyers emphasized the need to determine whether the mandible, on closure, is in centric relation or in a "convenient" anterior position. Anterior positioning generally results from tooth contact relationships which "force" the mandible into a forward position. In contrast, centric relation is determined by the muscles, the ligaments, and the temporomandibular joint (TMJ) anatomy under the control of the nervous system.

FREQUENCY OF CLASS III MALOCCLUSION

The **frequency** of Class III malocclusion varies among different ethnic groups. The incidence in Caucasians ranges between 1% and 4% depending on the method of classifying the malocclusion and the age group evaluated.[9-19] In a study of Swedish children between 7 and 13 years of age, the frequency was found to be 4.2% when classified according to the molar relationships. However, only one third of these children were found to have an anterior crossbite.[17] In older children between 14 and 18 years, the percentage of Class III malocclusion was found to be higher (9.4%).[13]

In African Americans the frequency of Class III malocclusion ranges between 5% and 8%.[20-24] However, one study showed that the incidence of Class III malocclusion in the rural and suburban Nigerian children was only 1%.[24]

In Asian societies the frequency of Class III malocclusion is higher because of a large percentage of patients with maxillary deficiency. The incidence of

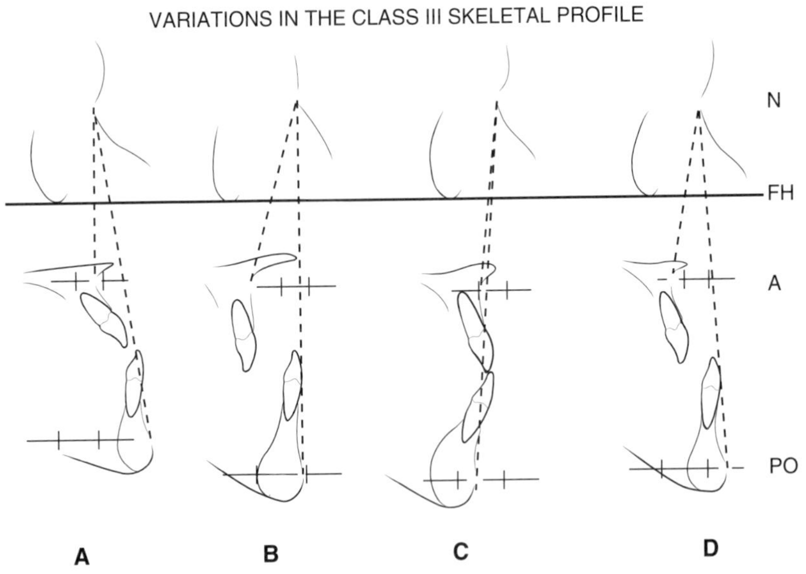

VARIATIONS IN THE CLASS III SKELETAL PROFILE

Figure 21-1 Tracings of four different types of Class III facial skeletal profiles. **A,** Normal maxilla and mandibular prognathism. **B,** Maxillary retrusion and normal mandible. **C,** Normal maxilla and mandible. **D,** Maxillary retrusion and mandibular prognathism. (From Ngan P et al: *Am J Orthod Dentofacial Orthop* 109:38-49, 1996.)

this malocclusion ranges between 4% and 13% among the Japanese[25] and 4% and 14% among the Chinese.[26-29] Few studies separate skeletal Class III malocclusion from pseudo Class III malocclusion. According to a study by Lin[29] on the prevalence of malocclusion in Chinese children age 9 to 15 years, the incidence of pseudo and true Class III malocclusion was 2.3% and 1.7%, respectively.

ETIOLOGY OF CLASS III MALOCCLUSION

The few studies of human inheritance and its role in the **etiology** of Class III malocclusion support the belief that growth and the size of the mandible are affected by heredity.[30,31] McGuigan[32] described the most well-known example of inheritance, the Hapsburg family, having the distinct characteristics of a prognathic lower jaw. Of the 40 members of the family for whom records were available, 33 showed prognathic mandibles. In 1970 Litton et al[30] studied the families of 51 individuals with Class III anomalies and concluded that the dental Class III characteristics were related to genetic inheritance in offspring and siblings.[30]

In addition, Rakosi and Schilli[33] suggested a role for environmental influences such as habits and mouth breathing in the etiology of Class III malocclusion. They hypothesized that excessive mandibular growth could arise as a result of abnormal mandibular posture because constant distraction of the mandibular condyle from the fossa may be a growth stimulus.

COMPONENTS OF CLASS III MALOCCLUSION

Individuals with Class III malocclusion may have combinations of skeletal and dentoalveolar components (Figure 21-1). Consideration of the various components is essential so that the underlying cause of the discrepancy can be treated appropriately. Taking into account the position of the maxilla, the mandible, the maxillary alveolus, the mandibular alveolus, and the vertical development and giving to each three possible values (plus, zero, and minus), Ellis and McNamara[34] have calculated 243 possible combinations of Class III malocclusion. Figure 21-2 shows examples of Class III malocclusion associated with various combinations of anteroposterior and vertical problems. Guyer et al[35] conducted a cephalometric study to identify the various types of skeletal Class III patterns between 13- and 15-year-old children. They found that approximately 57% of the patients with either a normal or prognathic mandible showed a deficiency in the maxilla. Masaki,[36] in a comparative study of native Japanese and Americans of Northern European ancestry, reported that maxillary skeletal retrusion occurred more often in Asians. In a sample of Chinese patients, Wu, Peng, and Lin[37] found the percentage of skeletal Class III malocclusion with maxillary retrusion to be as high as 75%. The Asian patients with Class III malocclusion typically had a more retrusive facial profile and a longer lower anterior facial height. A backward rotation of the mandible was often observed to accommodate the relatively smaller maxilla.

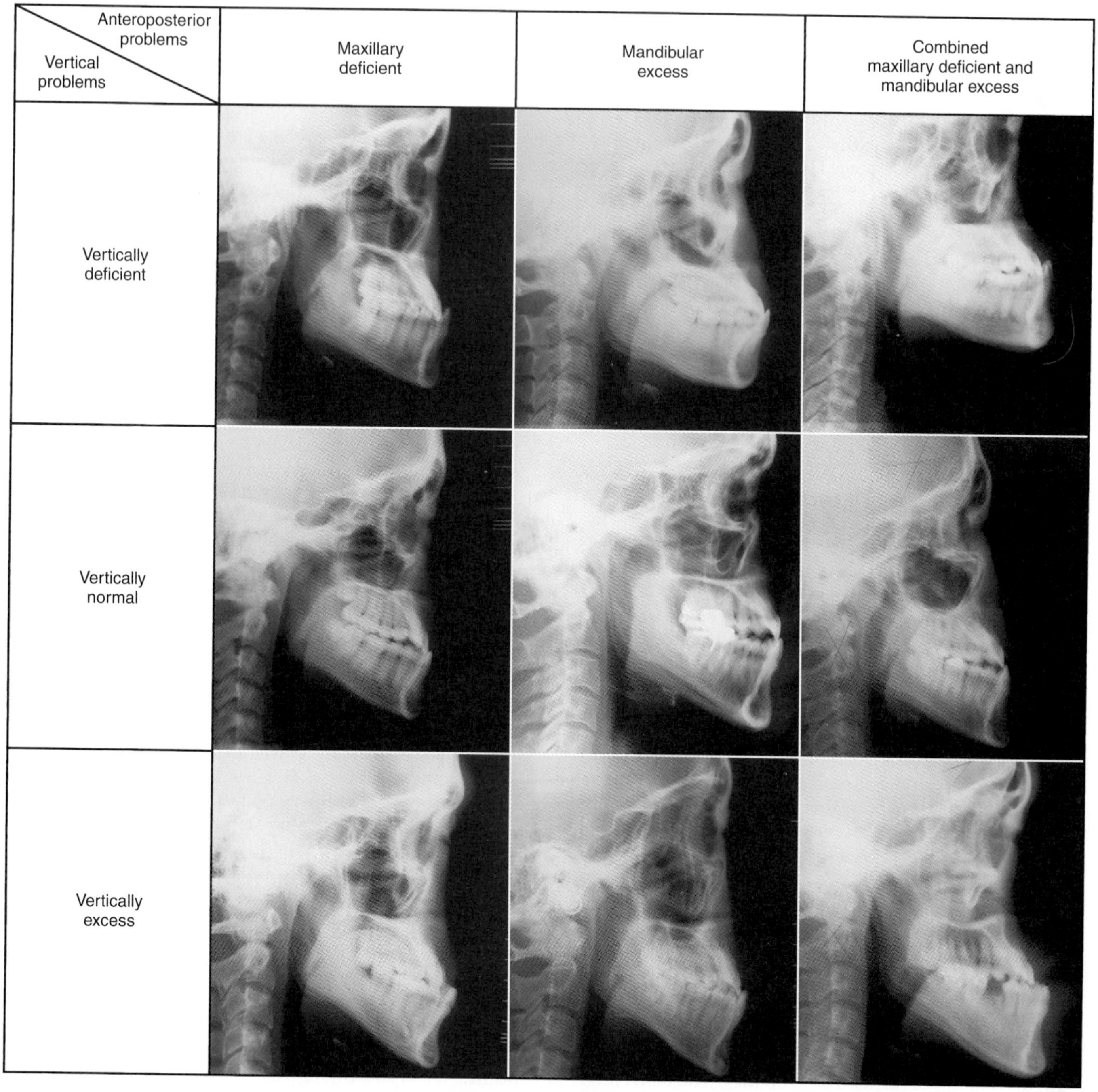

Figure 21-2 Examples of Class III malocclusion caused by various combinations of anteroposterior and vertical problems.

DIFFERENTIAL DIAGNOSIS OF CLASS III MALOCCLUSION

In evaluating the Class III relationship during the primary or mixed dentition period, it is important to consider whether the problem is dentoalveolar or skeletal in origin (Box 21-1). The possibility of treatment at this time must be weighed carefully for certain cases. In the **diagnosis** of Class III malocclusions, patients may present with Class III symptoms such as multiple teeth in anterior crossbite, minimal overjet, or lingually inclined lower incisors. In summary, anterior crossbites may be caused by the improper inclination of the maxillary and mandibular incisors, occlusal interferences (functional), or skeletal discrepancies of the maxilla or the mandible.

BOX 21-1	Differentiating a Dental Crossbite from a Skeletal Crossbite (Figure 21-3)

I. Dental assessment: Check if the Class III molar relationship is accompanied by a negative overjet. If a positive overjet or end-to-end incisal relationship is found with retroclined mandibular incisors, a compensated Class III malocclusion is suspected (i.e., upper incisors are proclined and lower incisors are retroclined to compensate for the skeletal discrepancy). If a negative overjet is found, proceed to functional assessment.

II. Functional assessment: Assess the relationship of the mandible to the maxilla to determine whether a centric relation(CR) or centric occlusion (CO) discrepancy exists. Anterior positioning of the mandible may result from an abnormal tooth contact that forces the mandible forward. Patients with a forward shift of the mandible on closure may have a Class I skeletal pattern, normal facial profile, and Class I molar relationship in CR but a Class III skeletal and dental pattern in CO—a situation referred to as *pseudo Class III malocclusion*. Elimination of CO-CR shift should reveal whether it is a simple Class I malocclusion or a compensated Class III malocclusion. On the other hand, a patient with no shift on closure most likely has a true Class III malocclusion.

III. Profile assessment: A profile evaluation involves an analysis of the facial proportions, chin position, midface position, and vertical proportion.[38] Figure 21-4 shows a method of evaluating the facial profile of patients with a Class III malocclusion.

A. Is the overall profile convex, straight, or concave? Patients with maxillary deficiency usually have a concave profile, evidenced by a flattening of the infraorbital rim and the area adjacent to the nose.

B. By blocking out the upper and lower lips, evaluate the chin position with reference to the nose, upper face, and forehead. Is the chin retruded or protruded? The chin should not be positioned anterior to a vertical line extending down from soft tissue glabella. However, it is important to remember that facial convexity decreases as the patient matures. A degree of chin prominence that would be normal for an adult may suggest a Class III skeletal pattern in a young child.

C. By blocking out the lower lip and chin, evaluate the midface. There should be a convexity to an imaginary line extending from the inferior border of the orbit, through the alar base of the nose, and down to the corner of the mouth. A straight or concave tissue contour indicates a midface deficiency.

D. Vertical proportion should be checked in CO and CR. The normal ratio of lower facial height to total facial height is approximately 0.55. This ratio is decreased in patients with functional shift and overclosure of the mandible.

IV. Cephalometric assessment: Cephalometric measurements can be used to confirm the contributions of the maxilla and mandible as well as the maxillary and mandibular incisors to the Class III skeletal and dental relationships. Class III malocclusion can, therefore, be categorized into dentoalveolar malrelationship, skeletal malocclusion, and pseudo Class III malocclusion.

Class III Malocclusion Caused by a Dentoalveolar Malrelationship (Figure 21-5)

In the dentoalveolar Class III malocclusion, there is no apparent sagittal skeletal discrepancy. The ANB angle is within normal limits. The problem is primarily caused by lingual tipping of the maxillary incisors and labial tipping of the mandibular incisors.

Skeletal Class III Malocclusion with Mandibular Protrusion, Maxillary Retrusion, or a Combination of Both (see Figure 21-2)

The ANB angle in the patients with skeletal Class III malocclusion is generally negative with a smaller-than-normal SNA angle or greater-than-normal SNB angle. Unfortunately, individual variations in cranial base flexure and anteroposterior displacement of nasion alter the ANB angle.[39] Alternative cephalometric values can be used to assess the anteroposterior relationship of the maxilla and mandible. These measurements include Nasion perpendicular to "A point," Wits appraisal, and effective maxillary and mandibular length. Vertically, patients with a long mandibular base usually have a large gonial angle. The incisal inclination in this type of Class III malocclusion is the opposite of that seen in the dentoalveolar Class III problem (i.e., the upper incisors are tipped labially, and the lower incisors are tipped lingually).

Pseudo Class III Malocclusion

Kwong and Lin[40] conducted a cephalometric study comparing the characteristics of patients with Class I, pseudo Class III, and skeletal Class III malocclusion (Table 21-1). Most of the cephalometric mea-

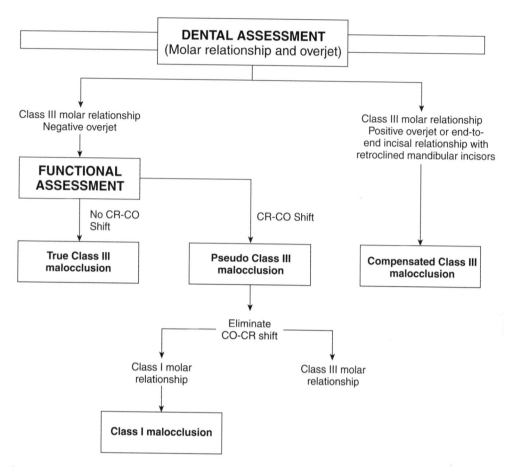

Figure 21-3 Diagnostic scheme for dental and skeletal anterior crossbites. (From Ngan P, Hu AM, Fields HW: *Pediatr Dent* 19:386-395, 1997.)

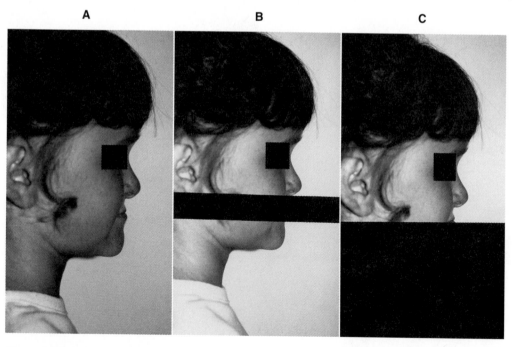

Figure 21-4 Profile evaluation of patients with Class III malocclusion. **A,** Facial profile of an 8-year-old patient with a Class III malocclusion showing concave profile and overclosure of the mandible. **B,** By blocking out upper and lower lips, the chin position should be evaluated with reference to the nose and upper face. In this patient the chin is retrusive. **C,** By blocking out the lower lip and chin, the midface should be evaluated. In this patient the maxilla is retrusive.

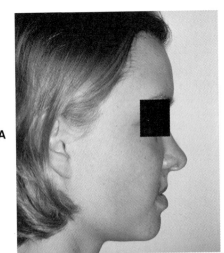

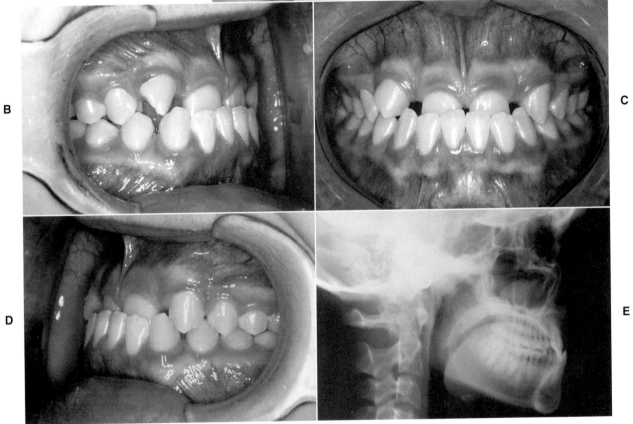

Figure 21-5 Clinical and cephalometric characteristics of a patient with dentoalveolar Class III malocclusion. **A,** Facial profile. **B** to **D,** Intraoral photographs. **E,** Lateral cephalometric radiograph.

TABLE 21-1	Cephalometric Characteristics of Patients with Class I, Pseudo Class III, and True Class III Malocclusions (in Degrees)						
		SNA	SNB	SN-MP	Gonial Angle	U1-SN	L1-MP
Class I	Mean	83.28	80.55	30.66	121.67	107.28	94.38
	SD	3.29	3.09	4.30	5.47	6.14	5.55
Pseudo Class III	Mean	81.43	81.15	33.02	120.46	109.41	91.73
	SD	3.90	3.57	4.86	5.66	5.81	6.87
True Class III	Mean	80.33	81.76	36.08	124.28	111.02	87.65
	SD	3.64	3.27	4.28	14.32	5.49	6.76

From Lin JJ: Proceedings from Advanced Symposium Mid-America Orthodontic Society, 1994.

surements suggested that pseudo Class III malocclusion is an intermediate form between Class I and skeletal Class III malocclusion. The only exception was the gonial angle, which was generally more obtuse in the skeletal Class III sample. Measurement of the gonial angle in the pseudo Class III sample was found to be rather similar to the Class I sample, making this measurement a key diagnostic feature in the differential diagnosis between pseudo and skeletal Class III malocclusions.

CLASS III SKELETAL GROWTH PATTERN

Cranial Base

Battagel[41] found the linear and angular measurements of the cranial base were decreased in patients with Class III malocclusion. Patients with a Class III malocclusion exhibited a cranial base angle (Ba-S-N) that was more acute and exhibited a more anteriorly positioned articulare compared with patients with a Class I malocclusion. In addition, the middle cranial fossa in the patient with a Class III malocclusion had a posterior and superior alignment. This alignment positions the nasomaxillary complex in a more retrusive relationship in the patient with a Class III malocclusion and contributes to a forward rotation of the mandible.

Maxilla

Patients with a Class III malocclusion commonly exhibit a decreased horizontal maxillary growth when compared with the patients with a Class I malocclusion. The horizontal "A Point" movement is approximately 0.4 mm/yr compared with 1.0 mm/yr in patients with a Class I malocclusion.

Mandible

The individual with a Class III malocclusion exhibits an increased length of the mandible, whereas the mandibular articulation is more anteriorly positioned, resulting in a more prominent lower law. The ascending ramus tends to be shorter with a steeper mandibular plane angle. The gonial angle is more obtuse in Class III malocclusions than in Class I malocclusions. The mandibular prominence along with the decreased length of the maxillary complex may accentuate the typical straight to concave profile in these cases. Typically, patients with Class III malocclusions display dentoalveolar compensation in the form of proclination of the maxillary incisors accompanied with retroclination of the mandibular incisors.

Growth Increments

Sugawara and Mitani[42] reported similar mandibular growth increments between patients with Class III and Class I malocclusions during the prepubertal, pubertal, and postpubertal growth periods. The authors concluded that Class III skeletal pattern was established at a young age and does not change fundamentally. However, the total increase in posterior cranial base in patients with prognathic mandibles was less than that in the Class I group. There was also a significant difference in the total change of the Wits appraisal between Class III and Class I individuals.

Facial growth changes in male and female patients with Class III malocclusions are different. Battagel[41] found that the largest increment of facial growth for males occurred between the ages of 14 and 16 years, whereas in female patients the maximum increment of facial growth occurred between the ages of 9.5 to 12 years, although active growth continued in the nasal area and both jaws after the age of 15 years. Female patients with Class III malocclusion possessed a more prominent mandible and an increased proclination of the maxillary incisors when compared to male patients.

CLASS III GROWTH PREDICTIONS

In 1970 Dietrich[43] reported that Class III skeletal discrepancies worsened with age. Children with a negative ANB angle were examined in three stages—stage 1, primary; stage 2, mixed; and stage 3, permanent dentition. The percentage of children with mandibular protrusion increased from 23% to 30% to 34% as the dentition progressed from stage 1 through stage 3, respectively. Maxillary anteroposterior deficiency problems went from 26% to 44% to 37%. These results indicate that the abnormal skeletal characteristics can become more pronounced with time.

Several investigators[44-46] attempted to predict the growth of Class III malocclusion. Their aim was to determine if **growth prediction** can be used to differentiate children with Class III tendency and identify a specific skeletal morphologic pattern in patients with Class III malocclusions. Certain cephalometric measurements such as cranial flexure, porion location, and ramus position have been used to predict normal or abnormal growth.[46] Unfortunately, the accuracy of these computer predictions was only 70% to 80%. Williams and Anderson[47] concluded that the diversity of skeletal patterns that result in Class III relationships explains the shortcomings of numeric predictive systems based on average incremental growth and a single formula.

Houston[48] reviewed the current status of facial growth prediction and stated, "In view of the variability of growth of most facial dimensions, detailed and accurate individualized growth prediction is not possible. The best that can be done is to base treatment planning on the existing facial pattern, allowing for average growth changes for the group to which the patient belongs." Thompson[49] pointed out the individuality in skeletal growth and that no two persons are identical—each person grows with a unique facial growth pattern.

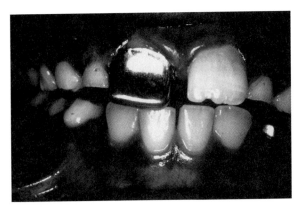

Figure 21-6 Intraoral photograph of a reverse stainless steel crown used to correct a single tooth in anterior crossbite.

INDICATIONS AND CONTRAINDICATIONS FOR EARLY CLASS III TREATMENT

The objective of early Class III treatment is to create an environment in which a more favorable dentofacial development can occur.[50] The goals of early interceptive treatment may include (1) preventing progressive, irreversible, soft tissue, or bony changes; (2) improving skeletal discrepancies and providing a more favorable environment for future growth; (3) improving occlusal function; (4) simplifying phase II comprehensive treatment and minimizing the need for orthognathic surgery; and (5) providing more pleasing facial esthetics, thus improving the psychosocial development of a child.

Turpin[51] developed a list of positive and negative factors to aid in deciding when to intercept a developing Class III malocclusion. The positive factors include good facial esthetics, mild skeletal disharmony, no familial prognathism, anteroposterior functional shift, convergent facial type, symmetric condylar growth, and growing patients with expected good cooperation. The negative factors include poor facial esthetics, severe skeletal disharmony, familial pattern established, no anteroposterior shift, divergent facial type, asymmetric growth, growth complete, and expected poor cooperation. The author recommends that early treatment should be considered for a patient that presents with characteristics listed in the positive column. For individuals who present with characteristics in the negative column, treatment can be delayed until growth is completed. Patients should be aware of the fact that surgery may be necessary at a later date, even when an initial phase of treatment may be successful.

TREATMENT OF PSEUDO CLASS III MALOCCLUSION

Patients with pseudo Class III malocclusion often present with anterior crossbites that are caused by a premature tooth contact or improper positioning of the maxillary and mandibular incisors and the temporomandibular joint. Elimination of the CO-CR discrepancy may avoid abnormal wear and traumatic occlusal forces to the affected teeth, avoid potential adverse growth influences in the maxilla and mandible, improve maxillary lip posture and facial appearance, and avoid abnormal posterior occlusion, which may develop as a result of habitual posturing of the mandible to accommodate the abnormal anterior occlusal contacts.

Early on, reverse stainless steel crown was used to correct a single tooth in anterior crossbite (Figure 21-6).[52] An oversized permanent lateral incisor preformed crown form is trimmed and contoured at the gingival margin to fit snugly over the maxillary primary tooth or teeth in crossbite. The crown is cemented in reverse (i.e., facial to lingual) with polycarboxylate cement. One drawback of this method is the nonesthetic appearance of the stainless steel crowns. With the advent of bonded resin composite, the stainless steel crown can be replaced by bonded composite resin slopes for anterior tooth crossbite correction.[53]

A tongue blade has also been used for the correction of a single tooth in anterior crossbite. This method is unpredictable and its effect is dependent on the frequency of patient use and the patient's tolerance of discomfort. This approach is best applied to teeth with some mobility or when the maxillary incisors are erupting.

Correction of multiple teeth in anterior crossbite has been accomplished by using a fixed or removable appliance with an inclined plane (Figure 21-7). This appliance can correct the malocclusion rapidly with little patient compliance when the inclined plane is cemented.[52] On the other hand, this appliance has several disadvantages[54]:
1. The force exerted on the ramp is unpredictable.
2. Patients may experience speech difficulty during treatment.

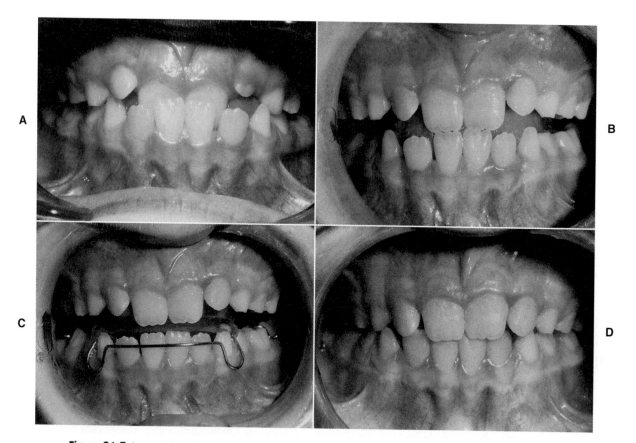

Figure 21-7 Removable inclined plane used to correct pseudo Class III malocclusion with one or more teeth in anterior crossbite. **A,** Intraoral photograph of an 8-year-old patient presenting with multiple teeth in anterior crossbite. **B,** Intraoral photograph of teeth in centric relation. Incisors in end-to-end position, indicating a pseudo Class III malocclusion. **C,** Intraoral photograph showing a removable inclined plane used to correct anterior crossbite. Note the angulation of the inclined plane. **D,** Posttreatment intraoral photograph.

3. A potential for root damage exists because of the heavy irregular forces placed on the tooth.

Other more reliable appliances and approaches are recommended. The removable appliance with auxiliary springs can be used successfully to move one or two teeth in the mixed dentition. However, patient cooperation is required for successful treatment. The maxillary lingual arch with finger springs is recommended when patient cooperation is questionable (Figure 21-8). The appliance is fabricated using an indirect technique. Bands are fitted on the maxillary second primary molars or the permanent first molars. An impression of the maxillary arch with the bands is taken. Bands are transferred to the impression before pouring. A lingual arch is fabricated and soldered to the molar bands. Finger springs with helices are soldered to the lingual arch. Anterior crossbite can usually be corrected in 2 to 3 weeks with little patient compliance. In patients presenting with a deep overbite, a mandibular Hawley appliance with an anterior labial bow can be used to prevent forward movement of the lower incisors during bite jumping. In most cases crossbite correction is maintained by the overbite, and no retention appliance is necessary (see Chapters 17 and 19).

TREATMENT OF SKELETAL CLASS III MALOCCLUSION

Functional Appliance Therapy

The Frankel III (FRIII) regulator is a functional appliance designed to counteract the muscle forces acting on the maxillary complex. According to Frankel,[55] the vestibular shields in the depths of the sulcus are placed away from the alveolar buccal plates of the maxilla to stretch the periosteum and allow for forward development of the maxilla. The shields are fitted closely to the alveolar process of the mandible to hold or redirect growth posteriorly. The effectiveness of each appliance is dependent on patient cooperation and wearing them full time.

Treatment with an FRIII and other types of functional appliances is more successful in patients with a Class III malocclusion presenting with a functional

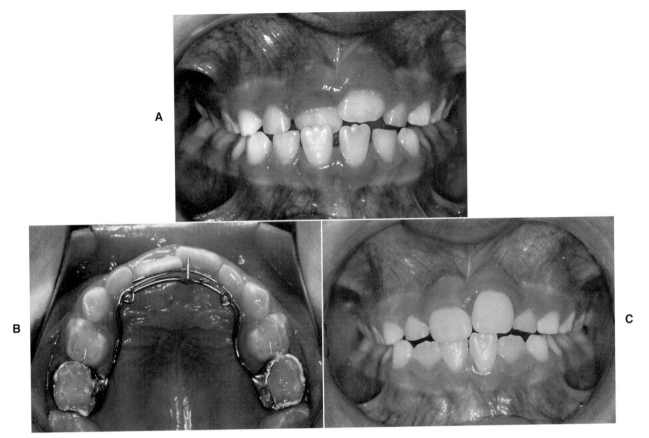

Figure 21-8 A maxillary lingual arch with finger springs used for anterior crossbite correction. **A,** Intraoral photograph of a 7-year-old patient with a single tooth in anterior crossbite. **B,** Intraoral photograph of a maxillary lingual arch constructed with 0.036-inch stainless steel base wire with soldered 0.020-inch stainless steel finger spring. A guide wire was placed between the incisors to keep the spring from moving incisally. **C,** Posttreatment photograph showing adequate overbite to maintain the anterior crossbite correction.

shift on closure. In two separate studies the FRIII appliance appears to effect occlusal changes (i.e., introducing dental compensations) by proclination of upper incisors and retroclination of lower incisors.[56,57] The mandible was repositioned downward and backward, decreasing the prognathism of the mandible and increasing the lower facial height. Changes in the position of the maxilla were minimal. The best response to FRIII treatment was noted in patients with Class III malocclusions with an increased overbite of 4 to 5 mm in the early mixed dentition.

The FRIII appliance can also be used as a retentive device following maxillary protraction treatment. Figure 21-9 shows a 6-year-old patient presenting with a mild Class III skeletal malocclusion and crossbites in the anterior and posterior segments. The patient was treated with maxillary expansion and a protraction headgear. A positive overjet was obtained after 8 months of maxillary protraction. An FRIII appliance was constructed to maintain the anteroposterior and transverse corrections until the maxillary incisors were fully erupted with sufficient overbite to maintain the Class III correction.

Chin Cup Therapy

Skeletal Class III malocclusion with a relatively normal maxilla and a moderately protrusive mandible can be treated with the use of a chin cup. This treatment modality is popular among the Asian populations because of its favorable effects on the sagittal and vertical dimensions. The objective of early treatment with the use of a chin cup is to provide growth inhibition or redirection and posterior positioning of the mandible.

Effects on Mandibular Growth
The orthopedic effects of a chin cup on the mandible include (1) redirection of mandibular growth vertically, (2) backward repositioning (rotation) of the mandible, and (3) remodeling of the mandible with closure of the gonial angle. To date, there is no agreement in the literature as to whether chin cup therapy may or may not inhibit the growth of the mandible.[58-60] However, chin cup therapy has been shown to produce a change in the mandible associated with a downward and backward rotation and a decrease in the angle of the mandible.[59-61] In addition, there is less incremental

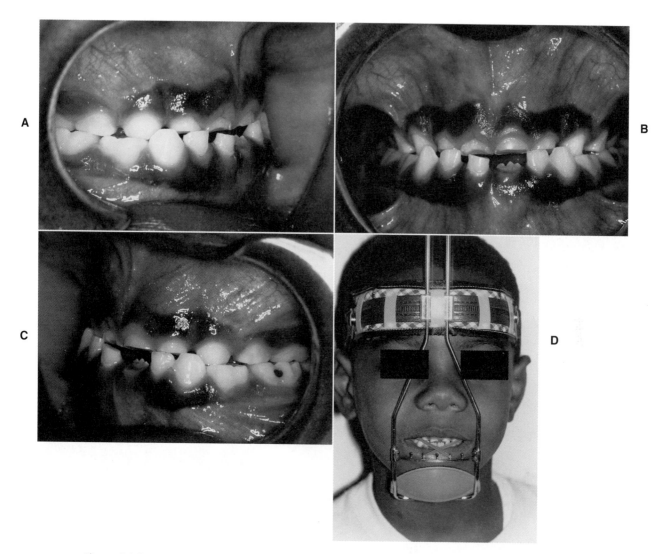

Figure 21-9 **A** to **C,** Pretreatment photographs of a 6-year-old patient presenting with a mild Class III malocclusion and crossbites in the anterior and posterior segments. **D,** Extraoral photograph showing protraction face mask.

Continued

increase in mandibular length together with posterior movement of "B point" and pogonion. Because of the backward mandibular rotation, control of the vertical growth during chin cup treatment is difficult to manage.

Effects on Maxillary Growth

Some studies have indicated that a chin cup appliance has no effect on the anteroposterior growth of the maxilla.[60-62] However, Uner, Yuksel, and Ucuncu[63] showed that early correction of an anterior crossbite with a chin cup appliance prevents retardation of anteroposterior maxillary growth. Sugawara et al[64] compared the growth changes of patients after chin cup treatment with control subjects and reported that, at age 17, the midface is more deficient in patients of the control groups than in those of the treatment groups.

Force Magnitude and Direction

Chin cups are divided into two types: the occipital-pull chin cup (Figure 21-10) that is used for patients with mandibular protrusion and the vertical-pull chin cup that is used in patients presenting with a steep mandibular plane angle and excessive anterior facial height. Most of the reported studies recommended an orthopedic force of 300 to 500 g per side.[25,63,65] Patients are instructed to wear the appliance 14 hr/day. The orthopedic force is usually directed either through the condyle or below the condyle.

Treatment Timing and Duration

Patients with mandibular excess can usually be recognized in the primary dentition despite the fact that the mandible appears retrognathic in the early years for most children. Evidence exists that treatment to

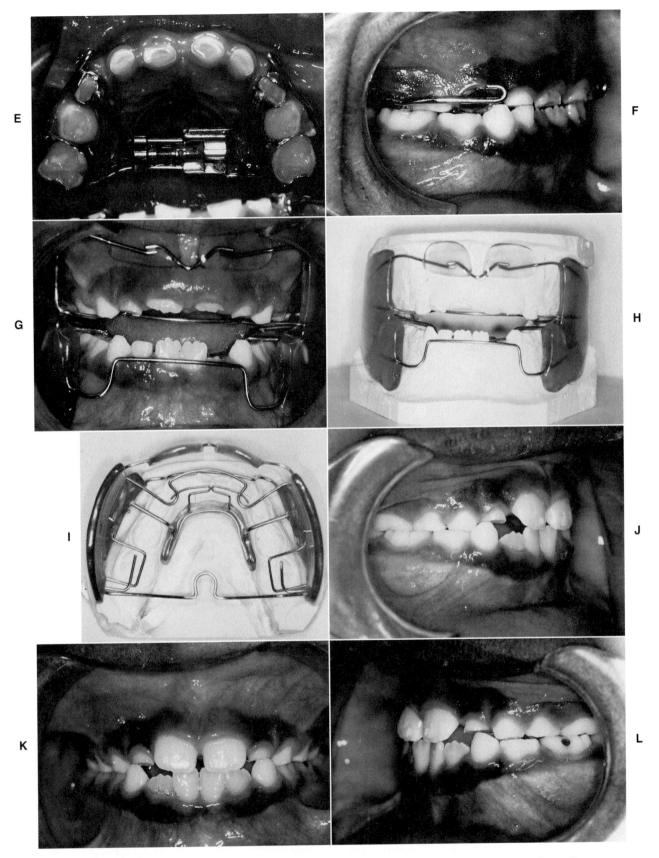

Figure 21-9, cont'd E, Intraoral photograph showing maxillary expansion appliance used as anchorage for maxillary protraction. **F,** Intraoral photograph showing protraction at the canine region to minimize anticlockwise rotation of the maxilla. **G,** A FRIII appliance was used as retention device after protraction. **H,** Design of the FRIII appliance (anterior view). **I,** Design of the FRIII appliance (occlusal view). **J** to **L,** Posttreatment intraoral photographs.

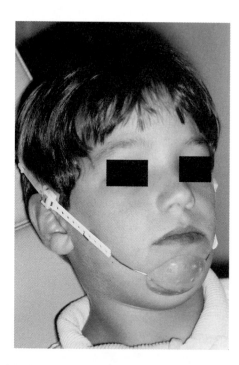

Figure 21-10 Occipital chin cup used for patients with mandibular protrusion. Note the direction of orthopedic force is directed through the condyle.

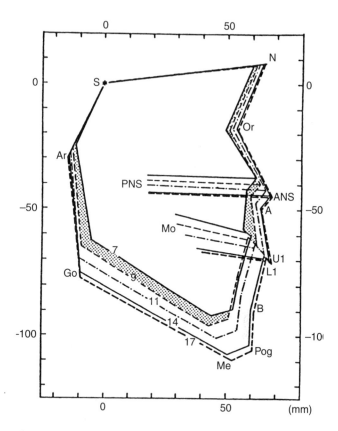

Figure 21-11 Longitudinal changes of skeletal profiles on patients who began chin cup therapy at age 7 and were observed at ages 9, 11, 14, and 17 years. Note the mandible grew downward and backward during treatment and resumed a forward and downward growth pattern during observation. (From Sugawara J et al: *Am J Orthod Dentofacial Orthop* 98:127-133, 1990.)

reduce mandibular protrusion is more successful when it is started in the primary or early mixed dentition.[61,63] The treatment time varies from 1 year to as long as 4 years depending on the severity of the original malocclusion.

Stability of Treatment The stability of chin cup treatment remains unclear. Several investigators reported stability in horizontal maxillary and mandibular changes associated with chin cup treatment.[65,66] However, few studies reported a tendency to return to the original growth pattern after the chin cup is discontinued.[58,60,63] Sugarwara et al[64] published a report on the long-term effects of chin cup therapy on three groups of Japanese girls who started chin cup treatment at 7, 9, and 11 years (Figure 21-11). All 63 patients were followed with serial lateral head films taken at the ages of 7, 9, 11, 14, and 17 years. The authors found that the skeletal profile was greatly improved during the initial stages of chin cup therapy, but these changes were often not maintained. Patients who started treatment at an earlier age had a catch-up mandibular displacement in a forward and downward direction before growth was completed. The authors concluded that chin cup therapy did not necessarily guarantee a positive correction

of the skeletal profile after completion of growth, which suggests the need for the extended use of the chin cup over the growth period.

Effects on the Temporomandibular Joint
There is some concern on the adverse effect of chin cup appliance on the TMJ. In a study by Deguchi and Kitsugi,[65] several patients complained of temporary soreness of the TMJ during the retention period. Of 40 patients, 2 continued to have TMJ pain and some degree of difficulty in opening the mouth after the end of active treatment. Several studies indicated that the chin cup affects the growth of not only the mandible, but also the cranial base structures as well.[62] However, a recent study failed to support the hypothesis that a chin cup appliance induces the posterior displacement of the glenoid fossa.[67]

Protraction Face Mask Therapy

Protraction face mask has been used in the treatment of patients with Class III malocclusion and a maxillary deficiency. In 1944 Oppenheim[68] believed that one could not control the growth or anterior displacement of the mandible and suggested moving the maxilla forward in an attempt to counterbalance mandibular protrusion. In the 1960s Delaire and others[69] revived the interest in using a face mask for maxillary protraction. Petit[70] later modified Delaire's basic concept by increasing the amount of force generated by the appliance, thus decreasing the overall treatment time. In 1987 McNamara[71] introduced the use of a bonded expansion appliance with acrylic occlusal coverage for maxillary protraction. Turley[38] improved patient cooperation in wearing the appliance by fabricating customized face masks. To date, short-term results show promising skeletal, dental, and profile improvements with treatment. The long-term benefits of early face

mask treatment need further substantiation, awaiting results from prospective clinical trials. The protraction face mask is made of two pads that contact the soft tissue in the forehead and chin region. The pads are connected by a midline framework and are adjustable through the loosening and tightening of a set screw.

The Protraction Face Mask An adjustable anterior wire with hooks is also connected to the midline framework to accommodate a downward and forward pull on the maxilla with elastics (Figure 21-12). To minimize the opening of the bite as the maxilla is repositioned, the protraction elastics are attached near the maxillary canines with a downward and forward pull of 30 degrees to the occlusal plane. Maxillary protraction generally requires 300 to 600 g of force per side,

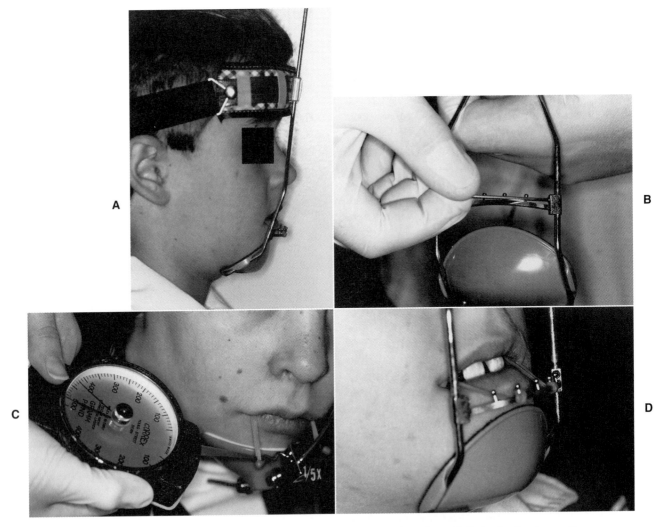

Figure 21-12 A, Extraoral photograph showing a protraction face mask appliance. **B,** Protraction headgear with adjustable anterior wire and hooks to accommodate a downward and forward pull of the maxilla with elastics. **C,** Protraction elastics of 300 to 600 g measured with a tension stress gauge. **D,** Protraction elastics attached near the maxillary canines with a downward and forward pull of 30 degrees to the occlusal plane.

depending on the age of the patient. Tension of the elastics can be estimated using a tension stress gauge. Patients are instructed to wear the face mask for 12 hours a day.

Design and Construction of the Anchorage System

Metallic Banded Palatal Expansion Appliance In the mixed dentition the banded palatal expansion appliance is constructed by using bands fitted on the maxillary primary second molars and permanent first molars (Figure 21-13). In the primary dentition the bands are fitted on the primary first and second molars. Taking a compound impression of the bands and maxillary teeth is recommended to improve the accuracy of transferring the bands to the impression. The impression is then poured up. Molar bands are joined by soldering a heavy wire (0.043-inch) to the palatal plate, which had a Hyrax-type screw (Palex expansion screw, Great Lakes Orthodontic Products, Tonawanda, NY) in the midline. A 0.045-inch wire is soldered bilaterally to the buccal aspects of the molar bands and extended anteriorly to the canine area for protraction with elastics. The appliance is activated twice daily (0.25 mm per turn) by the patient or parent for 1 week. In patients with a more constricted maxilla, activation of the expansion screw is carried out for 2 weeks or more depending on the discrepancy.

Acrylic Bonded Palatal Expansion Appliance The acrylic bonded palatal expansion appliance incorporates a Hyrax-type screw into a wire framework made from 0.040-inch stainless steel (Figure 21-14). The framework extends around the buccal and lingual surfaces of the dentition. A separate 0.040-inch stainless steel wire is bent to cross the occlusion between the primary first and second molars and ends with a hook

for protraction with elastics. Acrylic is then added on all the occlusal surfaces of the primary molars and permanent first molars using a "salt and pepper" application of methyl methacrylate monomer and polymer. The appliance is bonded to the teeth using a chemical-cure adhesive (Excel, Reliance Orthodontic Products, Itasca, IL) that is specially formulated for the bonding of large acrylic appliances.

Skeletal Effects of Maxillary Protraction Several circummaxillary sutures play an important role in the development of the nasomaxillary complex (Figure 21-15): frontomaxillary, nasomaxillary, zygomaticotemporal, zygomaticomaxillary, pterygopalatine, intermaxillary, ethmomaxillary, and the lacrimomaxillary sutures. Animal studies have shown that the maxillary complex can be displaced anteriorly with significant changes in the circummaxillary sutures and the maxillary tuberosity.[72] Maxillary protraction, however, does not always result in forward movement of the maxilla. Nanda[73] showed that with the same line of force, different midfacial bones were displaced in different directions depending on the moments of force generated at the sutures. Jackson, Kokich, and Shapiro[74] found that anterior positioning of the maxillary complex was accompanied with a small amount of counterclockwise rotation during the treatment period. The center of resistance of the maxilla was found to be located at the distal contacts of the maxillary first molars one half the distance from the functional occlusal plane to the inferior border of the orbit.[75] Protraction of the maxilla below the center of resistance produces counterclockwise rotation of the maxilla (Figure 21-16). Using human skulls, Hata and colleagues[76] also found that protraction forces at the level of the maxillary arch produced forward but counterclockwise rotation of the maxilla unless a heavy downward vector of force was applied.

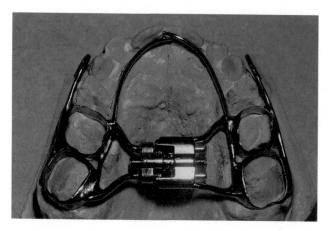

Figure 21-13 Banded palatal expansion appliance as anchorage for maxillary protraction. Note that the bands are joined by a heavy wire (0.043-inch) to the Hyrax-type expansion screw. A 0.045-inch wire is soldered bilaterally to the buccal aspects of the molar bands and extended anteriorly to the canine area for protraction with elastics.

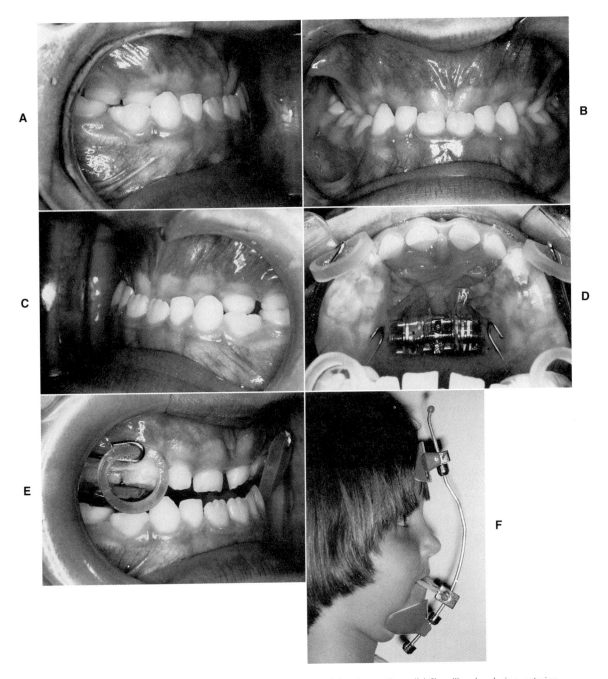

Figure 21-14 **A** to **C,** Pretreatment photographs of a 6-year-old patient with a mild Class III malocclusion, anterior crossbite, and a deep overbite. **D,** Intraoral photograph showing a bonded acrylic expansion appliance used as anchorage for maxillary protraction. **E,** Intraoral photograph showing the hook extended from the acrylic at the canine region for protraction with elastics. **F,** Maxillary protraction with a forward and downward pull 30 degrees to the occlusal plane.

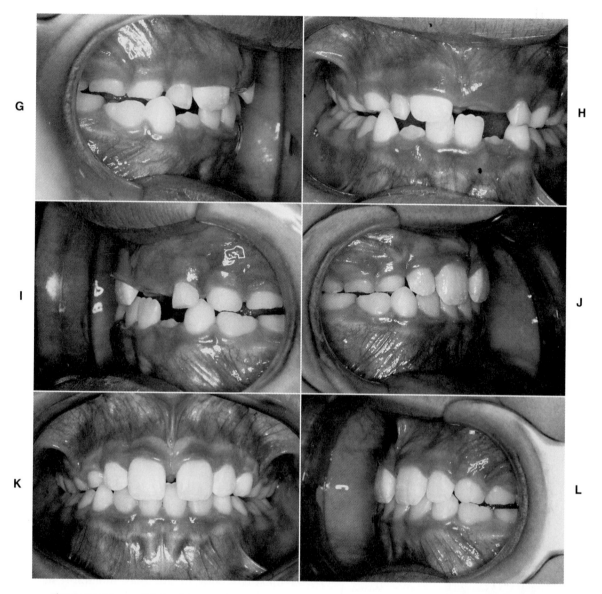

Figure 21-14, cont'd G to **I,** Posttreatment intraoral photographs. **J** to **L,** Intraoral photographs 2 years posttreatment.

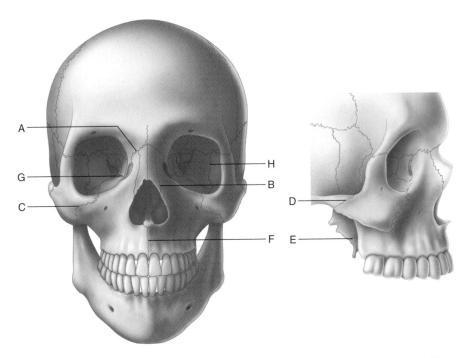

Figure 21-15 Circummaxillary sutures complex. *A,* Frontomaxillary suture. *B,* Nasomaxillary suture. *C,* Zygomatico-maxillary suture. *D,* Zygomaticotemporal suture. *E,* Pterygopalatine suture. *F,* Intermaxillary suture. *G,* Ethmomaxillary suture. *H,* Lacrimomaxillary suture.

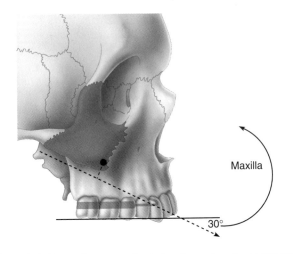

Figure 21-16 Maxillary protraction below the center of resistance produces anticlockwise rotation of the maxilla *(arrow).* Protraction elastics attached near the maxillary canine with a downward and forward pull of 30 degrees to the occlusal plane minimize bite opening. (From Ngan P et al: *Semin Orthod* 3:255-264, 1997.)

Clinical Response to Maxillary Protraction Clinically, anterior crossbites can be corrected with 3 to 4 months of maxillary expansion and protraction depending on the severity of the malocclusion. Improvement in overbite and molar relationship can be expected with an additional 4 to 6 months of maxillary protraction. In a prospective clinical trial,[77] overjet correction was found to be the result of forward maxillary movement (31%), backward movement of the mandible (21%),

labial movement of the maxillary incisors (28%), and lingual movement of the mandibular incisors (20%) (Figure 21-17). Molar relationship was corrected to a Class I or Class II dental relationship by a combination of skeletal movements and differential movement of the maxillary and mandibular molars (Figure 21-18). Anchorage loss was observed during maxillary protraction with mesial movement of the maxillary molars. Overbite was improved by eruption of the maxillary and mandibular molars. The total facial height was increased by inferior movement of the maxilla and downward and backward rotation of the mandible.

Patients with skeletal Class III malocclusion often present with a concave facial profile, a retrusive nasomaxillary area, and a prominent lower third of the face. The lower lip is often protruded relative to the upper lip. Treatment with maxillary expansion and protraction can straighten the skeletal and soft tissue facial profiles and improve the posture of the lips (Figure 21-19). It is important to note that the profile and occlusion of Class III patients usually become worse with no treatment because of deficient horizontal maxillary growth and excess mandibular growth. These changes often lead to dental compensations and overclosure of the mandible. Figure 21-20 compares the overjet changes in Class III patients with and without treatment. In patients treated with 8 months of maxillary protraction, the maxilla came forward an average of 2.1 mm. In control patients without treatment, the maxilla came for-

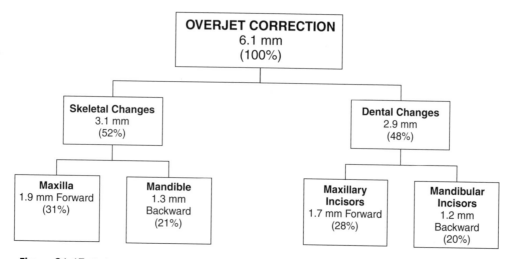

Figure 21-17 Skeletal and dental contributions to overjet correction with maxillary expansion and protraction.

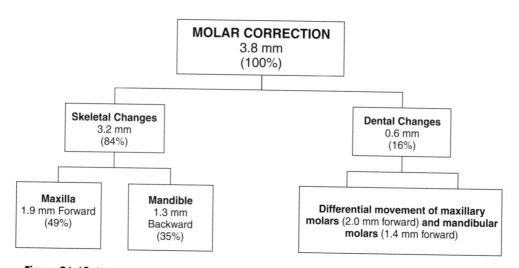

Figure 21-18 Skeletal and dental contributions to molar correction with maxillary expansion and protraction.

ward only 0.5 mm. On average, the mandible positioned back 1.0 mm with treatment. With no treatment the mandible came forward 1.7 mm. In addition, without treatment, the incisors compensated to the skeletal discrepancy by the proclination of the maxillary incisors and retroclination of the mandibular incisors. In general, the direction of these changes is similar to those occurring with treatment.

Variability in Clinical Response

Clinically, the maxilla can be advanced 2 to 4 mm over an 8- to 12-month period of maxillary protraction. The amount of forward maxillary movement is influenced by a number of factors including age of the patient, the use of anchorage system (with or without an expansion appliance), the force level,

direction and point of application, and treatment time (Table 21-2).[25,79-89]

Age of Patient Several studies have examined the effect of age on maxillary protraction therapy.[78-82] Although some studies[80,82] suggest that face mask/ expansion therapy may be most effective in the primary and early mixed dentitions, other studies[78,79,81] also suggest that it is a viable option for older children before the onset of puberty.

Design of Anchorage System The design of anchorage system for maxillary protraction varies from palatal arches to rapid maxillary expansion (RME) appliances (see Table 21-2). The need to expand the maxilla before protraction is not entirely clear. Most of the studies[77,79,83,85,87-89] utilize palatal expansion to "dis-

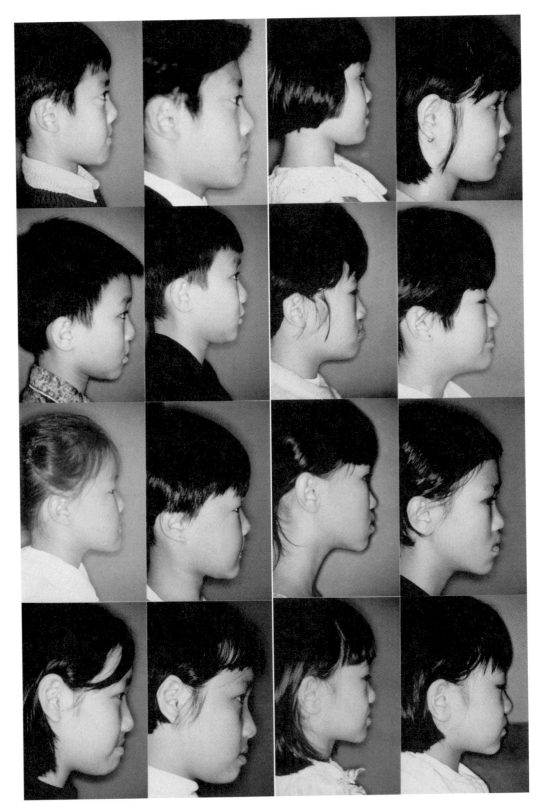

Figure 21-19 Improvement of facial profile in eight patients treated with maxillary expansion and protraction. Pretreatment facial profile *(left)*. Posttreatment facial profile *(right)*.

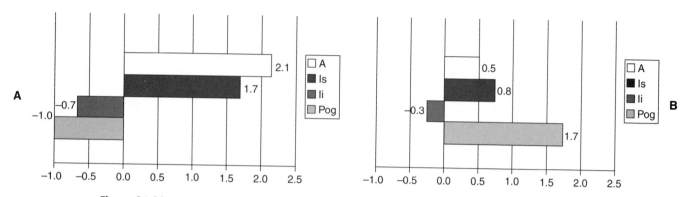

Figure 21-20 Comparison of overjet changes in patients with Class III malocclusion with or without treatment. **A,** Changes with treatment at the maxilla *(A)*, maxillary incisors *(Is)*, mandibular incisors *(Ii)*, and pogonion *(Pog)* with 8 months of maxillary protraction (effect of treatment). **B,** Changes with no treatment (control).

TABLE 21-2	Factors Influencing the Forward Movement of the Maxilla (A Point) with Protraction Face Mask				
Author	Year	Expansion	Force Level (g)	Treatment Time (Months)	Movement of A Point
Nanda[83]	1980	Haas	500	4	1.5 mm
Ishii[25]	1987	No expansion	250	11-24	2.7 mm
Tindlund[84]	1989	Quad helix	700	12	3.0 mm
Merwin[80]	1997	Hyrax	400	6	2.0 mm
Nartallo-Turley[87]	1997	Hyrax	200-450	11	3.3 mm
da Silva[85]	1998	Haas	350	12	1.5 mm
Gallagher[86]	1998	Slow expansion	600-800	8-9	1.6 mm/yr
Baik[79]	1998	Hyrax	300-400	6-8	2.1 mm
Pangrezio-Kulbersh[88]	1998	Bonded RME	400-600	7-8	1.8 mm
Kapust[81]	1998	Hyrax	300-400	9-10	2.8 mm
Bacetti[80]	1998	Bonded RME	400	11	2.1 mm
Ngan[77]	1998	Hyrax	400	8.9	2.1 mm
Sung[89]	1998	Hyrax	300-400	8-9	2.1 mm

RME, Rapid maxillary expansion.

articulate" the maxilla and initiate cellular response in the circummaxillary sutures, allowing a more positive reaction to protraction forces. Few studies have adequate control groups to determine whether it makes a difference if maxillary protraction was used in conjunction with RME. In a study by Baik,[79] 60 patients treated with a protraction face mask were divided into two groups with or without RME. The author found significantly greater forward movement of the maxilla (+2.0 mm) when protraction was used in conjunction with RME compared with protraction without RME (+0.9 mm). Does it make a difference if protraction was initiated during palatal expansion or after expansion? In the same study, greater forward movement of the maxilla (+2.8 mm) was found when protraction was initiated during maxillary expansion compared with protraction after expansion (+1.85 mm).

Force Level, Direction, and Point of Application Orthopedic effects require greater forces than do orthodontic movements. Successful maxillary protraction has been reported using 300 to 500 g of force per side in the primary and mixed dentitions (see Table 21-2). Most of these studies recommended wearing the headgear for 10 to 12 hr/day.

Hata et al[76] suggested that an effective forward displacement of the maxilla can be obtained clinically from a force applied 5 mm above the palatal plane. In deep overbite cases in which an opening of the bite is desired, a forward pull from the level of the maxillary arch with a concomitant anterior rotation of the maxilla aids in the treatment of these malocclusions. In several clinical studies a 30- to 45-degree forward and downward protraction force applied at the canine region produced an acceptable

A   B   C   D

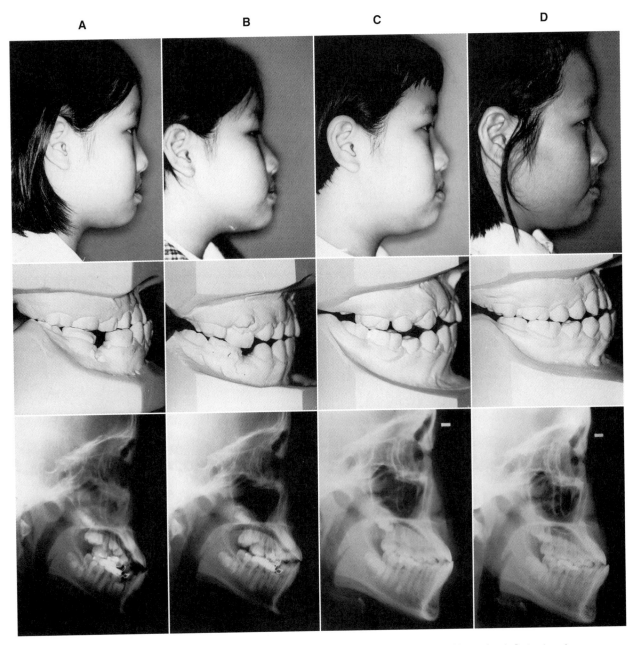

Figure 21-21 A 10-year, 10-month-old patient treated with protraction face mask for 12 months. **A,** Pretreatment model and lateral cephalometric radiograph. **B,** Immediately posttreatment model and lateral cephalometric radiograph. **C,** Two years posttreatment model and lateral cephalometric radiograph. **D,** Four years posttreatment model and lateral cephalometric radiograph.

clinical response with one degree of counterclockwise rotation of the palatal plane.[77,87]

Length of Treatment Time There is no consensus on the length of treatment with protraction headgear. A review of the literature shows that treatment time varies from 3 to 16 months (see Table 21-2). Most of the orthopedic changes are observed within the first 3 to 6 months after maxillary expansion. Prolonged use of protraction force results in dentoalveolar changes including mesial movement of maxillary molars and proclination of maxillary incisors. The benefit of repeated maxillary expansion

and protraction has not been reported in the literature. Increased treatment time may compromise patient oral hygiene and cooperation.

Posttreatment Stability Animal and human studies have shown that the effects on the maxilla remained stable for 1 to 2 years after treatment. In a few studies[77,84,86-91] in which patients were followed after maxillary expansion and protraction were completed, it was found that, in general, the anterior position of the maxilla was maintained posttreatment. It is interesting to note that during this growth period the maxilla and mandible reverted back to the original growth pattern

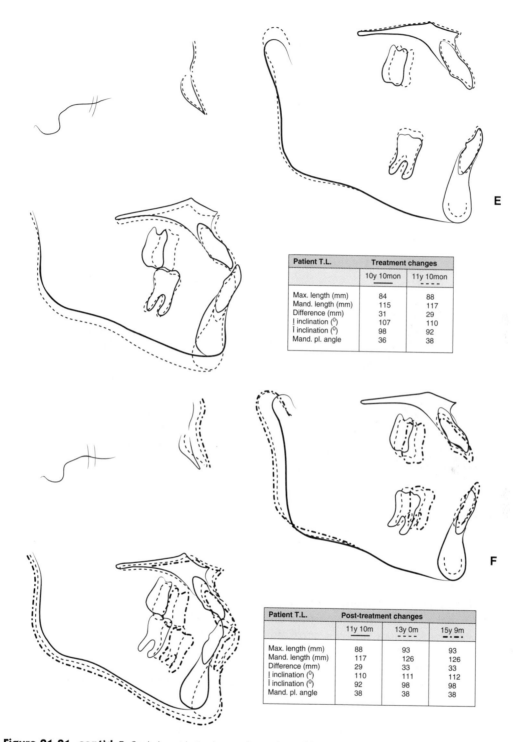

Patient T.L.	Treatment changes	
	10y 10mon	11y 10mon
Max. length (mm)	84	88
Mand. length (mm)	115	117
Difference (mm)	31	29
I inclination (⁰)	107	110
Ī inclination (⁰)	98	92
Mand. pl. angle	36	38

Patient T.L.	Post-treatment changes		
	11y 10m	13y 0m	15y 9m
Max. length (mm)	88	93	93
Mand. length (mm)	117	126	126
Difference (mm)	29	33	33
I inclination (⁰)	110	111	112
Ī inclination (⁰)	92	98	98
Mand. pl. angle	38	38	38

Figure 21-21, cont'd E, Cephalometric tracings and superimposition of treatment changes. Note the positive overjet after treatment. **F,** Cephalometric tracings and superimposition of posttreatment growth changes. Note the overjet reverted back to an anterior crossbite because of excessive forward mandibular growth.

and, in some cases, Class III correction was lost because of excess mandibular growth.

Fewer studies followed the early treatment patients through the pubertal growth period. In a prospective clinical trial, a group of Chinese patients were overtreated to a Class I or II relationship with maxillary expansion and protraction and then retained with a Class III functional appliance for 1 year.[77] The treatment was found to be stable 2 years after the removal of the appliances. When these patients were followed for another 2 years, 15 of the original 20 patients maintained a positive overjet. In patients that relapsed back to a negative overjet, the mandible outgrew the maxilla in the horizontal direction. Figure 21-21 illustrates

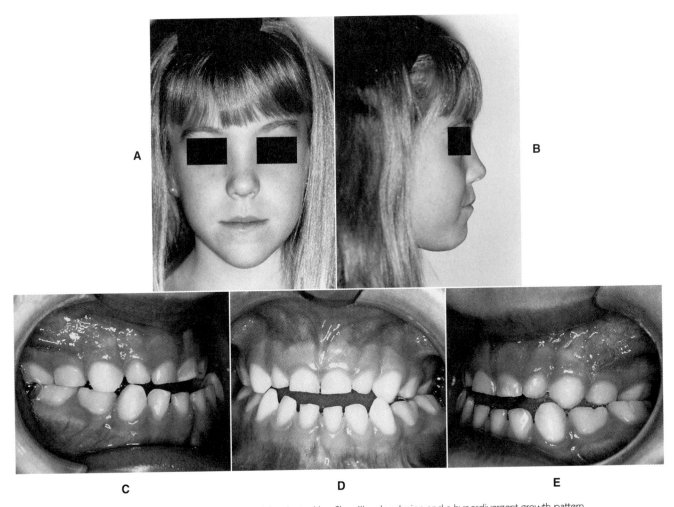

Figure 21-22 Treatment of a 6-year-old patient with a Class III malocclusion and a hyperdivergent growth pattern. **A** and **B,** Pretreatment facial profile. **C** to **E,** Pretreatment intraoral photographs.

unfavorable growth changes in a patient 4 years after treatment with maxillary expansion and protraction. The overjet reverted back to an anterior crossbite because of excessive forward mandibular growth. As a result, the authors recommend overcorrection of the overjet and molar relationships in anticipation of the subsequent horizontal mandibular growth. It is also advisable to use a retention device such as a mandibular retractor or a functional appliance following maxillary protraction.

Treatment Indications for Face Mask Therapy The face mask is most effective in the treatment of mild to moderate skeletal Class III malocclusions with a retrusive maxilla and a hypodivergent growth pattern. Patients presenting initially with some degree of anterior mandibular shift and a moderate overbite have a more favorable prognosis. In these cases correction of the anterior crossbite and the mandibular shift results in a downward and backward rotation of the mandible

that diminishes its prognathism. The presence of an adequate overbite helps maintain the immediate dental correction after treatment. For patients presenting with a hyperdivergent growth pattern and a minimal overbite, a bonded acrylic palatal expansion appliance to control vertical eruption of molars has been recommended. However, a study comparing the use of banded or bonded expansion appliances as anchorage devices for maxillary expansion and protraction showed little differences in the skeletal and dental changes following the use of either appliance.[92] Specifically, vertical eruption of the posterior molars and an increase in lower facial height were observed in both groups. Figure 21-22 shows the treatment of a 6-year-old patient presenting with a Class III malocclusion and a hyperdivergent growth pattern. An upper transpalatal arch and a lower lingual holding arch were used as retentive devices. The patient wore a vertical chin cup appliance at night to control mandibular growth and vertical eruption of the posterior teeth.

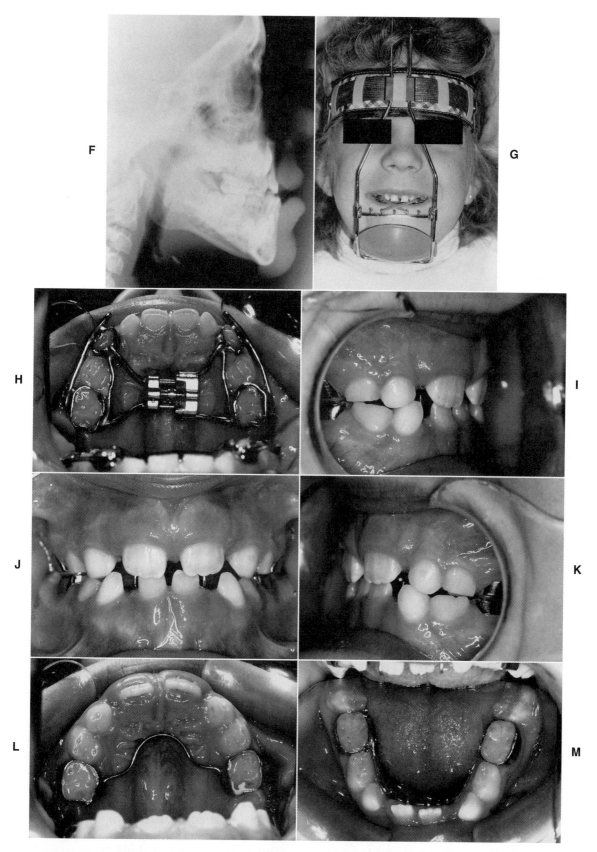

Figure 21-22, cont'd F, Pretreatment lateral cephalometric radiograph showing a combination of maxillary deficiency, mandibular prognathism, and a vertical growth pattern. **G,** Protraction face mask. **H,** Intraoral photograph of anchorage device used for maxillary protraction. **I** to **M,** Posttreatment intraoral photographs showing upper transpalatal arch and lower lingual holding arch as a retentive device.

Continued

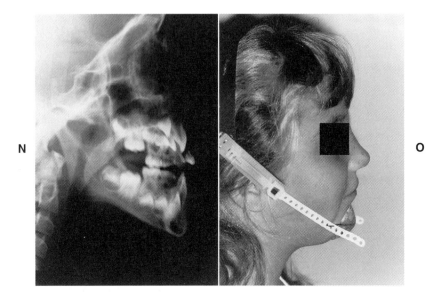

Figure 21-22, cont'd N, Posttreatment lateral cephalometric radiograph. **O,** Chin cup to control mandibular growth and vertical eruption during retention.

Treatment Timing for Face Mask Therapy The optimal time to intervene in a patient with early Class III malocclusion is at the time of initial eruption of the upper central incisors. A positive overjet and overbite at the end of face mask treatment appears to maintain the anterior occlusion after treatment. There is some evidence that better skeletal and dental response can be obtained in the primary and early mixed dentition.[82] The erupted maxillary first molars provides better anchorage for maxillary protraction. More recent clinical studies indicate that maxillary protraction is effective through puberty with diminishing skeletal response as the sutures mature.[78-81]

TREATMENT APPROACH IN ADOLESCENCE AND NONGROWING PATIENTS WITH CLASS III MALOCCLUSION

Treatment to Camouflage the Class III Skeletal Discrepancy

Skeletal discrepancies that cannot be resolved during mixed dentition by growth modification may require comprehensive appliance therapy or surgical correction. Patients treated during childhood may have the malocclusion recur during adolescence. Treatment of Class III malocclusion in adolescence is indicated in many instances to alleviate the potential psychosocial problems and perhaps reduce the need for surgery.[93,94]

Malocclusions with a mild mandibular prognathism and a moderate overbite can be corrected by dentoalveolar movements. Class III elastics with or without extraction of teeth have been used to camouflage the skeletal discrepancy, resulting in an acceptable facial profile. Figure 21-23 shows an 8-year-old patient with a mild mandibular prognathism and retroclined mandibular incisors. The patient was treated with maxillary expansion and a protraction face mask for 12 months to increase the overjet and allow for the proper alignment of the mandibular incisors. Figure 21-24 shows the cephalometric changes of the same patient after face mask treatment. Growth of the maxilla during this period was downward with little forward movement. It was decided to wait until adolescence before initiating phase II comprehensive orthodontic treatment. Figure 21-25 shows the pretreatment records of the same patient before fixed appliance therapy. The treatment plan included a nonextraction comprehensive orthodontic treatment with the use of a lip bumper and Class III elastics. Figure 21-26 shows the posttreatment result and the cephalometric tracings of the camouflaged treatment.

Class III cases with mild mandibular prognathism and crowding can be treated by various extraction schemes including four premolars, two lower premolars, or a mandibular incisor. Figure 21-27 shows an adult patient with mild mandibular prognathism and moderate crowding of the mandibular incisors. The treatment plan included comprehensive orthodontic treatment with extraction of the maxillary second premolars and the mandibular first premolars.

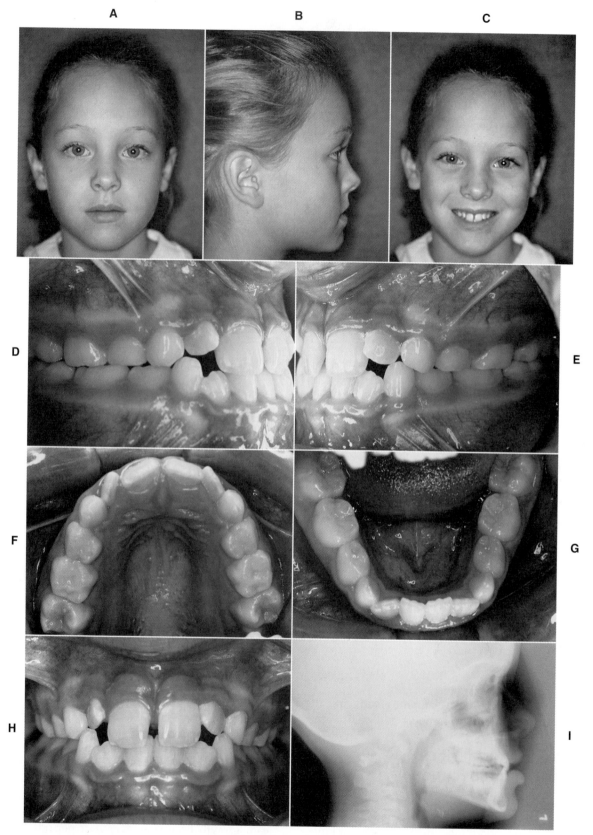

Figure 21-23 An 8-year-old patient presenting with mild mandibular prognathism and retroclined mandibular incisors. **A** to **C,** Pretreatment facial photographs. **D** to **H,** Pretreatment intraoral photographs. **I,** Pretreatment lateral cephalometric radiograph.

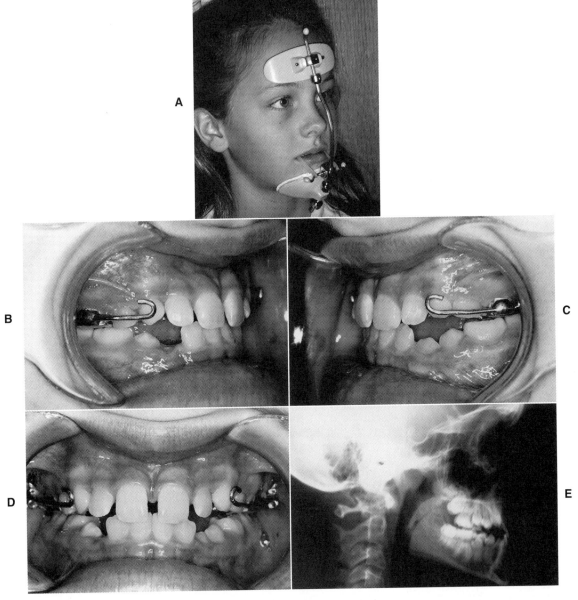

Figure 21-24 **A** to **D,** Intraoral and extraoral photographs of the same patient in Figure 21-23 during treatment with protraction face mask. **E,** Cephalometric radiograph taken after protraction face mask treatment.

Figure 21-28 shows the posttreatment results and the cephalometric tracing of the camouflaged treatment.

Combined Orthodontics and Orthognathic Surgery

Patients with continued disproportionate sagittal and vertical growth or with Class III malocclusion and maxillary retrusion or mandibular prognathism combined with a divergent facial pattern have few nonsurgical treatment options. Such patients are outside the "envelope of discrepancy" that Proffit and Ackerman[95] used to define the limit of orthodontic treatment. Early

surgery is a possible alternative solution, but surgical intervention in the maxilla in a young child may further adversely influence the growth potential that is probably already deficient.[96] Patients with true mandibular prognathism may continue to grow for several years beyond puberty. Therefore continued mandibular growth must be assumed until two lateral cephalograms taken at least 1 year apart demonstrate no significant growth occurring over that period. The current surgical methods for correcting skeletal Class III problems include ramus osteotomy to set back a prognathic mandible, mandibular inferior border osteotomy to reduce chin height or prominence,[97] or a Le Fort I

Text continued on p. 411

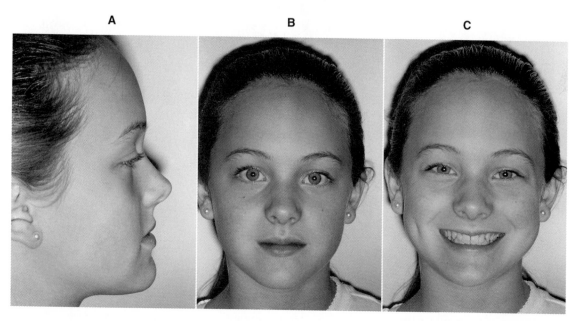

Patient: A.T.
——— Pre-Tx (10-19-93)
– – – Post-facemask Tx (6-7-95)

F

Figure 21-24, cont'd F, Cephalometric tracing and superimposition of changes with maxillary protraction.

A   B   C

Figure 21-25 A to C, Pretreatment facial photographs of the same patient in Figure 21-23 before fixed appliance therapy.

Continued

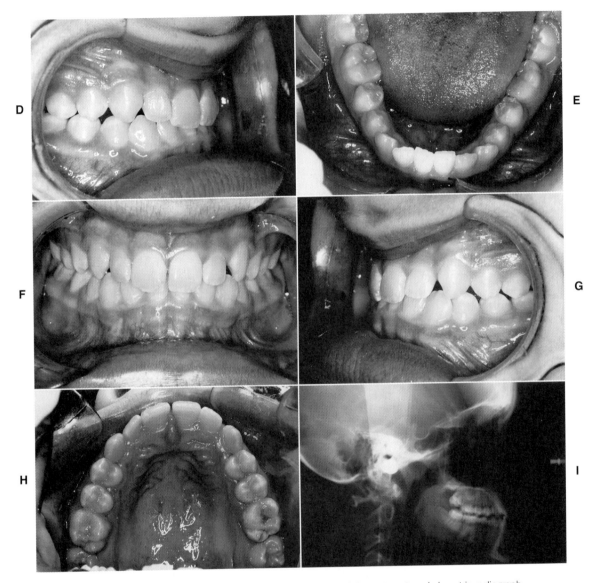

Figure 21-25, cont'd D to **H,** Pretreatment intraoral photographs. **I,** Pretreatment cephalometric radiograph.

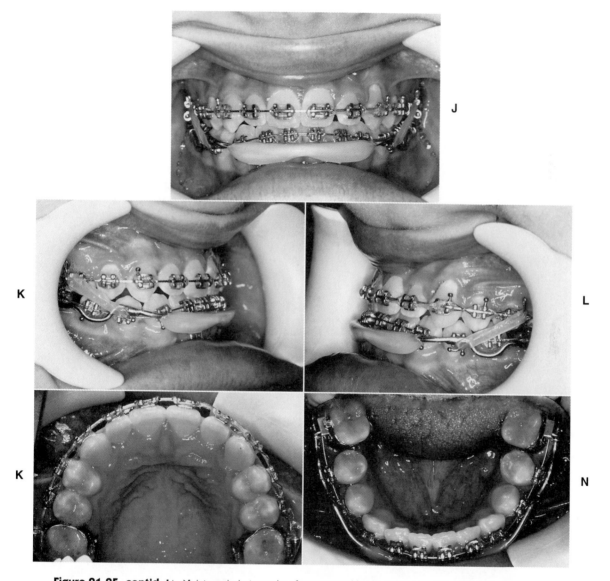

Figure 21-25, cont'd **J** to **N,** Intraoral photographs of treatment with a lip bumper and Class III elastics.

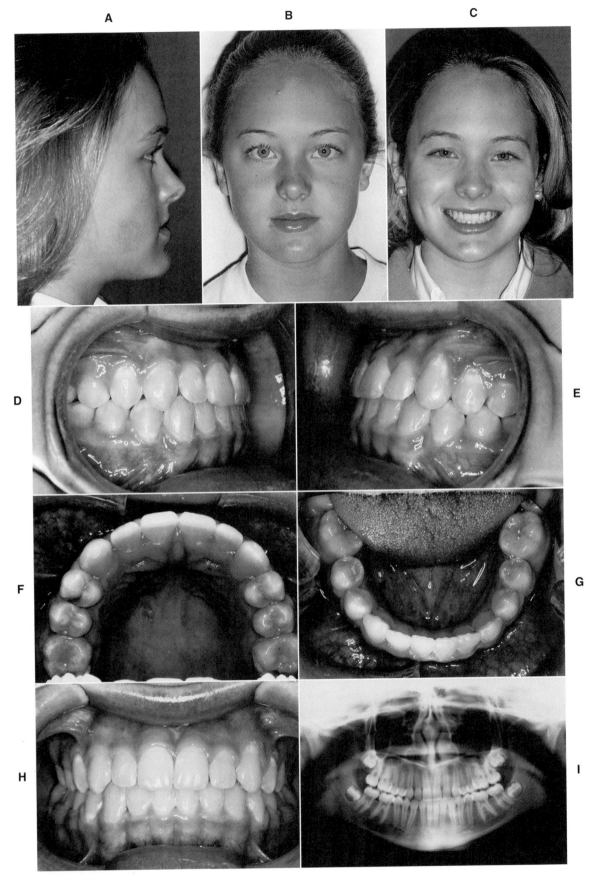

Figure 21-26 A to **C,** Posttreatment facial photographs of the same patient in Figure 21-23. **D** to **H,** Posttreatment intraoral photographs. **I,** Posttreatment panoramic radiograph.

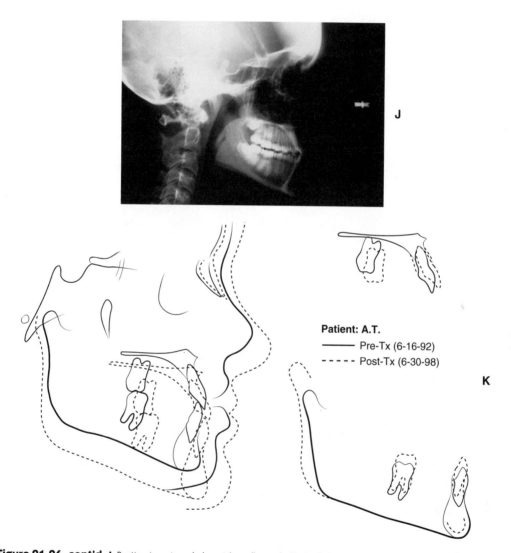

Patient: A.T.
—— Pre-Tx (6-16-92)
- - - - Post-Tx (6-30-98)

J

K

Figure 21-26, cont'd J, Posttreatment cephalometric radiograph. **K,** Cephalometric tracing and superimposition of treatment changes.

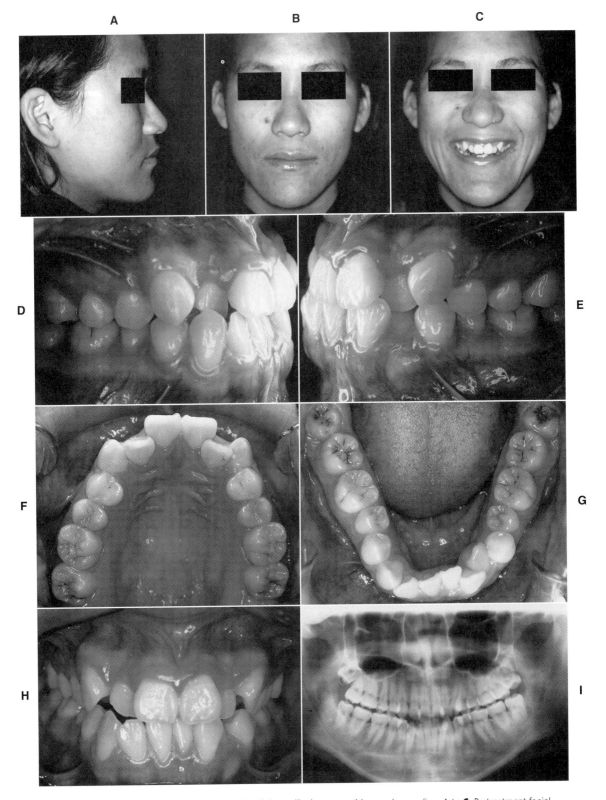

Figure 21-27 Adult patient presenting with mild mandibular prognathism and crowding. **A** to **C,** Pretreatment facial photographs. **D** to **H,** Pretreatment intraoral photographs. **I,** Pretreatment panoramic radiograph.

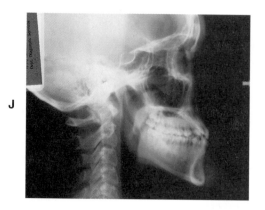

Figure 21-27, cont'd J, Pretreatment cephalometric radiograph.

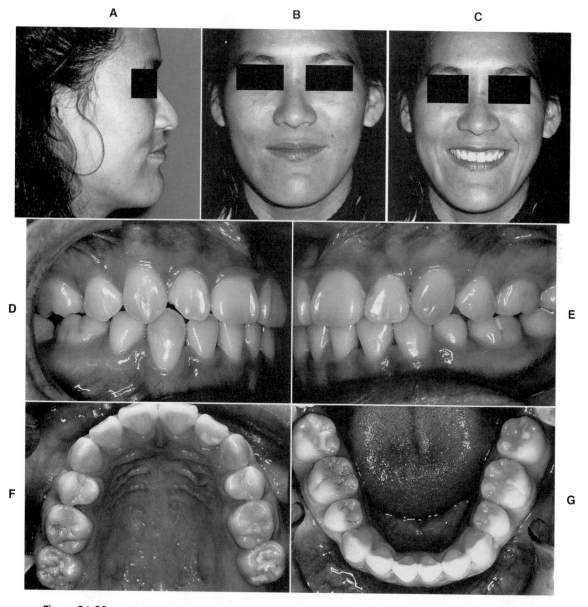

Figure 21-28 A to **C,** Posttreatment facial photographs of the same patient in Figure 21-27. **D** to **H,** Posttreatment intra-oral photographs.

Continued

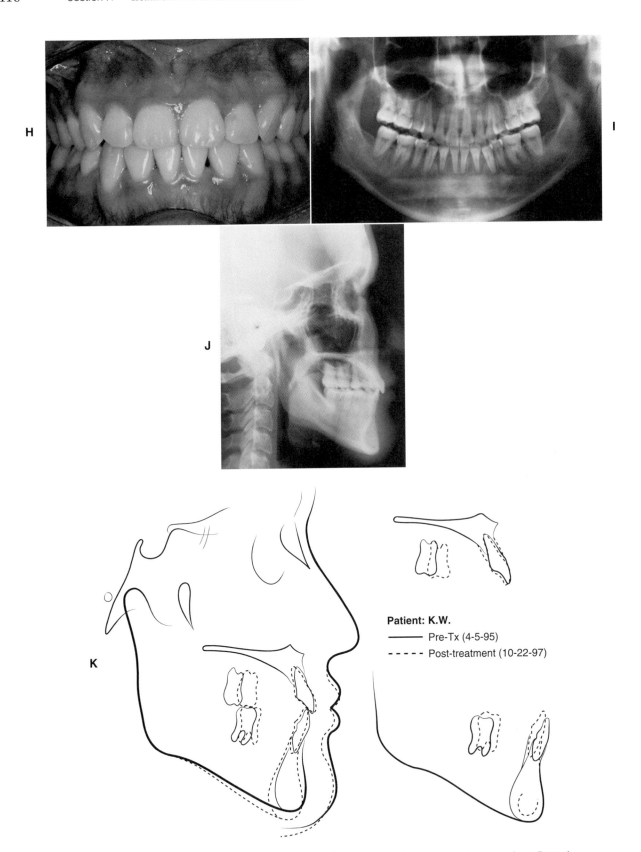

Figure 21-28, cont'd D to **H,** Posttreatment intraoral photographs. **I,** Posttreatment panoramic radiograph. **J,** Posttreatment cephalometric radiograph. **K,** Cephalometric tracings and superimposition of treatment changes.

osteotomy to advance a deficient maxilla, often segmented to allow for transverse expansion if indicated.

FUTURE INNOVATIVE TECHNIQUES FOR CLASS III TREATMENT

Distraction Osteogenesis to Advance the Maxilla

Distraction osteogenesis has recently been used to simulate a Le Fort I maxillary advancement and anterior segmental repositioning. Moline and Monasterio[98] distracted the entire maxilla in 36 patients with cleft lip and palate. An incomplete osteotomy placed above the canine and molar roots was performed through a vestibular incision. Pterygomaxillary disjunction and dissection of the nasal floor and septum were not performed. Distraction forces were placed on the maxilla by a reverse-pull headgear and an intraoral orthopedic appliance to advance the maxilla 8 to 12 mm. Figueroa and Polley[99] evaluated the cephalometric changes on 14 patients with cleft palate who were treated with a rigid external distraction technique. A complete Le Fort I osteotomy was performed, including pterygomaxillary and septal dysjunction, with mobilization. A cranially fixed rigid external distraction device was placed after surgery. Distraction was performed by turning the activating screw at a rate of 1 mm/day. The average predistraction ANB was −1.2 degrees and postdistraction was 7.3 degrees with an increase of 8.6 degrees. The average horizontal advancement of "A point" after distraction was 8.3 mm. Compared with the amount of forward maxillary movement that can be obtained from maxillary protraction with a face mask (average 2 to 4 mm), distraction osteogenesis, once perfected, has a far greater impact in treating patients with more severe Class III maxillary deficiencies.

Dental Onplants to Provide Absolute Anchorage for Maxillary Protraction

One of the limitations in maxillary protraction with tooth-borne anchorage devices such as expansion appliances and palatal arches is the loss of dental anchorage (i.e., compensatory dental changes), especially with prolonged maxillary protraction. These undesirable effects include the loss of arch length, forward movement of maxillary molars, and proclination of the maxillary incisors. These dental changes can be minimized or even eliminated with the use of a novel device called *maxillary onplants.*[100] The onplant comes as a disk, textured and coated with hydroxylapatite on one side and with an internal thread on the other side. The onplant can be placed on the palatal bone. After osseointegration is complete, forces can be applied to the teeth from the onplant palatal anchorage. Apart from providing a stationary orthopedic anchorage, this device can be used in patients with multiple missing teeth. The onplant device has been shown in animal studies to provide sufficient anchorage to successfully move and anchor teeth. To date, this new device has been placed on four orthodontic patients to distalize the maxillary posterior segments with no anchorage loss and minimal morbidity. The potential for using this new device as anchorage for maxillary orthopedics is promising.

REFERENCES

1. Angle EH: Classification of malocclusion, *Dent Cosmos* 41:248, 1899.
2. Goddard CL: *Orthodontia,* Philadelphia, 1900, Lea Brothers.
3. Dewey M *Practical orthodontia,* ed 4, St Louis, 1919, Mosby.
4. Hellman M: A study of some etiological factors of malocclusion, *Dent Cosmos* 56:1017, 1914.
5. Moore GR: Heredity as a guide in dentofacial orthopedics, *Am Assoc Orthod 42nd annual meeting,* 1944.
6. Broadbent BH: A new x-ray technique and its application to orthodontia, *Angle Orthod* 1:45-46, 1931.
7. Tweed CH: *Clinical orthodontics,* vol 2, St Louis, 1966, Mosby.
8. Moyers R: *Handbook of orthodontics,* ed 3, Chicago, 1997, Year-Book Medical.
9. Ainsworth NJ: The incidence of dental disease in the children. In Medical Research Council: Reports of the committee for the investigation of dental disease, Special Report Series, No 97, 1925.
10. Bjork A: The face in profile: an anthropological x-ray investigation of Swedish children and conscripts, *Lund: Berlingska Boktrycheriet* 40:58, 1947.
11. Enrich RE, Brodie AG, Blayney JR: Prevalence of Class I, Class II, and Class III malocclusions (Angle) in an urban population: an epidemiological study, *J Dent Res* 44:947-1014, 1964.
12. Humphreys HF, Leighton BC: A survey of anteroposterior abnormalities of the jaws in children between the ages of two and five and a half years of age, *Br Dent J* 88:3-15, 1950.
13. Massler M, Frankel JM: Prevalence of malocclusion in children aged 14-18 years, *Am J Orthod* 37:751-768, 1951.
14. Newman GV: Prevalence of malocclusion in children 6-14 years of age and treatment in preventable cases, *J Am Dent Assoc* 52:566-575, 1956.
15. Goose DH, Thompson DG, Winter FC: Malocclusion of school children of the West Midlands (England), *Br Dent J* 102:174-178, 1957.
16. Hill IN, Blayney JR, Wolf W: The Evanston dental caries study, XIX: prevalence of malocclusion of children in a fluoridated and control area, *J Dent Res* 38:782-794, 1959.
17. Thilander B, Myrberg N: The prevalence of malocclusion in Swedish school children, *Scan J Dent Res* 81:12-20, 1973.

18. Magnusson TE: An epidemiologic study of occlusal anomalies in relation to the development of the dentition in Icelandic children, *Community Dent Oral Epidemiol* 4:121-128, 1976.

19. Tschill P, Bacon W, Sonko A: Malocclusion in the deciduous dentition of Caucasian children, *Eur J Orthod* 19:361-367, 1997.

20. Altemus LA: Frequency of the incidence of malocclusion in American Negro children aged 12-16, *Angle Orthod* 29:189-200, 1959.

21. Horowitz HS, Doyle BS: Occlusal relations in children born and reared in an optimally fluoridated community, *Angle Orthod* 40:104, 1970.

22. Isiekwe MC: Malocclusion in Laso, Nigeria, *Community Dent Res* 1:59-62, 1983.

23. Garner LD, Butt MH: Malocclusion in black American and Nyeri Kenyans, *Angle Orthod* 55:139-146, 1985.

24. Otuyemi OD, Abidoye RO: Malocclusion in 12-year-old suburban and rural Nigerian children, *Community Dent Health* 10:375-380, 1993.

25. Ishii H et al: Treatment effect of combined maxillary protraction and chincap appliance in severe skeletal Class III cases, *Am J Orthod Dentofacial Orthop* 92:304-312, 1987.

26. Allwright WC, Burndred WH: A survey of handicapping dentofacial anomalies among Chinese in Hong Kong, *Int Dent J* 14:505-519, 1964.

27. Imudom S: *Occlusal characteristics of 5 year old Southern Chinese children*, Unpublished masters thesis, Hong Kong, 1994, University of Hong Kong.

28. Wang G: The prevalence of malocclusion in young Chinese population and their need and demand for orthodontic treatment, Unpublished PhD thesis, Faculty of Dentistry, Hong Kong, 1994, University of Hong Kong.

29. Lin JJ: Prevalence of malocclusion in Chinese children age 9-15, *Clin Dent (Chinese)* 5:57-65, 1985.

30. Litton SF et al: A genetic study of Class III malocclusion, *Am J Orthod* 58:565-577, 1970.

31. Harris JE, Kowalski CJ, Watnick SS: Genetic factors in the shape of the craniofacial complex, *Angle Orthod* 43:109-111, 1973.

32. McGuigan DG: *The Hapsburgs*, London, 1966, WH Allen.

33. Rakosi T, Schilli W: Class III anomalies: a coordinated approach to skeletal, dental, and soft tissue problems, *J Oral Surg* 39:860-870, 1981.

34. Ellis E, McNamara JA: Components of adult Class III malocclusion, *J Oral Maxillofacial Surg* 42:295-305, 1984.

35. Guyer EC et al: Components of Class III malocclusions in juveniles and adolescents, *Angle Orthod* 56:7-30, 1986.

36. Masaki F: Longitudinal study of morphological differences in the cranial base and facial structure between Japanese and American whites, *J Jpn Orthod Soc* 39:436-456, 1980.

37. Wu TF, Peng CJ, Lin JJ: Components of Class III malocclusion in Chinese young adults, *Clin Dent (Chinese)* 6:233-241, 1986.

38. Turley P: Orthopedic correction of Class III malocclusion with palatal expansion and custom protraction headgear, *J Clin Orthod* 22:314-325, 1988.

39. Latham RA: The sella point and postnatal growth of the human cranial base, *Am J Orthod* 61:156-162, 1972.

40. Kwong WL, Lin JJ: Comparison between pseudo and true Class III malocclusion by Veterans' General Hospital cephalometric analysis, *Clin Dent* 7(2):69-78, 1987.

41. Battagel J: The aetiological factors in Class III malocclusion, *Eur J Orthod* 15:347-370, 1993.

42. Sugawara J, Mitani H: Facial growth of skeletal Class III malocclusion and the effects, limitations, and long-term dentofacial adaptations to chin cap therapy, *Semin Orthod* 3:244-254, 1997.

43. Dietrich UC: Morphological variability of skeletal Class III relationships as revealed by cephalometric analysis, *Rep Congr Eur Orthod Soc* 131-143, 1970.

44. Enlow DH: *Handbook of facial growth,* ed 2, Philadelphia, 1982, WB Saunders.

45. Aki T et al: Assessment of symphysis morphology as a predictor of the direction of mandibular growth, *Am J Orthod Dentofacial Orthop* 106:60-69, 1994.

46. Schulof RJ, Nakamura S, Williamson WV: Prediction of abnormal growth in Class III malocclusions, *Am J Orthod* 71:421-430, 1977.

47. Williams S, Anderson CE: The morphology of the potential Class III skeletal pattern in the growing child, *Am J Orthod* 89:301-311, 1986.

48. Houston WJ: The current status of facial growth prediction: a review, *Br J Orthod* 6:11-17, 1979.

49. Thompson JR: The individuality of the patient in facial skeletal growth. Part 2. *Am J Orthod Dentofacial Orthop* 105:117-127, 1994.

50. Joondeph DR: Early orthodontic treatment, *Am J Orthod* 104:199-200, 1993.

51. Turpin DL: Early Class III treatment, unpublished thesis presented at 81st session, *Am Assoc Orthod* San Francisco, 1981.

52. Croll TP, Riesenberger RE: Anterior crossbite correction in the primary dentition using fixed inclined planes. I. Technique and examples, *Quintessence Int* 18:847-853, 1987.

53. Croll TP: Correction of anterior tooth crossbite with bonded resin-composite slopes, *Quintessence Int* 27:7-10, 1996.

54. Payne RC, Mueller BH, Thomas HF: Anterior crossbite in the primary dentition, *J Pedod* 5:281-294, 1991.

55. Frankel R: Maxillary retrusion in Class III and treatment with the functional corrector III, *Trans Eur Orthod Soc* 46:249-259, 1970.

56. Loh MK, Kerr WJS: The function regulator III: effects and indications for use, *Br J Orthod* 12:153-157, 1985.

57. Ulgen M, Firatli S: The effects of Frankel's function regulator on the Class III malocclusion, *Am J Orthod* 105:561-567, 1994.

58. Sakamoto T et al: A roentgenocephalometric study of skeletal changes during and after chin cup treatment, *Am J Orthod* 85:341-350, 1984.

59. Wendell P et al: The effects of chin cup therapy on the mandible: a longitudinal study, *Am J Orthod* 87:265-274, 1985.

60. Mitani H, Fukazawa H: Effects of chincap force on the timing and amount of mandibular growth associated with anterior reverse occlusion (Class III malocclusion) during puberty, *Am J Orthod Dentofacial Orthop* 9:454-463, 1986.

61. Graber LW: Chin cup therapy for mandibular prognathism, *Am J Orthod* 72:23-41, 1977.

62. Ritucci R, Nanda R: The effect of chin cup therapy on the growth and development of the cranial base and midface, *Am J Orthod Dentofacial Orthop* 85:341-350, 1984.

63. Uner O, Yuksel S, Ucuncu N: Long-term evaluation after chin cup treatment, *Eur J Orthod* 17:135-141, 1995.

64. Sugawara J et al: Long-term effects of chin cup therapy on skeletal profile in mandibular prognathism, *Am J Orthod Dentofacial Orthop* 98:127-133, 1990.

65. Deguchi T, Kitsugi A: Stability of changes associated with chin cup treatment, *Angle Orthod* 66:139-146, 1996.

66. Ohyama Y: A longitudinal cephalometric study on craniofacial growth of the orthodontically treated patient with mandibular prognathism, *J Osaka Univ Dental School* 26:270-294, 1981.

67. Deguchi T, McNamara JA: Craniofacial adaptations induced by chin cup therapy in Class III patients, *Am J Orthod Dentofacial Orthop* 115:175-182, 1999.

68. Oppenheim A: A possibility for physiologic orthodontic movement, *Am J Orthod Oral Surg* 30:277-328, 345-368, 1944.

69. Delaire VJ, Verdon P, Floor J: Ziele und ergebnisse extraoraler Zuge in postero-anteriorer Richtung in anwendung einer orthopadischen Maske bei der Behandlung von Fallen der Klasse III, *Fortschr Kiefer Orthop* 37:246-262, 1976.

70. Petit H: Adaptations following accelerated facial mask therapy in clinical alteration of the growing face. In McNamara JA Jr, Ribbens KA, Howe RP (eds): Monograph 14, Craniofacial Growth Series, Center for Human Growth and Development, Ann Arbor, Mich, 1983, University of Michigan.

71. McNamara JA Jr: An orthopedic approach to the treatment of Class III malocclusion in growing children, *J Clin Orthod* 21:598-608, 1987.

72. Kambara T: Dentofacial changes produced by extraoral forward force in Macaca irus, *Am J Orthod* 71:249-277, 1977.

73. Nanda R: Protraction of maxilla in rhesus monkeys by controlled extraoral forces, *Am J Orthod* 74:121-141, 1978.

74. Jackson GW, Kokich VG, Shapiro PA: Experimental and postexperimental response to anteriorly directed extraoral force in young Macaca nemestrina, *Am J Orthod* 75:318-333, 1979.

75. Lee K et al: A study of holographic interferometry on the initial reaction of the maxillofacial complex during protraction, *Am J Orthod Dentofacial Orthop* 111:623-632, 1997.

76. Hata S et al: Biomechanical effects of maxillary protraction on the craniofacial complex, *Am J Orthod Dentofacial Orthop* 91:305-311, 1987.

77. Ngan PW et al: Treatment response and long-term dentofacial adaptations to maxillary expansion and protraction, *Semin Orthod* 3:255-264, 1997.

78. Takada K, Petdachai S, Sakuda M: Changes in dentofacial morphology in skeletal Class III children treated by a modified maxillary protraction headgear and a chin cup: a longitudinal cephalometric appraisal, *Eur J Orthod* 15:211-221, 1993.

79. Baik HS: Clinical results of the maxillary protraction in Korean children, *Am J Orthod Dentofacial Orthop* 108:583-592, 1995.

80. Merwin D et al: Timing for effective application of anteriorly directed orthopedic force to the maxilla, *Am J Orthod Dentofacial Orthop* 112:292-299, 1997.

81. Kapust AJ, Sinclair PM, Turley PK: Cephalometric effects of face mask/expansion therapy in Class III children: a comparison of three age groups, *Am J Orthod Dentofacial Orthop* 113:204-212, 1998.

82. Baccetti T et al: Skeletal effects of early treatment of Class III malocclusion with maxillary expansion and face-mask therapy, *Am J Orthod Dentofacial Orthop* 113:333-343, 1998.

83. Nanda R: Biomechanical and clinical considerations of a protraction headgear, *Am J Orthod* 78:125-139, 1980.

84. Tindlund RS: Orthopaedic protraction of the midface in the deciduous dentition: results covering 3 years out of treatment, *J Craniomaxillofac Surg* 17:17-19, 1989.

85. da Silva Filho OG, Boas MC, Capelozza Filho L: Rapid maxillary expansion in the primary and mixed dentitions: a cephalometric evaluation, *Am J Orthod Dentofacial Orthop* 100:171-179, 1991.

86. Gallagher RW, Miranda F, Buschang PH: Maxillary protraction: treatment and posttreatment effects, *Am J Orthod Dentofacial Orthop* 113:612-619, 1998.

87. Nartallo-Turley P, Turley P: Cephalometric effects of combined palatal expansion and facemask therapy on Class III malocclusion, *Angle Orthod* 68:217-223, 1998.

88. Pangrazio-Kulbersh V, Berger J, Kersten G: Effects of protraction mechanics on the midface, *Am J Orthod Dentofacial Orthop* 114:484-491, 1998.

89. Sung SJ, Baik HS: Assessment of skeletal and dental changes by maxillary protraction, *Am J Orthod Dentofacial Orthop* 114:492-502, 1998.

90. Wisth PJ et al: The effect of maxillary protraction on front occlusion and facial morphology, *Acta Odontol Scand* 45:227-237, 1987.

91. Ngan P et al: Cephalometric and occlusal changes following maxillary expansion and protraction, *Eur J Orthod* 20:237-245, 1998.

92. Ngan P et al: Comparison of protraction headgear response with banded and bonded appliances, *J Dent Res* 77:112 (abstract #92), 1998.

93. Graber LW: Psycho-social implications of dentofacial appearance, Unpublished thesis, Ann Arbor, Mich, 1880, University of Michigan.

94. Proffit WR, White RP: The need for surgical-orthodontic treatment. In Proffit WR, White RP (eds): *Surgical orthodontic treatment*, St Louis, 1991, Mosby.

95. Proffit WR, Ackerman JL: A systematic approach to orthodontic diagnosis and treatment planning. In Graber TM, Vanarsdall RL (eds): *Current orthodontic concepts and techniques*, ed 3, St Louis, 2000, Mosby.

96. Kokich V, Shapiro P: The effects of LeFort I osteotomies on the craniofacial growth of juvenile Macaca nemestrina. In McNamara JA Jr, Carlson DS, Ribbens KA (eds): *The effect of surgical intervention on craniofacial growth*, Monograph 12, Craniofacial Growth Series, Center for Human Growth and Development, Ann Arbor, Mich, 1982, University of Michigan.

97. Sinclair PM, Proffit WR: Class III problems: mandibular excess/maxillary deficiency. In Proffit WR, White RP (eds): *Surgical orthodontic treatment,* St Louis, 1990, Mosby.

98. Moline F, Monasterio FO: Maxillary distraction: three years of clinical experience, *Plas Surg Forum* 16:54 (abstr), 1993.

99. Figueroa AA, Polley JW: Management of severe cleft maxillary deficiency with distraction osteogenesis: procedures and results, *Am J Orthod Dentofacial Orthop* 115:1-12, 1999.

100. Block MS, Hoffman DR: A new device for absolute anchorage for orthodontics, *Am J Orthod Dentofacial Orthop* 107:251-258, 1995.

CHAPTER 22

Interaction of the Sagittal and Vertical Dimensions in Orthodontic Diagnosis and Treatment Planning

Marla J. Magness, Shiva V. Shanker, and Katherine W.L. Vig

KEY TERMS

prevalence	diagnosis	adult	preadjusted appliance
development of the vertical	preadolescence	Class II elastics	stability
dimension	adolescent		

Since the 1890s classification of malocclusion has traditionally focused on the sagittal dimension only. This reflects the strong influence of Edward Angle[1] whose classification of occlusal relationships included normal occlusion and Class I, Class II, and Class III malocclusion. Angle's sagittal classification has stood the test of time, although contemporary interpretation includes an understanding of malocclusion in all three dimensions.

It is well recognized that there is an interrelationship between the sagittal and vertical dimensions with discrepancies in one plane affecting the other. Correction of the sagittal discrepancy is a common goal for both the patient and the orthodontist, but a successful clinical outcome is also dependent on an accurate diagnosis and clinical management of the vertical dimension. An increase or decrease in the patient's anterior vertical dimension also impacts the dental and skeletal relationships in the sagittal dimension.

The interaction of the vertical and sagittal dimensions in orthodontic diagnosis and treatment planning forms the basis for this chapter with a focus on Class II malocclusion.

PREVALENCE OF MALOCCLUSION

In the 1970s the United States Public Health Service (USPHS) surveyed 8000 representative children and adolescents between the ages of 6 and 11 and 12 and 17 years to determine the **prevalence** of malocclusion and reported that 75% of these individuals had some noticeable deviation from ideal occlusion. It was also reported that the severity of the malocclusions appeared to increase in the older age group.[2,3] An excessive overjet of greater than 6 mm was found in 15% to 17% of the group, and this was associated with a Class II dysplasia.[4] Class II dysplasia was found to be the second most prevalent type of malocclusion after Class I malocclusion with dental crowding (see Chapter 8).

THE SAGITTAL DIMENSION

An Angle Class II malocclusion may be the result of a maxillary protrusion or mandibular retrusion (see Chapter 20). Proffit and White[5] estimated that 40% of the United States population who have a Class II malocclusion caused by a skeletal mandibular deficiency has a normal to decreased facial height, and 25% of the mandibular-deficient population were found to have an increased facial height.[5] An evaluation of 253 adults with Class II malocclusion indicated that 25% exhibited an open bite component in the malocclusion.[6-8]

An Angle Class III malocclusion affects less than 1% of the population (see Chapter 21). It may reflect an underlying skeletal discrepancy of maxillary deficiency or mandibular excess. The latter tends to increase in severity with later growth of the mandible. Vertical discrepancies may also coexist with the Class III condition and, in many instances, significantly affect the clinical presentation of the patient because the vertical rotation of the mandible downward and backward may mask the severity of the sagittal component (Figure 22-1).

The Vertical Dimension

Increased vertical dimension is typically manifested dentally as an anterior open bite, whereas a decreased vertical dimension is manifested as an anterior deep overbite. When considering a discrepancy in the vertical dimension, a definite racial predilection was found (see Chapter 8). The USPHS reported the following frequency of anterior open bite malocclusion of 2 mm or greater:

Ages 6 to 11	Whites 1.4%	Blacks 9.6%
Ages 12 to 17	Whites 1.2%	Blacks 10.1%

Anterior open bite is more common in African Americans, whereas a deep bite malocclusion is seen most frequently in European Americans.

The Cause of Vertical and Sagittal Discrepancies

Malocclusion is a condition reflecting an expression of normal biologic variability. The greater the deviation from the accepted ideal or normal occlusion as classified by Angle, the more severe the expression of the malocclusion. Because malocclusion is not a pathologic entity, a specific cause for the developmental condition may not be obvious. Heredity and familial characteristics of facial pattern represent the influence of genetic factors, which contribute significantly to skeletodental

development. However, other influences may affect the proportionality of the facial skeleton and position of the teeth. Regardless of the severity or type of malocclusion, a specific cause can typically only be identified in less than 5% of malocclusions because the development of the dentition and craniofacial skeleton are the result of an interaction of genetic and nongenetic or environmental factors (see Chapter 8).

Factors Affecting the Development of the Vertical Dimension

The envelope of discrepancy is a three-dimensional concept that explains the limits of the maxillary and mandibular dentition in three planes of space.[9] The **development of the vertical dimension** is determined by the equilibrium between the tongue, lips, cheeks, and opposing dentition on the developing dentofacial complex. This equilibrium of the biologic system is determined more by the duration of a force than the magnitude of the force.

The muscles of mastication produce heavy, intermittent forces of short duration for chewing food.[10] The occlusal forces serve to maintain equilibrium in the vertical dimension of the orofacial complex, although pathologic (parafunctional) habits such as clenching, nocturnal bruxism, or hyperactive muscles of mastication have the potential to influence the vertical equilibrium. This may result in the incomplete eruption of posterior teeth and a decreased vertical development of the posterior maxillary and mandibular alveolar processes producing an increased anterior overbite. This interaction of facial development and tooth eruption was well described by Bjork and Skeiller[11] in their explanation of the facial pattern differences between the brachyfacial (short face) and dolicofacial (long face) development.

Additionally, soft tissue influences that include *tongue thrust* habits have been attributed to the development of an open bite, with the tongue having a direct cause and effect relationship. However, the tongue has a remarkable capacity to adapt to the confines of the intermaxillary space as seen in the outcome of orthognathic surgery. Superior repositioning of the maxilla to close a skeletal open bite results in autorotation of the mandible with a decrease in the intermaxillary space with the resultant adaptation of the position of the tongue resulting in normal speech and function.[12] Therefore the role of the tongue in relation to the initial open bite may not be causative but adaptive.

Prolonged *digit sucking,* also referred to as *nonnutritive sucking,* has been attributed to the development of malocclusion. The effects of a nonnutritive sucking habit on skeletal and dental development are usually not permanent if the habit ceases during the primary dentition stage. However, the amount of tooth displacement is dependent on the duration of hours per

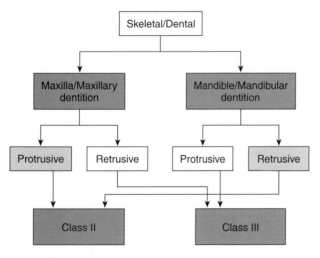

Figure 22-1 Components of the sagittal dimension.

day of sucking and not only on the magnitude of the pressures created. A thumb or finger routinely placed in an asymmetric position may result in the development of an asymmetric increase in overjet and open bite.

As the mandible relates to the maxilla on a hinge axis, vertical skeletodental effects have been attributed not only to soft tissue and habit influences but also to physiologic causal factors. *Nasal obstruction* and the resultant mouth breathing has been implicated in causing overeruption of the posterior teeth and an increase in the vertical lower face dimension caused by the mouth open posture.[13] However, evidence to demonstrate significant alterations in facial growth in humans as a result of mouth breathing secondary to nasal obstruction is still inconclusive.[14-16] Minimal increase in eruption of the posterior dentition has a greater effect on the anterior vertical dimension and hence the overbite because of the wedge geometry of the maxillomandibular occlusal plane. Differences in anterior facial height have been generalized to result from two different types of *mandibular rotation* by Bjork and Skeiller.[17] The differences impact the vertical and sagittal dimensions. Forward mandibular rotation tends to allow more horizontal expression of mandibular growth, thus improving a Class II correction, and results in a normal to decreased anterior vertical dimension. Backward mandibular rotation expresses mandibular growth in a more vertical direction, and thus compromises Class II correction and increases the chance of the patient developing a long face or an open bite malocclusion (Figure 22-2).

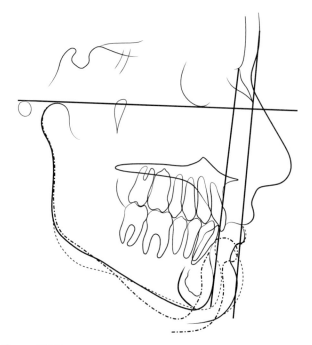

Figure 22-2 Lateral cephalometric tracing illustrating mandibular forward (-----) and backward (-·-·-·-) rotation and their affect on the sagittal position of the chin.

When Isaacson et al[18] compared the facial morphology of high-, average-, and low-angle subjects, they found that the vertical height from palatal plane to maxillary molars was increased in the high-angle subjects compared with the other two groups, indicating an increased posterior maxillary vertical dental development. High-angle subjects also displayed increased lower anterior facial height measurements (Boxes 22-1 and 22-2).

DIAGNOSTIC AND TREATMENT PLANNING CONSIDERATIONS

To develop a treatment plan and provide the patient with appropriate options requires a systematic approach to **diagnosis** (see Section II). The treatment plan is dependent on the age of the patient and also the severity of the malocclusion. For example, a child in the mixed dentition may benefit from growth modification if there is a skeletal discrepancy. On the other hand, an adolescent or adult patient who is past their peak height velocity of growth may benefit from camouflage procedures if the skeletal discrepancy is mild or a combination of orthodontics and surgery if the skeletal discrepancy is severe (see Chapters 20 and 21).

The Clinical Examination

The initial patient interview elicits the chief complaint and any relevant medical or dental history. A clinical evaluation of the patient considers the proportionality of the vertical, sagittal, and transverse facial and dental dimensions (Figure 22-3). Full-face evaluation should include the relation of patient's facial height to the facial width. As the lower facial height decreases, the facial form becomes more square. With an increase in lower facial height there is a more oval facial appearance. An increase in lower facial height may also result in a lip-apart posture and an excessive gingival display on full smile. Any vertical facial disproportion in the upper, middle, and lower facial thirds should also be detected. The lateral facial profile permits the sagittal dimension to be evaluated (Figure 22-4). This may be confirmed radiographically with the lateral cephalogram (Figure 22-5), which provides two-dimensional information in the vertical and sagittal dimensions. A Class I skeletal pattern with clockwise mandibular rotation assumes that the patient has a normal mandible that has rotated open and created the appearance of mandibular deficiency as illustrated in Figure 22-2.

The intraoral examination reveals an increase in overbite and overjet with a Class II Division 1 incisal relationship (Figure 22-6). The maxillary right canine is erupting, and the left maxillary primary canine is retained and mobile. The presence of the permanent canine is confirmed from the Panorex radiograph (Figure 22-7).

BOX 22-1 — Clinical and Cephalometric Characteristics of an Increased Vertical Dimension

Clinical Examination

Extraoral Characteristics
Steep mandibular plane angle
Increased lower anterior facial height
Lip incompetence usually with mentalis strain (resting lip separation >4 mm)
Shallow mentolabial sulcus
Class II malocclusion with the appearance of mandibular deficiency
Excessive gingival display on full smile

Dental Characteristics
Upright and supraerupted maxillary and mandibular incisors
Excessive eruption of posterior teeth
Anterior open bite
Narrow maxilla and posterior crossbite

Cephalometric Evaluation

Skeletal Characteristics
Rotation of the palatal plane down posteriorly
Inferiorly tipped occlusal plane secondary to maxillary rotation and elongation of maxillary posterior teeth
Short mandibular ramus height/decreased posterior facial height
Steep mandibular plane angle
Increased height of the anterior mandibular alveolus
Increased craniofacial flexure angle (saddle angle)
Increased maxillary or mandibular dentoalveolar height
Inferiorly tipped posterior palatal plane

BOX 22-2 — Clinical and Cephalometric Characteristics of a Decreased Vertical Dimension

Clinical Examination

Extraoral Characteristics
Acute nasolabial angle
Decreased lower facial height
No teeth showing at repose
Flat mandibular plane angle
Deep mentolabial fold
Well-developed pogonion

Dental Characteristics
Deep overbite

Cephalometric Evaluation

Skeletal Characteristics
Increased mandibular ramus height/increased posterior facial height
Flat mandibular plane angle
Acute gonial angle
Decreased anterior lower facial height
Shorter than normal dentoalveolar height

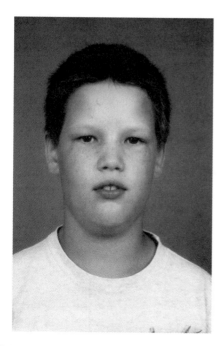

Figure 22-3 Full-face photograph of an 11-year-old boy with facial symmetry, balanced facial proportions, and a lip-apart posture.

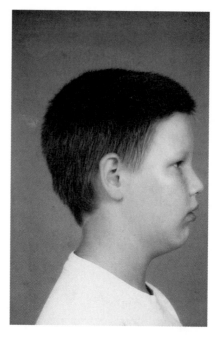

Figure 22-4 Profile facial photograph confirms the balanced vertical proportions with facial convexity and sagittal mandibular deficiency.

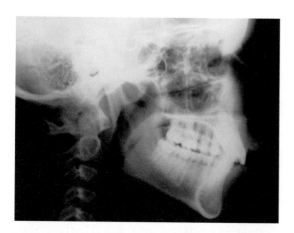

Figure 22-5 Lateral cephalogram in occlusion confirms balanced vertical proportions with facial convexity and sagittal mandibular deficiency.

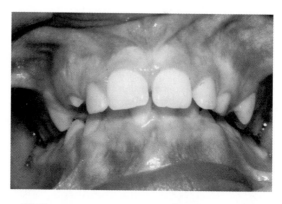

Figure 22-6 Anterior view in occlusion illustrates the increase in overjet and overbite.

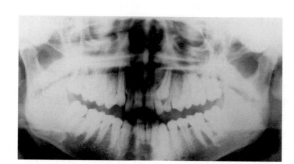

Figure 22-7 Panorex radiograph confirms the presence of the retained maxillary left primary canine and the unerupted permanent canine.

Ref	Sean 11y 8m	Norm
SNA	88	81
SNB	83	77
ANB	5	4
MxUL (mm)	97	87
MnUL (mm)	120	107
Unit Diff (mm)	23	22
A–NV (mm)	−1	+1
Pg–NV (mm)	−11	0
MP/SN	26	32
MP/FH	21	25
% Nasal	44	43
LFH (mm)	68	62
U1/SN	113	102
U1/NA	25	23
U1/NA (mm)	5	4
U1/Exp. (mm)	9	2
L1/MP	97	91
L1/NB	26	26
L1/NB (mm)	4	5

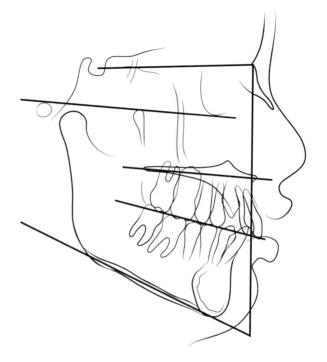

Figure 22-8 Lateral cephalometric tracing confirms the Class II skeletal mandibular deficiency and the Class II Division 1 malocclusion.

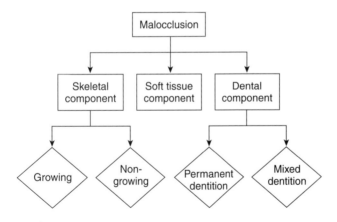

Figure 22-9 Skeletal and dental components of malocclusion.

The lateral cephalometric tracing and analysis illustrated in Figure 22-8 confirms the clinical evaluation of the skeletal and dental components of the malocclusion in the sagittal and vertical dimensions (Figure 22-9).

THE PRIORITIZED PROBLEM LIST

An evaluation of the diagnostic information obtained from the clinical evaluation and the selected diagnostic orthodontic records typically includes study models, photographs, and radiographs. Information from

these records and the clinical evaluation, including the patient's chief concern, are synthesized to produce a ranking of the patient's orthodontic problems. This systematic approach is based on the concept of a prioritized problem list suggested by Weed[19] and has been adapted to a problem-oriented approach in dentistry.

The skeletal component of malocclusion may be assessed clinically during the extraoral examination and confirmed by cephalometric analysis. The cephalometric analysis provides linear and angular measurements defining the sagittal and vertical skeletodental morphology, which was originally recognized by Sassouni and Nanda[20,21] who used constructed horizontal planes based on anatomic features of the craniofacial skeleton (Figure 22-10). In a vertically well-proportioned face, the five constructed planes should converge to a single point located posterior to the face at the occiput (see Figure 22-10, *B*). If the lines do not converge at a single point but are parallel, it is likely that there is a decrease in the vertical dimension (see Figure 22-10, *A*). Alternatively, convergence of the planes close to the external ear in front of the occiput indicates an increase in the anterior vertical dimension (see Figure 22-10, *C*). Other measures associated with the assessment of the vertical dimension include a steep mandibular plane angle, an increased anterior facial height, a short posterior face height, and supereruption of maxillary molars (see Chapter 20). Frost et al[22] concluded that a skeletal difference between long-faced and normal sub-

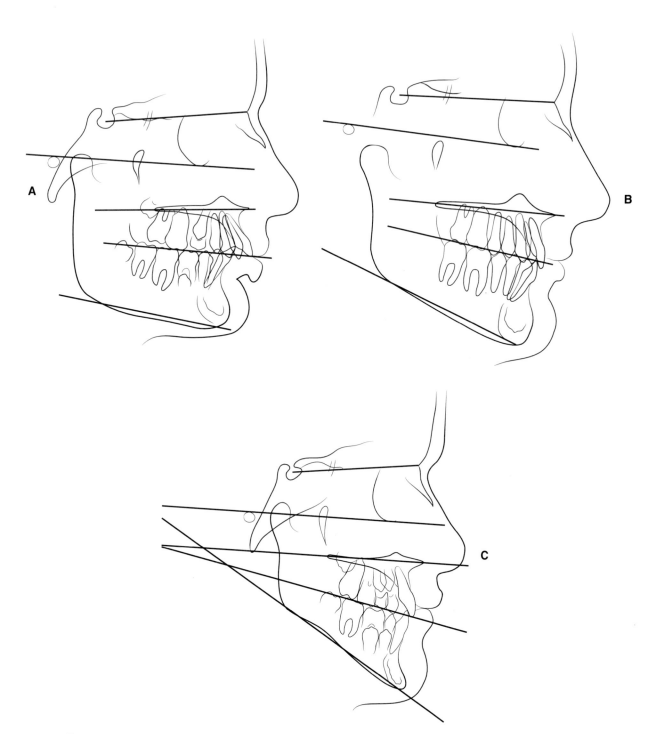

Figure 22-10 A, Tracing of a cephalogram with short anterior lower facial height with the Sassouni planes running almost parallel to each other. **B,** Tracing of a cephalogram with Sassouni planes converging closer to the occiput (back of the head) associated with normal vertical anterior facial height. **C,** Tracing of a cephalogram with the Sassouni planes converging closer to the external ear, in front of the occiput, indicating an increase in the anterior vertical dimension.

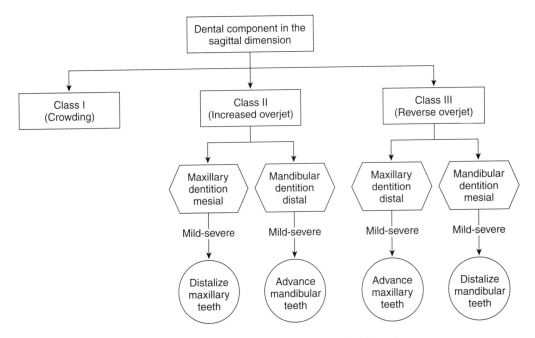

Figure 22-11 Treatment considerations in the sagittal dimension.

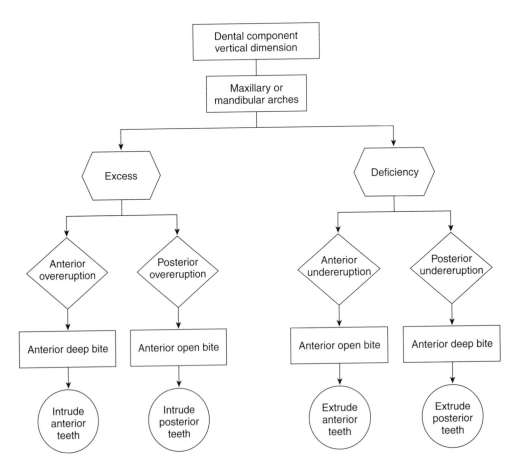

Figure 22-12 Treatment considerations in the vertical plane.

jects exists below the palatal plane and involves the mandibular plane angle secondary to maxillary dentoalveolar excess. Fields et al[23] concluded that differences between normal and long-faced subjects were located below the palatal plane. Specifically, mandibular morphology was determined to be the cause of the disproportionate lower face in long- and short-faced people. In long-faced children, the gonial angle increased, and in long-faced adults, the mandibular ramus height is short. Conversely, a low convergence angle of the mandibular, occlusal, palatal, and supraorbital planes indicated a decreased vertical dimension. Lack of ideal, equidistant convergence of one or more of the five planes indicates whether the maxilla or the mandible is contributing to the vertical disproportionality.

A rational approach to planning treatment for a patient with a sagittal discrepancy begins with identification of the dental and skeletal components contributing to the malocclusion in both the sagittal and vertical dimensions (Figures 22-11 and 22-12).

The skeletal vertical dimension needs to be recognized during diagnosis because its contribution to the malocclusion impacts treatment decisions. When the mandible tends to rotate open in a clockwise direction it appears more sagittally deficient with an increased anterior vertical dimension. When the mandible tends to rotate counterclockwise into a more sagittally protrusive position, there is a reduced anterior vertical dimension. Therefore, given two mandibles of the same size, one tends to appear more retrusive on a long-faced patient and the other more protrusive on a short-faced patient (see Figure 22-2).

TREATMENT OPTIONS RELATED TO AGE AND SEVERITY

It is normal to observe some degree of facial convexity in a patient in **preadolescence.** However, a moderate to severe skeletal discrepancy warrants consideration of modification or redirection of growth. The orthodontic management of a growing patient with a Class II malocclusion who also has an increased anterior vertical dimension or open bite tendency, necessitates an understanding of the interaction of the vertical and sagittal dimensions (see Box 22-1). Two anatomic characteristics that predispose to a skeletal open bite malocclusion are (1) a discrepancy between the vertical growth of the mandibular ramus and the eruption of posterior teeth and (2) the vertical orientation (cant) of the maxilla. Furthermore, correction of increased vertical dimension with growth modification requires prolonged orthodontic treatment because the last stage of growth to be completed is the vertical dimension.[24,25]

One major limitation of growth modification and redirection with a high-pull headgear is that it does not deliver a vertical force without a sagittal component. This may present a problem in the correction of Class III malocclusions with open bite tendencies.

Schudy[26] also emphasized the impact of the vertical dimension on the correction of anteroposterior discrepancies. His work and that of Bjork and Skeiller[17] resulted in considerable attention being directed toward the clockwise growth pattern with an increased vertical dimension and an anterior open bite. In contrast, the opposite growth pattern with the mandible rotating counterclockwise causes a decreased lower anterior facial height and may result in a deep impinging overbite (see Box 22-2). Because either an open bite or a compensated deep bite can occur in high-angle skeletal malocclusions, the results of treatment intervention on the skeletodental pattern have often been contradictory.[27,28]

TREATMENT OF CASES WITH MILD TO MODERATE SKELETAL DISCREPANCIES

Preadolescents with Growth Potential

Preadolescents with growth potential may benefit from modification and redirection of growth. The case illustrated in Figures 22-3 through 22-8 was diagnosed as a Class II malocclusion with associated skeletal mandibular deficiency but with a normal anterior lower facial height and an increased overbite. The prognosis for reduction of the overbite was, therefore, good if the growth pattern was maintained, but control of the vertical position of the maxillary incisors was a priority (Figure 22-13). Comprehensive orthodontic treatment therefore included the provision of a vertical intrusive

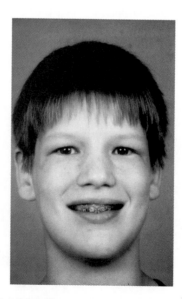

Figure 22-13 Full face photograph with the patient smiling, indicating an increase in gingival display.

force from a high pull headgear to the hooks soldered to the maxillary arch wire (Figure 22-14). Superimposition of the final cephalometric result represented a 2-year growth period (Figure 22-15). The maxillary incisors were held vertically while the increase in the intermaxillary vertical dimension and the growth of the lips continued during this period. This resulted in an excellent Class 1 occlusal relationship with balanced vertical and sagittal facial proportions (Figures 22-16 and 22-17).

The focus of Chapter 20 and of this chapter is the sagittal and vertical diagnosis and treatment planning of Class II malocclusion (Figure 22-18). On the other hand, the indications for a protraction face mask in the modification and redirection of growth in preadolescent skeletal maxillary deficient Class III malocclusion (Figure 22-19) are discussed in Chapter 21.

Adolescents with Minimal Growth Potential

Because the vertical skeletal and dentoalveolar growth is the last to be completed, the **adolescent** with an increased vertical dimension and minimal growth potential will not significantly improve from appliances that would only control any residual eruption potential of both the maxillary and mandibular dentition. Therefore, in these cases, if growth modification has been attempted unsuccessfully, orthognathic surgery should be considered once growth has stabilized.

For those borderline patients who benefited from growth modification but still exhibit the long face syndrome, any camouflage of the sagittal skeletal dimension with reduction of the overjet and extraction of maxillary first premolars is unlikely to be esthetically satisfactory. Wearing Class II elastics tends to rotate the mandible down and back with further eruption of the mandibular posterior dentition, whereas the retrusion and extrusion of the maxillary incisors increases the already obtuse nasolabial angle (see Chapter 20).

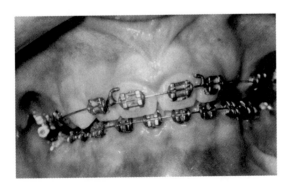

Figure 22-14 Hooks soldered on the arch wire for placement of an anterior high-pull J-hook headgear for incisor intrusion.

Adults with Little to No Growth Potential

If there is a mild skeletal discrepancy, orthodontic camouflage may be the optimal treatment choice. On the other hand, orthognathic surgery is an option that should be presented to **adult** patients with severe skeletal discrepancies. The severity of the skeletal and dental components of the malocclusion and esthetic needs of the patient must be taken into consideration in formulating a treatment plan for the patient (Figures 22-20 and 22-21).

The Effect of Class II Mechanics

Camouflage treatment for patients who have both functional and esthetic needs should meet specific selection criteria including mild vertical dentoalveolar discrepancies, protrusive maxillary incisors, and normal to mild sagittal problems. The orthodontic mechanics used to close spaces following premolar extraction facilitates the closure of open bites by two basic mechanisms: (1) mesial movement of molar teeth resulting in reduction of the mandibular plane angle and (2) retraction and retroclination of the maxillary incisors resulting in uprighting and relative extrusion. The use of **Class II elastics** to achieve a Class I molar relationship result in extrusion of the mandibular molars, which cause a clockwise mandibular rotation. Such a movement increases the mandibular plane angle, lengthens the lower facial height, and decreases the mandibular sagittal projection, making the patient appear even more mandibular deficient. If the resulting dental correction is satisfactory, reduction in the lower facial height and sagittal chin augmentation may be achieved with a genioplasty. Inferior mandibular border osteotomy (genioplasty) is a useful adjunctive procedure for the treatment of facial vertical excess, particularly when the discrepancy is manifested in the anterior part of the mandible.[29]

The Effect of Using Pretorqued and Preangulated Brackets

Patients with a severe skeletal open bite are not good candidates for orthodontic camouflage because most orthodontic mechanotherapy results in some extrusion of teeth. The **preadjusted appliance,** used routinely in the clinical practice of orthodontics, was designed to produce ideal dental relationships on normally positioned jaws. If the underlying skeletal features of a vertical problem are present, orthodontic alignment and leveling with such an appliance will often produce an open bite malocclusion. Orthodontic correction of open bite deformities is prone to failure because it does not address the underlying skeletal discrepancy. Therefore

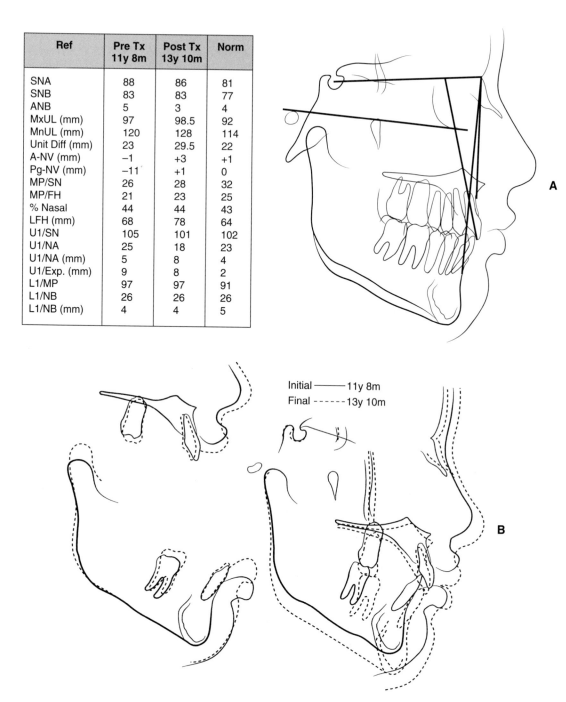

Ref	Pre Tx 11y 8m	Post Tx 13y 10m	Norm
SNA	88	86	81
SNB	83	83	77
ANB	5	3	4
MxUL (mm)	97	98.5	92
MnUL (mm)	120	128	114
Unit Diff (mm)	23	29.5	22
A-NV (mm)	−1	+3	+1
Pg-NV (mm)	−11	+1	0
MP/SN	26	28	32
MP/FH	21	23	25
% Nasal	44	44	43
LFH (mm)	68	78	64
U1/SN	105	101	102
U1/NA	25	18	23
U1/NA (mm)	5	8	4
U1/Exp. (mm)	9	8	2
L1/MP	97	97	91
L1/NB	26	26	26
L1/NB (mm)	4	4	5

Initial ———— 11y 8m
Final - - - - - 13y 10m

Figure 22-15 **A,** Posttreatment cephalogram indicating reduction in overjet and overbite with Class I molar relationship. **B,** Superimposition of pretreatment and posttreatment cephalograms with regional maxillary and mandibular superimpositions. Note the predominant vertical growth of the mandible during the 2-year treatment period.

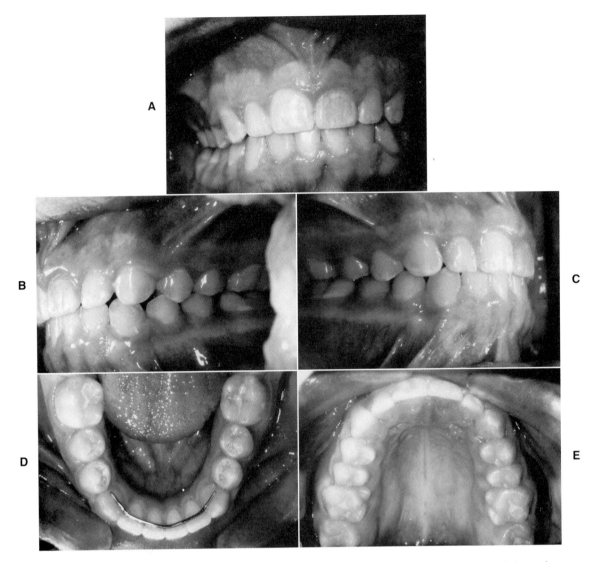

Figure 22-16 A, Anterior view of the occlusion showing reduction of overjet and overbite posttreatment. **B,** Intraoral view of the left buccal occlusion posttreatment. **C,** Intraoral view of the right Class I buccal occlusion posttreatment. **D,** Occlusal view of the mandibular arch with a bonded lower anterior retainer. **E,** Occlusal view of the well-aligned maxillary arch posttreatment.

successful correction of a moderate or severe vertical skeletal problem is more effectively treated with a combined orthodontic/orthognathic surgical approach.

Class III Malocclusions

Although the Class II vertical and sagittal components have been discussed in some detail, the Class III malocclusion has the opposite set of problems. The Class II skeletal malocclusion with mandibular deficiency may be treated with a mandibular surgical advancement in late adolescence, whereas mandibular excess with a resulting Class III malocclusion should be delayed until mandibular growth has stabilized. This requires an understanding of normal growth and development of the

craniofacial complex in which a cephalocaudal gradient exists so that those components more caudal to the brain, such as the mandible, continue growing after the maxillary complex has stabilized.

Retention

Stability of orthodontic correction of the vertical dimension depends more on the patient's posttreatment growth pattern than on the completed treatment result. Continued growth in an undesirable direction, which initially resulted in the development of a vertical dysplasia, may be the major cause of relapse after orthodontic treatment. An understanding of the individual's growth pattern and the anticipated residual

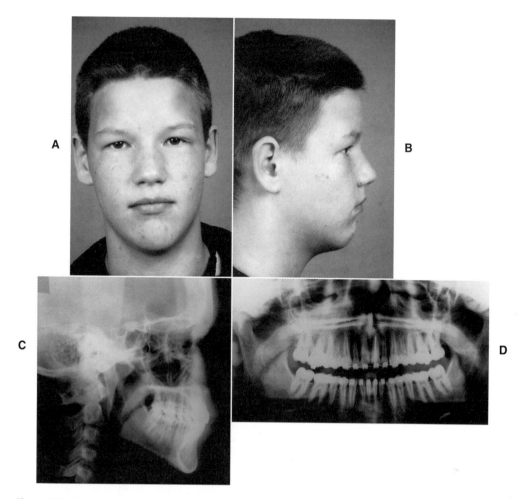

Figure 22-17 A, Frontal facial photograph following treatment. **B,** Profile facial photograph posttreatment illustrating well-balanced vertical and sagittal proportions. **C,** Posttreatment cephalometric radiograph. **D,** Panorex radiograph taken before appliance removal. The traumatized maxillary left central incisor was endodontically treated.

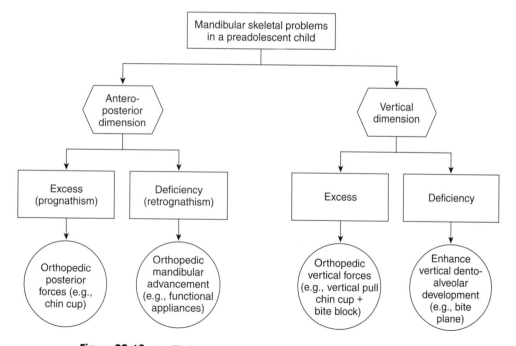

Figure 22-18 Mandibular treatment considerations (Class II and III malocclusions).

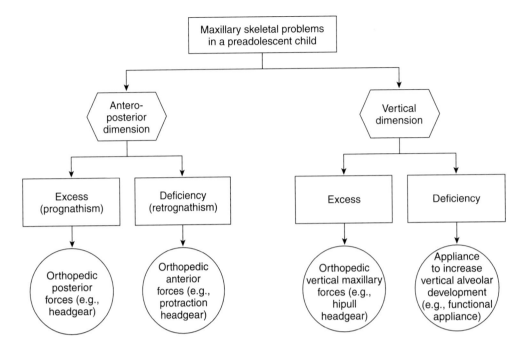

Figure 22-19 Maxillary treatment considerations (Class II or III malocclusion).

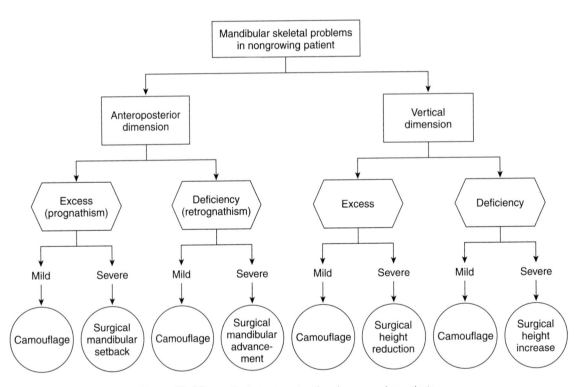

Figure 22-20 Mandibular treatment options in nongrowing patients.

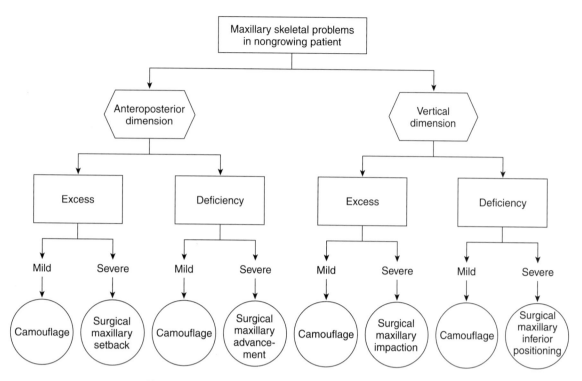

Figure 22-21 Maxillary treatment options in nongrowing patients.

growth should be considered in the design of a retainer. One of the most effective methods of controlling eruption of the posterior dentition, especially the maxillary molars, is a maxillary retainer with a high-pull headgear. Because growth is expressed primarily in the vertical dimension until early adulthood, a longer retention period should ideally be considered, although no reliable predictor of posttreatment stability has been identified.[30]

SUMMARY

The purpose of this chapter has been to relate the interdependence of the vertical and sagittal dimensions to the treatment of Class II malocclusion with decisions based on the age and severity of the patient. The skeletal and dental components contributing to the sagittal dimension in Class II and Class III malocclusion types are summarized in Figure 22-1. The dental anteroposterior or sagittal component is further summarized in Figure 22-11, which also considers treatment related to malocclusion severity. The dental component of malocclusion in the vertical dimension needs to be identified when treatment considerations are planned for open bite and deep overbite incisal relationships. In considering the mandibular skeletal contribution to the malocclusion in the preadolescent child, the interrelationship between the anteroposterior and vertical di-

mensions in mandibular skeletal discrepancies is crucial in treatment planning. Also discussed is the maxillary skeletal component in the preadolescent stage, which should relate the vertical and sagittal dimensions to the treatment options. When considering the nongrowing patient with a mandibular or maxillary skeletal discrepancy in the vertical and sagittal dimensions, the options of either camouflage or orthognathic surgery are important to discuss before a patient can make an informed decision. To the novice, the technical aspects of orthodontic treatment planning and delivery of care may seem deceptively simple with pretorqued and preangulated appliances, whereas the systematic approach to diagnosis and the development of a prioritized problem list are the critical foundation for a successful outcome. If the clinician fails to understand and identify the components contributing to the initial malocclusion, the process in providing treatment will surely fail.

REFERENCES

1. Angle EH: *Treatment of malocclusion of the teeth and fractures of the maxillae: Angle's systems,* ed 6, Philadelphia, 1900, SS White Dental Mfg.
2. Kelly JE, Sanchez M, Van Kirk LE: *An assessment of the occlusion of teeth of children,* DHEW pub no HRA 74-1612, Washington, DC, 1973, National Center for Health Statistics.

3. Kelly J, Harvey C: An assessment of the teeth of youths 12-17 years, DHEW pub no HRA 77-1644, Washington, DC, 1977, National Center for Health Statistics.

4. Proffit WR, Fields HW: The orthodontic problem. In Proffit WR, Fields HW (eds): *Contemporary orthodontics*, ed 3, St Louis, 2000, Mosby.

5. Proffit WR, White RP Jr: Long-face problems. In Proffit WR, White RP Jr (eds): *Surgical-orthodontic treatment*, St Louis, 1991, Mosby.

6. Ellis E III: The nature of vertical maxillary deformities: implications for surgical intervention, *J Oral Maxillofac Surg* 43:756-762, 1985.

7. Ellis E III, McNamara JA Jr, Lawrence TM: Components of adult Class II open-bite malocclusion, *J Oral Maxillofac Surg* 43(2):92-105, 1985.

8. Popovitch F, Thompson GW: Craniofacial templates for orthodontic case analysis, *Am J Orthod* 71:406-420, 1977.

9. Proffit WR, Ackerman JL: Diagnosis and treatment planning in orthodontics. In Graber TM, Vanarsdall RL (eds): *Orthodontics: current principles and techniques*, ed 3, St Louis, 2000, Mosby.

10. Ackermann JL, Proffit WR: Soft tissue limitations in orthodontics: treatment planning guidelines, *Angle Orthod* 67(5):327-336, 1997.

11. Bjork A, Skeiller V: Facial development and tooth eruption: an implant study at the age of puberty, *Am J Orthod* 62:339-383, 1972.

12. Proffit WR, Phillips C: Adaptations in lip posture and pressure following orthognathic surgery, *Am J Orthod Dentofacial Orthop* 93:294-302, 1988.

13. Linder-Aronson S: Respiratory function in relation to facial morphology and the dentition, *Br J Orthod* 6:59-71, 1979.

14. Vig KW: Nasal obstruction and facial growth: the strength of evidence for clinical assumptions, *Am J Orthod Dentofacial Orthop* 113(6):603-611, 1998.

15. Kluemper GT, Vig PS, Vig KW: Nasorespiratory characteristics and craniofacial morphology, *Eur J Orthod* 17:491-495, 1995.

16. Shanker S et al: Dentofacial morphology and upper respiratory function in 8-10-year-old children, *Clin Orthod Res* 2:19-26, 1999.

17. Bjork A, Skeiller V: Normal and abnormal growth of the mandible: a synthesis of longitudinal cephalometric implant studies over a period of 25 years, *Eur J Orthod* 5(1):1-46, 1983.

18. Isaacson JR et al: Extreme variation in vertical facial growth and associated variation in skeletal and dental relations, *Angle Orthod* 41:219-229, 1971.

19. Weed LL: *Medical records, medical education, and patient care: the problem-oriented record as a basic tool*, Cleveland, 1969, Case Western Reserve Press.

20. Sassouni VA: A classification of skeletal facial types, *Am J Orthod* 55(2):109-123, 1969.

21. Sassouni VA, Nanda S: Analysis of dentofacial vertical proportions, *Am J Orthod* 50(11):801-823, 1964.

22. Frost DE et al: Cephalometric diagnosis and surgical orthodontic correction of apertognathia, *Am J Orthod* 78(6):657-669, 1980.

23. Fields HW et al: Facial pattern differences in long face children and adults, *Am J Orthod* 85(3):217-223, 1984.

24. Behrents RG: *An atlas of growth in the aging craniofacial skeleton*. Monograph #18, Craniofacial Growth Series, Center for Human Growth and Development, Ann Arbor, Mich, 1985, University of Michigan.

25. Bishara SE et al: Changes in dentofacial structures in untreated Class II division 1 and normal subjects: a longitudinal study, *Angle Orthod* 67(1):55-66, 1997.

26. Schudy FF: The control of vertical overbite in clinical orthodontics, *Angle Orthod* 38(1):19-39, 1968.

27. Sarver DM, Weissman SM: Nonsurgical treatment of open bite in nongrowing patients, *Am J Orthod Dentofacial Orthop* 108(6):651-659, 1995.

28. Hering K, Ruf S, Pancherz H: Orthodontic treatment of openbite and deepbite high-angle malocclusions, *Angle Orthod* 69(5):470-477, 1999.

29. Fridrich KL, Casko JS: Genioplasty strategies for anterior facial vertical dysplasias, *Int J Adult Orthodon Orthognath Surg* 12(1):35-41, 1997.

30. Lopez-Gavito G et al: Anterior open-bite malocclusion: a longitudinal 10-year postretention evaluation of orthodontically treated patients, *Am J Orthod* 87(3):175-186, 1985.

CHAPTER 23

Skeletal and Dental Considerations in the Transverse Dimension

Katherine W.L. Vig, Shiva V. Shanker, and Marla J. Magness

KEY TERMS

posterior crossbite
orthodontic treatment

palatal expansion
malocclusion

surgically assisted rapid palatal
expansion

The transverse dimension is often interrelated with the sagittal and vertical dimensions. However, the transverse dimension relates primarily to the posterior occlusion, and any discrepancy is usually manifest as a crossbite of the buccal occlusion.

A **posterior crossbite** in the centric occlusal relationship may have skeletal and dental components and clinically may present as a unilateral or bilateral crossbite involving single or multiple teeth. In the functioning occlusal position this may be associated with a mandibular shift from centric relation (CR) to centric occlusion (CO). Although patients seeking **orthodontic treatment** do so for esthetic and functional reasons, the detection of a posterior crossbite is typically first noticed by the family dentist or pediatric dentist and brought to the parents' or patient's attention. If treatment is recommended, the intervention is designed to correct the transverse discrepancy and so provide a normal interocclusal relationship, which will be stable in its new position of equilibrium and occlusal interdigitation.

The purpose of this chapter is to consider the diagnosis and treatment planning of the posterior crossbite in the context of relating the cause to the age of the patient and the stage of dental development. Considerations in the primary, mixed, and permanent dentitions are discussed and illustrated.

In the young child a posterior crossbite is typically the result of a constricted maxillary dental arch. This is often associated with a thumb sucking habit (Figure 23-1). The habit is usually self-limiting with the child discontinuing the digit sucking habit as the result of peer pressure during the elementary school years. If the habit is discontinued, typically at a time when the permanent incisors are starting to erupt, the effect of an increased and asymmetric overjet in the primary dentition may be self-limiting in the early mixed dentition. However, although the digit sucking habit may be discontinued, the posterior crossbite, if present, may not self-correct. Alternatively, if the digit sucking habit persists but the child is ready to discontinue it, a quad helix type of appliance may effectively provide a reminder to the patient and provide interceptive correction of the crossbite (Figure 23-2).

UNILATERAL POSTERIOR CROSSBITE

Primary Dentition

If a CR/CO shift is associated with the posterior crossbite, the treatment recommended to expand the maxillary arch to correct the unilateral crossbite will also eliminate the mandibular shift. When using growth-modifying functional appliances to correct Class II malocclusions, the working bite is taken in a forward mandibular position to redirect mandibular growth and produce both skeletal and dental changes. This

431

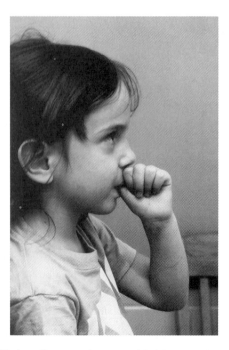

Figure 23-1 Profile view of a 3-year-old child with a thumb sucking habit that has an anterior protrusive effect on the maxillary primary incisors and often associated with lateral collapse of the posterior segments resulting in a posterior crossbite.

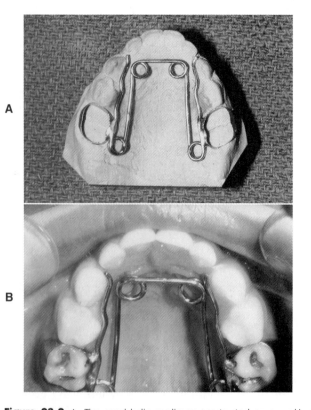

Figure 23-2 A, The quad helix appliance constructed on a working model for a patient in the primary dentition. Note the two anterior helices have been constructed anteriorly as a reminder to discontinue the digit sucking habit. **B,** The appliance intraorally cemented on to the primary second molars.

suggests that if the mandible is postured into an undesired position as a result of a functional shift, those factors that modify and redirect normal growth may cause the mandible to grow asymmetrically in an attempt to eliminate the CR/CO shift. The mandible is then no longer deflected into the unilateral crossbite position on closing into maximal occlusal interdigitation. This new occlusion is a result of the acquired mandibular skeletal asymmetry and the dental compensations that may occur in the untreated patient. Therefore a posterior unilateral crossbite associated with a mandibular shift should be treated in the primary dentition or early mixed dentition in an attempt to allow the permanent successors to erupt into a normal occlusal position after the CR/CO shift is eliminated.[1] Waiting for all the permanent successors to erupt before correcting the crossbite and the functional shift establishes the permanent dentition in a deflected occlusal position. On the other hand, if no CR/CO shift exists in the primary dentition, delaying treatment until the mixed dentition allows the first permanent molars to be included in the corrective appliance if they also erupt in a crossbite relationship.

Fixed or removable appliances, even those that deliver low-force magnitudes, have an effect on both skeletal and dental components during the correction in the primary dentition. The quad helix and W arch tend to be used extensively as interceptive corrective appliances for a posterior crossbite (Figure 23-3). The intermaxillary suture often responds to **palatal expansion** at this stage of development because the interdigitation of the midpalatal suture has not been established. Therefore a removable appliance with a jack screw, a W arch, or a quad helix appliance provides an increase in the transverse maxillary dentition with correction of the posterior crossbite (see Chapters 17 and 19).[2] In summary, the early correction of posterior crossbites by interceptive treatment is considered to result in a more stable, long-term occlusal correction.[3]

MIXED DENTITION

In the preadolescent patient, problems in the transverse dimension are generally identified as skeletal or dental and may range in severity. A common transverse problem is caused by skeletal maxillary constriction, which is manifest as a dental posterior crossbite. This may be unilateral or bilateral and usually includes multiple teeth. As with the primary dentition, the posterior crossbite is diagnosed in CO, but it should also be assessed in CR to identify if a mandibular shift exists (Figure 23-4). If there is no CR/CO mandibular shift then a true unilateral posterior crossbite exists. The cause may be from maxillary constriction or mandibular expansion and may involve one tooth or multiple teeth in a posterior crossbite relationship. A systematic diagnostic approach

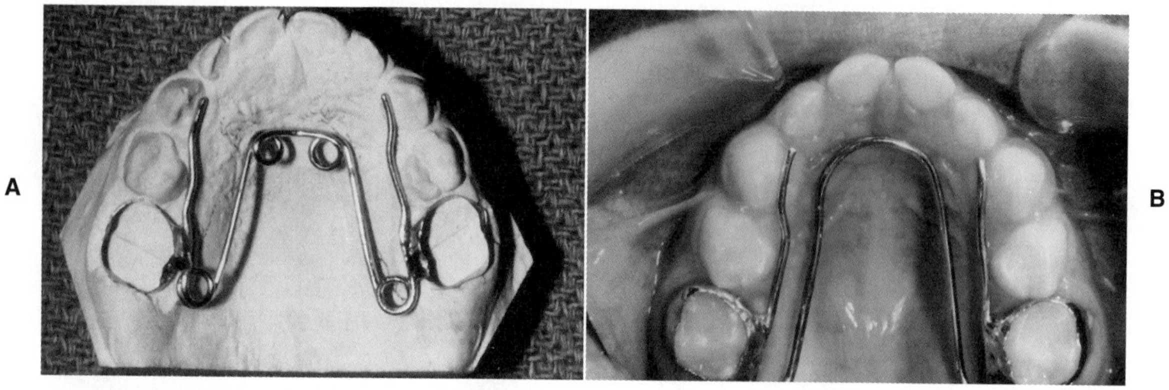

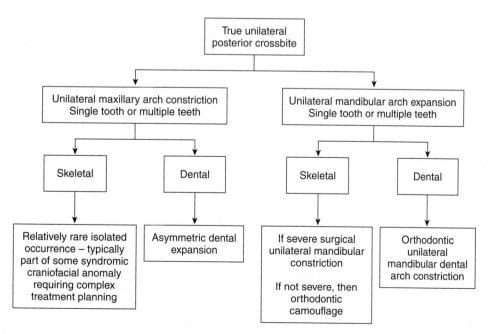

Figure 23-3 **A,** Quad helix appliance in the primary dentition to correct a posterior crossbite. **B,** W arch in the primary dentition as an alternative palatal expansion device.

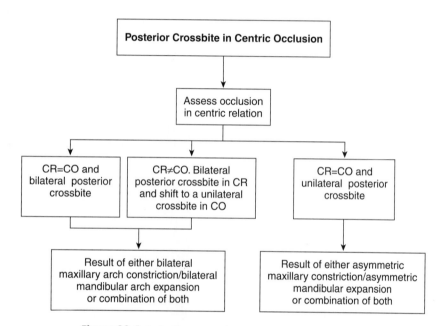

Posterior Crossbite in Centric Occlusion

Assess occlusion in centric relation

CR=CO and bilateral posterior crossbite

CR≠CO. Bilateral posterior crossbite in CR and shift to a unilateral crossbite in CO

CR=CO and unilateral posterior crossbite

Result of either bilateral maxillary arch constriction/bilateral mandibular arch expansion or combination of both

Result of either asymmetric maxillary constriction/asymmetric mandibular expansion or combination of both

Figure 23-4 Evaluating a posterior crossbite in centric occlusion.

True unilateral posterior crossbite

Unilateral maxillary arch constriction Single tooth or multiple teeth

Unilateral mandibular arch expansion Single tooth or multiple teeth

Skeletal

Dental

Skeletal

Dental

Relatively rare isolated occurrence – typically part of some syndromic craniofacial anomaly requiring complex treatment planning

Asymmetric dental expansion

If severe surgical unilateral mandibular constriction

If not severe, then orthodontic camouflage

Orthodontic unilateral mandibular dental arch constriction

Figure 23-5 Clinical flow chart with pathways for differential diagnosis and treatment planning for a true unilateral posterior crossbite.

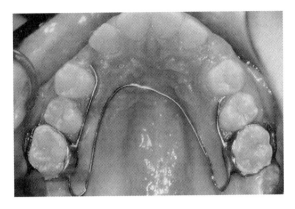

Figure 23-6 Late mixed dentition stage with a W arch designed asymmetrically to produce unilateral forces for dental correction.

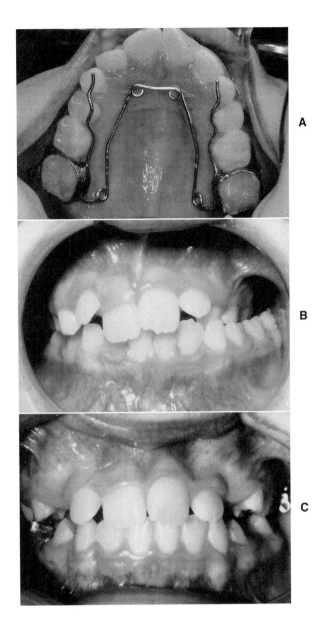

Figure 23-7 A, Quad helix appliance cemented to the first permanent molars in the early mixed dentition. **B,** Patient in the early mixed dentition with centric relation (CR)/centric occlusion (CO) shift into a left occlusal posterior crossbite with deviation of lower midline to the left. **C,** Same patient following palatal expansion with quad helix to eliminate the CR/CO shift, correct the posterior crossbite, and almost correct the dental midline discrepancy.

should identify the contribution of the dental and skeletal components so that the appropriate treatment may be selected based on the severity and the ability of the dentoalveolar component to compensate or camouflage the skeletal pattern (Figure 23-5). If individual teeth need to be repositioned asymmetrically, the anchorage requirements can be balanced by extending the palatal arm in a W type arch (Figure 23-6). This design maximizes the tooth movements on the opposite side.

An important caveat in recognizing a transverse problem is to ensure that the diagnosis has defined the skeletal and dental components of the **malocclusion.** A progressive skeletal asymmetry caused by early condylar fracture[4] or a craniofacial developmental anomaly such as hemifacial microsomia will result in asymmetric mandibular growth with adaptive maxillary dental arch compensation. These cases should be diagnosed and treated early to avoid creating severe skeletal discrepancies.[5] If the skeletal component of the malocclusion is treated solely by dental compensations, the correction of the crossbite may not be stable and could relapse to the initial unilateral crossbite relationship. True skeletal unilateral crossbites may require surgical as well as orthodontic corrections.

UNILATERAL POSTERIOR CROSSBITE IN CLEFT LIP AND PALATE

Maxillary skeletal asymmetry in unilateral complete clefts of the lip and palate may also be reflected in a unilateral posterior crossbite, which may be expanded with a quad helix type of appliance in the mixed dentition (Figure 23-7). Unlike those cases in the late mixed dentition for which rapid palatal expansion is the treatment of choice, the cleft maxilla does not have a midpalatal suture, which requires orthopedic forces to open. Instead there is a midpalatal cleft covered with

repaired and scarred palatal tissues limiting the rate and amount of expansion. The slower rate of expansion and the lower force magnitude provided by a quad helix appliance allows the soft tissue of the palate to stretch and adapt to the increasing maxillary width, avoiding a breakdown of the scar tissue that can result in an oronasal fistula (Figure 23-8). This type of orthodontic expansion treatment is often timed to precede the surgical placement of an alveolar bone graft in the mixed dentition stage.[6]

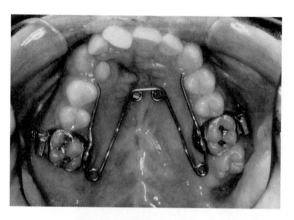

Figure 23-8 Unilateral repaired cleft lip and palate with quad helix to provide expansion of the posterior segments before an alveolar bone graft is placed and the fistula is closed.

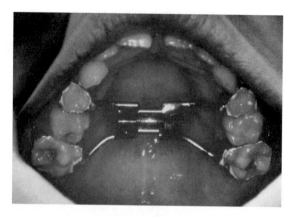

Figure 23-9 Rapid palatal expander cemented to maxillary first premolars and molars. Note the median diastema that has developed as a consequence of the expansion.

BILATERAL POSTERIOR CROSSBITE

Correction of a posterior crossbite in children and preadolescents may involve the whole buccal segment or may be localized to one or more teeth. If the crossbite or transverse discrepancy has a dental cause, cross elastics or coordinated upper and lower arch wires may change the dental relationship by tipping the teeth into their correct axial positions. Similarly, if there is a mild skeletal transverse discrepancy, camouflage by dental compensation may be the treatment of choice.

A bilateral posterior crossbite may result from either maxillary constriction or mandibular expansion or be the resultant of a combination of both.

In the older child more dental and less skeletal change occurs with the quad helix or W arch appliances. Typically, skeletal correction involves orthopedic maxillary arch expansion. If a CR/CO shift has resulted in an end-on occlusal relationship with an associated mandibular shift, the bilateral skeletal expansion of the maxilla will also eliminate the shift and correct the unilateral crossbite in the centric occlusal position.

Rapid palatal expansion provides an orthopedic force capable of expanding the midpalatal suture and requires a fixed appliance with bands cemented on the first permanent molars and either the first premolars or primary second molars depending on the stage of development of the occlusion. This may be accomplished with a hyrax type appliance screw (Figure 23-9). The patient turns the screw twice a day (each turn of the screw expands ¼ mm) to produce 0.5 mm of opening per day and delivering 2000 to 3000 g of force. In the initial phase of treatment there is more skeletal than dental movement and the force is directed to the maxillary midline over a 7- to 10-day period (Figure 23-10). Some overexpansion is indicated to compensate for the relapse tendency and to help stabilize the increased trans-

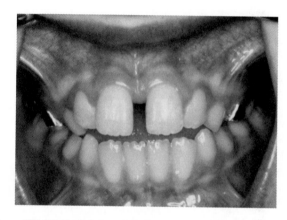

Figure 23-10 Anterior view of the same patient in Figure 23-9. The posterior crossbite is corrected. Further expansion for overcorrection will result in an increase in the median diastema and opening of the bite caused by cuspal interference.

verse skeletal width of the maxilla. During this period there may be some dental compensation as the skeletal transverse expansion settles. Following this active palatal expansion, the appliance remains in place for 3 months to allow bone to fill in the separated midpalatal suture and for the residual pressure to dissipate from the displaced structures. During this time the median diastema, which normally opens during the active phase of expansion, closes as the central incisors move spontaneously toward the midline. As the teeth are held rigidly by the appliance, the transverse relationship that has been overexpanded at least 2 to 3 mm maintains the correction. Radiographically, the midline suture opens more anteriorly than posteriorly, resulting in the V-shaped midline translucency (Figure 23-11).

Adding of palatal flanges of acrylic to the appliance may add to the skeletal expansion effect and has been advocated by Haas.[7] The Minne-expander (Figure 23-12) is another appliance that delivers orthopedic force to

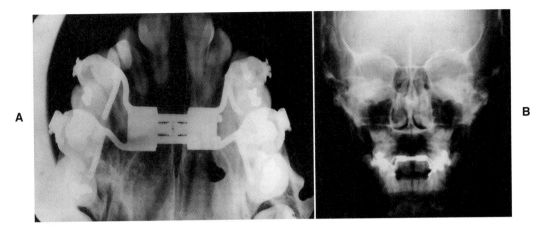

Figure 23-11 A, Occlusal radiograph with hyrax appliance following activation. Note the V-shaped midpalatal radiolucency associated with opening of the midpalatal suture more anteriorly than posteriorly. **B,** Posteroanterior radiograph showing midline translucency extending into the floor of the nasal cavity.

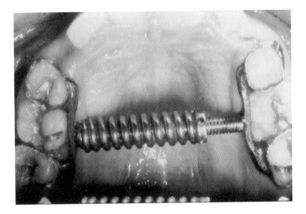

Figure 23-12 The Minne-expander cemented onto primary first molars and first permanent molars. The compressed spring has been considered to apply a more constant and physiologic expansion force.

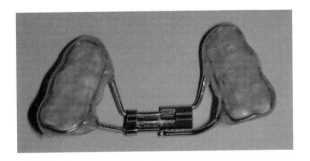

Figure 23-13 Posterior bite blocks on the maxillary molars provide control of the vertical dimension and reduce cuspal interference during the active expansion phase and during retention.

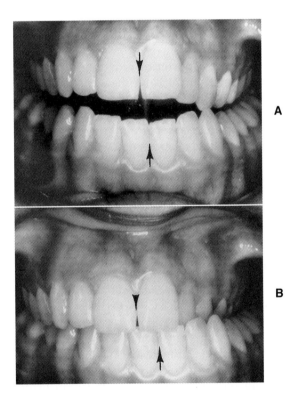

Figure 23-14 A, Occlusal interference on the left permanent canines that was not treated earlier in the development of the occlusion. Note mild midline discrepancy in centric relation (CR) and cant of maxillary occlusal plane. **B,** Occlusal relationship following CR/CO shift of the mandible to the left (CO). Note severe dental midline discrepancy and left unilateral complete posterior crossbite.

affect skeletal transverse growth modification. It provides a more constant but much stronger force through the compressed spring. Both these orthopedic expansion appliances may have posterior bite blocks added to control cuspal interference (Figure 23-13).

Permanent Dentition

Age and Maxillary Expansion
Expansion of the maxillary arch is the most common treatment intervention to correct posterior crossbite, and the treatment approach is related to the age of the patient. Before midpalatal suture fusion, orthopedic forces

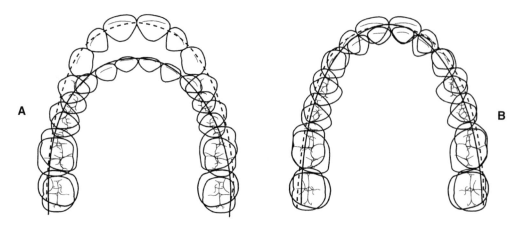

Figure 23-15 Representation indicating the effect on the transverse relationship by moving the mandibular arch anteriorly to create a Class I molar relationship (*dotted arch form*) with reduction of overjet. **A,** Class II occlusograms before movement. **B,** Occlusograms after movement. Note that the lower arch is now in posterior crossbite.

may be applied to separate the suture and allow bone to fill in the expanded midpalatal area. However, once the suture closes, usually at about 16 years of age, a decline in the ability (and stability) of rapid palatal expansion occurs as a result of the progressive interdigitation and fusion of the various sutures as well as the resistance of the skeletal and soft tissue structures, which, in turn, become less responsive to the expansion forces.[8] Although it is relatively easy to widen the maxilla by opening the midpalatal suture during adolescence, it becomes gradually more difficult during late adolescence. As a result, the effectiveness of rapid palatal expansion decreases and after 16 years of age is usually not recommended.[9] Some evidence supports the concept that early transverse expansion in the mixed dentition is more stable than when the expansion is performed later, following the eruption of the permanent dentition.[10] However, failing to recommend interceptive treatment may result in an established occlusal relationship in the permanent dentition associated with a CR/CO shift and possible skeletal asymmetry (Figure 23-14).

Surgically Assisted Expansion   The ability to increase the skeletal transverse dimension in the adult may be accomplished with a **surgically assisted rapid palatal expansion** or during orthognathic surgery when a two- or three-piece maxillary osteotomy widens the maxilla.

RELATIONSHIP OF THE TRANSVERSE DIMENSION WITH THE SAGITTAL DIMENSION

Often a posterior crossbite is associated with a sagittal Class II malocclusion in which a constricted maxillary arch is in a Class II molar relationship with an increased

overjet (see Chapter 20). This constricted maxillary arch width may result in a unilateral or bilateral crossbite. When the patient is asked to posture the mandible forward into a Class I molar relationship to eliminate the overjet the posterior crossbite becomes more apparent clinically (Figure 23-15). In the adult patient for whom growth modification is not an option, a surgical procedure to lengthen the mandible may also require presurgical transverse expansion of the maxilla. Children with sagittal maxillary deficiency reflected as a Class III malocclusion may benefit from growth modification by maxillary protraction, which is often accompanied by palatal expansion (see Chapter 21).[11] In skeletal Class III malocclusions, which require surgical correction, the change in the sagittal dimension might also correct the clinical transverse discrepancy if one exists. Therefore a mandibular skeletal Class II or Class III malocclusion in which intervention is primarily targeted at correcting the sagittal dimension alone may either improve or exaggerate the transverse discrepancy. This relationship should be taken into consideration during the treatment planning of these cases.

Other Factors to Consider

Crowding has been suggested as a reason to perform rapid palatal expansion to avoid the extraction of premolars. This approach may be successful in creating adequate space (Figure 23-16). Palatal expansion should probably be considered primarily as the correction of posterior crossbites rather than for a means for generating space to relieve crowding. This especially applies if there is a satisfactory posterior occlusion with no crossbite relationship.

Mandibular arch expansion may occur in cases of macroglossia with spacing of the teeth or in severe skeletal discrepancies between the maxilla and mandible. Alternatively, a bilateral buccal posterior cross-

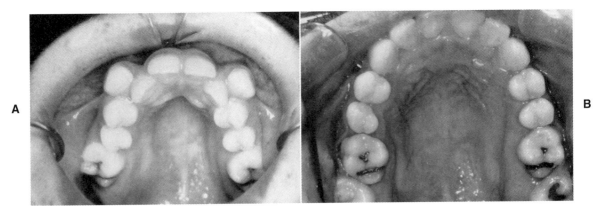

Figure 23-16 **A,** Early permanent dentition with maxillary canines excluded from the arch buccally. **B,** Maxillary expansion and comprehensive orthodontic treatment to align the maxillary arch with alignment of the maxillary canines.

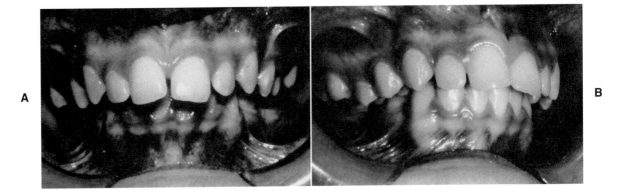

Figure 23-17 Anterior view of Brodie bite with the maxillary arch in a bilateral posterior crossbite telescoping the mandibular arch. **B,** Lateral occlusal view to show complete buccal crossbite.

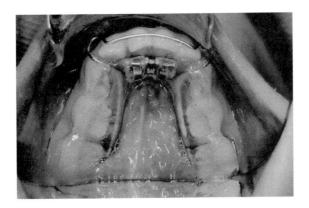

Figure 23-18 Schwartz type of lower expansion device with midline hyrax screw and posterior bite blocks.

bite may occur when the maxillary dentition telescopes the lower dental arch to produce a Brodie bite (Figure 23-17). Correction of this type of malocclusion requires opening the bite to allow expansion of the mandibular arch, which may be achieved with a Schwartz type of active appliance (Figure 23-18), a functional appliance, or a surgical intervention. Expansion of the lower arch is difficult to achieve in many cases, and the need for prolonged retention to stabilize the lower expansion will be necessary.

Another physiologic association that has been observed to impact the transverse dimension is the presence of a posterior crossbite attributed to a mouth-breathing habit as a result of upper respiratory obstruction.[12] The rationale assumes that the open mouth posture allows an oral airway to be maintained, which results in the tongue being lower in the inter-maxillary space and simultaneously increasing the relative influence of the buccal musculature on the unsupported maxillary posterior teeth.

SUMMARY

The objectives of this chapter have been to systematically consider the cause and treatment of discrepancies in the transverse dimension as a function of the age and

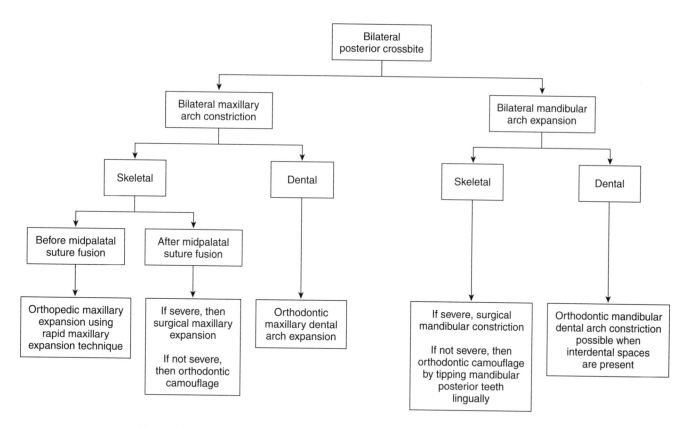

Figure 23-19 Clinical flow chart for the diagnosis and treatment of bilateral posterior crossbite.

the dental development of the child. The clinical consequence of a transverse skeletal or dental discrepancy is the development of a unilateral or bilateral posterior crossbite in the primary, mixed, and permanent dentitions. Selected contemporary appliances illustrate methods of treating the skeletal and dental components of the posterior crossbite relationships.

REFERENCES

1. Christensen JR, Fields HW: Treatment planning and treatment of orthodontic problems. In Pinkham JR et al (eds): *Pediatric dentistry: infancy through adolescence,* ed 3, Philadelphia, 1999, WB Saunders.
2. Hicks E: Slow maxillary expansion: a clinical study of the skeletal versus the dental response to low magnitude force, *Am J Orthod* 58:1-20, 1970.
3. Thilander B, Wahlund S, Lennartsson B: The effect of early interceptive treatment in children with posterior crossbite, *Eur J Orthod* 6:25-34, 1984.
4. Proffit WR, Vig KW, Turvey TA: Early fracture of the mandibular condyles: frequently an unsuspected cause of growth disturbances, *Am J Orthod* 78(1):1-24, 1980.
5. Vig KW: Orthodontic perspectives in craniofacial dysmorphology. In Vig KW, Burdi AR (eds): *Craniofacial morphology and dysmorphology,* Ann Arbor, Mich, 1988, Center for Human Growth and Development.
6. Vig KW, Turvey TA: Orthodontic surgical interaction in the management of cleft lip and palate. In Trier WC: *Clinics in plastic surgery,* Philadelphia, 1985, WB Saunders.
7. Haas AJ: The treatment of maxillary deficiency by opening the midpalatal suture, *Angle Orthod* 35:200-217, 1965.
8. Melsen B: Palatal growth studied on human autopsy material, *Am J Orthod* 68:42-54, 1975.
9. Proffit WR: The first stage of comprehensive treatment: alignment and leveling. In Proffit WR, Fields HW Jr (eds): *Contemporary orthodontics,* ed 3, St Louis, 2000, Mosby.
10. McNamara JA, Brudon WL: Treatment of tooth size/arch size discrepancy problems. In McNamara JA, Brudon WL (eds): *Orthodontic and orthopedic treatment in the mixed dentition,* Ann Arbor, Mich, 1993, Needham Press.
11. Williams MD et al: Combined rapid maxillary expansion and protraction facemask in the treatment of Class III malocclusions in growing children: a prospective long-term study, *Semin Orthod* 3:265-274, 1997.
12. Vig KW: Nasal obstruction and facial growth: the strength of evidence for clinical assumptions, *Am J Orthod Dentofacial Orthop* 113:603-611, 1998.

SECTION V

OTHER ASPECTS RELATED TO TREATMENT

CHAPTER 24

Periodontal Considerations during Orthodontic Treatment

Robert L. Boyd

KEY TERMS

fixed orthodontic appliances	synergistic response	routine dental examinations	stannous fluoride
plaque accumulation	mobility	compliance	Listerine rinse
gingiva	removable appliances	toothpaste	tryclosan
alveolar bone	decalcification	posttreatment report	chlorhexidine
pocket	diagnosis	bonding of molars	antiplaque agents
pseudopocket	referral	conventional toothbrushes	gingival recession
periodontal breakdown	brushing instructions	electric toothbrush	oral irrigator
bone loss	plaque removal effectiveness		

In the United States there are approximately four million patients undergoing treatment with **fixed orthodontic appliances.** These patients have an increased risk for **plaque accumulation** because of the increased difficulty of plaque removal with fixed appliances. A number of studies have documented the potential damage to teeth, **gingiva,** and **alveolar bone** associated with fixed appliances.[1-29] This chapter describes the various types of damage that may occur during orthodontic treatment and provides recommendations that clinicians may use to prevent these problems from occurring. The general dentist plays an important role in the oral health of their patients undergoing orthodontic treatment and should see these patients who need operative or periodontal treatment at regular intervals during orthodontic treatment for examinations. In addition, general dentists may also perform some orthodontic treatment on their patients and thus should be aware of appropriate measures needed to prevent any damage to the teeth and periodontal tissues.

ACTUAL DAMAGE TO PERIODONTAL TISSUES AND TEETH IN ORTHODONTIC PATIENTS

In a classic study Ericsson et al[18] in 1977 found that orthodontic appliances could potentially cause gingivitis and progress to periodontitis, especially during tipping and intrusive movements. This is because the gingival **pocket** tends to deepen when teeth are tipped or intruded, resulting in the development of a **pseudopocket.** A pseudopocket is caused when tissue becomes bunched up or positioned higher on the surface of the crown as the teeth tip and leads to an increased pocket depth (Figure 24-1). When this occurs, the deepened pocket provides an opportunity for subgingival bacteria to become colonized and initiates **periodontal breakdown.** In another classic study Wennstrom et al[29] demonstrated in an animal model that active moderate to advanced periodontitis during treatment with fixed appliances can potentially cause

442

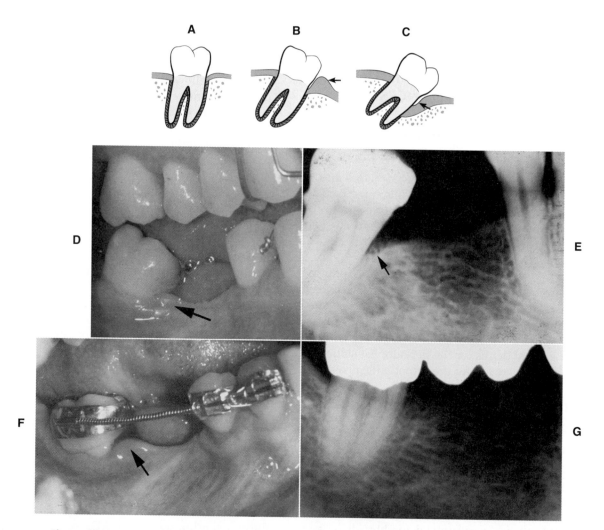

Figure 24-1 Tooth tipping and its effects on soft tissue and bone. **A,** The tooth is initially upright and in a normal position. **B,** The molar has tipped *(arrow)* and the soft tissue has piled up on the mesial surface forming a pseudopocket. **C,** As the pseudopocket deepens, subgingival bacteria accumulate and, in a susceptible patient, bone loss from periodontitis may be initiated *(arrow)*. **D,** Clinical example of a mesially tipped molar. Note height of tissue on the mesial side *(arrow)*. **E,** Radiograph of the tipped molar. Note vertical intraosseous periodontal defect *(arrow)*. **F,** Fixed uprighting appliance with changes in the soft tissue height on the mesial surface. Note gingival bleeding from repeated scaling during treatment, which is necessary to keep the mesial pocket healthy *(arrow)*. **G,** Radiographic appearance of the tooth after it was moved to an upright position and stabilized by a fixed bridge. Notice that the infrabony pocket on the mesial side of this tooth that was present before orthodontic treatment has been eliminated via molar uprighting.

accelerated **bone loss** beyond that which could be explained from plaque accumulation only. This accelerated bone loss is apparently a **synergistic response** in patients who have both active moderate to advanced periodontitis and orthodontic treatment with fixed appliances. This exaggerated response is the result of a synergistic response of orthodontic treatment with the inflammatory disease caused by plaque. The most likely mechanism for this synergistic, accelerated response is that orthodontic forces cause widening of the periodontal ligament with subsequent clinical mobility. This process is synonymous with other types of occlusal traumas that are usually caused by occlusal interferences, clenching, or grinding because both have mobility as their mutual pri-

mary clinical sign. **Mobility** has long been considered a potential aggravating factor for periodontal breakdown in untreated moderate to advanced periodontitis. **Removable appliances** have not been shown to cause such a periodontal liability, most probably because of the absence of significant plaque accumulation.[30]

On the other hand, it is important to emphasize that the longitudinal studies performed by Alstad and Zachrisson[31] and Boyd et al[19] have shown that if patients comply with effective preventive dentistry recommendations during orthodontic treatment with fixed appliances, no clinically significant damage will occur to either the periodontal tissues or the teeth **(decalcification).**

MAJOR COMPONENTS OF AN EFFECTIVE PREVENTIVE PROGRAM FOR ORTHODONTIC PATIENTS WITH FIXED APPLIANCES

Components before Orthodontic Treatment

The following steps need to be followed before any orthodontic treatment is rendered to minimize periodontal damage during treatment as well as to encourage patients to maintain proper dental hygiene.

1. Initial **diagnosis** and **referral** for treatment to control active periodontal disease and caries
2. Informed consent of the risks during orthodontic treatment and responsibilities of the patients and clinician
3. All general dental and periodontal treatment completed before orthodontic treatment (request a letter from the general dentist or the periodontist stating that the patient is ready for the orthodontic phase)

Components during Orthodontic Treatment

Once the orthodontic appliances are placed, the patient needs to be instructed in how to manage the new oral environment and how to maintain the health of the dental and periodontal structures.

1. Provide the patient with initial **brushing instructions** with either a conventional toothbrush or a powered toothbrush when the appliances are first placed. The patient should use a fluoride toothpaste with the American Dental Association (ADA) seal on it that also has an antigingivitis effect. If plaque removal is ineffective after 3 to 4 visits with a conventional toothbrush, the patient should be instructed to use a powered toothbrush.
2. Check **plaque removal effectiveness** at the beginning of every nonemergency visit by giving the patients a mirror to jointly determine if plaque removal is effective. Have the patient brush until the appliances are clean. This increases the length of the visit for poor compliance patients, which acts as a form of negative reinforcement.
3. Record plaque removal effectiveness in the patient's chart.
4. Use a positive reinforcement approach (praise) and avoid criticism.
5. Introduce additional methods to improve oral hygiene such as flossing only when success is established with simple brushing.
6. Check to see if the patient has had **routine dental examinations** and record the information in the patient's chart. These examinations are usually performed every 6 months unless the patient has poor plaque control or periodontal disease. Then the examinations and prophylaxis should be more frequent.
7. If poor **compliance** persists (more often in adolescents), the following steps may be considered:
   a. Schedule more frequent orthodontic visits (every 3 to 4 weeks) when the assistant can spend more time with the patient. Consider adding a contingency fee and alert parents of the increased professional time needed to manage the child's case.
   b. Schedule the patient with an auxiliary who has the best motivational skills.
   c. Send a letter describing the problems to the patient or parents as well as the general dentist.
   d. If all this fails, consider the use of a chlorhexidine rinse treatment for 12 weeks. Let the patient know and send a letter to the patient and parents indicating that this is the final effort by the clinician before appliance removal.
   e. Check carefully the progress of periodontal disease and decalcification.
   f. Refer back to the general dentist for more frequent examinations and prophylaxis.

Components after Orthodontic Treatment

At the completion of orthodontic treatment the clinician should encourage the patient to maintain proper oral hygiene habits.

1. Make sure all children and adolescents are using a fluoride **toothpaste** with an ADA seal of approval at least twice daily to promote remineralization.
2. Make sure that the patient has resumed routine dental care with the general dentist.
3. Send a **posttreatment report** to the patient and to the general dentist. Outline future responsibilities and how well the goals of treatment have been achieved.

Suggestions That Will Improve Plaque Removal Efficiency during Treatment with Fixed Appliances

- **Bonding of molars** results in better periodontal health than banding.[23] This approach is especially important in adults who are in periodontal maintenance (Figure 24-2).
- Use single arch wires whenever possible.
- Remove excess composite around brackets, especially at the gingival margin (see Figure 24-2).
- Avoid using lingual appliances whenever possible.
- Minimize the length of the second phase of treatment with fixed appliances by correcting significant skeletal and alignment problems in the mixed dentition.

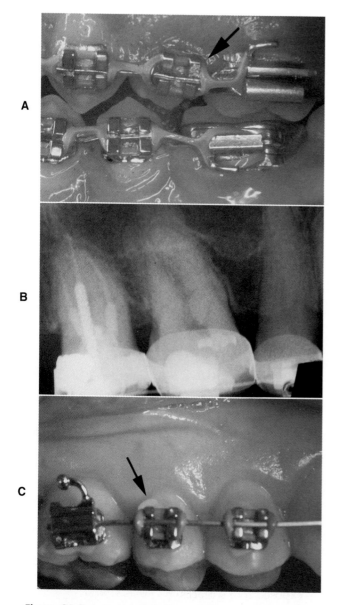

Figure 24-2 A, Typical gingival appearance of a banded molar. Note that the gingiva is enlarged and inflamed around the margin of the band *(arrow).* **B,** Radiograph of a tooth with bands in place. Note that there is a large overhang, which is typically at the apical margin of the band. This occurs because the band must be wider than the widest part of the tooth at the height of convexity to be seated. Thus there will usually be an overhang at the gingival margin when a band is used. **C,** Typical gingival appearance of a bonded molar. Note healthy gingiva and ease of access for plaque removal, especially in the interproximal area. It is important to be sure to remove excess composite material, especially if it approaches the gingival margin *(arrow)* because this causes plaque to accumulate and initiates gingival inflammation.

Important Considerations in Understanding Benefits of Oral Hygiene Products on the Market

The clinician should be aware of and share with the patient the following facts:

1. Plaque is not a disease! It must be present for 72 hours before gingival inflammation is initiated and for 3 weeks before gingivitis is established.

2. Methods that can result in short-term plaque reduction in nonorthodontic patients may not result in similar reduction of gingivitis in orthodontic patients.

3. To be reliably effective, products should show reduction of gingivitis in orthodontic patients over significant periods of time (more than 6 months) (Figure 24-3).

4. Beware of new product claims showing significant reduction of periodontal disease in orthodontic patients without clinical studies published in refereed journals.

PRODUCTS AND METHODS OF PLAQUE REMOVAL FOR ORTHODONTIC PATIENTS

Conventional Toothbrushes

Because there are few well-controlled, long-term studies comparing toothbrushes, the following should be taken into consideration:

1. Brushes should have soft bristles with rounded ends to minimize gingival and tooth abrasion.

2. Orthodontic designs (with the middle row of bristles shorter than the outer rows) may be more effective.

3. Motivated patients usually develop a high personal preference to brush head size and shape, handle design, etc.

4. Because the strength of the professional recommendations (of the doctor and staff) is usually the guiding force for most patients, these opinions must be based on scientific evaluations of their effectiveness.

Tooth Brushing Instructions

The presence of the brackets, arch wires, and ligatures, and other appliances make it more difficult for the patient to maintain proper oral hygiene. Therefore it is important for the clinician to do so.

1. Emphasize cleaning behind arch wires (i.e., interproximal areas [blind spots]) by attempting to get the bristles into these areas (Figure 24-4).

2. The modified bass method (i.e., with the bristles at 45 degrees to sulcus) is only necessary for adults with deepened pockets.

3. Vibrate gently in one place and avoid scrubbing, which can cause cervical abrasion and gingival recession.

4. Let the toothbrush air-dry for 24 hours between uses.

5. Let patients demonstrate the efficiency of brushing at each regular visit until they have mastered the technique. The patient must know when appliances are clean (shiny) by looking in the mirror.

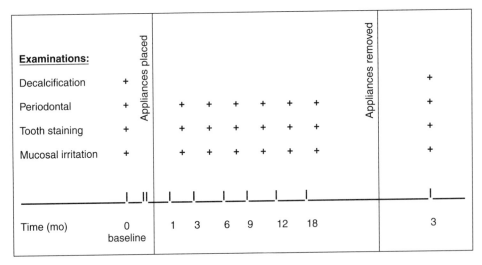

Figure 24-3 Optimal study design for a controlled, prospective, longitudinal clinical study of orthodontic patients. The patients to be studied are matched for age, gender, and periodontal status. Groups are then formed from subjects randomly selected from this pool of matched subjects. In this manner treatment groups can be assigned to use a particular product or technique during the treatment to determine if the response is different from another group that had a different treatment or no treatment (control group). In a study that spans the entire length of orthodontic treatment, any resistant forms of bacteria that might emerge, product breakage, or lack of compliance would be reflected in the data throughout the treatment. This study design is the best way to determine actual decalcification that might occur during treatment as opposed to only studying fluoride release via in vitro models or their short-term effects (4 to 12 weeks) on decalcification of patients during orthodontic treatment.

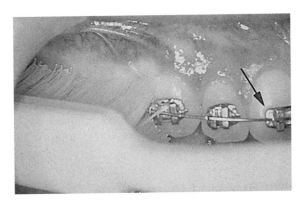

Figure 24-4 Standard technique for a conventional toothbrush in removing plaque from orthodontic appliances. It is important to educate the patient that the most important area to clean is the blocked out area behind the arch wire at the interproximal area. This is especially important because periodontal disease is generally initiated in interproximal areas. Clean, shiny, fixed appliances should be recognizable by the patient (*arrow*) and used as a goal. For routine orthodontic treatment the patient should be given a hand mirror and should be asked at each visit if their appliances are clean and shiny. If the appliances are not clean and shiny and the patient states that they are, instructions must be repeated to educate the patient as to what plaque-free appliances look like in the mirror.

Electric Toothbrushes

Previous studies have demonstrated that 20% to 40% of orthodontic patients with fixed appliances will show less than ideal plaque removal with conventional toothbrushes even with repeated instructions.[19,31]

1. Because 20% to 40% of orthodontic patients will not effectively remove all plaque using a conventional toothbrush, these patients may benefit from the use of electric toothbrushes.

2. The Rotadent **electric toothbrush** with the short pointed bristles is most effective for orthodontic patients (Figure 24-5).[25,28] Its advantages include the following:
   a. Most effective toothbrush for interproximal plaque removal[32]
   b. Least abrasion because of smaller diameter bristles (especially important for implants or exposed root surfaces)[33]
   c. Lower cost for replacement brush heads (needed only every 6 to 8 weeks)

3. Oral B-Braun and Interplak are more effective than the conventional toothbrush but have higher costs for replacement brush heads, which are needed usually every 2 to 3 weeks for Braun and every 4 to 6 weeks for Interplak.

In addition to the toothbrushes, patients can use a number of agents to help improve their gingival situation. These agents include **stannous fluoride** gels, **Listerine rinse, tryclosan, chlorhexidine** rinses, and other **antiplaque agents.**

Stannous Fluoride Gels

1. Stannous fluoride (SnF_2) gels have been shown to be effective against gingivitis, provided they contain >90% available stannous ions (Sn^{++}). The ADA seal ensures that the gel has the proper Sn^{++} concentration.

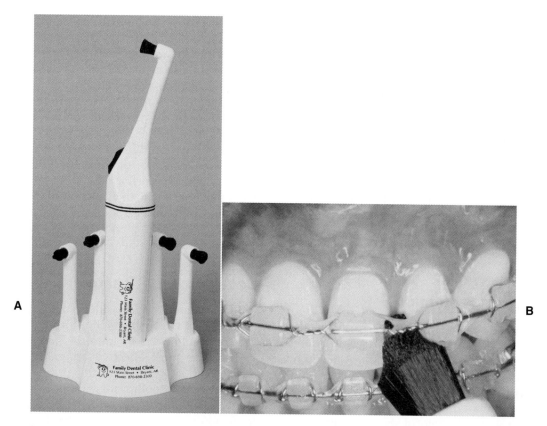

Figure 24-5 A, The Rotadent electric toothbrush. **B,** Note the short pointed brush, which has been shown in several studies to be more effective at interproximal plaque removal because the brush tips actually displace the papilla slightly as the bristles reach into the interproximal area.

2. Of the patients using SnF$_2$, 15% to 20% will develop mild staining in 3 to 6 months.[34,35]
3. The main problem is that additional compliance by the patient is needed for the twice-daily applications of the gel.

Listerine Rinse (Active Ingredient Is Essential Oils)

1. Contains 26% alcohol (precludes use by adolescents) and becomes ineffective if diluted
2. Should be used as a rinse twice daily for 1 minute
3. Mild antigingivitis effect
4. Approved by the ADA but not the Food and Drug Administration (FDA) as antigingivitis product
5. Does not contain fluoride (no effect on caries)
6. Mint flavor usually preferred
7. Can use generic brands, which are less costly
8. Listerine toothpaste not established as effective against gingivitis

Tryclosan

Another important new antigingivitis agent now formulated in some toothpastes is tryclosan (only available in Colgate Total toothpaste). This product has important advantages including having mild antigingivitis effects, good taste and supragingival calculus control equivalent to tartar control toothpastes.[36] This is the only currently ADA- and FDA-approved toothpaste with an antigingivitis effect. For this reason, tryclosan toothpaste should be the standard toothpaste for all orthodontic patients with fixed appliances.

Chlorhexidine Rinses

The best product for optimum management of severe gingivitis in adolescent orthodontic patients is chlorhexidine. A recent study showed a dramatic reduction in plaque (−65%) and gingival bleeding (−77%) with a 3-month use of 0.12% chlorhexidine (Figure 24-6).[37] Chlorhexidine is available as Peridex (Proctor & Gamble) or Periogard (Colgate) products. One of the main problems with chlorhexidine rinses is that they can potentially stain the margins of composite restorations that cannot be easily removed. Chlorhexidine is also useful for patients after orthognathic surgery, especially if intermaxillary fixation is used. It usually requires a prescription for three 16-ounce bottles sufficient for a 2-ounce (a capful) twice-daily use for a 6-week supply. The orthodontist should refill the prescription as needed.

Other Antiplaque Agents

Other products such as baking soda toothpastes (which may also contain peroxide) are marketed as antiplaque agents. Studies are equivocal as to their efficacy against gingivitis.[38] These products should contain fluoride if used for orthodontic patients. Unfortunately, most adolescents do not like their taste.

Another antiplaque product is the alkaloid sanguinaria, which is used in Viadent rinse and toothpaste. In some published studies this product showed mild antigingivitis effects, but, unfortunately, the rinse has no fluoride and must be used with Viadent toothpaste (which does have fluoride) for best results.[39,40] Many adolescents and some adults may not like the taste. Sanguinaria, baking soda, and peroxide are not FDA or ADA approved as antigingivitis agents.

Decalcification Protection

The literature indicates that the best way to prevent decalcification in orthodontic patients is by using a daily, self-applied, topical, low-concentration of 0.05% or 0.4% SnF_2 gels.[21,22,26,27] However, recent studies have shown a likely equivalent effect from the use of a fluoride toothpaste without rinsing with water after use.[41-43] The fluoride rinse or gel protocol should continue for 6 months after appliance removal to remineralize areas

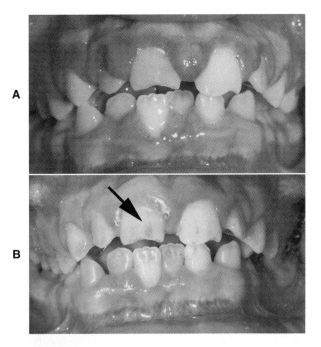

Figure 24-6 **A,** A patient with severe gingivitis present before orthodontic treatment. Because the gingivitis was so severe, the patient was placed on twice daily 0.12% chlorhexidine rinse before treatment is initiated to obtain healthy periodontal tissues. **B,** Note the dramatic difference at the end of 3-months use of chlorhexidine. The tissue is no longer as hyperplastic, which now allows the placement of fixed orthodontic appliances. Note the light-brown stain that has formed on the teeth from the chlorhexidine rinse (arrow).

of decalcification that may have occurred during treatment (Figure 24-7).

In addition, a light-cured sealant containing fluoride should also be used on the entire labial surface.[44] This can also be reapplied during treatment if demineralized areas appear. Other products that contain fluoride such as cements, elastomeric chains, or sealants may reduce decalcification; however, most studies of these products do not show an actual reduction in the incidence of decalcification but only that there is a short-term fluoride release (4 to 8 weeks).[45-47] On the other hand, in vitro studies of glass ionomer cements have demonstrated a more sustained fluoride release (1 to 2 years), and evidence exists that these cements may reduce decalcification.[48-50]

Decalcification Treatment

Mild decalcification is evidenced by a clinical color change (white or white-yellow stains) with possible surface roughness (see Figure 24-7). As explained previously, the most effective approach is to prevent decalcification from occurring during treatment by using a fluoride toothpaste without rinsing with water or by using a topical fluoride rinse or gel twice daily for 6 months until the surface is hard. With such a regimen there is approximately a 50% reduction in the discoloration. For stains still present after 6 months, a rotary green stone or a tungsten finishing bur may be used to remove a thin outer layer of decalcified enamel. This method may remove as much as an additional 25% of the stains.

Moderate postorthodontic decalcification is usually seen as larger areas of color changes (yellow-brown stain) with definite surface roughness (Figure 24-8).

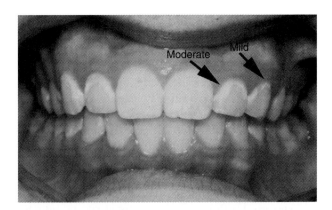

Figure 24-7 A patient who has experienced mild decalcification in the form of white, or white-yellow spots on the teeth. Mild areas may represent a slightly rough surface to the movement of a sharp explorer (arrow) or have greater surface roughness and size that indicates moderate decalcification (arrow). These areas will generally be remineralized within 3 to 4 months by the daily low levels of fluoride in the saliva. This frequently leads to an improved appearance. After remineralization, a finishing burr can also be used to remove the most superficial layer of stain.

The treatment is the same as mild decalcification but is less likely to successfully remove all stains. In some instances the patient may need to have a restoration placed.

Severe postorthodontic decalcification is characterized by large areas of darker, yellow-brown stains with lost enamel. It is important to send the patient to the general dentist as soon as possible for evaluation, especially if the teeth are symptomatic (e.g., thermal sensitivity) for the placement of a restoration, if needed.

Gingival Recession

Patients who undergo orthodontic treatment may experience greater **gingival recession** than untreated patients.[4,12-15,51] However, other studies have not found increased recession.[52-57] On an individual case basis the clinician should be aware of the potential for an increase in the amount of gingival recession and plan this into the treatment plan.[58,59] Areas of thin gingiva are usually noted as having a washboard appearance of prominent roots and a narrow width of attached gingiva (usually less than 1 mm) (Figure 24-9, A). If tooth movement is in a labial direction, this area may require a soft tissue graft. For best esthetics in the anterior areas, a connective tissue graft is preferred (see Figure 24-9, B and C). If teeth that have thin tissue are going to be moved lingually, there is a potential for the tissue to move coronally and become thicker.[58] In this case any grafting of soft tissue should be postponed until after tooth movement is completed.[51,58,59] If no orthodontic treatment is planned for children or adolescents, areas of thin gingival tissue should be monitored only periodically as the width of the attached gingiva generally increases with normal growth from the mixed to the permanent dentition.[60]

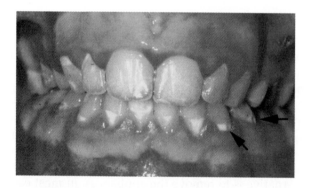

Figure 24-8 Severe postorthodontic decalcification *(arrows)*. The areas of decalcification have an actual break in the surface of the enamel as well as large, darkened spots on the teeth. These areas require placement of restorations as soon as possible.

PREVENTIVE ORAL HYGIENE RECOMMENDATIONS FOR ORTHODONTIC PATIENTS

All Patients

All patients (adolescents and adults with full fixed appliances) should have their plaque control effectiveness checked and recorded in the chart at the beginning of each visit (positive reinforcement is the preferred approach, then negative reinforcement only as a last resort, but never punishment). Patients should be able to look at their appliances and determine weather or not they are clean.

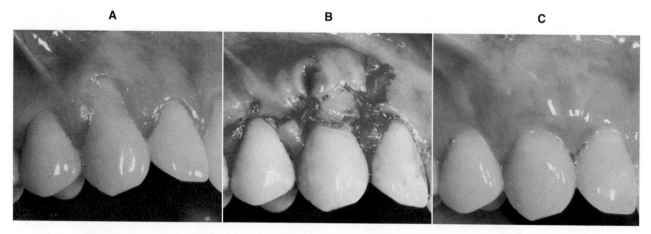

A   **B**   **C**

Figure 24-9 **A,** Pretreatment view of an upper canine that has experienced gingival recession. The patient was unhappy with the esthetics of this recession because she had a high lip-line that showed the area of recession when she smiled. **B,** A connective tissue graft taken from the palate has been surgically placed in the area of recession. The tissue flap, which has a keratinized border, is sutured over the top of the connective tissue graft to form new gingiva. **C,** One year postoperative appearance of the grafted area. Note the complete root coverage and favorable esthetic appearance of the tissue.

Children in the Mixed Dentition

Children should be treated with removable appliances when feasible. Treatment goals in the first phase should be clear and limited so as to cut down on treatment time. Treatment time should not exceed 12 to 16 months. Following these suggestions will minimize patient burnout. If fixed appliances are used, the clinician should remove the appliances between the two phases of treatment (Figure 24-10). Finally, the use of an ADA-approved fluoride toothpaste with a special flavor should be considered for children. Antigingivitis activity of tryclosan toothpastes is not as important because the gingivitis in children usually does not progress to periodontitis as it does in adolescents and adults.

Compliant Adolescents

Of adolescent patients, 40% to 60% are compliant. They can use soft, conventional toothbrushes with round-ended bristles and dental floss (waxed tape is best). However, the Rotadent electric brush with the short pointed brush is more effective.[25,28] All patients should also use a tryclosan toothpaste twice daily without rinsing with water.

Less Compliant Adolescents

Of adolescent patients, 20% to 40% are less compliant. For these patients the Rotadent toothbrush with the short pointed brush is best. They should also use a tryclosan toothpaste twice daily without rinsing with water.[25,28]

Noncompliant Adolescents

About 2% to 5% of adolescent patients are noncompliant. They should first be informed that they need to have their appliances removed. Most patients will not want to do this and will ask what else can be done. If they want to continue, they should be told that they can be enrolled in a 6- to 12-week chlorhexidine (Peridex or Periogard) program during which they have to rinse with chlorhexidine twice daily. If they elect to do this, a letter should be sent home to the family with a copy to the general dentist explaining this treatment. The main problem with the chlorhexidine rinse program is that compliance may continue to be an issue because the chlorhexidine rinse has a strong aftertaste and contains 15% alcohol. If the patient elects to be on this program, he or she should be given a prescription that indicates that it can be refilled as necessary. The orthodontist should explain to the patient that a prophylaxis at the end of treatment will be performed to remove any stains. There should be an additional fee for this program. Because of the

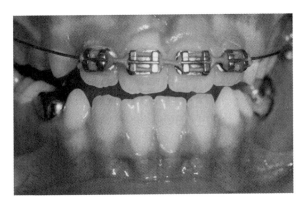

Figure 24-10 A typical patient during the first phase of orthodontic treatment using fixed appliances. These appliances present the same liability for the occurrence of decalcification as in full-appliance therapy during the second phase of treatment. Fortunately, the gingivitis that occurs during the mixed dentition ages (8 to 11 years) rarely converts to periodontitis until the onset of puberty. Removable retainers should be used after the first phase of treatment. It is a good idea to remove appliances between the first and second phases to minimize the possibility of decalcification and to give the patient a break in treatment and to avoid cooperation burnout during the second phase.

extended treatment time, the patient should be checked at 2 weeks and then at 3- to 4-week intervals thereafter to ensure that the patient continues to use the rinse. Approximately 60% of adolescents develop a light-brown stain, especially around the edges of bonded brackets. Almost 100% of adults will develop significant stains. Patients should understand that this stain will be removed periodically. If this approach fails to improve the lack of compliance, the only other alternative is to remove the appliances. In most cases, if appliances are removed because of cooperation problems, it is best to have the patient sign a release that explains that they understand that the treatment has not been completed.

For adults with healthy periodontal tissues and with either low or elevated caries, the best approach is to stick with conventional methods using a soft-bristle toothbrush with rounded ends supplemented by flossing. Usually the best type of floss is the waxed tape because it can pass between the teeth more easily without a floss threader. Another approach for these patients is to use the Rotadent electric toothbrush with the short pointed brush. All of these patients should use a tryclosan toothpaste (Colgate Total) without rinsing with water to promote remineralization. Adults with low caries susceptibility could rinse with water.

Adults in Periodontal Maintenance

Adults should be carefully monitored to ensure that they are regularly keeping their visits for periodontal maintenance. Usually these visits are done every 3 months but may increase in frequency to every 1 or 2 months if poor plaque removal persists or pocket depths increase. Usually the hygienist or general dentist should enter the pocket depths on the patient's chart at every other recall visit. Any pockets found to increase in depth should be retreated with additional scaling, root planing, or soft tissue curettage. The patient should also be made aware of areas of increasing pocket depth to enable the patient to more effectively focus on these areas each day.

It is also important to remember that when a patient completes treatment with a periodontist, it is wise not to change any of the methods that the patient has been taught to perform during their treatment with the periodontist. Unneeded change tends to confuse the patient and undermine the recommendations that both the hygienist and the periodontist have given to the patient.

Patients in periodontal maintenance will frequently be following a home-care protocol of conventional methods such as using round-ended toothbrushes, toothpicks or toothpick-holding devices, interproximal brushes, and dental floss. The only additional recommendation that should be made for the patient is to use waxed tape floss that can be threaded under the arch wire without fraying.

Another method that works well for patients in periodontal maintenance is to use the Rodatent with either a short or long pointed brush.[61,62]

Patients in periodontal maintenance can also rinse once or twice daily with a chlorhexidine rinse. The problem with this approach is that almost all adults will get a light to dark-brown stain in only 3 to 4 weeks. The main reason chlorhexidine rinses are effective for patients who are in periodontal maintenance is that it retards the formation of supragingival plaque, which then retards the formation of subgingival plaque. It is the subgingival plaque that contains the bacteria that most commonly causes bone loss. It is also important to realize that staining can occur under composite restorations, which may necessitate the restoration to be replaced. Also, if the patient smokes or drinks coffee, the staining will be even more problematic. Other adverse affects with the use of chlorhexidine include increased supragingival calculus formation, occasional loss of taste, or a black coating on the tongue.

A final effective method for home care for patients in periodontal maintenance is the use of an **oral irrigator** with regular tap water at high pressure with a conventional irrigator tip.[63-66] If gingival bleeding on probing persists, a way of enhancing the effect of oral irrigation would be to add two capfuls of chlorhexidine rinse to approximately 150 ml of water and irrigate the pockets directly using a specially modified irrigating tip called the *Pik Pocket* (Teledyne Corporation) at a medium level of pressure.[67,68]

REFERENCES

1. Sjolien T, Zachrisson BU: Periodontal bone support and tooth length in orthodontically treated and untreated persons, *Am J Orthod* 64:28-37, 1973.
2. Zachrisson BU, Alnaes L: Periodontal condition in orthodontically treated and untreated individuals. I. Loss of attachment gingival pocket depth and clinical crown height, *Angle Orthod* 43:402-411, 1973.
3. Hamp S, Lundstrom F, Nyman S: Periodontal conditions in adolescents subjected to multiband orthodontic treatment with controlled oral hygiene, *Eur J Orthod* 4:77-86, 1982.
4. Hollender L, Ronnerman A, Thilander B: Root resorption, marginal bone support and clinical crown length in orthodontically treated patients, *Eur J Orthod* 2:197-205, 1980.
5. Artun J, Urbye KS: The effect of orthodontic treatment on periodontal bone support in patients with advanced loss of marginal periodontium, *Am J Orthod Dentofacial Orthop* 93:143-148, 1988.
6. Zachrisson BU: Cause and prevention of injuries to teeth and supporting structures during orthodontic treatment, *Am J Orthod* 69:285-300, 1976.
7. Eliasson L et al: The effects of orthodontic treatment on periodontal tissues in patients with reduced periodontal support, *Eur J Orthod* 4:1-9, 1982.
8. Baxter DH: The effect of orthodontic treatment of alveolar bone adjacent to the cement-enamel junction, *Angle Orthod* 37:35-47, 1976.
9. Kloehn JS, Pfeifer JS: The effect of orthodontic treatment on the periodontium, *Angle Orthod* 44:127-134, 1974.
10. Boyd R: Longitudinal evaluation of a system for self-monitoring plaque control effectiveness in orthodontic patients, *J Clin Periodontol* 10:380-388, 1983.
11. Polson AM, Reed BE: Long-term periodontal status after orthodontic treatment, *Am J Orthod Dentofacial Orthop* 93:51-58, 1988.
12. Trosello V, Gianelly A: Orthodontic treatment and periodontal status, *J Periodontol* 50:665-671, 1979.
13. Coatoam GW et al: The width of keratinized gingiva during orthodontic treatment: its significance and impact on periodontal status, *J Periodontol* 52:307-313, 1981.
14. Artun J, Krogstad O: Periodontal status of mandibular incisors following excessive proclination, *Am J Orthod Dentofacial Orthop* 91:225-232, 1987.
15. Sadowsky C, BeGole E: Long-term effects of orthodontic treatment on periodontal health, *Am J Orthod* 80:156-172, 1981.
16. Dorfman HS, Turvey TA: Alterations in osseous crestal height following interdental osteotomies, *Oral Surg* 48:120-125, 1979.
17. Kwon H, Pihlstrom B, Waite DE: Effects of the periodontium of vertical bone cutting for segmental osteotomy, *J Oral Maxillofac Surg* 43:952-955, 1985.
18. Ericsson IB et al: The effect of orthodontic tilting movements on the periodontal tissues of infected and noninfected dentitions in dogs, *J Clin Periodontol* 4:278-293, 1977.

19. Boyd RL et al: Periodontal implications of orthodontic treatment in adults with reduced or normal periodontal tissues versus those of adolescents, *Am J Orthod Dentofacial Orthop* 96:191-199, 1989.

20. Strateman MW, Shannon IL: Control of decalcification in orthodontic patients by daily self-administered application of a water-free 0.4% stannous fluoride gel, *Am J Orthod* 66:273-279, 1974.

21. Gorelick L, Geiger AM, Gwinnett AJ: Incidence of white spot formation after bonding and banding, *Am J Orthod* 81:93-98, 1982.

22. O'Reilly MM, Featherstone JBD: Demineralization and remineralization around orthodontic appliances: an in vitro study, *Am J Orthod Dentofacial Orthop* 92:33-40, 1987.

23. Boyd RL, Baumrind S: Periodontal considerations in the choice between banded or bonded molars in adults and adolescents, *Angle Orthod* 62:117-126, 1992.

24. Ogaard B: Prevalence of white spot lesions in 19-year-olds: a study on untreated and orthodontically treated persons 5 years after treatment, *Am J Orthod Dentofacial Orthop* 96:423-427, 1989.

25. Boyd RL, Murray P, Robertson PB: Effect of rotary electric toothbrush versus manual toothbrush on periodontal status during orthodontic treatment, *Am J Orthod Dentofacial Orthop* 96:342-347, 1989.

26. Boyd RL: Two-year longitudinal study of the effects of a peroxide-fluoride rinse on decalcification in adolescent orthodontic patients, *J Clin Dent* 3:83-87, 1992.

27. Boyd RL: Comparison of three self-applied topical fluoride preparations for control of decalcification during orthodontic treatment, *Angle Orthod* 63:25-30, 1993.

28. Boyd RL, Rose CM: Effect of rotary electric toothbrush versus manual toothbrush on decalcification during orthodontic treatment, *Am J Orthod Dentofacial Orthop* 105:450-456, 1994.

29. Wennstrom JL et al: Periodontal tissue response to orthodontic movement of teeth with infrabony pockets, *Am J Orthod Dentofacial Orthop* 103:313-319, 1993.

30. Eliasson LA et al: The effects of orthodontic treatment on periodontal tissues in patients with reduced periodontal support, *Eur J Orthod* 4:1-9, 1982.

31. Alstad S, Zachrisson BU: Longitudinal study of periodontal condition associated with orthodontic treatment in adolescents, *Am J Orthod* 76:277-286, 1979.

32. Sarker S, McLey L, Boyd RL: Clinical and laboratory evaluation of powered electric toothbrushes: laboratory determination of relative interproximal cleaning efficiency of four powered toothbrushes, *J Clin Dent* 8:81-85, 1997.

33. McLey L, Boyd RL, Sarker S: Clinical and laboratory evaluation of powered electric toothbrushes: laboratory determination of relative abrasion of three powered toothbrushes, *J Clin Dent* 8:76-80, 1997.

34. Boyd RL, Leggott P, Robertson PB: Effects on gingivitis of two different 0.4% SnF$_2$ gels, *J Dent Res* 67:503-507, 1988.

35. Boyd RL, Chun Y: Eighteen-month evaluation of the effects of a 0.4% SnF$_2$ gel on gingivitis, *Am J Orthod Dentofacial Orthop* 105:35-41, 1994.

36. Volpe AR et al: A review of plaque, gingivitis, calculus and caries clinical efficacy studies with a fluoride dentifrice containing triclosan and PVM/MA copolymer, *J Clin Dent* 7(suppl):1-14, 1996.

37. Brightman LJ et al: The effects of a 0.12% chlorhexidine gluconate mouthrinse on orthodontic patients aged 11 through 17 with established gingivitis, *Am J Orthod Dentofacial Orthop* 100:324-329, 1991.

38. Marshall MV, Cancro LP, Fischman SL: Hydrogen peroxide: a review of its use in dentistry, *J Periodontol* 66:786-796, 1995.

39. Hannah JJ, Johnson JD, Kuftinec MM: Long-term clinical evaluation of toothpaste and oral rinse containing sanguinaria extract in controlling plaque, gingival inflammation, and sulcular bleeding during orthodontic treatment, *Am J Orthod Dentofacial Orthop* 96(3):199-207, 1989.

40. Harper DS et al: Clinical efficacy of a dentifrice and oral rinse containing sanguinaria extract and zinc chloride during 6 months of use, *J Periodontol* 61:352-358, 1990.

41. Chesters RK: Effect of oral care habits on caries in adolescents, *Caries Res* 26:299-304, 1992.

42. Sjogren K, Birkhed D: Effect of various post-brushing activities on salivary fluoride concentration after toothbrushing with a sodium fluoride dentifrice, *Caries Res* 28:127-131, 1994.

43. Attin T, Hellwig E: Salivary fluoride content after toothbrushing with a sodium fluoride and an amine fluoride dentifrice followed by different mouthrinsing procedures, *J Clin Dent* 7:6-8, 1996.

44. Frazier M, Southard TE, Doster PM: Prevention of enamel demineralization during orthodontic treatment: an in vitro study using pit and fissure sealants, *Am J Orthod Dentofacial Orthop* 110:459-465, 1996.

45. Basdra EK, Huber H, Komposch G: Fluoride released from orthodontic bonding agents alters the enamel surface and inhibits enamel demineralization in vitro, *Am J Orthod Dentofacial Orthop* 109:466-472, 1996.

46. Bishara, S, Swift EJ, Chan DCN: Evaluation of fluoride release from an orthodontic bonding system, *Am Orthod Dentofacial Orthop* 100:106-109, 1991.

47. Ogaard B et al: Fluoride level in saliva after bonding orthodontic brackets with a fluoride containing adhesive, *Am J Orthod Dentofacial Orthop* 111:199-202, 1997.

48. Vorhies AB et al: Enamel demineralization adjacent to orthodontic brackets bonded with hybrid glass ionomer cements: an in vitro study, *Am J Orthod Dentofacial Orthop* 114:668-774, 1998.

49. Chung C, Cuozzo PT, Mante FK: Shear bond strength of a resin-reinforced glass ionomer cement: an in vitro comparative study, *Am J Orthod Dentofacial Orthop* 115:52-54, 1999.

50. Millett DT et al: Decalcification in relation to brackets bonded with glass ionomer cement or a resin adhesive, *Angle Orthod* 69(1):65-70, 1999.

51. Dorfman HS: Mucogingival changes resulting from mandibular incisor tooth movement, *Am J Orthod* 74:286-297, 1978.

52. Kloehn JS, Pfeifer JS: The effect of orthodontic treatment on the periodontium, *Angle Orthod* 44:127-134, 1974.

53. Busschop JL et al: The width of the attached gingiva during orthodontic treatment: a clinical study in human patients, *Am J Orthod* 87:244-249, 1985.

54. Pearson LE: Gingival height of lower central incisors, orthodontically treated and untreated, *Angle Orthod* 38:337-339, 1968.

55. Zachrisson BU, Alnaes L: Periodontal condition in orthodontically treated and untreated individuals. I. Loss of attachment, gingival pocket depth and clinical crown height, *Angle Orthod* 43:402-411, 1973.

56. Alstad S, Zachrisson BU: Longitudinal study of periodontal condition associated with orthodontic treatment, *Am J Orthod* 76:277-286, 1979.

57. Ruf S, Hansen K, Pancherz H: Does orthodontic proclination of lower incisors in children and adolescents cause gingival recession? *Am J Orthod Dentofacial Orthop* 114:100-106, 1998.

58. Boyd RL: Mucogingival considerations and their relationship to orthodontics, *J Periodontol* 49(2):67-76, 1978.

59. Wennstrom JL: Mucogingival considerations in orthodontic treatment, *Semin Orthod* 2:46-54, 1996.

60. Andlin-Sobocki A, Bodin L: Dimensional alterations of the gingiva related to changes of facial/lingual tooth position in permanent anterior teeth of children: a 2-year longitudinal study, *J Clin Periodontol* 20:219-224, 1993.

61. Boyd RL, Murray P, Robertson PB: Effect on periodontal status or rotary electric toothbrushes vs. manual toothbrushes during periodontal maintenance. I. Clinical results, *J Periodontol* 60:390-395, 1989.

62. Boyd RL, Murray P, Robertson PB: Effect on periodontal status or rotary electric toothbrushes vs. manual toothbrushes during periodontal maintenance. II. Microbiological results, *J Periodontol* 60:396-401, 1989.

63. Greenstein G: *The role of supra- and subgingival irrigation in the treatment of periodontal diseases,* Committee on Research, Science and Therapy. The American Academy of Periodontology Scientific, Clinical and Educational Affairs Department, 1995.

64. Boyd RL et al: Effect of self-administered daily irrigation with 0.02% SnF$_2$ on periodontal disease activity, *J Clin Periodontol* 12:420-431, 1985.

65. Newman MG et al: Effectiveness of adjunctive irrigation in early periodontitis: multi-center evaluation, *J Periodontol* 65:224-229, 1994.

66. Eakle W, Ford C, Boyd RL: Depth of penetration in periodontal pockets with oral irrigation, *J Clin Periodontol* 13:39-44, 1986.

67. Eakle W et al: Penetration of periodontal pockets with irrigation by a newly designed tip, *J Dent Res* 67(special issue):400, 1998 (abstract).

68. Boyd RL, Hollander BN, Eakle WS: Comparison of subgingivally placed cannula oral irrigator tip with a supragingivally placed standard irrigator tip, *J Clin Periodontol* 19:340-344, 1992.

CHAPTER 25

Behavioral Considerations in Orthodontic Treatment

Robert G. Keim

KEY TERMS

behavioral sciences	educational psychology	patient compliance	experiential learning theory
social psychology of orthodontics	self-concept	personality test	sensitivity threshold
orthodontic motivational psychology	self-esteem	doctor-patient interaction	patient-oriented approach
	body images	rapport	

The **behavioral sciences** have played a significant role in orthodontics, both in clinical practice and research, since the early part of this century. All of the scenarios that follow are based on actual occurrences. In each of these cases the patient's or the doctor's individual behavior dictated an eventual course of action in an orthodontic practice. These scenarios, and countless others like them, illustrate the role of the behavioral sciences in modern orthodontic practice.

❖Scenario 1: The Adolescent Patient❖

An ordinarily perky and outgoing seventh grader stares into a mirror sobbing mournfully. Her eyes are red and puffy from hours of crying. During lunch break in the school cafeteria several of her classmates had teased her about being buck toothed. Mocking the way her lower lip was trapped behind her upper incisors, they laughed at the way she bit and chewed her sandwich. The teasing was ignorantly cruel. The hurt was deep and lasting. It precipitated the present crisis of tears and insecurities. Like all 12-year-old children she is confused and a little frightened by the physical and emotional changes brought on by puberty. Social acceptance has become of paramount importance to her. In her mind her own physical appearance plays a big role in that acceptance.

Racked by self-doubt and insecurities, she questions whether she is pretty or not. She wonders if she will ever be accepted. She wonders if she will ever be popular.

❖Scenario 2: The Compliant Adult Patient❖

A young executive ponders the factors that can help him move up in his firm. His professional competence, individual credentials, and technical skills are absolutely outstanding, but so are those of the other 17 rising stars in his office. He is determined that it is the other little things that will contribute to his success. He has read all of the self-help manuals suggesting that certain shirts and ties are absolute musts. He knows that the cut of his suit must be just so. He has spent countless hours working on his all-important golf game. His crooked teeth have bothered him for years. He has now convinced himself that if he could get them straightened, it would be one more rung up the ladder. He seeks out a good orthodontist and assures her that he will follow her instructions to the "t."

❖Scenario 3: The Orthodontist❖

An orthodontist notices that the patients who follow her instructions regarding using their headgear, maintaining their oral hygiene, and showing up for their regularly scheduled appointments get remarkably better final results than do the patients who are less fastidious, or less compliant, in following her doctor's orders. Many of her treatment planning decisions are based on whether or not she thinks the patients will comply with her instructions. She gets the feeling that she could probably guess which patients will be compliant and which ones will not be, but her years of college, dental school, and graduate specialty schooling have left her well trained in the empirical sciences. Based on this scientific background, her instincts tell her that there must be a more reliable scientific way of predicting patient compliance. She reviews the literature for any papers that have addressed the issue of using standardized personality tests to predict orthodontic patient compliance. Finding several papers in the orthodontic literature that address this very issue, she orders a supply of personality inventories from a large psychologic publisher.

The areas of behavioral research and the applications of practical psychology to the clinical practice of orthodontics can be divided into two broad categories. The first category could be loosely termed the **social psychology of orthodontics.** This encompasses such divergent fields as why patients seek orthodontic care, the psychosocial outcomes of orthodontic therapy, and the use of standardized psychologic instruments to assess prospective orthodontic patients. The second broad category of orthodontic behavioral science could be termed **orthodontic motivational psychology.** This field involves the area of motivating patients to follow doctors' orders, thus achieving patient compliance. Here again, standardized psychologic instruments have been used to assess patients, this time to predict patient compliance as a part of the overall diagnosis and treatment planning process. A relatively new area of application of the behavioral sciences in orthodontics is the use of **educational psychology** to achieve patient compliance. Herein the role of doctor as teacher rather than doctor as healer is explored further.

This chapter highlights the relationship of each of these areas of the behavioral sciences to the clinical practice of orthodontics.

SOCIAL PSYCHOLOGY OF ORTHODONTICS

Why Patients Seek Orthodontic Treatment

The majority of orthodontic patients who seek care under their own initiative (i.e., adult patients) do so to improve their facial appearance. Most adolescents, on the other hand, seek care because, "my mom thinks I need braces." When their mothers are asked why they are bringing their children in for treatment, most respond that they want their children to look better. So answer-

ing why most patients seek orthodontic care becomes a matter of answering the question, "Why do people want to look better?"

Obviously, the question of why patients seek orthodontic care is vested in the social psychology of personal appearance. The phenomenon of "looking better" has been explored extensively in social psychology. One of the landmark works relative to orthodontics was the book *The Social Psychology of Facial Appearance* by Bull and Rumsey.[1] Reporting on the research they conducted throughout the 1960s and 1970s, the authors conclude that facial appearance is a key determinant of whether or not a person was believed to be attractive. They found facially disfigured people, such as orthodontic patients with significant skeletal discrepancies, had a more difficult time in school. They also noted that such disfigured people were less likely to do well in employment, politics, or advertising. Clearly, a person's dentofacial appearance can have a significant effect on their overall quality of life. Many patients seek orthodontic care to improve that quality of life.

Adams[2] suggested a developmental perspective for examining the social psychology of beauty. He argued that the following four central assumptions about the developmental relationship between outer attractiveness and inner behavioral processes and outcomes could be extracted from the research literature:

1. Physical attractiveness stimulates differential expectations toward another.
2. An individual's attractiveness appears to elicit differential social exchanges from others.
3. An important developmental outcome results from this social exchange. As a consequence of receiving relatively constant positive or negative social reactions from others, physically attractive or unattractive persons are likely to internalize differing social images, self-expectations, and interpersonal personality styles.
4. Because of their greater experience with positive social interaction, attractive people are more likely to manifest confident interpersonal behavior patterns than lesser attractive individuals.

In short, a person's attractiveness has a lot to do with that person's self-confidence in social settings.

Early research into the social psychology of orthodontics revealed that dentofacial appearance has a lot to do with the way people are perceived. Personal adjustment can be difficult for a person with malocclusion. Secourd and Jourard[3] evaluated the importance of dentognathic conditions as clues to personality impressions when compared with all other body clues. Judges were found to associate some personality traits with selected dentally related conditions. Four attributes (sincerity, intelligence, conscientiousness, and good looks) were attributed to persons with more correctly aligned teeth. Crookedness of teeth was related to warmheartedness, esthetic appearance, and intelligence. Secourd and Jourard's studies[3] show that malocclusions can give an observer various impressions of an individual's personality. If the malocclusion is highly visible, it can evoke aversion, thereby interfering with social interaction and acceptance. According to Klima, Wittemann, and McIver[4] people attribute personal "worth, good, etc." to others on a basis of facial characteristics.

Adolescents with significant dentofacial disharmonies are frequently considered to be at risk for negative self-esteem and social maladjustment. Phillips, Bennett, and Broder[5] stated that dentofacial anomalies, such as crooked teeth and skeletal disharmonies, have been reported as the "cause of teasing and general playground harassment among children and are associated with lowered social attractiveness." It is not uncommon for an orthodontist to have a young patient request to have braces so that "the other kids will stop teasing me!" This is a rather blunt answer to the question of why certain patients seek orthodontic treatment.

Psychologic Outcomes of Orthodontic Treatment

The precise role that dentofacial esthetics plays in the development of a child's **self-concept** and **self-esteem** remains controversial. A number of authors have explored this topic. Dann et al[6] found that children with serious malocclusions did not necessarily have poor self-concepts or poor **body images** of themselves at the outset of orthodontic care. They also noted that the patients' self-concept and body image scores did not improve significantly with orthodontic treatment. Albino[7] also explored the psychologic and social effects of orthodontic treatment. He investigated the hypothesis that dentofacial disharmonies may well indeed have important social consequences and significant psychologic effects on the patient in question. Contrary to Dann et al,[6] Albino[7] found that parent-, peer-, and self-reported evaluations of dentofacial specific self-image items improved significantly after the patients received orthodontic treatment. In other words, the children who received orthodontic treatment felt better about their facial appearance after braces than they did before them. Their parents and friends felt the same way. Interestingly enough, Albino[7] reported that the parent- and self-reported evaluations of social competency or social goals did not improve after braces, nor did the subjects' self-esteem. So why the apparent discrepancy between Dann's and Albino's findings? The answer lies in the patients' attitudes at the outset of treatment. If patients feel bad about the way they look at the outset of treatment, the therapist is more likely to notice an improvement in their feelings about themselves than if they felt good about themselves from the beginning.

Are the psychologic outcomes of orthodontic treatment different for adult and adolescent populations? It is fairly safe to say that a normal occlusion is generally perceived as being more attractive and as having more positive outcomes relative to the patient's self-image development, whether the patient is an adolescent or an adult. Varela and Garcia-Camba[8] evaluated the extent to which this perception affects self-image and self-esteem in adult patients. They recognized that there are considerable controversies about the psychologic repercussions of malocclusions on affected persons. With the aid of standardized psychologic tests, these researchers found a significantly positive effect of orthodontic treatment on adult patients' body image and self-concept. Rephrased in simpler terms, orthodontic treatment made these adult patients feel better about themselves, regardless of their state of mind at the outset of treatment.

Developmental Psychology of Orthodontics

If dentofacial appearance is important to both children and adults, does the way a person feels about their dentofacial appearance in childhood affect the way they feel about themselves as an adult? Shaw et al[9] evaluated the risk/benefit appraisal for orthodontic treatment with an emphasis on the developmental outcomes of orthodontics. The authors discussed the benefit of social psychologic well-being in terms of three subgroups. First, the authors looked at nicknames and teasing and stated that the contribution of orthodontic treatment should not be underestimated where conspicuous dentofacial deviation has attracted the hurtful mockery of peers. Secondly, they evaluated dental appearance and social attractiveness. Here, they found that faces displaying a range of dental conditions affected perception of social characteristics such as perceived friendliness, social class, popularity, and intelligence. Lastly, the authors discussed self-esteem and popularity. They found an association between dental attractiveness and self-esteem and other factors. Shaw et al[9] concluded that when personal dissatisfaction with dental appearance is felt in childhood, it might well remain for a lifetime.

Tung and Kiyak[10] reported on the psychologic influences on patients relative to the timing of orthodontic treatment (Figure 25-1). They suggested that the developing child's psychologic well-being may be as much of an indication for early orthodontic treatment as are anatomic or physiologic considerations. Their research also suggests that there may be racial differences in the psychologic influences of orthodontics. They state, "Although white and minority children were similar in their self-ratings and expectations from orthodontics, the former were more critical in their es-

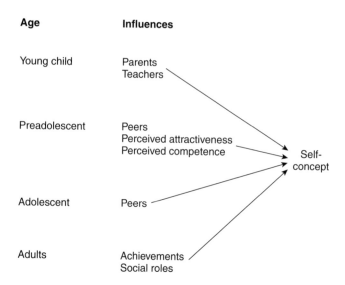

Age	Influences
Young child	Parents Teachers
Preadolescent	Peers Perceived attractiveness Perceived competence
Adolescent	Peers
Adults	Achievements Social roles

Self-concept

Figure 25-1 Social factors affecting self-concept. (From Tung AW, Kiyak HA: *Am J Orthod Dentofacial Orthop* 113[1]:29-39, 1998.)

thetic judgments." They rated faces with crowded teeth, overbite, and diastemata more negatively than did ethnic minorities. These results suggest that younger children are good candidates for Phase I orthodontics, have high self-esteem and body image, and expect orthodontics to improve their lives. White children who have been referred for Phase I orthodontics appear to have a narrower range of esthetic acceptability than minority children.

PATIENT COMPLIANCE

The success of orthodontic therapy frequently depends on **patient compliance.** Headgear effects, functional appliance treatment, oral hygiene, and keeping treatment on schedule by keeping appointments are all dependent on the patient complying with the doctor's instructions. Egolf and others[11] described a compliant patient as one who practices good oral hygiene, wears appliances as instructed without abusing them, follows an appropriate diet, and keeps appointments. Adult patients are generally in the orthodontist's office because they want to be. They have sought out care on their own, they have made the financial commitment to complete care, and they generally have specific outcomes in mind. Adults are generally, but not always, very compliant patients. Adolescents, who represent the majority of orthodontic patients, are another matter. They are generally in the orthodontist's office because a parent has brought them there. They have little or no financial interest vested in the outcome, and their own goals for treatment are frequently nonspecific. Southard et al[12] pointed out that the assurance of good compliance can be difficult in the case of adolescents. Adolescents are

expected to be responsible for much of their care during what can be a lengthy treatment. Compliance by the patient helps achieve the treatment objectives in a minimum treatment time. Improved cooperation by the patient can also reduce expenses of orthodontic treatment. According to Sinha, Nanda, and McNeil,[13] the efficiency of care and improved oral hygiene can decrease damage to the periodontal tissues and limit the effects of enamel decalcification and caries.

Understanding the Adolescent Patient

Peterson and Kuipers[14] described adolescence as a period in life between childhood and adulthood when considerable change is occurring. The personal and social changes provide the adolescent with developmental opportunities to choose to engage in health-risking behaviors or to adopt a healthy lifestyle. The most important concern for adolescents is appearance, particularly facial appearance.[15] Changes in their appearance can affect how adolescents perceive themselves, contributing to anxiety on one hand or positive self-confidence on the other.

Physical changes in the adolescent can be stressful. Females reach puberty between 8 and 13 years old, whereas males start puberty between 9½ and 13½ years old.[14] Differences in timing and tempo of puberty have serious effects on adolescent experiences. For example, early-maturing females may succumb to eating disorders as a result of body changes (e.g., weight gain). Conversely, early-maturing boys enjoy higher self-esteems that are related to their competence in sports and increased strength.

Cognitively, adolescents become capable of thinking hypothetically, applying logic, and using abstract concepts.[14] They become aware of future consequences for their actions. However, their cognitive abilities can break down when faced with emotional situations that can lead to impulsive actions without considering the alternative.

Peterson and Kuipers[14] also note that psychosocial changes in adolescence shape their sense of self. Adolescents feel pressure to conform to the norms and do so by comparing themselves to others. Adolescents spend a majority of their time with their peers and withdraw from adults. The peer group may play a role in identity development, but parents can help guide their child in selecting a peer group with positive influences. Understanding adolescent development can allow the orthodontist to help overcome obstacles in treating patients in this age group.

Motivating the Adolescent Patient

Cooper and Shapiro[16] looked at patients' values on health pitted against competing values that were not health-specific motivation. They elucidated a few features of adolescent behavior that can be used to ascertain a particular behavior. First, adolescents are concerned with self-image and identity, which can be useful in motivating them. Second, independence and autonomy are important to an adolescent; therefore achieving an adult-like status could motivate the adolescent. Third, peer relationships are important, so this feature may motivate behaviors that meet social needs. For example, an adolescent will lose weight based on perceived social pressure to be thin rather than because of health risks associated with obesity.

Cooper and Shapiro[16] suggested taking time to identify an adolescent's concerns and then to treat them as individuals. This approach reduces compliance barriers. Orthodontic patients may have difficulty complying for various reasons; Cooper and Shapiro[16] suggested that more successful motivation can be accomplished by individualizing the patient and recognizing adolescent values and issues. The orthodontist should understand that adolescents are not influenced strongly by health-specific goals.

Personality Testing and Compliance

Major orthodontic treatment decisions are based on an anticipated level of patient compliance. The orthodontist may or may not decide to extract teeth or may lean toward using fixed appliances based on expectations of patient compliance. In one study over 80% of the orthodontists surveyed responded that they had no particular method for assessing compliance.[15] Southard et al[12] examined the feasibility of using a commercially available adolescent **personality test,** the Millon Adolescent Personality Inventory ([MAPI] Millon, Green, and Meagher, 1982), to predict the behavior of adolescent patients in an orthodontic practice. The results of the MAPI were then correlated to the results of an ordinal assessment of the patients' compliance over 2 years of orthodontic treatment. The authors concluded that the MAPI is a useful instrument for predicting adolescent orthodontic patient compliance behavior.

Cucalon and Smith[17] studied 252 adolescent orthodontic patients between the ages of 11 and 17 years. Patient compliance was rated as good, fair, or poor after 1 year in treatment. Three questionnaires were given: (1) the Comprehensive Personal Assessment System: Self-Report Inventory, (2) the Adolescent Alienation Index, and (3) the Home Index. They found that females were significantly more compliant than males. No significant differences were found for age or race. Patients with low self-esteem scores proved not to be compliant, whereas higher self-esteem scores were associated with higher levels of compliance. Overall, the authors found that females from higher socioeconomic backgrounds can be expected to exhibit good compliance, whereas males with low socioeconomic status generally show lower compliance scores.

Orthodontist and Patient Communication

Several studies have shown that the way the doctor and the patient interact can have profound effects on patient compliance. Klages, Sergl, and Burucker[18] studied the characteristics of doctor-patient communication by means of audiotaping patients' office visits. They stated that, ideally, the adolescent patient should offer information, initiate light conversation, and give positive responses to the doctor. They found strong relationships between clinician's encouraging behavior and patient communication cooperation, which they described as communication that includes the patient taking an active part in communication, such that they answer questions in detail and take initiative to change the subject to a matter of special interest to themselves. They concluded that the orthodontist's behavior may be relevant for patient verbal cooperation. Similarly, Barsch et al[19] found that **doctor-patient interaction** was the best predictor of how well a patient could be expected to comply with the doctor's instructions.

Nanda and Kierl[20] conducted an extensive prospective study of patient compliance in a university graduate orthodontic clinic. Their study was perhaps the most extensive in the literature to date. They investigated numerous variables that had been suggested to affect patient compliance in prior literature. The variables they looked at included parent-child relationship, psychosocial characteristics of the parent, psychosocial characteristics of the patient, the patient's attitude and opinions about orthodontics, the parents' attitudes and opinions about orthodontics, the parents' perceptions of the child's degree of social compromise, the child's perceptions of their own degree of social compromise, patient demographics, and the parents and child's relationship with the orthodontist. Of all of these possible predictors of compliance, the authors found that the variables assessing the orthodontist's perception of the doctor-patient relationship had the strongest association with patient compliance. In a follow-up study, Sinha, Nanda, and McNeil[13] concluded that the orthodontist's behavior influences patient satisfaction, the orthodontist-patient relationship, and patient cooperation in orthodontic treatment. Overall, if the doctor wants good cooperation from a patient, the most important factor in obtaining it is the establishment of good **rapport** with that patient.

Educational Psychology: Patient Learning Styles

One of the most promising areas of current research in patient cooperation is the area of educational psychology, notably the application of **experiential learning theory** and patient learning styles. It is often assumed that the word *doctor* implies healer. In reality, the word comes from the Latin *docere,* which means to teach. Originally, the word *doctor* meant someone who teaches. Steed-Veilands[15] was the first to explore the orthodontist-patient relationship from the perspective of a teacher-student relationship rather than that of healer-patient relationship. Through the application of experiential learning theory, significant advances have been made in diverse areas of education including diabetic patient education,[15] smoking cessation programs,[15] corporate personnel training,[21] and classroom management for adolescent students.[21] Steed-Veilands[15] reasoned that if the orthodontist was trying to teach the adolescent patient how to cooperate for treatment success rather than dictating a set of doctor's orders, the application of experiential learning theory to clinical or-

thodontics may meet with success similar to that achieved in the areas previously mentioned.

The Learning Styles Inventory—IIa that was developed by Kolb[21] categorized 135 orthodontic patients into the four **learning styles** described by Kolb: accommodator, diverger, assimilator, and converger (Figures 25-2 and 25-3 and Box 25-1).[21] Significant differences were found in the patients' individual learning styles and in their level of cooperation with oral hygiene, headgear/elastic wear, and appliance maintenance. One of the key tenets of experiential learning theory is that students learn the material presented to them in a style unique unto themselves. It is up to the teacher—the doctor—to teach to that unique style of learning. Studies of exactly which patient education

---

BOX 25-1   Learning Strengths and Preferred Learning Situations of the Four Modes of Learning

Learning Mode	Learning Strengths	Preferred Learning Situations
Concrete experience	Learning by intuition Learning from specific experiences Relating to people	Learning from new experiences Role playing, games Personalized counseling Doctor as coach
Reflective observation	Learning by perception Careful observations before making judgments	Lectures Opportunities to take an observer role Doctor as guide or taskmaster
Abstract conceptualization	Learning by thinking Understanding a situation	Readings Doctor as communicator of information
Active experimentation	Learning by doing Ability to get things done	Opportunities to practice Doctor as role model

From Kolb DA: *Experiential learning: experience as the source of learning and development,* Englewood Cliffs, NJ, 1984, Prentice-Hall.

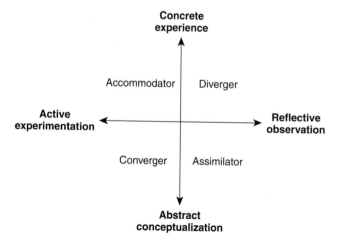

Figure 25-2 Kolb's learning styles. Kolb divides learning into two dimensions: prehension and transformation. Prehension is how a learner internalizes information. Transformation is how the learner changes the raw information that was gathered into useful knowledge. These processes are explained by two learning dialectics. These may be best understood as two opposite poles of a learning dimension. For prehension, a learner may use concrete experience *(CE)* or abstract conceptualization *(AC)*. For transformation, a learner may use active experimentation *(AE)* or reflective observation *(RO)*. Exactly how a learner mixes these dialectics in their own learning process defines their learning style. An accommodator learns best by combining AE with CE, a diverger learns best by combining CE and RO, an assimilator learns best by combining RO and AC, and a converger learns best by combining AC and AE. (From Kolb DA: *Experiential learning: experience as the source of learning and development,* Englewoods Cliffs, NJ, 1984, Prentice-Hall.)

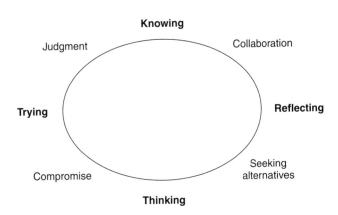

Figure 25-3 Ego states in combination with Kolb's learning cycle. (From Woods MF: *Trans Anal J* 12:153-158, 1982.)

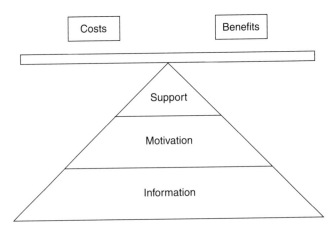

Figure 25-4 Patient-centered model of compliance to therapeutic regimens. (From Rosen DS: Creating the successful adolescent patient: a practical patient-oriented approach. In McNamara JA, Trotman C [eds]: *Creating the compliant patient,* Ann Arbor, Mich, 1996, Center for Human Growth and Development.)

and consultation technique work best for each learning style are currently under way.

Achieving Patient Compliance

White[22] proposed a new way to look at motivation for the typical orthodontic patient. He and others for many years have believed that positive reinforcement for good behavior is the key to conditioning patients to cooperate. Little success was found with various reward schemes for patient cooperation, such as a free bicycle for keeping all appointments or token economies for rewarding the wearing of headgear. In this situation, if the patient wears the gear for the prescribed time each month, they would get a token to shop for goodies in the office store. White[22] proposed that diversity in human personalities almost guarantees the impossibility of finding any universal reinforcement scheme that works for everyone.

White[22] observed that compliance was unpredictable in his practice. Frequently, he found broken appliances or gingivitis in patients in fixed appliances or patients simply failing to wear removable appliances such as headgear or functionals. He noted that these problems were always seen in the same patients. There seemed to be some influence of their personality beyond the positive and negative reinforcers. He increasingly came to realize that compliance seemed to be related to the patients' **sensitivity threshold,** which relates to a patient's pain tolerance.[23] Chase and Thomas[23] proposed that this threshold is an unchangeable characteristic of the patient's genetically determined personality. White[22] reasoned that if the patient's sensitivity threshold is unchangeable, the doctor's treatment strategies are not. He offered several suggestions to lessen patient discomfort and to encourage cooperation throughout the course of orthodontic therapy:

1. Use a soft-bristle toothbrush and, if necessary, chlorhexidine rinses.

2. Use the simplest appliance necessary to achieve treatment objectives with forces that are continuous and of low magnitude.
3. Prescribe analgesics when needed.
4. Expedite treatment time.
5. Let the fees reflect the challenge of a difficult patient.

Rosen[24] provided a practical **patient-oriented approach** to creating a compliant patient. He stated that health care providers should collaborate with patients by designing an individualized compliance plan. In other words, they should develop a compliance model that is patient-centered rather than clinician-centered (Figure 25-4). In this case the patients are able to decide the scope and limits of the care they choose to receive based on their own analyses of the costs and benefits of the treatment plan. Rosen[24] suggests that the orthodontist should first provide the patient with the information necessary to educate them about their malocclusion. Next, the orthodontist should motivate the patient by being open and straightforward and by building a relationship of mutual respect. Third, patients need support from family and peers to be compliant. Family provides encouragement, supervision, and assistance as well as a means to get to the office. Rosen[24] also states that the orthodontist should not coerce compliance through brute force. It is more productive to appreciate the patient's perspective and to work with him or her in overcoming barriers to achieve a good treatment outcome.

SUMMARY

Psychology and the behavioral sciences have been an integral part of orthodontics both in research and in clinical practice since the early days of this century. Numerous studies have explored the psychologic outcomes of orthodontics, and it can be stated safely that, for most patients, the effect on their own self-image is positive. In broad terms, straight teeth make for more attractive smiles. More attractive smiles make for more positive self-images. Although orthodontics has numerous other benefits for the patient's health and well-being, perhaps the most import effect is that it makes patients feel better about themselves. Throughout the course of orthodontic therapy, the orthodontist would do well to keep in mind the fact that the psychologic outcomes of treatment are every bit as important as the occlusal and functional outcomes of treatment. The therapist should make every effort to build the self-confidence of their patients. They should point out the patient's stepwise successes and honestly seek out reasons for small but significant failures as treatment progresses. They should make every effort to understand just why the patient is seeking care and just what the patient expects in terms of the effect of orthodontics on their lifestyle. It is important to point out unrealistic expectations before treatment ever begins.

For the orthodontist to provide a patient with a pleasing outcome, patient cooperation is essential. This chapter has reviewed a great deal of the information available on orthodontic patient cooperation and has suggested several approaches the clinician may take in achieving that goal. The therapist should understand the patient's individualized learning style and adjust the doctor's teaching style accordingly. Treatment should be made as expeditious and comfortable as possible. If the doctor expects the patient to comply with his or her wishes, those wishes should be easy and comfortable to follow. One golden thread that runs throughout the literature of orthodontic psychology is the importance of the doctor-patient relationship. Once the orthodontist has earned the trust and respect of the patient by establishing a good rapport, the task of achieving a good treatment result is made remarkably easier.

Orthodontics is, in many ways, one of the most rewarding professions. One of the greatest rewards in the clinical practice of orthodontics comes in watching timid young patients who believe themselves to be ugly because of crooked or "buck" teeth develop into self-confident, beautiful young ladies or handsome young men. Knowing that the orthodontist has played a major role in that development is a reward in and of itself that defies description.

REFERENCES

1. Bull R, Rumsey N: *The social psychology of facial appearance,* New York, 1988, Springer-Verlag.

2. Adams G: Physical attractiveness, personality, and social reactions to peer pressure, *J Psych* 96:287-296, 1977.

3. Secourd PF, Jourard SM: The appraisal of body cathexis: body cathexis, and self, *J Consult Psychol* 17-25, 1968.

4. Klima RJ, Wittemann JK, McIver JE: Body image, self-concept, and the orthodontic patient, *Am J Orthod* 75(5):507-516, 1979.

5. Phillips C, Bennett ME, Broder HL: Dentofacial disharmony: psychological status of patients seeking treatment consultation, *Angle Orthod* 68(6):547-556, 1998.

6. Dann C et al: Self-concept, Class II malocclusion, and early treatment, *Angle Orthod* 65(6):411-416, 1995.

7. Albino JE: Psychological reasons for orthodontic treatment explored, *J Am Dent Assoc* 98:1002-1003, 1979.

8. Varela M, Garcia-Camba JE: Impact of orthodontics on the psychologic profile of adult patients: a prospective study, *Am J Orthod Dentofacial Orthop* 108(2):142-148, 1995.

9. Shaw WC et al: Quality control in orthodontics: risk/benefit considerations, *Br Dent J* 170: 33-37, 1991.

10. Tung AW, Kiyak HA: Psychological influences on the timing of orthodontic treatment, *Am J Orthod Dentofacial Orthop* 113(1):29-39, 1998.

11. Egolf RJ, BeGole EA, Upshaw HS: Factors associated with orthodontic patient compliance with intraoral elastic and headgear wear, *Am J Orthod Dentofacial Orthop* 97:336-348, 1990.

12. Southard KA et al: Application of the Millon adolescent personality inventory in evaluating orthodontic compliance, *Am J Orthod Dentofacial Orthop* 100:553-561, 1991.

13. Sinha PK, Nanda RS, McNeil DW: Perceived orthodontist behaviors that predict patient satisfaction, orthodontist-patient relationship, and patient compliance in orthodontic treatment, *Am J Orthod Dentofacial Orthop* 100:370-377, 1996.

14. Peterson AC, Kuipers KS: Understanding adolescence: adolescent development and implications for the adolescent as a patient. In McNamara JA, Trotman CF (eds): *Creating the compliant patient,* Ann Arbor, Mich, 1996, Center for Human Growth and Development.

15. Steed-Veilands A: Patient compliance as a function of learning styles, Masters thesis, University of Tennessee, Memphis, 1998.

16. Cooper ML, Shapiro ML: Motivations for health behaviors among adolescents. In McNamara JA, Trotman C (eds): *Creating the compliant patient,* Ann Arbor, Mich, 1996, Center for Human Growth and Development.

17. Cucalon A, Smith RJ: Relationship between compliance by adolescent orthodontic patients and performance on psychological tests, *Angle Orthod* 60:107-113, 1989.

18. Klages U, Sergl HG, Burucker I: Relations between verbal behavior of the orthodontist and communicative cooperation of the patient in regular orthodontic visits, *Am J Orthod Dentofacial Orthop* 102:265-269, 1992.

19. Barsch A et al: Correlates of objective patient compliance with removable appliance wear, *Am J Orthod Dentofacial Orthop* 104:378-386, 1993.

20. Nanda RS, Kierl MJ: Prediction of cooperation in orthodontic treatment, *Am J Orthod Dentofacial Orthop* 102:15-21, 1992.

21. Kolb DA: *Experiential learning: experience as the source of learning and development*, Englewood Cliffs, NJ, 1984, Prentice-Hall.

22. White LW: A new paradigm of motivation. In McNamara JA, Trotman C (eds): *Creating the compliant patient*, Ann Arbor, Mich, 1996, Center for Human Growth and Development.

23. Chase S, Thomas A: *Know your child*, New York, 1987, Basic Books.

24. Rosen DS: Creating the successful adolescent patient: a practical patient-oriented approach. In McNamara JA, Trotman C (eds): *Creating the compliant patient*, Ann Arbor, Mich, 1996, Center for Human Growth and Development.

CHAPTER 26

Root Resorptions and Tissue Changes during Orthodontic Treatment

Vicki Vlaskalic and Robert L. Boyd

KEY TERMS

root resorption	bone loss	mononuclear giant cells	force magnitude
external apical resorption	sequelae	advanced stages of root resorption	jiggling movements
external resorption	spatial and temporal tissue changes	exposed mineralized root surface	continuous versus intermittent forces
apical root resorption	pressure sites	cessation	dental anomalies
incidence	hyalinization		types of tooth movement
prevalence	tissue necrosis		
risk			

SIGNIFICANCE OF THE PROBLEM

The external resorption of roots has perplexed the orthodontic specialty since the early reports of Ottolengui in 1914.[1] Many types of **root resorption** exist; physiologic resorption of primary teeth, as well as internal and external inflammatory resorption often associated with dental trauma and pulpal inflammation. The loss of tooth substance has been referred to by many names; root absorption, **external apical resorption, external resorption,** and, simply, root resorption.

External apical resorption associated with orthodontic treatment is diagnosed clinically via a radiograph by a detectable shortening of the roots at the apex (Figure 26-1). Detection of resorption radiographically is most obvious in the apical area; however, histologic investigation provides evidence that the same resorptive process also occurs on other areas of the root surface.

Although **apical root resorption** occurs in individuals who have never experienced orthodontic tooth movement, the incidence among treated individuals is

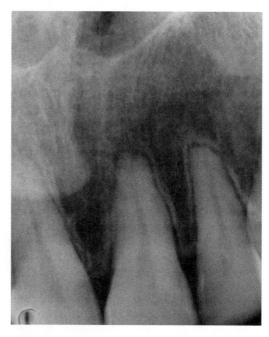

Figure 26-1 External apical root resorption observed after orthodontic treatment.

TABLE
26-1

Root Resorption Data from Published Articles

Study (Reference)	Year	Patients Number	Average Age Range	Number of Teeth	Teeth Examined	Treatment Type	Extractions/ Nonextractions	Source	Patients with Resorption (%)	Teeth with Resorption (%)	Resorption Amount	Treatment Time (yr:mo)
Stenvik and Mjor[52]	1970	—	10-13	35	PM	INTR	—	HIST	—	93	—	35 days
Stenvik and Mjor[52]	1970	—	10-13	35	PM	NT	—	HIST	—	0	—	—
Rosenberg[81]	1972	—	—	—	3,5	Begg	EXT	PANO	—	37	—	—
Stolien and Zachrisson[101]	1973	59	12:0	1180	5-5	EW	EXT	PA	—	—	0.5-1.8 mm	2:2
Plets et al.[87]	1974	50	16:8	100	1	NT	—	PA	27.5	27.5	—	—
Plets et al.[87]	1974	45	12:8	45	1	Fixed	—	CEPH	46	46	1.78 mm	2:3
Goldson and Henrikson[88]	1975	42	11-19	924	5-5	Begg	EXT	PA	100	77	—	1:8
Goldson and Henrikson[88]	1975	42	11-19	924	5-5	NT	—	PA	—	4	—	—
Hollender et al.[102]	1980	12	13:3	120	All	EW	EXT	PA	—	50	< 2 mm in 88%	1:6
Ronnerman and Larsson[112]	1981	23	11-14:8	—	21/12	ACT/EW	—	PA	39	—	1-3 mm	2:4-3:2
Harry and Sims[51]	1982	10	11-18	18	PM	INTR	—	PA/HIST	100	100	—	70 days
Harry and Sims[51]	1982	10	11-18	18	PM	NT	—	PA/HIST	0	0	—	—
Linge and Linge[75]	1983	719	12:8	2451	21/12	Varies	—	PA	—	—	0.7/mm	0:11

Study	Year	N										
Kennedy et al.[67]	1983	32	—	—	All	EW	EXT	PA	26.5	—	—	1:9
Kennedy et al.[67]	1983	32	—	—	All	SER 1 EW	EXT	PA	20.5	—	—	1:1
Kennedy et al.[67]	1983	32	—	—	All	SER	EXT	PA	6	—	—	—
Copland and Green[113]	1986	45	13:1	45	1	Fixed	—	CEPH	—	—	2.93 mm	2:10
Dermaut and Munck[89]	1986	20	15	66	21/12	INTR	—	PA	—	86	2.5 mm	0:7
Dermaut and Munck[89]	1986	15	22	58	21/12	NT	—	PA	0	0	—	—
Sharpe et al.[104]	1987	18	11:4	323RTS	All	EW	—	PA	89	20.1	—	3:7
Sharpe et al.[104]	1987	18	12:7	323RTS	All	EW	—	PA	83	13.3	—	2:7
Levander and Malmgren[92]	1988	98	15	390	21/12	B/EW	EXT/NONEXT	PA	—	34	—	0:6-0:9
Levander and Malmgren[92]	1988	98	15	390	21/12	B/EW	EXT/NONEXT	PA	—	56	—	1:75
Levander and Malmgren[92]	1988	55	14	22	21/12	B/EW	EXT	PA	—	—	—	1:8
Levander and Malmgren[92]	1988	153	14:4	610	21/12	B/EW	EXT/NONEXT	PA	—	56	—	1:8
Goldin[82]	1989	17	8-15:5	17	1	EW	—	CEPH	—	—	1.36 mm/yr	1:7
McFadden et al.[69]	1989	38	13:1	152	21/12	INTR	EXT/NONEXT	PA/CEPH	—	—	1.84 mm upper 0.61 lower	2:4

From Brezniak N, Wasserstein A: Am J Orthod Dentofacial Orthop 103(1):62-66, 1993.

RTS, Roots; ALL, all teeth; 1 maxillary central incisors; 21/12 maxillary incisors; PM, premolars; 3,5, canines and second premolars; 5-5, maxillary and mandibular incisors, canines, and premolars; Fixed, fixed appliances; NT, no treatment; LL, labiolingual; EW, edgewise; ACT, Activator; INTR, intrusion; Varies, fixed and removable; SER, serial extractions; B/EW, Begg/edgewise; PA, periapical; CEPH, lateral headfilm; HIST, histology; PANO, Panoramic film.

significantly higher.[2-5] The difficulty in accurately assessing the **incidence** (number of new cases) and **prevalence** (number of existing cases in a given population) of apical root resorption in the general population lies in the fact that, presently, radiographs or histologic sections are required to detect the condition. Orthodontic patients are screened specifically for the occurrence of apical root resorption, thus it is this population that demonstrates a higher prevalence. Compounding the problem of accurate epidemiologic data gathering are the variations in identification techniques used.

Despite the difficulty in conducting such surveys, the incidence and prevalence of apical root resorption in treated and untreated subjects have been reported and summarized in table form by Brezniak and Wasserstein (Table 26-1).[2] Depending on the source of information, the range of prevalence of root resorption is large. If the source is histologic, up to 100% of subjects are found to be affected, with figures between 0% to 100% for those diagnosed via radiographs.[6-8] The results of the histologic surveys in untreated populations suggest that a certain amount of apical root resorption may be a normal physiologic process.

Among treated populations the increase in the incidence of root resorption reported also varies greatly (see Table 26-1). Lupi, Handelman, and Sadowsky[3] used periapical radiographs of maxillary and mandibular incisors to measure apical root resorption. They reported from their sample of 88 ethnically and racially diverse adults that 15% of teeth had resorption before treatment and that this increased to 73% after at least 12 months of fixed appliance treatment. Although only 2% of the teeth showed moderate (beyond blunting and up to one third of root length) to severe (beyond one third of root length) resorption before treatment, 24.5% displayed this severity after treatment. Of patients, 2% experienced resorption beyond one third of the original root length. However, because no periapical radiographs were evaluated before the pretreatment periapical radiographs in this study, the presence of actual root shortening over time (apical root resorption) may have been difficult to distinguish from blunting, indistinct borders, or short roots.

Incidence of Root Resorption in Different Teeth

Most studies in which radiographs were used to detect loss of root structure focus on the apices of the maxillary central and lateral incisor teeth. This may be because of the fact that loss of cementum and dentine can be more easily detected at the root apex. In addition, these teeth are more often documented radiographically, and the incisors have been found to be more often affected by root resorption.[9] Finite element analysis of

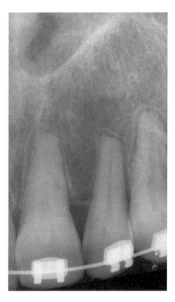

Figure 26-2 External apical root resorption observed during orthodontic treatment.

the stress response in the periodontium suggests that anatomic differences may be responsible for the variation in **risk** between teeth. During tooth movement, stress concentration is found to be the highest at the furcation level of the first maxillary molar.[10] In contrast, the area of highest stress concentration of an incisor during tooth movement is found at the apex.[9,11] In reality, the root resorption process is active at many sites around the root surface but is commonly detectable radiographically at the apex.

Root Resorption and Orthodontic Treatment

Although most orthodontically treated patients may lose a portion of tooth root during treatment, they do not appear to experience consequential additional risk of future tooth loss (Figure 26-2).[12-15] However, some patients experience an amount of root structure loss to the point where treatment plans need to be reviewed to avoid the presumed possibility of negative sequelae such as excessive tooth mobility and eventual tooth loss.[16] These severe cases are exacerbated when alveolar **bone loss** occurs in conjunction or subsequent to root loss, thus further minimizing tooth attachment.[17] It has been reported, however, that no correlation exists between root resorption and subsequent bone loss.[18]

Analyzing the amount of periodontal attachment area loss secondary to apical root resorption via a computer graphics system, Kalkwarf, Krejci, and Pao[17] calculated the amount of periodontal attachment area remaining after various lengths of root loss that was experienced on a central incisor tooth. Results indicated that up to 4 mm of apical root loss results in approximately 20% attachment loss. Investigators have stressed the fact that apical root resorption is less critical in terms of periodontal support than is crestal bone loss, particularly in the initial stages (3 mm or less) of root resorption.[3,17]

Surprisingly little literature has been devoted to the **sequelae** of root resorption associated with orthodontic treatment. No articles have reported tooth loss caused by severe apical root resorption after orthodontic treatment where no other form of trauma or infection was involved. The few studies and case reports that have looked specifically at the long-term outcome of teeth affected by apical root resorption reveal no instances of tooth loss.[12-15] Remington et al[13] found that, out of a total of 100 cases, the worst outcome was hypermobility (found in only two cases). Tooth vitality was not compromised in resorbed teeth. In VonderAhe's study[12] of 57 patients experiencing mild, moderate, and severe degrees of apical root resorption with an average postretention period of 6.5 years, there were no cases of hypermobility or other negative sequelae detected.

Of the long-term treatment outcome studies that were not specifically investigating the effects of apical root resorption but included its evaluation, the findings revealed the frequent detection of minor resorption and with no discernible clinical significance.[19,20]

It must be concluded from the body of evidence existing in the literature that the sequelae of orthodontically related resorption does not pose a long-term threat to the patient. It should be realized, however, that the combined long-term effects of apical root resorption and crestal alveolar bone loss might not have such seemingly innocent sequelae.

ORTHODONTIC TOOTH MOVEMENT AND THE BIOLOGY OF ROOT RESORPTION

Periodontal Ligament Changes during Tooth Movement

Alterations in the periodontal tissues during orthodontic tooth movement specifically affect the alveolar bone, periodontal ligament, and the root surface. **Spatial and temporal tissue changes** during orthodontic tooth movement have been documented in many studies pioneered in the early 1950s by Reitan and many others.[21-35] From the observed histologic and coincident biochemical analysis, researchers have been able to extrapolate relationships between these tissue changes and clinically detectable root resorption. Experimental variables that should be taken into account include differences in the species tested, tooth moving mechanics, force level and duration, as well as analytic techniques.

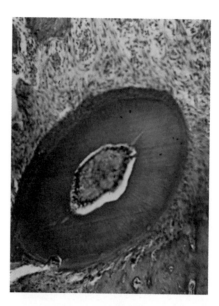

Figure 26-3 Canine/premolar exhibiting initial reaction of periodontal ligament following orthodontic tooth movement. A small resorption lesion is observed in the lower left corner. (Courtesy Dr. Birte Melsen.)

Orthodontic force initiation stimulates the remodeling of alveolar bone, which results in tooth movement.[21-28] Before this remodeling, initial changes in response to a local compression of the periodontal ligament include a reduction in width and vascular changes.

Periodontal ligament changes occur most noticeably at **pressure sites** during tooth movement (Figure 26-3). Tissue reactions observed include early proliferation of blood vessels, cellular extravasation, extravascular coagulation, and tissue necrosis.[29,30] Some histologic sections may show areas devoid of cellular elements, commonly referred to as **hyalinization.** Cellular elements observed initially at pressure sites adjacent to the bone interface and subsequently throughout the periodontal ligament are largely comprised of multinucleated giant cells. Other cellular elements found include monocytes, macrophages, and neutrophils. **Tissue necrosis** is evident at all stages and at varying degrees of progression during orthodontic tooth movement.[29] It is hypothesized that vascular changes such as stasis, ischemia, thrombosis, degeneration, and obliteration contribute to this necrotic process.

Results of histologic studies strongly suggest that root resorption occurs in response to damage initiated by orthodontic treatment to the periodontal ligament.[26,29,31,32] The innermost cells of the periodontal ligament have particularly been implicated in this process.[36] When the protective nature of these cells is lost, clast type cells may resorb not only necrotic tissue, but also the root surface indiscriminately. Trauma to the periodontal ligament initiated by orthodontic treatment has been found to occur with even a light orthodontic force (50 to 100 g).[29]

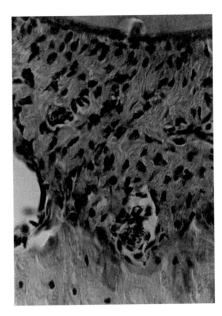

Figure 26-4 Initial resorption lesion on root surface following orthodontic tooth movement on canine/premolar. (Courtesy Dr. Birte Melsen.)

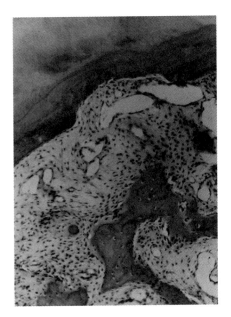

Figure 26-5 More extreme external apical root resorption defect. (Courtesy Dr. Birte Melsen.)

Root Surface Changes during Tooth Movement

Root surface change does not become apparent before cellular change occurs in adjacent periodontal ligament and bone. In human teeth, changes are observed in the 3- to 5-week period after initiation of a light force. Initial change is manifested histologically as congregation of **mononuclear giant cells** along the root surface with some of these cells associated with areas of damaged periodontal ligament (Figure 26-4). **Advanced stages of root resorption** are typified by odontoclast-like cells with ruffled borders, numerous resorption defects, and clear zones on the root surface (Figure 26-5). The residual matrix covering the surface of the resorption defects consists of exposed collagen fibrils. It has been suggested that a relationship, other than geographic, exists between resorption of the root surface and periodontal ligament injury.*

A significant finding is that both the healing process and early stages of root resorption involve a high percentage of mononuclear giant cells.† This has led to the suggestion that the mononuclear giant cells nonselectively remove the precementum layer together with adjacent necrotic periodontal ligament.[31] Other cells such as TRAP-negative macrophage and fibroblast cells have also been implicated in this process.[40,41] This exposed mineralized matrix is capable of inducing the cytodifferentiation of preodontoclasts and preosteoclasts.[42-47] These multinucleated cells displaying ruffled borders

and clear zones are responsible for the resorption of mineralized structures.[48] Researchers have suggested that mononuclear giant cells may also be induced to transform into odontoclasts by the **exposed mineralized root surface** because these cells all belong to the hemopoietic monocyte-macrophage lineage.

Root Resorption Initiation, Cessation, and Repair

Reports on the timing of the first histologic detection of root resorption vary from 1 week to a few weeks. This may be because of such variables as the species tested, magnitude and duration of force, and the analytic procedure involved. The progression of root resorption in terms of depth and number of lacunae has been found to increase with continuation of force.[29]

Controversy also exists as to the **cessation** of the root resorption process. Some investigations have concluded that root resorption ceases with termination of force application, whereas other studies have shown that the process continues even after force termination.[26,29] This last finding has been used to support the hypothesis that cessation is more likely linked to complete removal of necrotic tissue than force application despite an earlier finding of continued root resorption after the removal of necrotic tissue by Rygh and others.[26,29]

Repair of resorption lacunae has been observed as early as 3 to 5 weeks after the initiation of light orthodontic tooth movement. No distinct matrix layer has been detected between the residual resorption matrix

---

*References 25, 26, 29, 32, 33, 37-41.
†References 25, 26, 32, 33, 38-41.

and those collagen fibrils of the precementum repair matrix. The formation and attachment of the repair matrix resembles that of either acellular extrinsic fiber cementum or cellular intrinsic fiber cementum. The restoration of a dentinocemental junction corresponding to that formed at odontogenesis implies that a repetition of the initial cementogenesis occurring at the advancing root edge takes place when a root has previously been resorbed.[29,49,50]

Clinical Implications of the Repair Process

The extent to which the process of repair of resorption lacunae impacts the vitality and longevity of affected teeth is unknown. Previous investigators have observed that treatment interruption[51,52] or appliance removal with relapse of tooth position will initiate repair and cause the resorptive process to cease.[26,53] It has been postulated that repaired cementum and dentine may actually provide increased resistance to root resorption, substantiating the perceived beneficial effect of a 3-month pause in treatment mechanics.[52]

Several studies have shown that the repair of apical root resorption is temporally linked to root resorption.[31,50] In their study on the effects of active force and force termination on rats teeth, Brudvik and Rygh[31] found that there seem to be several determinants of continued resorption or repair of an active root resorption process.[31] Their findings indicated that when active force is removed but passive stress of the periodontal ligament remains through retention of the tooth in its new position, resorption would continue as long as necrotic tissue is still present locally. In a later paper by the same authors, repair was reported to occur even in the presence of a light force. However, the length of the rest period necessary for repair of a resorption lacunae before reactivation of force was not resolved.[54] Additional research investigating the spatial and temporal repair patterns of orthodontically induced surface resorption patches reaffirms that the mechanism for deposition of an initial acellular cementum formation occurs within 2 weeks after force cessation and that a slower deposition of cellular cementum occurs at more advanced stages of healing.[55] Previous investigators have observed that treatment interruption[51,52] or appliance removal with relapse of tooth position will initiate repair and cause the resorptive process to cease.[26,53] Using this information, it may become possible to identify an optimum cycle of orthodontic force application versus orthodontic force release to minimize or even prevent radiologically evident apical root resorption. No significant differences have been found in the repair potential between the cervical, middle, and apical thirds of roots.[49]

The repair potential of teeth has clinical implication in relation to the prognosis of affected teeth.[56] It has been suggested that a final decision regarding prognosis should not be made for at least 6 months after active orthodontic treatment is completed. This is because, during treatment, the roots may still be resorbing with the inorganic portion not visible radiographically. If the teeth are allowed to stabilize, the radiolucent demineralized matrix will remineralize. This area then becomes radiopaque and may make the root appear longer. In addition, during regular orthodontic retention, the width of the periodontal ligament narrows and mobility decreases. Thus decisions regarding splinting should also be delayed to allow adaptation of the periodontal ligament to the occlusal forces. Patients who have bruxism or clenching habits should also be treated with night guards to eliminate this primary cause of mobility.

ETIOLOGY OF ROOT RESORPTION RELATED TO ORTHODONTIC TREATMENT

Potential Etiologic Factors

The relationship between orthodontics and external apical root resorption has traditionally been approached as a cause and effect model. As a result, studies of possible etiologic factors have been directed toward treatment variables. Treatment-related factors that have been investigated include the magnitude of orthodontic force,[35,57-60] treatment mechanics,[61-65] direction of tooth movement,[7,11,60,64,66-68] appliance type,[63,65] and treatment duration.[61,69,70]

Ambiguously, recent studies have disputed widely proposed causative factors such as increased **force magnitude**,[57,58,68,69] amount of tooth movement,[61,63,70] duration of treatment,[66] **jiggling movements** of teeth,[71] and **continuous versus intermittent forces**.[61,65,72]

Many studies have implicated certain **types of tooth movement** during orthodontic treatment, such as intrusion or retraction, as initiating root resorption.[2,59,64,68,73-75] To further clarify the relationship between the magnitude and direction of movement of the upper central incisor apex with apical root resorption in orthodontically treated adults, Baumrind, Korn, and Boyd[70] compared the magnitude of displacement measured on lateral cephalograms with resorption measured on standardized anterior periapical radiographs. Previous studies of this relationship have been based on radiographic measurement of the amount of root resorption on cephalometric radiographs only, which have almost four times the measurement error as standardized periapical radiographs.[76] Surprisingly, the regression coefficient for both the absence of apical movement and apical retraction were highly significant for root resorption;

however, those for extrusion, intrusion, and advancement were not. At the 95% confidence level, an average of 0.99 mm (standard error ± 0.34) of root resorption was implied in the absence of root displacement, and an average of 0.49 mm (standard error = ± 0.14) of resorption was implied per millimeter of apical retraction. Results from other investigators such as Dermaut and De Munck[7] and McFadden and others,[64] have also failed to find statistically significant correlations between root resorption and tooth intrusion.

Another finding is that resorption is likely to occur even when the apex of the tooth does not appear to move, which may be consistent with either apical root resorption occurring in untreated populations or with jiggling movements produced in treatment. Jiggling movements have long been identified as a potential risk factor for root resorption.[71]

It should be emphasized that the study of root resorption in adolescence requires additional caution because continued root growth may be occurring simultaneously. On the other hand, no confounding root length changes occur in the adult population.[77] Parker and Harris[78] found in their sample of 110 adolescent subjects that incisor intrusion and increase in proclination were strong predictors of root resorption. Baumrind, Korn, and Boyd[79] also studied a sample of orthodontically treated adolescents. Results showed that the intercept and intrusion were highly significant (p <0.001) for root resorption. However, the significance was contrary to conventional wisdom in that greater displacement of the apex resulted in *less* root resorption. To explain these findings, three hypotheses may be considered: (1) teeth with incomplete root formation may displace more readily, (2) incompletely formed roots may be "biologically protected" from root resorption, and (3) root growth may be accelerated by application of tooth-moving forces to teeth with incompletely formed roots. Four independent variables studied also showed statistical significance for root resorption. They were original overbite, change in original overbite, change in upper incisor angle, and clinician effect.

Despite rigorous investigation, neither a single factor nor a group of factors related purely to orthodontic treatment has been identified as directly causing external apical root resorption. The only consistent finding is that a wide individual variation of responses exists. The fact that research results are inconsistent and provide low R^2 scores implies that even if any of these factors alone or combined are etiologic for root resorption, other still unidentified factors are more significantly responsible for the resorptive response. This conclusion has focused attention on the identification of discriminating risk factors within patients' histories.

Predisposing Patient Factors

Patient-related etiologic factors that have been investigated include genetic predisposition,[80] age,[12,35,64,66,81] gender,[64,82] tooth vitality,[13] tooth type,[19] facial and dentoalveolar structure,[61,67] preexisting root resorption,[83] nutrition,[84] habits,[85,86] root form,[4,61,82] previous trauma,[66,83] and dense alveolar bone.[61] Mirabella and Artun[61] showed that patients with long roots may be more predisposed to root resorption than patients with normal root lengths.

Studies investigating the role of genetics and root resorption using large numbers of sibling pairs have identified that a significant amount of the variability in response to root resorption can be explained by heritability factors.[80] Harris, Kineret, and Tolley[80] found high heritability estimates averaging 70%. The variables of gender and age were not predictive of susceptibility. The results of this study indicated that revelation of the biochemical factors responsible for controlling familial factors may provide useful information in the quest for the control of root resorption.

PREVENTIVE MEASURES

Individual Risk Characterization

Within the context of the present understanding of the cause of apical root resorption, the concept of prevention is largely empirical and is often based on anecdotal evidence. Ideally, suggestions for prevention should arise from studies that demonstrate high correlational findings with root resorption in addition to the controlled study of strategies that result in a lower incidence of apical root resorption. Unfortunately such studies in humans are not yet available.

The literature is replete with papers suggesting preventive therapeutic approaches such as short duration of treatment,[4,68] decreased root movement,[61,70] avoidance of elastics,[60,87] the use of light intermittent forces,[26,35,60,68,88] and scrutinization of medical history and familial tendency records.[64,85,89] These papers, however, do not provide definitive preventive strategies that apply to most orthodontic patients. Furthermore, there is no data available that proves that any or all of these actions result in a lower incidence of apical root resorption.

Characterization of patients exhibiting long, narrow roots and abnormal root form,[61] various other dental anomalies,[82,90] finger and tongue habits,[85-87] and a history of previous traumatic injury[66,87] as "at risk" for external root resorption suggest that a preventive strategy may be possible in the form of early detection. The success of such a strategy was questioned by Mirabella and Artun,[61] who found that the variation in root resorption explained by the identification of such risk factors was as low as 20%. In addition, an investigation into the significance of a variety of **dental anomalies** such as tooth agenesis, small lateral incisors, dens invaginatus, taurodontism, ectopic eruption, and abnormally short roots as risk factors for root resorption did not identify any of these anomalies as predisposing factors.[90] Clearly, factors other than those identified are involved in the individual patient response in terms of resorption to orthodontic tooth movement.

Clinical Management of High-Risk Patients

Despite the findings of Mirabella and Artun,[61] the determination of the relative overall patient susceptibility to root resorption may be of use to the orthodontic clinician. By collectively identifying alleged genetic, morphologic, and treatment-related predisposing variables such as sibling experience of root resorption, prolonged treatment time, and long and narrow root forms, the clinician may recognize patients who may be at an increased risk for root resorption.

Clinical strategies such as visible labeling of these patients' charts and specific monitoring protocols may aid in the early identification of cases that may have otherwise become severely affected by root resorption. Because monitoring radiographic protocols remains strictly empiric with the formation of risk profiles, however, these protocols may be applied on a more selective basis. Patients at increased risk should have monitoring radiographs taken at least once within the first year of treatment and usually including an anterior periapical film. Caution by the clinician should be used when diagnosing from radiographs because resorption defects may be difficult to diagnose, even with the use of periapical films.[91] When the patient profile includes genetic, morphologic, and treatment variables such as a history of previous trauma to teeth and long treatment duration, monitoring radiographs should be taken at more frequent intervals such as every 3 to 4 months. The clinician must keep in mind that a patient without any identifiable risk factors for root resorption may still incur loss of root structure during orthodontic treatment. This has prompted researchers to recommend that it may be prudent to take monitoring radiographs at regular intervals for all orthodontic patients.

Protective Factors

Recently, several studies have indicated that some protective factors such as incomplete root formation,[66,81,88,92] endodontic treatment of otherwise nontraumatized teeth,[13,93] and aspirin therapy[94] may be associated with a lower incidence or severity of root resorption. The exact mechanism responsible for the re-

ported increased resistance to root resorption has not been elucidated.

The findings by Fenn, Boero, and Boyd[92] support the hypothesis that teeth with open apices may be more resistant to apical root resorption. This is particularly interesting in light of the trend toward mixed dentition treatment. Thus it may be prudent to begin treatment of moderate to severe malocclusions at or before the age of 9 years, when most incisors have open apices.[95] In addition, if a biochemical mechanism for this apparent immunity of teeth with open apices to root resorption can be identified, this knowledge may possibly be applied for the protection of fully formed teeth.

The clinical control of root resorption using chemotherapeutic agents is a potential strategy in the future. Investigators have found that agents such as tetracycline, doxycycline, and thyroxine have the potential to prevent or regulate molecular mechanisms contributing to root resorption.[96-98] Clinical screening for dentinal matrix proteins in periodontal ligament fluid may be an effective device in the future to aid the early detection of resorption in patients.[99] This may then allow the clinician to revise the treatment plan for any patient in whom resorption has been detected at an early stage.

TREATMENT MEASURES

Modification of Treatment Plans

Once root resorption has been detected by the clinician, a decision must be made regarding the potential impact on the patient so that possible evasive strategies may be employed. Treatment of external root resorption is limited to cessation of the biochemical events leading to further loss of structure and maintaining the compromised dentition.

To stop the resorption process, cessation of orthodontic tooth movement has been proposed.[52,100] This may not be a suitable solution for the patient if orthodontic objectives are far from being met. Modification of treatment plans with the aim of minimizing tooth movement has been suggested. This may include interproximal reduction rather than premolar extraction, orthognathic surgery, or, in severe cases, terminating treatment before all treatment objectives are met. If the resorption process is so advanced that teeth are hypermobile, wire and composite splints have been reported to be successful in providing a favorable long-term outcome.[100]

FUTURE RESEARCH DIRECTION

Previous investigators have illustrated histologic events occurring during orthodontic tooth movement, including those associated with external root resorption. Largely because of these efforts, it is possible to describe chronologically cellular and tissue changes that represent the progression of external root resorption. The question still remains, however, as to the molecular control and regulatory events associated with these histologic changes. As a result, efforts are being directed toward identification of the molecules involved in the sequence of events leading to root resorption.

By comparing the expression of mRNAs in the periodontium of rats subjected to orthodontic forces with those without applied force, characterization of molecular determinants of root resorption is possible.[101] Techniques involved include differential display of poly(A)-RNA, amplification and subcloning of cDNA fragments, and DNA sequence analysis. Such human genetic information may allow clinicians to identify individuals most susceptible to loss of root structure during orthodontic treatment before therapy begins. This information may allow alternative treatment plans to be implemented, consent procedures to be more accurate, and in-treatment monitoring to be specifically targeted to at-risk patients. All of these possibilities could potentially reduce the incidence of root resorption and the costs associated with nonspecific monitoring procedures.

Alternative diagnostic techniques for the detection of root resorption may be developed in the future. For reasons such as additional radiation exposure and the use of nonstandardized radiographic techniques, traditional radiographic detection of root resorption is not an ideal method. It may become possible to use other techniques such as monitoring of dentinal proteins in gingival crevicular fluids. Investigators have confirmed that two noncollagenous acidic phosphoproteins found in mineralizing dentine matrix (Dentin Matrix Protein 1 and Dentin Phosphophoryn) may act as markers for root resorption.[99]

It will become increasingly relevant to look at the long-term outcomes of patients experiencing all levels of apical root resorption after orthodontic treatment. This demand for data collection on treatment success is stimulated by the specialty's need to manage patients using objective rather than subjective decision making, as well as heightened medicolegal awareness. This long-term view should be accounted for in the planning of future studies. Until the cause of external root resorption related to orthodontic treatment is elucidated and falls under the control of the clinician, orthodontists are obligated to inform each of their patients of the possibility and implications of external root resorption.

ACKNOWLEDGMENTS

The authors would like to acknowledge Dr. Birte Melsen for supplying the photomicrographs used in this chapter.

REFERENCES

1. Ottolengui R: The physiological resorption of tooth roots, *Den Items Int* 36:332-362, 1914.
2. Brezniak N, Wasserstein A: Root resorption after orthodontic treatment. Part 1. Literature review, *Am J Orthod Dentofacial Orthop* 103:62-66, 1993.
3. Lupi JE, Handelman CS, Sadowsky C: Prevalence and severity of apical root resorption and alveolar bone loss in orthodontically treated adults, *Am J Orthod Dentofacial Orthop* 109:28-37, 1996.
4. Levander E, Malmgren O: Evaluation of the risk of root resorption during orthodontic treatment: a study of upper incisors, *Eur J Orthod* 10:30-38, 1988.
5. Sjolien T, Zachrisson B: Periodontal bone support and tooth length in orthodontically treated and untreated persons, *Am J Orthod* 64:28-37, 1973.
6. Henry JR, Weinman JP: The pattern of resorption and repair of human cementum, *J Am Dent Assoc* 42:270-290, 1951.
7. Dermaut LR, De Munck A: Apical root resorption of upper incisors caused by intrusive movement: a radiographic study, *Am J Orthod Dentofacial Orthop* 90:321-326, 1986.
8. Massler M, Perreault JG: Root resorption in the permanent teeth of young adults, *J Dent Child* 21:158-164, 1954.
9. Beck BW, Harris EF: Apical root resorption in orthodontically treated subjects: analysis of edgewise and light wire mechanics, *Am J Orthod Dentofacial Orthop* 105 (4):350-361, 1994.
10. Jeon PD et al: Analysis of stress in the periodontium of the maxillary first molar with a three-dimensional finite element model, *Am J Orthod Dentofacial Orthop* 115(3):267-274, 1999.
11. Cotsopoulos G, Nanda R: An evaluation of root resorption incident to orthodontic intrusion, *Am J Orthod Dentofacial Orthop* 109:543-548, 1996.
12. VonderAhe G: Postretention status of maxillary incisors with root-end resorption, *Angle Orthod* 3:247-255, 1973.
13. Remington DN et al: Long-term evaluation of root resorption occurring during orthodontic treatment, *Am J Orthod Dentofacial Orthop* 96:43-46, 1989.
14. Parker WS: Root resorption: long-term outcome, *Am J Orthod Dentofacial Orthop* 112:119-123, 1997.
15. Desai HM: Root resorption: another long-term outcome, *Am J Orthod Dentofacial Orthop* 116(2):184-186, 1999.
16. Lyndon Carman L: Arrested root resorption during orthodontic treatment, *Am Soc Orthod Tr* 171-175, 1936.
17. Kalkwarf KL, Krejci RF, Pao YC: Effect of apical root resorption on periodontal support, *J Prosthet Dent* 56:317-319, 1986.
18. Ogaard B: Marginal bone support and tooth lengths in 19-year-olds following orthodontic treatment, *Eur J Orthod* 10(3):180-186, 1988.
19. Tahir E, Sadowsky C, Schneider BJ: An assessment of treatment outcome in American Board of Orthodontics cases, *Am J Orthod Dentofacial Orthop* 111:335-342, 1997.
20. Ahlgren J: A ten-year evaluation of the quality of orthodontic treatment, *Swed Dent J* 17:201-220, 1993.

21. Reitan K, Kvam E: Comparative behavior of human and animal tissue during experimental tooth movement, *Angle Orthod* 41:1-14, 1971.

22. Rygh P: Ultrastructural vascular changes in pressure zones of rat molar periodontium incident to orthodontic tooth movement, *Scand J Dent Res* 80:307-321, 1972a.

23. Rygh P: Ultastructural cellular reactions in pressure zones of rat molar periodontium incident to orthodontic tooth movement, *Acta Odont Scand* 30:575-593, 1972b.

24. Rygh P: Ultrastructural changes of the periodontal fibers and their attachment in rat molar periodontium incident to orthodontic tooth movement, *Scand J Dent Res* 81:467-480, 1973.

25. Rygh P: Elimination of hyalinized periodontal tissues associated with orthodontic tooth movement, *Scand J Dent Res* 82:57-73, 1974.

26. Rygh P: Orthodontic root resorption studied by electron microscopy, *Angle Orthod* 47:1-16, 1977.

27. Davidovitch Z et al: Neurotransmitters, cytokines, and the control of alveolar bone remodeling in orthodontics, *Dent Clin North Am* 32:411-434, 1988.

28. Vandevska-Radunovic V et al: Changes in blood circulation in teeth and supporting tissues incident to experimental tooth movement, *Eur J Orthod* 16:361-369, 1994.

29. Bosshardt DD, Masseredjian V, Nanci A: Root resorption and tissue repair in orthodontically treated human premolars. In Davidovitch Z, Mah J (eds): *Biological mechanisms of tooth eruption, resorption and replacement by implants,* Boston, 1998, Harvard Society for the Advancement of Orthodontics.

30. Murrell EF, Yen EHK, Johnson RB: Vascular changes in the periodontal ligament after removal of orthodontic forces, *Am J Orthod Dentofacial Orthop* 110(3):280-286, 1996.

31. Brudvik P, Rygh P: Root resorption associated with combined orthodontic/experimental tooth movement: the initial attack and the resorption/repair sequence on root surfaces exposed to compression. In Davidovitch (ed): *Biological mechanisms of tooth eruption, resorption and replacement by implants,* Boston, 1994, Harvard Society for the Advancement of Orthodontics.

32. Kvam E: Cellular dynamics on the pressure side of the rat periodontium following experimental tooth movement, *Scand J Dent Res* 80:369-383, 1972.

33. Reitan K: The initial tissue reaction incident to orthodontic tooth movement as related to the influence of function, *Acta Odont Scand* 9(suppl):6, 1951.

34. Reitan K: Clinical and histologic observations on tooth movement during and after orthodontic treatment, *Am J Orthod* 53(10):721-745, 1967.

35. Reitan K: Initial tissue behavior during apical root resorption, *Angle Orthod* 44(1):68-82, 1974.

36. Andreasen JO: Review of root resorption systems and models: etiology of root resorption and the homeostatic mechanisms of the periodontal ligament. In Davidovitch Z (ed): *The biological mechanisms of tooth eruption and root resorption,* Boston, 1988, Harvard Society for the Advancement of Orthodontics.

37. Kvam E: A study of the cell-free zone following experimental tooth movement in the rat, *Trans Eur Orthod Soc* 45:419-434, 1970.

38. Williams S: A histomorphometric study of orthodontically induced root resorption, *Eur J Orthod* 6:35-47, 1984.

39. Tanaka T et al: Endocytosis in odontoclasts and osteoclasts using microperoxidase as a tracer, *J Dent Res* 69:883-889, 1990.

40. Brudvik P, Rygh P: The initial phase of orthodontic root resorption incident to local compression of the periodontal ligament, *Eur J Orthod* 15:249-263, 1993a.

41. Brudvik P, Rygh P: Non-clast cells start root resorption in the periphery of hyalinized zones, *Eur J Orthod* 15:467-480, 1993b.

42. Sasaki T et al: Cytodifferentiation of odontoclasts in physiological root resorption of human deciduous teeth. In Davidovitch Z (ed): *The biological mechanisms of tooth eruption and root resorption,* Birmingham, 1988, EBSCO Media.

43. Sasaki T et al: Multinucleated cells formed on calcified dentine from mouse marrow cells treated with 1 alpha, 25-dihydroxyvitamin D3 have ruffled borders and resorb dentine, *Anat Rec* 224:379-391, 1989.

44. Chambers TJ et al: Resorption of bone by isolated rabbit osteoclasts, *J Cell Sci* 66:383-399, 1984.

45. Chambers TJ, Darby JA, Fuller K: Mammalian collagenase predisposes bone surfaces to osteoclastic resorption, *Cell Tissue Res* 241:671-675, 1985.

46. MacDonald BR et al: Formation of multinucleated cells that respond to osteotropic hormones in long-term human bone marrow cultures, *Endocrinology* 120:2326-2333, 1987.

47. Takahashi N et al: Osteoclast-like cell formation and its regulation by osteotropic hormones in mouse marrow cultures, *Endocrinology* 122:1373-1382, 1988.

48. Marks SC, Popoff SN: Bone cell biology: the regulation of development, structure, and function in the skeleton, *Am J Anat* 183:1-44, 1988.

49. Bosshardt DD: Formation and attachment of new cementum matrix following root resorption in human teeth: a light- and electron microscopic study. In Davidovitch Z (ed): *Biological mechanisms of tooth eruption, resorption and replacement by implants,* Boston, 1994, Harvard Society for the Advancement of Orthodontics.

50. Owman-Moll P, Kurol J, Lundgren D: Repair of orthodontically induced root resorption in adolescents, *Angle Orthod* 65:403-408, 1995.

51. Schmid W: Root resorption after orthodontic treatment, *Dental Digest* 38:698-699, 1931.

52. Levander E, Malmgren O, Eliasson S: Evaluation of root resorption in relation to two orthodontic treatment regimes: a clinical experimental study, *Eur J Orthod* 16:223-228, 1994.

53. Reitan K: Biomechanical principals and reaction. In Graber TM, Swain BF (eds): *Orthodontic current principles and technique,* St Louis, 1985, Mosby.

54. Brudvik P, Rygh P: The repair of orthodontic root resorption: an ultrastructural study, *Eur J Orthod* 17:189-198, 1995.

55. Sismanidou C, Lindskog S: Spatial and temporal repair patterns of orthodontically induced surface resorption patches, *Eur J Oral Sci* 103:292-298, 1995.

56. Owman-Moll P, Kurol J: Root resorption pattern during orthodontic tooth movement in adolescents. In Davidovitch Z, Mah J (eds): *Biological mechanisms of tooth eruption, resorption and replacement by implants,* Boston, 1998, Harvard Society for the Advancement of Orthodontics.

57. Owman-Moll P, Kurol J, Lundgren D: The effects of a four-fold increased orthodontic force magnitude on tooth movement and root resorptions: an intra-individual study in adolescents, *Eur J Orthod* 3:287-294, 1996.

58. Kurol J, Owman-Moll P, Lundgren D: Time-related root resorption after application of a controlled continuous orthodontic force, *Am J Orthod Dentofacial Orthop* 110:303-310, 1996.

59. Reitan K: Effects of force magnitude and direction of tooth movement on different alveolar bone types, *Angle Orthod* 34:244-255, 1964.

60. Harry MR, Sims MR: Root resorption in bicuspid intrusion: a scanning electron microscopic study, *Angle Orthod* 52:235-258, 1982.

61. Mirabella AD, Artun J: Risk factors for apical root resorption of maxillary anterior teeth in adult orthodontic patients, *Am J Orthod Dentofacial Orthop* 108:48-55, 1995.

62. Mirabella AD, Artun J: Prevalence and severity of apical root resorption of maxillary anterior teeth in adult orthodontic patients, *Eur J Orthod* 17:93-99, 1995.

63. Alexander SA: Levels of root resorption associated with continuous arch and sectional arch mechanics, *Am J Orthod Dentofacial Orthop* 110:321-324, 1996.

64. McFadden WM, Engstrøm H, Anholm JM: A study of the relationship between incisor intrusion and root shortening, *Am J Orthod Dentofacial Orthop* 96:390-396, 1989.

65. Blake M, Woodside DG, Pharoah MJ: A radiographic comparison of apical root resorption after orthodontic treatment with the edgewise and Speed appliances, *Am J Orthod Dentofacial Orthop* 108:76-84, 1985.

66. Linge L, Linge BO: Apical root resorption in upper anterior teeth, *Eur J Orthod* 5:173-183, 1983.

67. Taithongchai R, Sookkorn K, Killiany DM: Facial and dentoalveolar structure and the prediction of apical root shortening, *Am J Orthod Dentofacial Orthop* 110:296-302, 1996.

68. Stenvik A, Mjor IA: Pulp and dentine reactions to experimental tooth intrusion: a histologic study of the initial changes, *Am J Orthod* 57:370-385, 1970.

69. Owman-Moll P: Orthodontic tooth movement and root resorption with special reference to force magnitude and duration: a clinical and histological investigation in adolescents, *Swed Dent J Suppl* 105:1-45, 1995.

70. Baumrind S, Korn EL, Boyd RL: Apical root resorption in orthodontically treated adults, *Am J Orthod Dentofacial Orthop* 110:311-320, 1996.

71. Stuteville OH: Injuries caused by orthodontic forces and the ultimate results of these injuries, *Am J Orthod Oral Surg* 24:103-116, 1938.

72. Owman-Moll P, Kurol J, Lundgren D: Continuous versus interrupted orthodontic force related to early tooth movement and root resorption, *Angle Orthod* 65:395-401, 1995.

73. Vlaskalic V, Boyd R, Baumrind S: Etiology and sequelae of root resorption, *Semin Orthod* 4:124-131, 1998.

74. Brezniak N, Wasserstein A: Root resorption after orthodontic treatment. Part 2. Literature review, *Am J Orthod Dentofacial Orthop* 103:138-146, 1993.

75. Killiany DM: Root resorption caused by orthodontic treatment: an evidence-based review of literature, *Semin Orthod* 5:128-133, 1999.

76. Boyd RL, Baumrind S: Root length and interproximal bone height changes associated with fixed orthodontic treatment in adults and adolescents: design and preliminary findings of a retrospective radiographic study. In Davidovitch Z (ed): *Biological mechanisms of tooth movement and craniofacial adaption,* Columbus, Ohio, 1992, The Ohio State University College of Dentistry.

77. Bishara SE, Vonwald L, Jakobsen JR: Changes in root length from early to mid-adulthood: resorption or apposition? *Am J Orthod Dentofacial Orthop* 115:563-568, 1999.

78. Parker RJ, Harris EF: Directions of orthodontic tooth movement associated with external apical root resorption of the maxillary central incisor, *Am J Orthod Dentofacial Orthop* 114(6):667-683, 1998.

79. Baumrind S, Korn E, Boyd RL: *Apical root resorption in orthodontically treated adolescents,* San Francisco, 1998, University of the Pacific, in preparation.

80. Harris EF, Kineret SE, Tolley EA: A heritable component for external apical root resorption in patients treated orthodontically, *Am J Orthod Dentofacial Orthop* 111:301-309, 1997.

81. Rosenberg HN: An evaluation of the incidence and amount of apical root resorption and dilaceration occurring in orthodontically treated teeth, having incompletely formed roots at the beginning of Begg treatment, *Am J Orthod* 61:524-525, 1972.

82. Kjaer I: Morphological characteristics of dentitions developing excessive root resorption during orthodontic treatment, *Eur J Orthod* 17:25-34, 1995.

83. Phillips JR: Apical root resorption under orthodontic therapy, *Angle Orthod* 25:1-22, 1955.

84. Becks H: Root resorption and their relation to pathologic bone formation, *Int J Orthod* 22:445-482, 1936.

85. Newman WG: Possible etiologic factors in external root resorption, *Am J Orthod* 67:522-539, 1975.

86. Odernick L: Nailbiting: frequency and association with root resorption, *Br J Orthod* 12:78-81, 1985.

87. Linge L, Linge BO: Patient characteristics and treatment variables associated with apical root resorption during orthodontic treatment, *Am J Orthod Dentofacial Orthop* 99:35-43, 1991.

88. Rudolph CE: An evaluation of root resorption occurring during orthodontic treatment, *J Dent Res* 19:367-371, 1940.

89. Jacobson O: Clinical significance of root resorption, *Am J Orthod* 38:687-696, 1952.

90. Lee RY, Artun J, Alonzo TA: Are dental anomalies risk factors for apical root resorption in orthodontic patients? *Am J Orthod Dentofacial Orthop* 116:187-195, 1999.

91. Andreasen FM et al: Radiographic assessment of simulated root resorption cavities, *Endod Dent Traumatol* 3:21-27, 1987.

92. Fenn K, Boero R, Boyd R: The effect of fixed orthodontic treatment on developing maxillary incisor root apices, master's thesis, San Francisco, 1997, University of the Pacific.

93. Wickwire NA et al: The effects of tooth movement upon endodontically treated teeth, *Angle Orthod* 44:235-242, 1974.

94. Kameyama Y et al: Inhibitory effect of aspirin on root resorption induced by mechanical injury of the soft periodontal tissue in rats, *J Period Res* 29:113-117, 1994.

95. Moorees CFA, Fanning EA, Hunt EE Jr: Age variation of formation stages for ten permanent teeth, *J Dent Res* 6:1490-1504, 1963.

96. Loberg EL, Engstrom C: Thyroid administration to reduce root resorption, *Angle Orthod* 64:595-599, 1994.

97. Christiansen RL: Commentary: thyroxine administration and its effects on root resorption, *Angle Orthod* 64:399-400, 1994.

98. Ramamurthy NS et al: In vivo and in vitro inhibition of matrix metalloproteinases including MMP-13 by several chemically modified tetracyclines (CMTs). In Davidovitch Z, Mah J (eds): *Biological mechanisms of tooth eruption, resorption and replacement by implants,* Boston, 1998, Harvard Society for the Advancement of Orthodontics.

99. Srinivasan R, Evans C, George A: Detection of dentin matrix protein and dentin phosphophoryn in gingival crevicular fluid, *J Dent Res* 77:1026, 1998 (abstract).

100. Bednar JR, Wise RJ: A practical clinical approach to the treatment and management of patients experiencing root resorption during and after orthodontic therapy. In Davidovitch Z, Mah J (eds): *Biological mechanisms of tooth eruption, resorption and replacement by implants,* Boston, 1998, Harvard Society for the Advancement of Orthodontics.

101. Grageda E et al: Gene expression induced by orthodontic forces and root resorption, *J Dent Res* 78:202, 1999 (abstract).

SECTION VI

ORTHODONTICS
AND ADJUNCT TREATMENT

CHAPTER 27

Orthodontics and Craniomandibular Disorders

Athanasios E. Athanasiou

KEY TERMS

craniomandibular disorders	occlusal acrylic splint	medications	orthodontic treatment
occlusion	physical therapy	malocclusions	

CRANIOMANDIBULAR DISORDERS

Craniomandibular disorders (CMDs) is a collective term embracing a number of clinical problems that involve the masticatory musculature, the temporomandibular joint (TMJ), or both. The term is synonymous with the term *temporomandibular disorders (TMDs)*.[1] Although traditionally viewed as one syndrome, current research supports the view that CMDs are a cluster of related disorders in the masticatory system that have many features in common.[2]

CMD can be associated with headaches, muscle hypertrophy without pain, abnormal occlusal wear, and osseous alterations of the TMJ. CMDs may also be related to stressful habits, emotional disorders, structural malrelationships, trauma to the face or head, occlusal disharmonies, and other medical problems. The most common clinical markers of CMDs in the general population are a limited range of mandibular motion, muscle and TMJ tenderness, and TMJ sounds.[3]

Despite the many textbooks, published articles, and continuing education activities concerning this topic, there continues to be a vast chasm between different dental professionals and groups who deal specifically with CMDs. These differences encompass everything from thoughts on etiology to treatment procedures.[4] A clear understanding of all facets of CMDs is currently lacking. However, this may be explained by the voluminous mass of literature on the subject. A National Library of Medicine literature search on CMDs uncovered 917 citations between January, 1990, and December, 1995.[5]

Prevalence and Frequency

The prevalence of CMDs may reach considerable numbers if nonspecific symptoms and moderate clinical signs are included. The frequency of severe disorders that are accompanied by headache and facial pain and that are characterized by urgent need of treatment is 1% to 2% in children, about 5% in adolescents, and 5% to 12% in adults. TMJ sounds are the most common clinical sign. However, because of its poor reliability and reproducibility, this clinical sign does not by itself indicate a necessity for treatment.[6]

Studies of the prevalence of the signs and symptoms of CMDs have found that mild problems are equally distributed among men and women of the general population. Severe problems are much more common among women in clinical populations, and more women than men seek care for CMDs by about 8:1.[7]

Independent studies of patients who requested care for CMDs at Scandinavian institutions concluded that there was a common peak in the age distribution of the patients, specifically during the period between 20 and 40 years (Figure 27-1).[8] Possible explanations for this

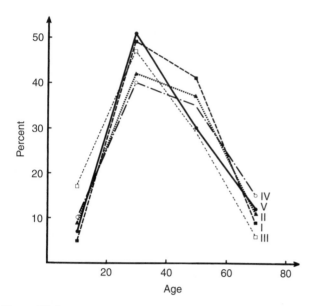

Figure 27-1 Age distribution of five samples of patients with temporomandibular joint dysfunction. *I*, Umea;[1] *II*, Goteborg;[2] *III*, Oslo;[3] *IV*, Malmo;[4] *V*, Goteborg.[5]

1. Agerberg G et al: Dysfunction of masticatory apparatus: a bite physiological, roentgenological and serological study, *Sver Tandlakarforb Tidn* 62:1192-1211, 1970.
2. Carlsson GE, Svardstrom G: A survey of the symptomatology of a series of 299 patients with stomathognatic dysfunction, *Sven Tandlak Tidskr* 64:889-899, 1971.
3. Heloe B, Heloe LA: Characteristics of a group of patients with temporomandibular joint disorders, *Community Dent Oral Epidemiol* 3:72-79, 1975.
4. Rosell CG, Oberg T: Referral: "Temporomandibular joint troubles": study of patients from a central polyclinic, *Tandlakartidningen* 67:941-950, 1975.
5. Carlsson GE, Magnusson T, Wedel A: Patient records at a department for occlusal physiology: an analysis of cause for referral, symptoms and treatment of 1,213 patients, *Sven Tandlak Tidskr* 69:115-121, 1976.

finding may relate to the emotional aspects and stressful lifestyles that characterize this age period.

There have been several studies on the prevalence of signs and symptoms of CMDs in different countries or ethnic groups, indicating a lack of great deviations in the findings. Ethnic origin should be no reason for expecting significant differences in the prevalence of CMDs between populations in the industrialized world where lifestyles, nutrition, and health delivery systems do not differ significantly.

Classification

Classification systems have been based on signs and symptoms, tissues of origin, etiology, structural and functional disorders, frequency, and medical classification. Currently there is a notable lack of consensus with regard to a classification of CMDs. Moreover, such a classification is unlikely to be uniformly accepted.[9] CMDs represent a broad range of conditions that involves medical, dental, and psychologic factors. From a clinical perspective, CMDs can be divided into five

main categories: (1) masticatory muscle disorders, (2) disk-interference disorders, (3) inflammatory disorders of the joint, (4) chronic mandibular hypomobilities, and (5) growth disorders of the joint.[2]

Etiology

CMDs do not constitute one particular and single abnormal condition, although the term embraces a number of clinical problems that involve the masticatory musculature, the TMJs, or both. Current research supports the view that CMDs are a cluster of related disorders in the stomatognathic system that has many features in common. In this sense, the cause of a CMD should be considered multifactorial.

CMDs may be associated with stressful activities, emotional diseases, structural malrelationships, trauma to the craniofacial region, malocclusion, and medical problems related to various types of arthritis or viral diseases.

Role of Occlusion

The role that **occlusion** plays in the development of CMDs is controversial. Today its role is widely considered as contributory by initiating, perpetuating or predisposing to CMDs.[1]

Initiating factors lead to the onset of the symptoms and are related primarily to trauma or adverse loading of the masticatory system.

In the perpetuating factors the following subcategories may be included:
1. Behavioral factors (grinding, clenching, abnormal oral behavior, and abnormal jaw and head posture)
2. Social factors (could affect perception and influence learned response to pain)
3. Emotional factors (characterized by prolonged, negative feelings such as depression and anxiety)
4. Cognitive factors (thoughts or attitudes that, when negative, can make resolution of the illness more difficult)

Predisposing factors are pathophysiologic, psychologic, or structural processes that alter the masticatory system sufficiently to increase the risk of CMD development.

The stomatognathic system, like any other part of the body, undergoes continuous structural and functional influences and changes that can be of importance to the physiology of all tissues involved. A dynamic model on the cause of CMDs presented by Parker[10] describes how a continuous interplay exists between factors that tend to increase the adaptability of the stomatognathic system or to produce hyperfunction (Figure 27-2). Morphologic, functional, and behavioral alterations, which influence factors such as general health, nutrition, stress, posture, and occlusion and induce physical trauma, can produce changes in the status of

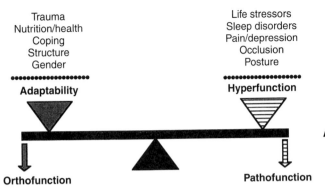

Figure 27-2 Model showing a balance in the stomatognathic system between destructive overloading that leads to craniomandibular disorders and homeostatic adaptability that promotes normal function. The model includes five factors that prescribe the potential for the system to adapt homeostatically and five factors that predispose to destructive hyperfunction. The five factors on each side of the model interrelate to determine whether the balance tilts toward dysfunction or normal function of the stomatognathic system. (Redrawn from Parker MW: *J Am Dent Assoc* 120:283-290, 1990.)

the stomatognathic system in either an orthofunctional or a pathofunctional direction.

Evaluation

The American Academy of Craniomandibular Disorders has published consensus-based guidelines that outline principles for CMD diagnosis and evaluation.[1] Of particular importance is the classification containing diagnostic criteria consistent with the International Headache Society's Classification of headache disorders, cranial neuralgias, and facial pain.[11]

The aim in evaluating CMDs is to determine the chief complaint, the diagnosis, the contributing factors, and the level of complexity.[1] All major textbooks dealing with the subject of CMDs extensively and systematically describe the screening evaluation, comprehensive history, comprehensive physical examination, behavioral and psychosocial assessment, and additional clinical or laboratory tests. Application of a well-organized, comprehensive, and systematic approach is absolutely mandatory for developing a problem list, differential diagnosis, treatment planning, management, and assessment of treatment.

With regard to the history, special attention should be given to inflammatory bone diseases, muscle disorders, face and head trauma, and chronic facial pain. The clinical examination must address the issues of pain, limitations, noises, and deviations in detail. The clinical examination should minimally include evaluation of mandibular mobility, impaired function of the TMJs, detection for masticatory and neck muscle pain, and TMJ pain as well as assessment of head and body posture.

The only available and logical gold standard that can presently be used to identify the presence or absence of

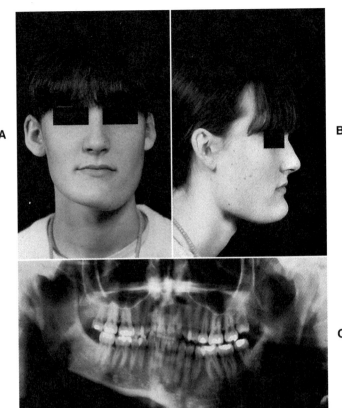

Figure 27-3 A 20-year-old female with severe facial asymmetry (**A** and **B**) resulting from a hyperplastic left condyle as it appears in a linear sagittal tomogram (**C**). The right condyle is normal.

CMDs is the evaluation of the patient's chief complaint, history, clinical examination, and, when indicated, radiographs. Thorough TMD and medical histories and head and neck clinical examinations are the first and, in most of the cases, only procedures that provide sufficient diagnostic information.[12]

Methodologic and clinical studies indicate that TMJ radiology and imaging should be used only when the patient presents with developmental facial asymmetries, continuously changing intermaxillary relationships, no response to conservative treatment, history of trauma, crepitation of the TMJ, and history of rheumatic disease (Figures 27-3 to 27-7).[13,14] A thorough knowledge of the diagnostic possibilities and limitations of the various radiographic techniques must always precede a decision for referring the patient for such an examination. Accumulation of unnecessary diagnostic data, overinterpretation of abnormal findings, excessive exposure to radiation, increased cost of treatment, and wrong diagnosis may be, otherwise, some of the resulting consequences of the routine application of imaging techniques of TMJ.[15] Simply said, clinicians should not refer a patient to the radiologist without first having formulated a diagnostic hypothesis and

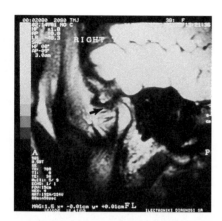

Figure 27-4 Magnetic resonance imaging (MRI) of the right temporomandibular joint (TMJ) of a 38-year-old female taken in maximal opening that confirms the presence of an anteriorly displaced and deformed disk without reduction *(arrow)*. The patient suffers from a systemic collagen disorder, regularly takes corticosteroids, and has undergone splint and physical therapy for 6 months before the MRI was taken. The therapy resulted in an increase of maximal interincisal opening from 22 to 34 mm and the disappearance of TMJ and muscle pain. However, the patient is unable to perform protrusive and laterotrusive mandibular movements. (From Athanasiou AE: *Prakt Kieferorthop* 7:269-286, 1993.)

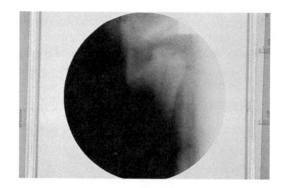

Figure 27-6 Degeneration on the right mandibular condyle is clearly visible in this linear sagittal tomogram of an adult male patient presenting with temporomandibular joint crepitus. (From Athanasiou AE: *Prakt Kieferorthop* 7:269-286, 1993.)

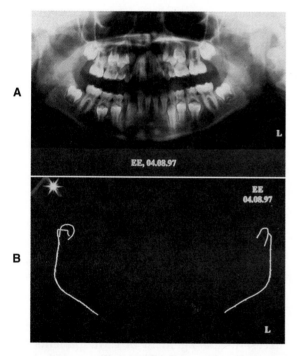

Figure 27-5 Panoramic radiograph of an 8-year-old girl **(A)** and tracing of the left and right condyles and rami **(B)**. The radiograph was taken and correlated with a history of recent face trauma that was reported during the visit of the patient at the orthodontic office. Condyle fractures are noted in both sides.

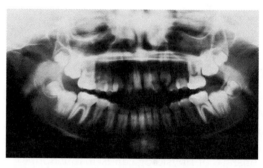

Figure 27-7 The panoramic radiograph of an 11-year-old boy with a history of juvenile rheumatoid arthritis indicates the presence of severe resorption of both condyles. (From Athanasiou AE: *Prakt Kieferorthop* 7:269-286, 1993.)

evaluated. Moreover, in most joints with internal derangements, the findings of conventional radiography are either noncontributory or nonspecific. On the other hand, plain films are an inexpensive method for nondetailed screening of degenerative alterations, traumatic abnormalities, or developmental deformities.

Computed tomography (CT) scanning is an excellent imaging modality and provides images with good bony details. CT scanning is of particular value in evaluating trauma and developmental abnormalities of the craniofacial region using three-dimensional technology. Unfortunately, CT scanning is inappropriate for imaging the soft tissues of the TMJ.

Both arthrography and magnetic resonance imaging (MRI) are of proven value in evaluating internal derangements of the TMJ. Arthrography has the advantages of providing a dynamic display of TMJ mechanisms and easy detection of disk perforation. However, its technical difficulties, invasive nature, and poor visualization of the disk in the mediolateral direction limit this method. An MRI of the TMJ provides excel-

knowing what they are looking for. The ideal imaging technique for the diagnosis of TMDs should provide information about the osseous structures, the articular disk, and the joint dynamics.

Conventional radiography is of limited value because only the osseous components of the TMJ can be lent soft tissue detail and demonstrates mediolateral disk displacements more readily than arthrography. MRI also enables both TMJs to be examined at the same time using dual superficial coil technology. MRI does not, however, usually reveal perforations of the disk or the ligaments, and the bony anatomy is not shown as clearly as on plain radiography or on a CT scan. In addition, real-time dynamic imaging of joint mechanics is impossible with MRI.

At present, the choice of TMJ imaging is based on the presence of a clearly understood diagnostic objective and the availability of arthrography and MRI.[16]

Caution should be exercised in using electronic devices for the interpretation of the recorded mandibular movements and TMJ sounds. Several of these instruments have not been adequately tested concerning their sensitivity, specificity, reliability, and validity. Furthermore, none of these magnetic jaw-tracking devices can produce a discrete clinical diagnosis of CMDs in the absence of a thorough history and physical examination.[17,18]

Management

Management of CMDs should primarily aim at eliminating or significantly reducing pain to improve mandibular motion and to address any other serious symptoms by establishing normal condyle-disk-fossa relationships or physiologic muscle function.

Some problems of internal TMJ derangements (e.g., disk displacement with reduction of mild character; disk displacement without reduction during the acute phase; and myofacial pain that is associated with parafunction or muscle hypertonicity or that is secondary to trauma) usually can be successfully managed by means of flat or repositioning occlusal acrylic splints (Figures 27-8 and 27-9).

However, it should be kept in mind that for controlling the pain of CMDs, multiple strategies may also be needed in addition to the use of splints. Such strategies may include biofeedback training; application of physical therapy; and exercises for restoring function, strengthening the muscles, or stopping stressful and traumatic habits. Occasionally, medication should be used. Of CMD patients with TMJ internal derangements or osseous degeneration, 3% to 5% may require surgery that can repair, remove, reconstruct, or reconfigure the joint.

The choice of one or more of the above-mentioned nonsurgical methods of management of CMDs may depend on the information collected by the clinical examination, the history of the case, and the findings of x-rays or imaging examinations, if any. A significant number of CMD symptoms are expressed as mainly muscular. In addition to the dental specialties, medical specialties may often significantly contribute to

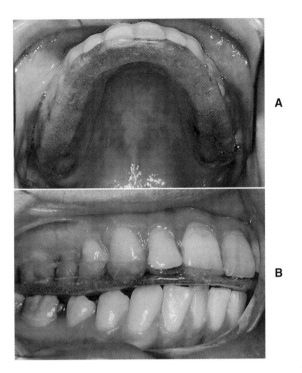

Figure 27-8 Full-coverage, flat, occlusal maxillary splint. **A,** Occlusal view. **B,** Lateral view. (From Athanasiou AE: *Prakt Kieferorthop* 7:269-286, 1993.)

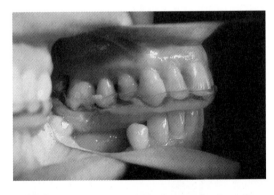

Figure 27-9 Full-coverage, repositioning, occlusal maxillary splint. (From Athanasiou AE: *Prakt Kieferorthop* 7:269-286, 1993.)

the successful management of CMD patients (i.e., Neurology; Ear, Nose, and Throat; Physical Medicine; Psychiatry; Rheumatology; and Ophthalmology). Chronic pain syndromes are also recognized to affect patients with orofacial pain, leading to the development of interdisciplinary teams for chronic orofacial pain management.[3]

With regard to the use of an **occlusal acrylic splint,** it is expected that by using it, disarticulation of the occlusion may take place, thereby eliminating existing occlusal interferences with implications on maxillomandibular relation, muscle function, and TMJ internal arrangements. There are also many opinions on how a

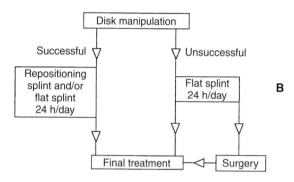

A

B

Figure 27-10 Charts of action in cases of temporomandibular joint internal derangements characterized by disk displacement with reduction (**A**) and displacement without reduction (**B**) during the acute phase. (From Athanasiou AE: *Prakt Kieferorthop* 7:269-286, 1993.)

splint works by including claims for changes in the position of tongue and other soft tissues as well as the placebo effect. The major theories covering the mechanism of action of splints include those of occlusal disengagement, alteration of vertical dimension, maxillomandibular realignment, TMJ repositioning, and cognitive awareness.[19]

No "cookbook" approach is available to using occlusal splints. The personal opinion of this author concerning the types and ways of the splints normally used in patients with a CMD has been described elsewhere and, in brief, follows.[13]

The acrylic splints are flat, full-coverage splints that are made in a way that allow the patients to move in all directions without any particular guidance (see Figure 27-8). There are some exceptions to this rule. For example, some patients present with signs of the acute phase of anterior disk displacement without reduction. In these cases a repositioning splint may be used at the beginning of the management (see Figure 27-9 and 27-10).

Depending on each patient's occlusal characteristics, maxillary or mandibular splints may be selected based on practicality, better function, stability, and esthetics. Maxillary splints are used more often. However, in cases of severe and extensive buccal crossbites, the use of a mandibular splint may be preferred to provide better stability (Figure 27-11). Some partially edentulous patients may have a dental arch with enough teeth and so will be selected because the arch can accommodate the splint.

With regard to the opening of the bite produced by the splint, there are many different opinions and of course it depends on the individual case. There are cases of excessive overclosure caused by the lack of adequate posterior occlusal support where increase of the vertical dimension even with a violation of the existing freeway space may be indicated. There are other cases in which the increase of vertical dimension by means of a splint should aim to restore proper internal TMJ function by reestablishing normal condyle-disk-fossa relationships. In such cases sometimes the amount of

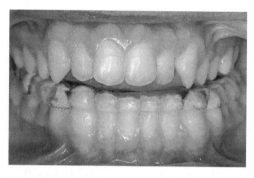

Figure 27-11 Full-coverage, flat, occlusal mandibular splint. (From Athanasiou AE: *Prakt Kieferorthop* 7:269-286, 1993.)

vertical increase can be problematic from the muscle point of view.

Splints are not required to be used on a full-time basis when the problems are masticatory muscle hyperactivity and dysfunction. However, in cases where signs and symptoms of TMJ internal derangements are dominant, it is recommended that the splints be used on a full-time basis, except for when the patient is brushing his or her teeth.

All patients undergoing CMD management by means of splints must be informed of the changes in occlusion that may occur and of the possibility of a second phase of treatment to reestablish optimum occlusion to the new maxillomandibular relationship, if any.

Hawley bite planes have been shown recently to be effective in decreasing ipsilateral masseter and anterior temporal muscle activities at rest and in maximum closure.[20]

Physical therapy and exercises are important supplements to splint therapy, or they can be applied independently. They can be used to restore function, strengthen weak muscles, instruct the patient how to alter oral habits, and reduce stress and anxiety. With regard to the application of physical therapy and muscle exercises, the patient may be referred to a physical therapist who can be fully responsible for this management, especially when, in some of these cases, strengthening of the muscles should not be limited to those of the stomatognathic region. However, equipment and instruments are available that can be used in the dental office environment during the time the patient is in the office or on a regular basis at home.[21]

Examples of these types of exercises include opening and closing, protrusion, and laterotrusive movements. In several of these patients with anterior disk displacement without reduction in whom it has been decided that the prognosis for recapturing the disk is low, priority may be given to how much, gradually, the patient can open the mouth. This goal can be accomplished by performing regular physical exercises toward this direction.[22]

Symptoms of CMDs and especially orofacial pain can be managed with **medications.** However, such a management is an important adjunct to other treatment modalities. As with all therapies, establishment of a proper diagnosis is crucial to determine the appropriate medication. Several categories of medications may be prescribed for patients with CMDs including antiinflammatory agents, muscle relaxants, antianxiety agents, antihistamines, opiate-narcotic analgesics, local anesthetics, and antidepressants. For example, when the use of medication is crucial, the use of antiinflammatory agents in patients with polyarthritis should be discussed.[23]

Conservative management of CMD problems in a clinic or private practice environment is reported to be the most logical approach. The same holds true for orthodontic practices.[24]

CMD AND OCCLUSION

In the present context, Amsterdam defined two types of occlusion. The physiologic occlusion is one that adapts to the stress of function and can be maintained indefinitely. The pathologic occlusion cannot function without contributing to its own destruction.[25]

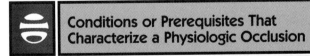

Conditions or Prerequisites That Characterize a Physiologic Occlusion

- The physiologic occlusion could be a malocclusion that is in a state of health.
- The physiologic occlusion has adapted well to its environment.
- The physiologic occlusion has no pathologic manifestations or dysfunctional problems.
- The physiologic occlusion is in a state of harmony and requires no therapy.

The relation between the functioning dentition and the TMJs has been addressed extensively during the last 100 years. An informative literature review has been presented recently by Perry.[26]

A significant debate concerning etiologic factors of CMDs involves the contribution of various **malocclusions** or occlusal factors. In most instances the methodological weaknesses of the studies, which aimed to correlate occlusal factors with CMD (i.e., lack of reliable measures or heterogeneous samples), have made the results inconclusive. Of course, sometimes occlusal abnormalities can be considered as predisposing or initiating factors to the occurrence of CMDs.

Signs of dysfunction may be the result of how the individual uses the occlusion and not a result of its structural features.[27] Thus the term *nonphysiologic occlusion* does not imply a cause and effect relationship.

For example, in subjects with increased overbite, minimal overjet, and palatal inclination of maxillary incisors, a precise mandibular muscular guidance in the closing phase of mastication is necessary to avoid incisal interferences. Such a response may be associated with strong action of the posterior temporal muscles by an increased overlap between the elevators and the lateral pterygoid and digastric muscles in the shift from opening to closing and vice versa (Figure 27-12).[28]

Although the role of occlusion in CMDs is muddled in disagreement, its potential effects on the biomechanics of the craniofacial complex cannot be ignored. McNeill et al[29] theorized that a broader array of biomechanical factors contributes to the development of CMDs rather than occlusal factors alone.

Pullinger, Seligman, and Gornbein[30] applied multiple factor analysis, which indicated the low correlation of occlusion to TMDs. However, the following occlusal factors did have a slight relation:
1. Apertognathia (open bite)
2. Overjets greater than 6 to 7 mm
3. Retruded contact position/intercuspal position with slides greater than 4 mm
4. Unilateral lingual crossbite
5. Five or more missing posterior teeth

With regard to the distribution of occlusal contacts, symmetry of their intensity (stress) rather than symmetry of their number in the posterior occlusion, per se, seemed to be important in relation to temporomandibular function.[31] Increased number and more frequent headaches in individuals with few occlusal contacts have also been noted.[32]

Pullinger and Seligman[33] estimate that occlusal factors contribute about 10% to 20% to the total spectrum of multifactorial factors, which differentiates between healthy persons and patients with TMDs.

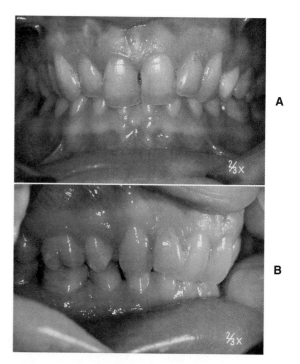

Figure 27-13 Frontal view (**A**) and right lateral view (**B**) of inappropriate posttreatment occlusal relationships in a 21-year-old female presenting with occlusal trauma, severe signs of temporomandibular joint internal derangements, and muscle hyperactivity. The patient had received orthodontic treatment by means of removable appliances and extractions of the four first premolars at an earlier age. In this case litigation process against the general practitioner was initiated by the patient who claimed that the signs of temporomandibular disease were related to the previous orthodontic treatment and led to the conviction of the dentist. (From Athanasiou AE: *Prakt Kieferorthop* 7:269-286, 1993.)

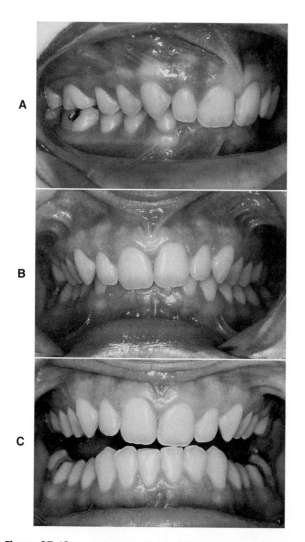

Figure 27-12 A and **B,** Malocclusion characterized by increased overbite, minimal overjet, and palatal inclination of maxillary incisors in a young adult female suffering from masticatory myalgia. **C,** This condition can be related to excessive muscle action necessary to produce mandibular muscular guidance and to avoid incisal interferences. (From Athanasiou AE: *Prakt Kieferorthop* 7:269-286, 1993.)

CMD AND ORTHODONTIC TREATMENT

Orthodontists have traditionally tried to improve esthetics and oral health, as well as the stability and function of the treated dentition. Brodie, Thompson, and Ricketts have been considered as the leaders in the American orthodontic community in emphasizing the interrelationship between occlusion and TMJ.[26]

In a malpractice trial in the United States, an orthodontist was found liable for a patient's suffering from CMD symptoms. This case provoked a response by the American Association of Orthodontists in supporting research related to orthodontic treatment and its effect on the TMJs. The results of numerous studies discounted orthodontic treatment as an etiologic factor and provided some noteworthy caveats for the orthodontic practitioner.

The overwhelming evidence supports the conclusion that orthodontic treatment performed on children and adolescents is generally not a risk for the development of CMDs at a later age.[34] Two main explanations have been advocated: (1) the multiplicity of factors that may be responsible for producing or exacerbating a CMD and (2) orthodontic mechanotherapy that produces gradual changes in an environment that is generally adaptive.

On the other hand, if orthodontic therapy or any other dental treatment compromises the ability of the stomatognathic system to adapt, it may well predispose to CMDs or it may perpetuate an existing dysfunction. Inappropriate posttreatment occlusal relationships that cause trauma, severe mandibular displacement, or muscle hyperactivity can be examples of iatrogenic origin related to the occurrence of CMDs (Figure 27-13). Significant orthodontic relapse that creates a functional imbalance between the TMJs, muscles, and occlusion, may

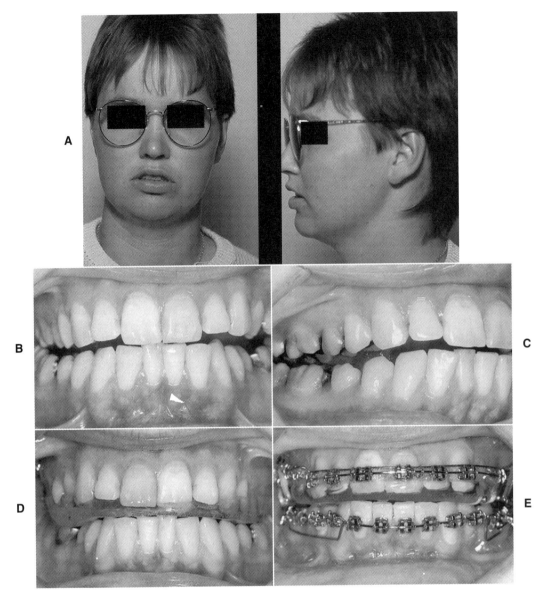

Figure 27-14 Frontal and profile photographs **(A),** frontal view **(B),** and right lateral view **(C)** of the occlusal relationships in a 25-year-old female patient. The patient used a full-coverage, flat, occlusal maxillary splint 24 hr/day **(D),** became symptom free, and was referred by a craniomandibular disorder clinic for orthodontic treatment to achieve final occlusal stabilization. Review of the history and the previous treatments of this patient revealed a diagnosis of anterior disk displacement with reduction of the right temporomandibular joint, unsuccessful splint therapy, unsuccessful surgical repositioning of the disk, surgical removal of the disk, and subsequent use of another splint to achieve occlusal stability and joint unloading. The patient was treated by means of fixed orthodontic appliances and with the splint in place **(E)** until stable interocclusal relationships were established **(F).** Optimum occlusal relationships were achieved posttreatment as they appear in the frontal view **(G)** and right lateral view **(H). I,** Overall superimposition of the cephalometric tracings indicates minor tooth movements in the sagittal plane. However, significant anterior rotation of the mandible, which occurred and contributed to bite closure, can be attributed mainly to the correction of the transverse occlusal malrelationships in the molar regions. (From Athanasiou AE: *Prakt Kieferorthop* 7:269-286, 1993.)

also contribute to the occurrence of signs and symptoms of CMDs in some patients. However, a clear distinction must be made between individual CMD cases caused by orthodontic misdiagnosis or treatment failure and unjustified attempts to systematically associate any orthodontic treatment with the cause of a CMD.

Furthermore, no scientific proof indicates that any particular method of orthodontic treatment, whether it involves extractions or not, has any causative effect on CMDs. On the contrary, studies have shown that individuals who had undergone orthodontic treatment during childhood had a significantly lower clin-

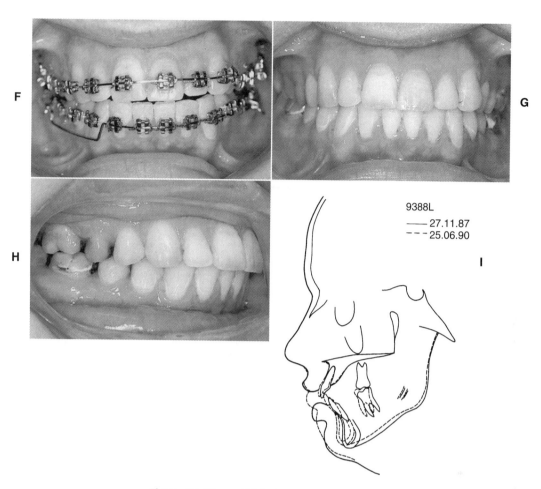

Figure 27-14, cont'd For legend see opposite page.

ical dysfunction index during adulthood than those who had not received orthodontic therapy.[34] Also there are many patients with CMDs who have been successfully managed and then had orthodontic treatment instituted to provide the final occlusal stabilization (Figure 27-14).

MANAGEMENT OF CMDs IN THE ORTHODONTIC CLINIC

More patients with CMDs are being seen in orthodontic offices. There may be several explanations for such a phenomenon. For example, **orthodontic treatment** is now routinely available to adults whose CMD prevalence is higher than that of children. Also, adjunctive orthodontic treatment is often used to facilitate other dental procedures necessary to control disease and restore function. Furthermore, orthodontists are able to better detect, diagnose, and manage CMDs as a result of better undergraduate and postgraduate training and continuing education programs.

Like any other health problem, CMDs can be present during the initial examination of the orthodontic patient, or they can occur during treatment, posttreatment, or postretention periods.

Before Orthodontic Treatment[13,35]

All patients, independent of their type of malocclusion and the reasons for seeking orthodontic treatment, must get the same attention during initial screening before the initiation of therapy. As mentioned before, this must include a thorough temporomandibular examination, medical history, and head and neck clinical examination. With regard to the history, special attention should be given to inflammatory bone or muscle disorders (e.g., rheumatoid arthritis), craniofacial trauma, and chronic facial pain (Figure 27-15).

If there is no evidence of CMDs, the orthodontist should proceed with the orthodontic treatment as planned. If there is evidence of CMDs, a differential diagnosis must be attempted and the severity of the disorder should be assessed. The first thing that should be

Examination Protocol

Patient's Name _____   Dr. _____

Address _____   Address _____

_____

Occupation: _____

Examination date: _____

Chief complaint: _____

_____

_____

CM–history

A

		yes
Pain:	face	☐
	head	☐
	ear	☐
	eye	☐
	neck	☐
	regular headache	☐
TMJ sounds:	clicking	☐
	other noises	☐
Disturbances of mandibular functions:	difficulties in opening, closing, chewing, muscular tiredness, stiffness of the jaw	☐
Oral habits	nail-lip biting, smoking etc.	☐
Previous extensive dental treatments:	prosthodontics	☐
	orthodontics	☐
	surgery	☐
	equilibration	☐

Are you comfortable with the way your teeth fit together?   yes ☐   no ☐

Medical history

Do you have or did you have a history of ?

	yes
infection (hepatitis)	☐
heart and cardiovascular diseases	☐
blood diseases	☐
respiratory tract diseases	☐
digestive tract diseases	☐
urinary and genital diseases	☐
neurological diseases	☐
metabolism	☐
allergies	☐
rheumatoid diseases	☐
psychological problems	☐
hormonal problems	☐
pregnancy	☐
trauma	☐
drugs _____	☐
general anaesthesia or surgery	☐

Figure 27-15 A standard history form **(A)** and a form to record clinical findings **(B)** are used in the examination of patients with craniomandibular disease. The forms were produced in 1985 by the European Academy of Craniomandibular Disorders. (From Athanasiou AE: *Prakt Kieferorthop* 7:269-286, 1993.)

Clinical Findings

Range of motion * opening (with overbite) [ ] mm   Deviation on movement R [ ] L [ ]

Laterotrusion to the right [ ]   Laterotrusion to the left [ ]

Protrusion [ ]

Auscultation TMJ clicking R [ ] L [ ]   TMJ crepitation R [ ] L [ ]

Tenderness to palpation

	R	L		R	L
TMJ laterally during movements	[ ]	[ ]	Temporalis M. insertion	[ ]	[ ]
Temporalis M.	[ ]	[ ]	Pterygoid M. complex	[ ]	[ ]
Masseter M.	[ ]	[ ]	Tongue	[ ]	[ ]

Provocation test positive [ ]   negative [ ]

Inspection Excessive facial asymmetries [ ]

Dentition Shiny facets [ ] —————   fractures [ ] —————

Manipulation of the mandible in CR (RP)
easy [ ]   difficult [ ]   impossible [ ]

Slide CR — CO (RCP — ICP)
sagittal [ ] mm   lateral [ ] mm   vertical [ ] mm

Contacts on movements
to the left   to the right   in protrusion

Conclusion Can you explain the chief complaint of the patient by your findings?   yes [ ]   no [ ]

Diagnosis (provisional) _____

Important If you cannot explain the chief complaint do not start to treat !
Refer your patient to a specialist !

X—rays are always to be taken when you suspect

- growing facial asymmetries
- continuously changing intermaxillary relationship
- no response to the treatment
- history of trauma
- crepitation of the joint

If you cannot interpret a X—ray do not take it !
Refer your patient to a X—ray specialist with your specific questions.

---

* Please fill the appropriate box with the amount of movement in mm. In the right hand diagramm draw deflections or deviations from the midline during the opening and/or closing movements as well as the position where TMJ sounds occur.

B

Figure 27-15, cont'd For legend see opposite page.

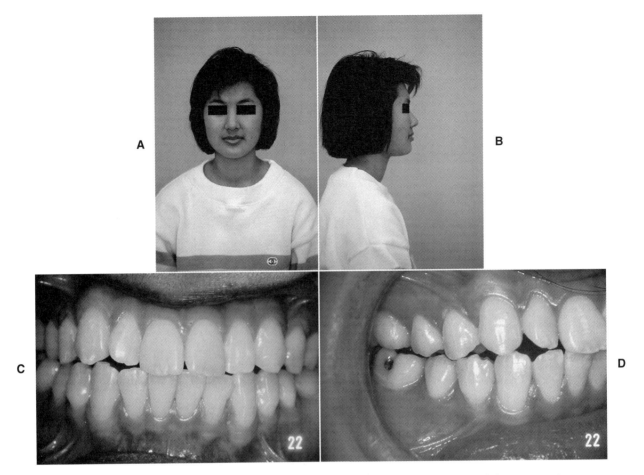

Figure 27-16 Frontal (**A**) and profile (**B**) photographs and frontal view (**C**) and right lateral view (**D**) of occlusal relationships of a 14-year old female patient. The patient presented with severe signs of anterior disk displacement with reduction. A partial-coverage, flat, occlusal mandibular splint was used during the first phase of treatment. After 4 months of splint therapy the patient became symptom free. Because the patient was unable to function in the maximum intercuspal position without reoccurrence of the symptoms, it was decided to proceed with orthodontic treatment to achieve final occlusal stabilization. Following articulator mounting, without and with the splint

done is to inform the patient accordingly and to document the findings in the patient's file. Then, depending on the preliminary diagnosis, it may be decided to manage the problem in the orthodontic office or to refer the patient to a colleague who is more specialized and involved in this field.

In general, orthodontic therapy must not be performed on patients presenting with acute and severe signs and symptoms of CMDs until these problems are under control. In cases of minor signs or symptoms (i.e., TMJ clicking with no pain), orthodontic treatment can be recommended and initiated, but the CMD should be observed and monitored.

Following the management of CMDs by means of one or a combination of the various therapeutic modalities discussed previously, orthodontic treatment should proceed only if the patient is free of pain, can function adequately, and has a stable mandibular position for at least 3 to 6 months. In ad-

dition, the patient should continue to be regularly observed by the clinician who initially treated the CMD.

Not every patient who undergoes CMD therapy requires orthodontic treatment for functional/occlusal reasons. There are cases when, following CMD therapy, the patient can have acceptable stomatognathic function utilizing the existing occlusal relationships without any orthodontic intervention. However, there are patients who present with minimal or no CMD symptoms after the initial splint therapy, but their attempts to discontinue the splint were unsuccessful because of a reoccurrence of discomfort. In these cases, when the patients cannot function in the existing occlusal relationships, occlusal treatment may be necessary to provide stability during function. Minor or major occlusal changes can be achieved by means of equilibration, resin or amalgam dental restorations, prosthodontics, orthodontics, and orthognathic surgery (Figure 27-16).

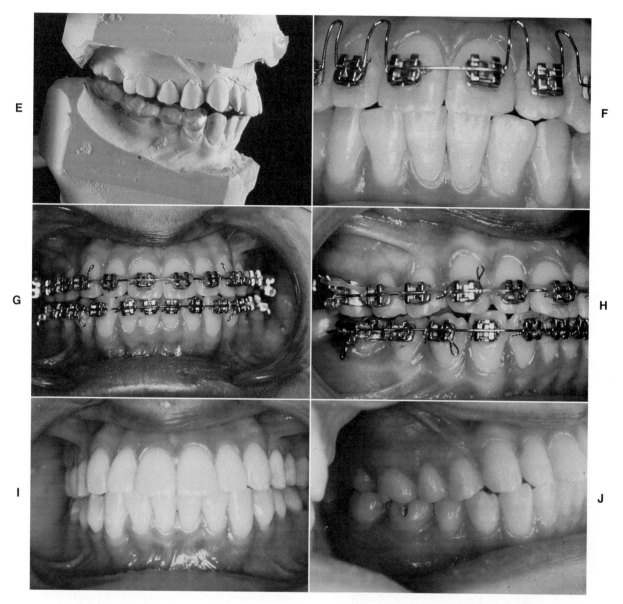

Figure 27-16, cont'd E, A three-dimensional assessment of the occlusal relationships was made, which detected premature interferences in the anterior occlusion. The patient was treated initially by means of fixed orthodontic appliances in the maxillary dental arch and with the splint in place in the mandible **(F)** until a stable interocclusal relationship was established **(G** and **H).** Optimum occlusal relationships were achieved posttreatment as they appear in the frontal view **(I)** and in the right lateral view **(J).**

Of course there may still be other reasons for seeking and performing orthodontic therapy after the initial phase of management of CMD including dental or facial esthetics and in preparation for restorative, prosthodontic, or periodontal dental work.

Following successful management of a CMD, the orthodontist should respect the new functional balance present between the TMJ, the masticatory muscles, and the therapeutic occlusal relationships. Subsequently, proper interocclusal registrations, articulator mounting of the case, and monitoring of all functional aspects are required (Figure 27-17).

During Orthodontic Treatment[13]

Clinical examinations of the function of the stomatognathic system should be done regularly during the entire period of orthodontic treatment. If severe signs and symptoms of a CMD occur during orthodontic therapy, the differential diagnosis will influence the decisions of the orthodontists to postpone treatment, alter occlusion with corrective orthodontic tooth movements, or discontinue treatment.

A differential diagnosis should be made before any decision concerning the continuation of orthodontic

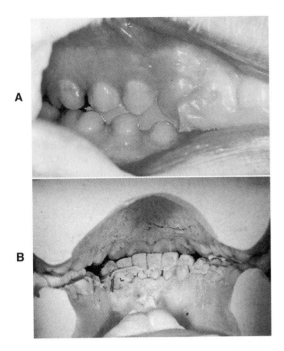

Figure 27-17 A, After the use of a splint, an interocclusal registration by means of Ramitec (Espe) or any other similar material has been made. **B,** Following articulator mounting, a three-dimensional assessment of the occlusal relationships, including evaluation for possible premature interferences, can be performed. (From Athanasiou AE: *Prakt Kieferorthop* 7:269-286, 1993.)

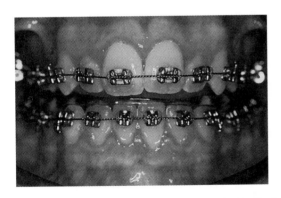

Figure 27-18 Frontal view of the occlusion with fixed orthodontic appliances placed in both dental arches and a full-coverage, flat, occlusal mandibular splint in a 14-year-old female. The patient presented with mild symptoms of craniomandibular disorders during orthodontic treatment. Following the full-time use of the splint for 2 months, the symptoms ceased. Subsequently the splint was discontinued and orthodontic therapy proceeded as it was initially planned.

treatment is made (i.e., cases in which the clinician considers postponing treatment until the CMD is under control). In these cases all CMD management modalities discussed previously need to be applied (Figure 27-18).

CMD symptoms that occur during orthodontic treatment may be associated with occlusal traumatic interferences associated with the movements of the teeth. In

these instances appropriate corrective orthodontic tooth movements may be required. In some cases the use of heavy intermaxillary elastics (Class II or Class III) may have to be discontinued if muscular and TMJ pain have developed following their use.

Orthodontic Posttreatment[13]

The retention procedures recommended for patients who had orthodontic treatment and also presented earlier with a CMD should have a dual purpose. The first purpose is to minimize the orthodontic relapse, and the second purpose is to preserve the existing functional balance between TMJs, the muscles, and the established occlusion. Retention appliances that incorporate a full-coverage acrylic splint for nighttime use may contribute to the reduction of detrimental influences of parafunctional activities on the occlusion, muscles, and TMJs.

Of course the occurrence of dysfunctional signs and symptoms in orthodontic patients posttreatment should be addressed by applying the same comprehensive diagnostic and management procedures as those used in patients with a CMD who did not receive orthodontic therapy.

SUMMARY

The development of CMDs cannot be predicted. Once a CMD is present, cure cannot be assumed or assured. No method of CMD prevention has been demonstrated.

The harmony of the interface between the teeth, muscles, nerves, supporting tissue, and TMJs must be established to provide health, functional efficiency, esthetics, and stability to the entire stomatognathic system.[26] An optimum condyle/disk position during optimum integrated muscle activity with maximal occlusal stability must constitute the functional goal of any orthodontist.[28]

As much as 50% of the population may resort to uncontrolled nocturnal parafunctional activity at one time or another as a stress-strain release mechanism, thus protection of the TMJs is essential. A simple splint worn at night may be all that is necessary. If there is functional impingement on the retrodiskal pad during the day, other measures must be taken by the clinician. Nature has provided an efficient mechanism for the multifunctional stomatognathic system. Understanding the physiologic aspects of this system is a prime requisite.[36]

According to existing literature, the relationship of the TMDs to occlusion and orthodontic treatment is minor. The important question that still remains in dentistry is how this minor contribution can be identified within the population of patients with TMDs.[37]

REFERENCES

1. McNeill C: *Craniomandibular disorders: guidelines for evaluation, diagnosis, and management,* Chicago, 1990, Quintessence.
2. Bell WE: *Temporomandibular disorders: classification, diagnosis, management,* Chicago, 1990, Year Book Medical.
3. Fricton JR: Recent advances in temporomandibular disorders and orofacial pain, *J Am Dent Assoc* 122:25-32, 1991.
4. National Institute of Health Technology Assessment Conference: *Mangement of temporomandibular disorders,* Washington, DC, NIH, April 29-May 1, 1996.
5. National Library of Medicine: *Mangement of temporomandibular disorders: current bibliographies in medicine,* CEM 96-2, Bethesda, Md, 1996, National Institute of Health, US Department of Health and Human Services.
6. Bakke M, Moeller E: Craniomandibular disorders and masticatory muscle function, *Scand J Dent Res* 100:32-38, 1992.
7. Rugh JD, Solberg WK: Oral health status in the United States: temporomandibular disorders, *J Dent Educ* 49:398-405, 1985.
8. Carlsson GE, Magnusson T, Wedel A: Patient records at a department for occlusal physiology: an analysis of cause for referral, symptoms and treatment of 1,213 patients, *Sven Tandlak Tidskr* 69:115-121, 1976.
9. Kaplan AS: Classification. In Kaplan AS, Assael LA (eds): *Temporomandibular disorders: diagnosis and treatment,* Philadelphia, 1991, WB Saunders.
10. Parker MW: A dynamic model of etiology in temporomandibular disorders, *J Am Dent Assoc* 120:283-290, 1990.
11. Okeson J (ed): International headache society classification of headache disorders, cranial neuralgias, and facial pain, *Cephalalgia* 8(suppl 7):1-96, 1988.
12. Greene CS: Can technology enhance TMD diagnosis? *Calif Dent Assoc J* 18:21-24, 1990.
13. Athanasiou AE: TM disorders, orthodontic treatment and orthognathic surgery, *Prakt Kieferorthop* 7:269-286, 1993.
14. Capurso U et al: Stomatognathic function in patients with chronic juvenile rheumatoid arthritis, *Kieferorthopaedie* 11:27-34, 1997.
15. Athanasiou AE: Use and misuse of radiographic imaging techniques in the diagnosis and treatment of temporomandibular joint disorders, *Orthod Rev* 4:24-25, 1990.
16. Elefteriadis JN, Athanasiou AE: Guidelines for temporomandibular joint imaging, *Eur Dent* 4:19-21, 1995.
17. Mohl ND et al: Devices for the diagnosis and treatment of temporomandibular disorders. Part I. Introduction, scientific evidence, and jaw tracking, *J Prosthet Dent* 63:198-201, 1990.
18. Mohl ND et al: Devices for the diagnosis and treatment of temporomandibular disorders. Part II. Electromyography and sonography, *J Prosthet Dent* 63:332-335, 1990.
19. Clark GT: A critical evaluation of orthopedic interocclusal appliance therapy: design, theory and overall effectiveness, *J Am Dent Assoc* 108:359-364, 1984.
20. Greco PM et al: An evaluation of anterior temporal and masseter muscle activity in appliance therapy, *Angle Orthod* 69:141-146, 1999.
21. Dunn J: Physical therapy. In Kaplan AS, Assael LA (eds): *Temporomandibular disorders: diagnosis and treatment,* Philadelphia, 1991, WB Saunders.
22. Capurso U, Marini I, Alessandri Bonetti G: *I Disordini Cranio-mandibolari fisioterapia speciale stomatognatica,* Bologna, Italy, 1996, Martina.
23. McMullen RD: Pharmacologic management of psychiatric disorders. In Kaplan AS, Assael LA (eds): *Temporomandibular disorders: diagnosis and treatment,* Philadelphia, 1991, WB Saunders.
24. Randolph CS: Conservative management of temporomandibular disorders: a posttreatment comparison between patients from a university clinic and from private practice, *Am J Orthod Dentofacial Orthop* 98:77-82, 1990.
25. Amsterdam M: Periodontal prosthesis: twenty-five years in retrospect. Part II. Occlusion, *Compend Contin Educ Dent* 5:325-334, 1984.
26. Perry HT: Orthodontics and TMD: past and present. In Sachdeva RCL et al (eds): *Orthodontics for the next millennium,* Gendora, Calif, 1997, Ormco.
27. Okeson J: *Fundamentals of occlusion and temporomandibular disorders,* St Louis, 1989, Mosby.
28. Moeller E: The myogenic factor in headache and facial pain. In Kawamura Y, Dubner R (eds): *Oral-facial sensory and motor functions,* Chicago, 1981, Quintessence.
29. McNeill C et al: Temporomandibular disorders: diagnosis, management, education, and research, *J Am Dent Assoc* 120:253-255, 257, 1990.
30. Pullinger AG, Seligman DA, Gornbein JA: A multiple regression analysis of risk and relative odds of temporomandibular disorders as a function of common occlusal features, *J Dent Res* 72:968-979, 1993.
31. Gianniri AI et al: Occlusal contacts in maximum intercuspation and craniomandibular dysfunction in 16- to 17-year-old adolescents, *J Oral Rehabil* 18:49-59, 1991.
32. Wanman A, Agerberg G: Etiology of craniomandibular disorders: evaluation of some occlusal and psychosocial factors in 19-year-olds, *J Craniomandib Disord* 5:35-44, 1991.
33. Pullinger AG, Seligman DA: Quantification and validation of predictive values of occlusal variables in temporomandibular disorders using a multifactorial analysis, *J Prosthet Dent* 83:66-75, 2000.
34. Sadowsky C: The risk of orthodontic treatment for producing temporomandibular disorders: a literature overview, *Am J Orthod Dentofacial Orthop* 101:79-83, 1992.
35. Gaynor G: Orthodontic therapy. In Kaplan AS, Assael LA (eds): *Temporomandibular disorders: diagnosis and treatment,* Philadelphia, 1991, WB Saunders.
36. Graber TM: The clinical implications of the unique metabolic processes in the human temporomandibular joint. In Sachdeva RCL et al (eds): *Orthodontics for the next millennium,* Gendora, Calif, 1997, Ormco.
37. McNamara JA, Seligman DA, Okeson JP: Occlusion, orthodontic treatment and temporomandibular disorders: a review, *J Orofacial Pain* 9:73-90, 1995.

CHAPTER 28

Adjunctive Orthodontic Therapy in Adults: Biologic, Medical, and Treatment Considerations

W. Eugene Roberts, William F. Hohlt, and James J. Baldwin

KEY TERMS

medical factors	adult orthodontic	adjunctive orthodontic	multidisciplinary treatment
biologic considerations	treatment	treatment	complications

Increasing numbers of adults, with a wide range of malocclusions, are referred for adjunctive orthodontic care. Some problems are limited in nature and respond well to relatively simple removable or fixed mechanics.[1,2] Other malocclusions require a comprehensive approach with full fixed appliances.[3-9] Currently, a most rapidly increasing group of patients is middle age and older adults with complex, partially edentulous malocclusions. The latter are often challenging problems requiring integrated multidisciplinary treatment. Compared with problems of children and adolescents, the acquired malocclusions of adults are usually more complex because of **medical factors**, periodontal compromise, and functional complications.[9,10]

In evaluating a new patient, the initial objective (Figure 28-1) is the collection of a thorough diagnostic database. To prevent overlooking significant problems, it is important to adhere to a disciplined evaluation process. Begin with an overall consideration of the patient's health (the "big picture"): history of the chief complaint, medical evaluation, psychological considerations and lifestyle. The next objectives are to progressively focus on the face, oral cavity, periodontium, teeth, and malocclusion (see Section II). In a thorough, well-ordered evaluation, the malocclusion is the last factor to be considered. A disciplined evaluation process is analogous to a target that represents all the health needs of the patient. The actual assessment of

the malocclusion is the ultimate focus of the diagnostic evaluation.

MEDICAL CONSIDERATIONS

Genetic and Acquired Health Problems

All adults, especially those who are partially edentulous, should be thoroughly screened for genetic and acquired health problems. Medical factors that may contraindicate elective dental treatment such as recent myocardial infarction, valvular prosthesis, severe renal compromise, chronic alcoholism and drug addiction must be respected. Furthermore, any disease that is resistant to treatment, for instance uncontrolled diabetes, osteoporosis or osteomalacia, may preclude a predictable result with bone manipulative therapy.[6,10] Adverse medical factors are **biologic considerations** that limit the potential of **adult orthodontic treatment**.

Advances in medical care have reduced the risks of elective dental treatment for many medically compromised adults. Potential patients with inherited disorders (Figure 28-2) or even a history of radiation therapy to the jaws (Figure 28-3) may be candidates for orthodontics. Chanavaz[10] reported that many "serious" medical problems are no longer considered to be "absolute" contraindications for invasive dental procedures such as endosseous implants, bone grafts and or-

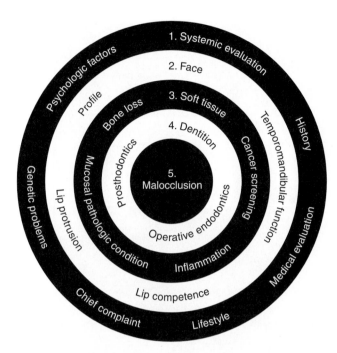

Figure 28-1 Target concept of diagnosis. A disciplined evaluation of an adult malocclusion is a progressive focus from the whole patient (systemic evaluation) down to the level of the chief complaint (malocclusion).

thognathic surgery. Among conditions that are currently considered to be manageable problems are acquired immunodeficiency syndrome, prolonged use of corticosteroids, metabolic bone disease, chemotherapy, endocrine disorders, and smoking. Renal and liver disorders are often manifest as bone problems. Significant disease of the liver or kidney may adversely affect vitamin D metabolism resulting in osteomalacia or osteopenia (Figure 28-4). Elective dental treatment is a viable option if calcium metabolism is stabilized.[10] In brief, the specific needs of each medically compromised patient should be discussed with his or her physician.

Calcium Metabolism and Bone Mass

Epidemiologic studies in the United States of adults over the age of 50 have documented a high incidence of osteopenia (asymptomatic low bone mass) and osteoporosis (symptomatic or potentially symptomatic low bone mass).[11] The World Health Organization (WHO) defines *osteopenia* as bone mass 1 to 2.5 standard deviations (SD) below the young adult mean (YAM). WHO defined *osteoporosis* as >2.5 SD below the YAM. Bone mineral density (BMD) measurements of adult women over age 50 indicated that 13% to 18% have osteoporosis and 37% to 50% have osteopenia. For men of the same age, 3% to 6% have osteoporosis and 28% to 47% have osteopenia.[11] For both genders, the ethnic order of prevalence for osteopenia and osteoporosis in the United States is White > Hispanic >

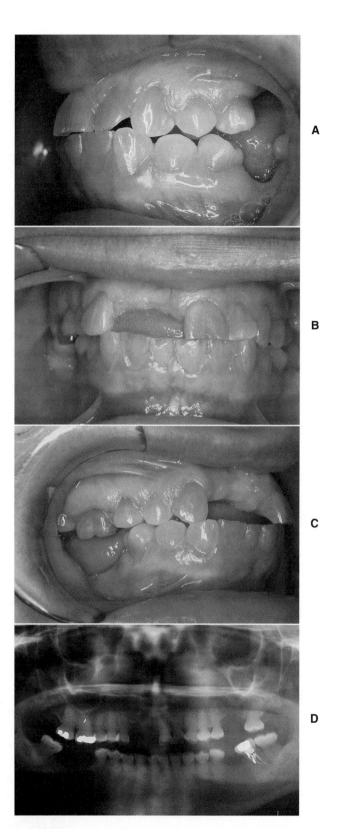

Figure 28-2 A to **C,** A young adult female presents with a partially edentulous malocclusion secondary to dentinogenesis imperfecta. She has a history of atraumatic fracture of multiple permanent teeth. The patient was referred by a prosthodontist for preprosthetic alignment. **D,** A panoramic radiograph reveals a fragile dentition with multiple missing teeth. The left mandibular molar is cracked and has a questionable prognosis. Preprosthetic alignment is indicated to optimize the functional loading of abutments for fixed prostheses.

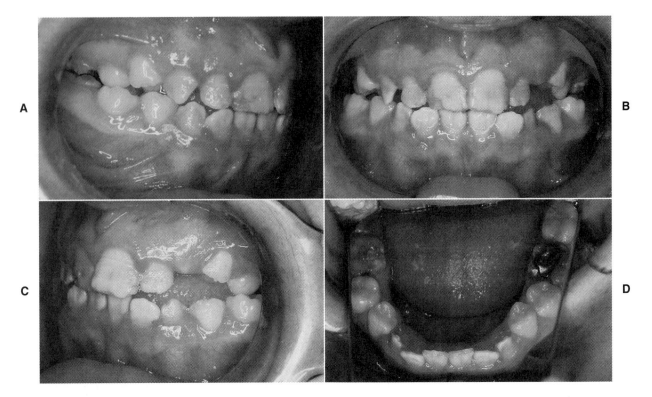

Figure 28-3 **A** to **C,** Facial views of the dentition of an adolescent female show enamel dysplasia of the permanent incisors, canines, and first molars. The patient received radiation therapy to the jaws at about 3 years of age to treat orofacial hemangioma. Premolars are unaffected. **D,** A mandibular occlusal photograph reveals that only the early transitional dentition (incisors, canines, and first molars) is affected. The late transitional dentition (premolars and second molars) is unaffected, apparently, because the enamel formed after the period of radiation therapy. There is delayed and incomplete eruption of multiple teeth. Because of the extensive restorative needs, this problem is classified as an adult malocclusion. (From Roberts WE: *Indiana Dent Assoc J* 76(2):33-41,1997.)

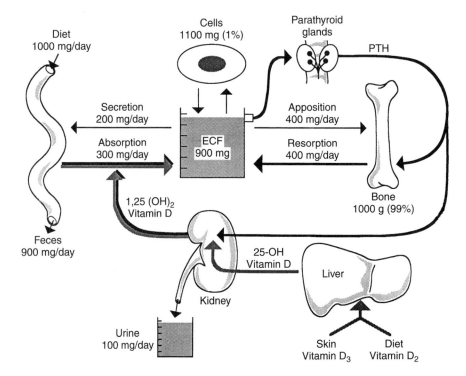

Figure 28-4 A schematic drawing of the principal elements of calcium metabolism demonstrates the delicate physiology associated with zero calcium balance. An aberration of one or more of the organs involved may be associated with negative calcium balance, which eventually manifests as osteopenia. (From Graber TM, Vanarsdall RL Jr (eds): *Orthodontics: current principles and techniques,* ed 3, St Louis, 2000, Mosby.)

Medical History Addendum: Bone Metabolism

- Do you have painful or deformed bones? Yes/No Which ones? _____
- Has anyone in your family had osteoporosis? Yes/No Who? _____
- Are you in sunlight regularly? Yes/No If not, why? _____
- Do you take calcium or vitamin D? Yes/No How much? _____
- Do you exercise regularly? Yes/No What type of exercise? _____
- Do you smoke? Yes/No Number of packs per day? _____
- Have you fractured any bones recently? Yes/No What bones and when? _____
- Have you decreased in height? Yes/No If so, how much? _____
- Have you noticed a more stooped posture? Yes/No If so, when? _____
- Do you consume dairy products? Yes/No How many servings per day? _____
- Do you drink alcoholic beverages? Yes/No How many drinks per day? _____

Women

- Are your menstrual periods regular? Yes/No If not, do you know why? _____
- Have you entered menopause? Yes/No If so, how many years ago? _____
- Do you take estrogen? Yes/No If so, how often and what dose? _____
- Do you take drugs to protect your bones? Yes/No If so, give drug and dose. _____
- Do you have children? Yes/No List your age at their birth. _____

Comments: _____

Figure 28-5 A supplementary health questionnaire used to elicit specific information about osteoporosis risk factors.

Black. Note that even for the lowest risk group, which is black men, the prevalence of osteoporosis is still about 3% and of osteopenia is 28%. Risk of low bone mass is not trivial for any group in modern society.[11] When evaluating adults for surgical procedures or orthodontics or both, a bone metabolic assessment is an essential part of the diagnostic workup.

Calcium homeostasis is a complex physiologic interaction of the skeletal, epidermal, endocrine, gastrointestinal, hepatic, and renal systems (see Figure 28-4). Typical health questionnaires for dental patients rarely provide adequate information for an assessment of calcium metabolism. A supplementary health questionnaire is recommended to collect information on physiologic factors and lifestyle deficits that may compromise bone health (Figure 28-5).[12]

Skeletal and dental health are related. Because loss of teeth is a risk factor for osteoporosis, the skeletal health of all partially edentulous adults is suspect.[13] Furthermore, an adequate restoration of dental esthetics and function depends on a positive bone response. All partially edentulous adult patients, particularly postmenopausal women, should be screened for osteoporosis risk factors and other bone-related metabolic problems.[14]

A clinical investigation was conducted on the prevalence of bone-related medical problems in partially edentulous adults over 50 years of age and who presented for orthodontic consultation as part of a multidisciplinary evaluation.[3] Using the osteopenic risk factor analysis (see Figure 28-5), 44% of the potential patients were referred for medical evaluation including a BMD measurement of the hip, spine, and wrist (Figure 28-6). This fraction of the orthodontic patient pool (44%) is comparable to the findings of Looker et al[11] that up to 47% of men and 50% of women over age 50 are osteopenic. Because BMD measurement involves a dose of radiation, it is not recommended as a routine assessment for all potential patients. As a result, screening for osteoporosis risk factors should be used as a reliable method for determining which dental patients to refer for a bone evaluation.[12,13,15]

In the previously mentioned study, all partially edentulous patients over 50 years of age who presented with one or more established risk factors proved to be osteopenic at one or more sites when BMD was measured.[3] Although osteopenic risk factor analysis is an effective clinical tool for screening dental patients, it has significant limitations in medical practice. Over 20% of patients who develop osteoporosis fail to demonstrate any recognized risk factors.[12] Furthermore, assessment of risk factors is of limited value for reducing future risk of osteoporosis.[16] Because of these limitations, dentists should also be alert for other signs

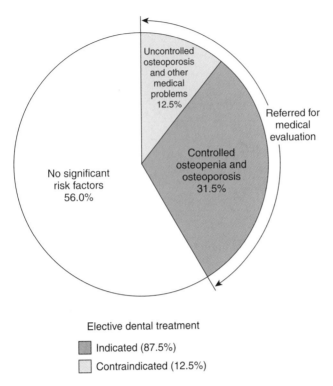

Elective dental treatment

■ Indicated (87.5%)

□ Contraindicated (12.5%)

Figure 28-6 Prevalence of osteopenia and osteoporosis in adults over 50 years of age. More than 40% of the sample were referred for medical evaluation because of one or more risk factors for osteoporosis. Following medical treatment and institution of preventive measures, all but 12.5% of the sample successfully completed orthodontic treatment. (From Roberts WE: *Indiana Dent Assoc J* 76[2]:33-41, 1997).

of metabolic bone problems that may be manifest in intraoral radiographs, including a bone image that has a ground glass or cotton wool appearance, poorly defined trabecular structure, and lack of a distinct lamina dura around roots of teeth (Figure 28-7, *A*).

For the sample of adult patients over 50 years of age with one or more risk factors for osteopenia and osteoporosis, 87.5% were sufficiently controlled to successfully complete multidisciplinary dental treatment including orthodontics.[3,13] The remaining 12.5% of the patients were inadequately stabilized from a medical perspective to justify pursuing extensive dental treatment; elective bone manipulative therapy was contraindicated (see Figure 28-6).The risk of complications is too great.

In brief, most osteopenic and osteoporotic adults are good candidates for **adjunctive orthodontic treatment** once the negative calcium balance is stabilized. However, clinicians must be alert for medical signs and symptoms that preclude extensive elective treatment.[3,9,10]

Endocrinology

The endocrine system is an important consideration for adult patients, many of whom are osteopenic, because hormones help control calcium metabolism and bone re-

modeling (turnover). Bone remodeling is a coupled sequence of cell activation (A), bone resorption (R), and bone formation (F). The ARF sequence to create a new secondary osteon or portion of trabecular bone is accomplished by the bone multicellular unit (BMU). The BMU is a coordinated group of precursor cells, osteoblasts, and osteoclasts that creates a new secondary osteon.[17] Regulation of the rate of bone resorption controls the flux of calcium into the extracellular fluid (see Figure 28-4).

The activation frequency of bone remodeling events, defined as the number of new secondary osteons generated per unit time, is enhanced by both parathyroid hormone (PTH) and thyroid hormone (TH). PTH is a specific hormone for increasing serum calcium. It acts by enhancing bone resorption, calcium reabsorption from the urine, and production of the active metabolite of vitamin D. TH increases bone remodeling by elevating the metabolic rate of the entire body. Estrogen tends to suppress the remodeling frequency, thus estrogen replacement therapy (ERT) is effective in preventing the high turnover of osteopenia that begins at menopause. Elevation of the remodeling (turnover) rate is a mechanism of skeletal atrophy because, for each remodeling event, slightly less bone is formed than was resorbed. Suppression of the metabolically driven remodeling rate is a physiologic mechanism for conserving bone that does not interfere with the mechanism of tooth movement.

Optimal Skeletal Health of Adults

Skeletal health of adult orthodontic patients is an important consideration because optimal treatment often requires extensive bone manipulative therapy including implants, orthodontics, and prostheses. Maintenance of normal bone resorption is important for healing, bone adaptation, orthodontic tooth movement, and maintenance of implant osseointegration. The rigid fixation of an implant within living bone (osseointegration) is maintained by the continuous remodeling of bone at the implant surface.[18,19] This mechanism maintains a layer of partially mineralized lamellar bone within 1 mm of the implant surface.[20] Estrogen and its analogs preserve bone mass without directly inhibiting bone resorption. Thus conservation of the skeleton, while maintaining a normal capability for bone resorption, is an advantage of ERT in osteopenic and osteoporotic women. Hormones and synthetic analogs may also be used to treat osteopenic and osteoporotic men.

Medications, Diabetes, and Orthodontic Treatment

Many adult patients have health problems that require prescription drugs. Others are substantial consumers of over-the-counter medications. Medications with an-

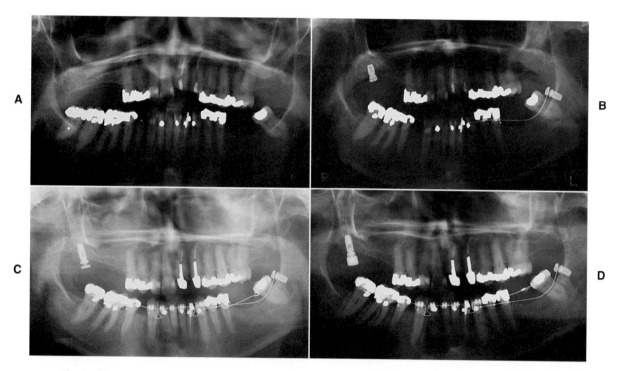

Figure 28-7 **A,** Pretreatment panoramic radiograph of a diabetic adult female shows an osseous morphology typical of high turnover metabolic bone disease: *1,* bone has a ground glass or cotton wool appearance; *2,* trabecular structure is poorly defined; and *3,* lack of a distinct lamina dura around teeth. This patient has a history of rampant caries and progressive renal failure. Medical referral for a bone mineral density measurement resulted in a diagnosis of osteopenia. **B,** Postoperative film shows a titanium implant in the ramus of the mandible distal to the left third molar and another implant distal to the right maxillary sinus. Note the titanium alloy anchorage wire extending from the retromolar implant to the canine and premolar region. After 7 months of orthodontic treatment with retromolar implant anchorage to intrude and upright the left mandibular third molar, the patient experienced rapidly declining renal function associated with progressive osteoporosis. Regular orthodontic visits were interrupted for 8 months while the patient received kidney and pancreas transplants. **C,** Six months after transplant surgery, orthodontic treatment progressed normally. Note improved bone trabeculation and cortical definition. The patient no longer requires insulin but is taking prednisolone to suppress transplant rejection and raloxifene to control the osteoporosis. A root spring tied down to the anchorage wire has been used to intrude the mandibular third molar and move it mesially. **D,** Nine months later bilateral space closure is accomplished with a 0.019 × 0.025-inch stainless steel arch with keyhole loops mesial to the canines. Radiographically, tooth movement is slow but normal.

tiinflammatory or immunosuppressive activity have the potential for interfering with the inflammatory nature of orthodontic tooth movement.[21-23] There is little specific pharmacologic information concerning the relationship between drug regimens and orthodontic therapy. A particular area of controversy is the use of nonsteroidal antiinflammatory drugs (NSAIDs) such as ibuprofen and aspirin. Some experimental studies in animals suggest that NSAIDs may inhibit the rate of tooth movement, but clinical studies have failed to consistently confirm a significant effect. In the absence of definitive data, it is best to assume there may be an effect on tooth movement that will negatively impact orthodontic treatment.

Centrally acting analgesics, such as acetaminophen (e.g., Tylenol) are preferred for controlling orthodontic pain. A short course of NSAIDs to control pain for the first day or two after an orthodontic adjustment is an acceptable alternative. However, long-term use of NSAIDs should be avoided because of high probability of gastrointestinal problems.

There are specific concerns with regard to medications that modify bone physiology. The most common medical problems with dentally significant bone effects are diabetes and osteoporosis. Periodontal disease in patients with uncontrollable diabetes can result in severe bone loss. Orthodontic treatment of diabetics with periodontal disease is a high-risk procedure likely to result in significant complications. Treatment should be carefully coordinated with a periodontist (see Chapter 24). On the other hand, if diabetes (insulin dependent or not) is well controlled and the patient's periodontium is healthy, multidisciplinary implant and orthodontic therapy can be accomplished in a routine manner.[10]

Common complications of diabetes are renal failure and osteoporosis resulting from compromised vitamin D metabolism and failure to reabsorb calcium from the

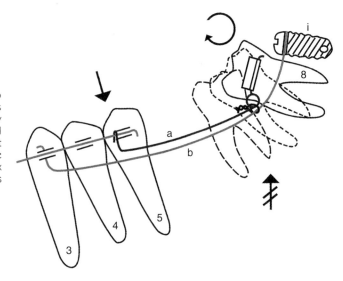

Figure 28-8 Free body diagram of the continuous mechanics used to align the third molar (8). The retromolar implant, anchorage mechanism was used continuously during the 21-month period of renal failure and kidney transplantation. Activation of the auxiliary spring (a) for a root mesial moment on the molar results in an intrusive force on the wire segment between the premolar brackets (4 and 5) and an extrusive force on the molar brackets. The extrusive force on the molar is negated by tying the helix of the root spring to the gingivally positioned anchorage wire (b), which is anchored by the implant (i).

urine. Renal failure was previously considered to be a contraindication for orthodontic care. However, if the patient is under good medical control and the periodontium is healthy, adjunctive orthodontic treatment can proceed. As shown previously, Figure 28-7, A, is a pretreatment film of a patient who suffered acute renal failure and received a kidney transplant. Figure 28-7, B to D, a series of panoramic films, demonstrates the progress of orthodontic treatment. Although the rate of tooth movement was inhibited, apparently by the intense antiinflammatory and immunosuppressive therapy, orthodontic treatment progressed throughout the period of renal failure and kidney transplantation. The principal active mechanics were a retromolar implant anchorage mechanism with a root spring to upright a molar. The root spring had a long range of activation to achieve mesial root movement of a mandibular third molar. Intrusion of the molar was accomplished with a steel ligature connecting the root spring inserted in the molar tube to the apically positioned implant anchorage wire (Figure 28-8). These are versatile mechanics for aligning potential abutments that probably would be extracted otherwise.[4,24]

As is discussed later, treatment of osteoporosis is potentially problematic during dental, surgical, or orthodontic therapy because drugs that inhibit bone resorption (bisphosphonates and calcitonin) may disturb bone modeling and remodeling dynamics. Careful coordination of medical and dental treatment is essential for medically compromised patients. Drugs that inhibit normal bone adaptation have negative biologic considerations for adjunctive orthodontic treatment.

Osteoporosis

Bone loss can be suppressed by decreasing the remodeling frequency with ERT or with selective estrogen re-

ceptor modulators (tamoxifen and raloxifene). The alternative is to directly inhibit bone resorption with calcitonin or bisphosphonates.[25] ERT is the most common long-term therapy for protecting the bones and cardiovascular systems of postmenopausal women. Unopposed estrogen is preferable for women who have had a hysterectomy. However, postmenopausal women with an intact uterus are usually treated with a combination of estrogen and progestin. Unopposed estrogen poses the risk of excessive endometrial stimulation, which is associated with an increased incidence of neoplasms.

Hormone replacement therapy is controversial primarily because of the increased risk of breast cancer. Long-term use of estrogen may increase the risk of breast cancer about 10%, but the combined use of estrogen and progestin increases the risk to about 30%.[26] In general, the bone, cardiovascular, dental, and other health benefits of ERT far outweigh the risks of breast cancer for most women. However, the risk/benefit ratio for the combined estrogen and progestin therapy is less certain.[27]

The principal alternatives to hormone replacement therapy for prevention and treatment of osteoporosis are calcitonin, bisphosphonates and the selective estrogen receptor modulators. Bisphosphonate treatment of low bone mass with drugs such as risedronate, etidronate, or alendronate (Fosamax) is a concern during bone-manipulative therapy because these drugs inhibit bone resorption.[28] The body's ability to remove bone is an essential element for wound healing and orthodontic tooth movement. An early-generation bisphosphonate (etidronate) has been associated with loss of implant integration.[29] However, at the doses currently recommended for the newer generations of bisphosphonates, no problems with maintaining implant integration have been reported.

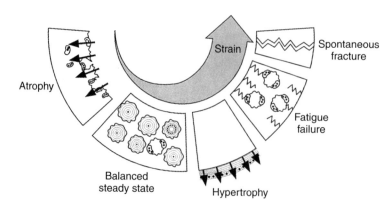

Figure 28-9 A schematic drawing demonstrating the strain-dependent relationship of common states of bone pathophysiology. Relative to the ultimate strength of bone (spontaneous fracture at 25,000 microstrain), the repetitive peak loading of living bone for each state is given as a percentage of ultimate strength. The relationship of strain to the level of bone adaptation in disuse atrophy (less than 2%), balanced steady state of remodeling (approximately 2% to 10%), subperiosteal hypertrophy (approximately 11% to 15%), fatigue failure (at least 16%) and spontaneous fracture (100%). (From Roberts WE: *Indiana Dent Assoc J* 78(3):24-32, 1999.)

There are no specific studies of orthodontic tooth movement, postoperative implant healing, or other forms of bone manipulative therapy in patients receiving the more commonly used bisphosphonates. Regardless, there are sufficient theoretic grounds on which to base the decision to avoid antiresorptive agents during elective bone manipulative therapy. Once the multidisciplinary restoration of occlusal function is complete, a bisphosphonate may be the drug of choice, especially for osteopenic males and for females who prefer to avoid estrogen therapy.

Oral Manifestation of Osteoporosis and the Effect of Estrogen Replacement Therapy

Osteoporosis is a systemic deterioration of the skeletal system that may have the following significant dental implications:
1. Decreased edentulous ridge height[30,31]
2. Decreased posterior maxillary arch width[32]
3. Progressive alveolar bone loss[33]
4. Loss of attachment and gingival recession[34]
5. Increased incidence of prosthetic units[35]
6. Loss of teeth[36]
7. Progressive decrease in numbers of teeth after menopause[13]

The degree of oral bone deterioration in osteoporotics is highly variable probably because of the superimposed variables of dental disease and disuse atrophy.[6] In the presence of a high rate of caries and periodontal disease, teeth are lost. Subsequent disuse atrophy associated with poor masticatory function may contribute to a higher rate of oral bone loss, particularly when superimposed on negative calcium balance. The relatively high rates of bone turnover in the jaws may enhance the loss of bone in edentulous and partially edentulous adults.[37-39]

In addition to its systemic benefits, ERT has a variety of oral health benefits, including a significant decrease in the loss of periodontal attachment and greater reten-

tion of teeth during the postmenopausal period.[13,40-44] As presently reviewed, many studies of medical and dental status suggest that women maintained on ERT are healthier than those who are not. However, ERT continues to be controversial because women who are compliant with ERT may be more health conscious in general. This group may have a better attitude toward aging and may pursue an overall healthier lifestyle than less health conscious women. Because it is difficult to adequately control clinical studies for lifestyle and psychologic variables, the ERT controversy is likely to continue. All considered, ERT is highly recommended for most postmenopausal orthodontic patients; however, orthodontists must stay abreast of the current literature because there will continue to be many questions about it.

In brief, the bone of patients with osteoporosis is normal; there is just not enough of it. There are no known deficits with regard to wound healing, response to orthodontic therapy, implant integration, or skeletal adaptation to altered functional loading. Once the negative calcium balance is stabilized, patients with osteoporosis are excellent candidates for orthodontics and other bone-manipulative therapy.[6,7] The critical factor is whether a potential patient has adequate residual bone to support treatment. If not, augmentation bone grafting may be needed. Once the osseous structure of the jaws is enhanced, it is important to adequately load the new bone. The most common procedures for improving the functional loading of edentulous alveolar bone are with implants, orthodontically repositioned teeth, or fixed prostheses. Treatment planning should be directed toward establishing optimal functional loading to avoid disuse atrophy of the alveolar process (Figure 28-9).

Osteoporosis Treatment during Bone-Manipulative Therapy

Osteoporosis, per se, presents no risk for dental implant therapy if residual bone is adequate.[45,46] As previously mentioned, some drugs used to treat osteoporosis may pose a problem.[29] If the periodontium is healthy, osteoporotic patients can be treated orthodontically.[3] Long-term corticosteroid treatment has long been associated with decreased rates of bone formation and osteoporosis.[47] However, elective orthodontic treatment is a viable option for patients under long-term corticosteroid therapy, but the rate of tooth movement may be slower.[48] Figure 28-7 demonstrates slow but otherwise normal tooth movement in a patient maintained on continuous prednisolone therapy. A diagram of the mechanics utilized during the period of intense medical and surgical treatment is illustrated in Figure 28-8.

Because its mode of action is to suppress the bone remodeling (turnover) frequency, estrogen treatment presents no risk for prospective orthodontic or dental implant patients. However, calcitonin, bisphosphonates (e.g., Fosamax), and other antiresorptive agents are a concern because bone resorption is an essential element of postoperative healing and long-term maintenance of integrated fixtures.[3,49] Devitalized, immature, and fatigued bone can only be removed by osteoclastic activity. Unfortunately, no clinical studies report the influence of bone resorption inhibitors on bone-manipulative therapy such as postoperative healing, osseointegration, or orthodontics. This is a significant problem because many osteoporotic adults are commonly treated with the bisphosphonate alendronate (Fosamax) to prevent fractures.[50]

Tamoxifen and raloxifene are selective estrogen receptors that suppress the rate of bone turnover. They are both effective in preserving the skeleton and protecting the cardiovascular system of postmenopausal women without increasing the risk of breast cancer. Raloxifene (Evista) is recommended for female patients with an intact uterus because it does not stimulate the endometrium and reduces the risk of breast cancer.[51] Estrogen, tamoxifen, and raloxifene are currently the therapies of choice for treating or preventing osteoporosis during active bone-manipulative therapy. Tamoxifen and raloxifene have been particularly useful in managing the osteopenia and osteoporosis of medically compromised orthodontic patients.

Medical and Dental Interactions

To effectively communicate with patients and physicians, all orthodontists should be aware of the critical issues and therapeutic alternatives for common health problems. As a general rule, medical conditions that are relatively stable and under adequate control do not preclude elective dental treatment. The specific treatment plan should be discussed with the patient's physician so that medical and dental care can be coordinated.

The medical problems that are most likely to impact orthodontic treatment of adults are metabolic bone diseases that manifest as osteopenia and osteoporosis. Bone metabolism problems are complex medical disorders that are best treated by specifically trained physicians experienced with appropriate diagnostic and treatment-monitoring equipment. Measurement of BMD at the hip, wrist, and spine with dual-energy photon absorptiometry is essential for the management of most patients with osteopenia or osteoporosis.[12] The dental practitioner should inquire in the local medical community to determine the most appropriate referral for dental patients with suspected bone metabolic disorders. Appropriate facilities are available in major medical centers.

Depending on the specific diagnosis, osteopenia and osteoporosis may be treated with exercise, dietary supplements (calcium or vitamin D or both), hormones, or specific drugs. However, as previously mentioned, there is considerable potential for medical treatment to interfere with optimal dental treatment and vice versa. Thus it is important to confer regularly with affected patients and their physicians. Everyone involved should be well informed about osteopenia, osteoporosis, hormonal considerations, and therapeutic measures. Because of the strong interaction of dental and bone physiology, it is important that medical and dental treatment be well coordinated.[33,52] A well-informed patient is a valuable asset in this regard.

Adults have an age-related risk of medical compromise that must be carefully considered as part of the diagnosis before beginning any elective dental treatment. Most patients with medical problems can be adequately controlled to pursue routine surgical and orthodontic options. Once the medical considerations have been appropriately addressed, the next step in an ordered diagnosis and treatment planning process is a careful evaluation of the face, oral cavity, and dentition.

Demographic Considerations

Demographics is an important consideration in evaluating the cause of adult malocclusions. The decreasing prevalence of caries and periodontal disease has substantially reduced the rate of edentulousness.[53,54] At age 50 the average adult has lost some teeth, usually molars or premolars, but retains an adequate dentition for fixed or removable prostheses. However, loss of occlusal antagonists and adjacent teeth often precipitates a cycle of functional compensation that results in extrusion, spacing, and axial inclination changes of the remaining teeth. Uncontrolled drift and extrusion of teeth may result in an acquired malocclusion that precludes routine restorative care (Figure 28-10). Adjunctive orthodontic treatment is essential for achieving an optimal restoration of function and esthetics.

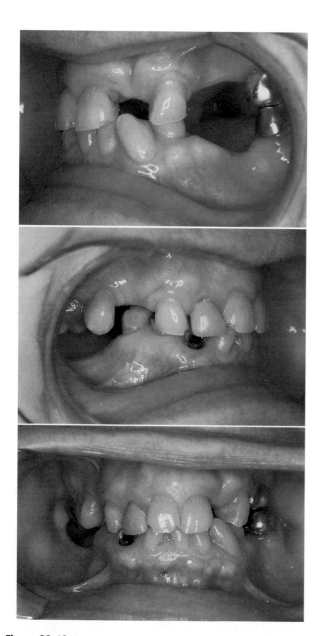

Figure 28-10 Pretreatment buccal and frontal intraoral views of a 78-year-old female show a severe compensated malocclusion that has resulted from long-term partial edentulousness and bruxism.

The proximal cause of most partially edentulous malocclusions is neglect. Failure to restore edentulous spaces may lead to dental compensations that result in poor orthognathic function, functional shifts in occlusion, microtrauma, and orthopedic instability of the temporomandibular joint.[55] When arch integrity and occlusal antagonists are lost, the remaining dentition extrudes and tips until a new stable equilibrium is achieved. This functional compensation can result in a severe acquired malocclusion. It may be difficult, if not impossible, to adequately restore esthetics and function without extensive orthodontic therapy as part of a **multidisciplinary treatment** plan (see Figure 28-10).

DIAGNOSIS AND TREATMENT PLANNING

The progressive focus of a disciplined orthodontic diagnosis of an adult is essential. To avoid overlooking significant problems, the practitioner should always begin with a systemic evaluation relative to the chief complaint: medical evaluation, history, lifestyle, genetic problems, and psychologic factors. The second consideration is the face: frontal symmetry, profile, and lip protrusion and competence. The third area of interest is the soft tissue: periodontium (inflammation and loss of attachment caused by pockets, recession, and bone loss), pathologic condition of the mucosa, and cancer screening. The fourth focus is the status of the dentition: operative, endodontic, and prosthodontic problems. The last consideration is an evaluation of the malocclusion. The appropriate perspective for evaluating a malocclusion ("bulls eye") is in the context of the entire patient (whole target [see Figure 28-1]).

Etiology

In the absence of congenital anomalies or significant trauma most people with a full complement of teeth have the genetic potential to develop and maintain a normal occlusion. Less than 10% of common malocclusions appear to be genetic problems.[24] Under optimal functional circumstances the jaws and dentition are highly adaptable and capable of developing and maintaining a normal occlusion over a lifetime.[6] Consequently, the cause of many malocclusions is environmental: habits, diet, functional compromises, soft tissue posture, caries, periodontal disease, developmental aberrations and trauma. Because each malocclusion is a manifestation of a unique set of environmental and genetic aberrations, it is, therefore, wise to carefully consider the cause of the malocclusion and then direct treatment at eliminating or controlling as many aberrant factors as possible.

Many malocclusions are esthetic problems caused by intermaxillary tooth size discrepancies. The most common problem is a mismatch in the size of the maxillary and mandibular incisors. The Bolton analysis is an important consideration in the evaluation of all malocclusions (Figure 28-11).[2,56] Complex, acquired malocclusions in partially edentulous adults may also have an underlying genetic component. This is an important etiologic distinction because true genetic problems are likely to be skeletal deficits requiring orthognathic surgery. On the other hand, acquired malocclusions are developmental compensations for aberrations such as ectopic eruption, premature loss of primary teeth, missing permanent teeth, and trauma.

Name: _____   D.O.B. _____

Sex: _____   Ethnicity: _____

Malocclusion: _____

Mesiodistal Tooth Measurements in Millimeters

Maxillary Tooth #	Trial 1	Mandibular Tooth #	Trial 1
3		19	
4		20	
5		21	
6		22	
7		23	
8		24	
9		25	
10		26	
11		27	
12		28	
13		29	
14		30	

Anterior ratio: $\dfrac{\text{Md. 6} \times 100}{\text{Mx. 6}}$ $\dfrac{\text{mm}}{\text{mm}} \times 100 =$ _____%

Posterior ratio: $\dfrac{\text{Md. 12} \times 100}{\text{Mx. 12}}$ $\dfrac{\text{mm}}{\text{mm}} \times 100 =$ _____%

Mean anterior ratio 77.2; mean posterior ratio 91.3.

A

Figure 28-11 A, Form for Bolton analysis of mesiodistal tooth width measurements.

Establishing the probable cause of an acquired malocclusion is important for cost-effective treatment. Therapeutic measures are directed at reversing the developmental compensations that created the problem. More severe acquired malocclusions may require osseointegrated implants for orthodontic anchorage to achieve an optimal result.

As seen in the following case study, many acquired malocclusions in adults are secondary to loss of permanent molars (Figure 28-12, *A* to *F*). The patient in Figure 28-12 lost all four permanent molars during childhood. The ensuing breakdown of arch integrity and loss of occlusal antagonists resulted in collapse of the vertical dimension of occlusion, a posterior vector of force on the mandible caused by the inclined plane of incisal guidance, and the physiologic drift of teeth into a compromised functional relationship. A common scenario for the development of such a condition is as follows:

1. First molars are extracted during childhood or adolescence.

2. Loss of posterior occlusal stops results in heavy occlusal contacts on the incisors.
3. The mandibular condyles are distally positioned in the fossa by the inclined plane of incisal guidance.
4. Mandibular growth is altered.
5. Maxillary and mandibular incisors tip labially.

In effect, a developing Class I occlusion may evolve into an asymmetric skeletal Class II malocclusion with a retrusive mandible (see Figure 28-12, *I*).

Functional compromises such as abnormal lip or tongue posture and occlusal shifts may disturb growth and mandibular posture. This scenario can result in a skeletal discrepancy (see Figure 28-12, *J*). A functional shift and distal vectors may occur in the occlusion, which tends to drive the condyles posteriorly in the articular fossa.

Asymmetry

Asymmetries are usually environmental problems because the genome is unilateral. In other words, hu-

Bolton Analysis Tooth Size Discrepancies

Overall Ratio: 12 Permanent teeth from first molar to first molar					
Sum mandibular "12" _____ mm		S.E.M.	0.26		
_____ ÷ _____ × 100 = _____%		Mean	91.3		
	Overall Ratio	SD	1.91		
		Range	87.5 to 94.8		

---------→ "12" ←---------

Max.	Mand.	Max.	Mand.	Max.	Mand.
85	77.6	94	85.8	103	94.0
86	78.5	95	86.7	104	95.0
87	79.4	96	87.6	105	95.9
88	80.3	97	88.6	106	96.8
89	81.3	98	89.5	107	97.8
90	82.1	99	90.4	108	98.6
91	83.1	100	91.3	109	99.5
92	84.0	101	92.2	110	100.4
93	84.9	102	93.1		

Anterior Ratio: 6 permanent teeth from canine to canine					
Sum mandibular "6" _____ mm		S.E.M.	0.22		
_____ ÷ _____ × 100 = _____%		Mean	77.2		
	Anterior Ratio	SD	1.65		
		Range	74.5 to 80.4		

---------→ "6" ←---------

Max.	Mand.	Max.	Mand.	Max.	Mand.
40.0	30.9	45.5	35.1	50.5	39.0
40.5	31.3	46.0	35.5	51.0	39.4
41.0	31.7	46.5	35.9	51.5	39.8
41.5	32.0	47.0	36.3	52.0	40.1
42.0	32.4	47.5	36.7	52.5	40.5
42.5	32.8	48.0	37.1	53.0	40.9
43.0	33.2	48.5	37.4	53.5	41.3
43.5	33.6	49.0	37.8	54.0	41.7
44.0	34.0	49.5	38.2	54.5	42.1
44.5	34.4	50.0	38.6	55.0	42.5
45.0	34.7				

Patient Analysis

If overall ratio exceeds 91.3:*

_____ Actual mand. "12" − _____ Correct mand. "12" = _____ Excess mand. "12"

If overall ratio is less than 91.3:

_____ Actual max. "12" − _____ Correct max. "12" = _____ Excess max. "12"

Patient Analysis

If anterior ratio exceeds 77.2:*

_____ Actual mand. "6" − _____ Correct mand. "6" = _____ Excess mand. "6"

If anterior ratio is less than 77.2:

_____ Actual max. "6" − _____ Correct max. "6" = _____ Excess max. "6"

*The discrepancy is excessive mandibular tooth mass. In the overall ratio chart above left, locate the patient's maxillary "12" measurement; opposite it is the ideal or "correct" mandibular measurement. The difference between the actual and correct mandibular measurement is the amount of excess mandibular tooth mass. The other calculations for excess mandibular and maxillary tooth size are performed similarly.

B

Figure 28-11, cont'd B, Form for Bolton analysis of the interarch tooth size discrepancy calculation.

mans have genes for only half of the body, thus opposite sides tend to be a mirror image of each other.[57] It follows that a variation in tooth size from side to side is an environmental effect. True genetic problems, such as mandibular prognathism and maxillary deficiency, tend to be symmetric while epigenetic problems like condylar hyperplasia are asymmetric (see Chapter 29). Some developmental (congenital) problems such as unilateral clefts are asymmetric because of the interaction of genetic and environmental (epigenetic) factors. Although an anomaly may be a genetic susceptibility, the actual expression of the trait may have strong epigenetic or environmental influence.[58]

Asymmetric Class II malocclusions are usually acquired problems reflecting abnormal occlusal development (Figure 28-13, *A*).

In planning orthodontic treatment it is wise to consider the cause of the malocclusion. For the patient illustrated in Figure 28-12, *A* to *G*, it appears the mandibular midline deviation and Class II canine relationship are probably a result of the following scenario:
1. Mandibular incisor crowding in the early mixed dentition
2. Ectopic eruption of the mandibular left lateral incisor
3. Premature exfoliation of the primary left canine.

This aberrant developmental sequence results in a midline deviation, lingual tipping of maxillary and mandibu-

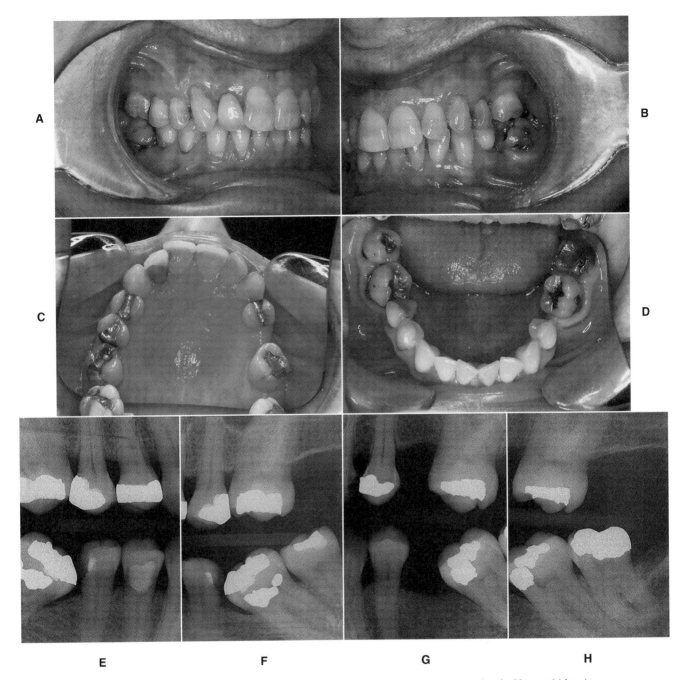

Figure 28-12 Pretreatment buccal (**A** and **B**) and occlusal (**C** and **D**) intraoral photographs of a 58-year-old female show a severe compensated malocclusion associated with loss of all four first permanent molars in childhood. **E** to **H,** Pretreatment bitewing radiographs illustrate severe mesial tipping of mandibular second and third molars. (**A** to **H** From Roberts WE, Baldwin JJ: *Case Studies in Orthod* 3[1]:1-6, 2000.)

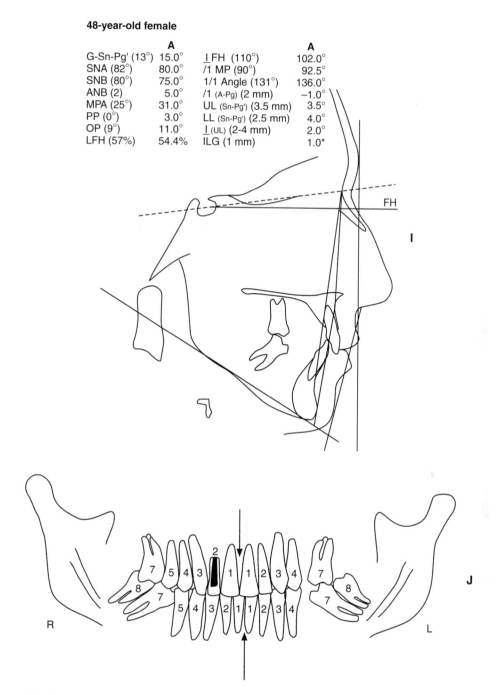

48-year-old female

	A		A
G-Sn-Pg' (13°)	15.0°	⊥FH (110°)	102.0°
SNA (82°)	80.0°	/1 MP (90°)	92.5°
SNB (80°)	75.0°	1/1 Angle (131°)	136.0°
ANB (2)	5.0°	/1 (A-Pg) (2 mm)	−1.0°
MPA (25°)	31.0°	UL (Sn-Pg') (3.5 mm)	3.5°
PP (0°)	3.0°	LL (Sn-Pg') (2.5 mm)	4.0°
OP (9°)	11.0°	⊥ (UL) (2-4 mm)	2.0°
LFH (57%)	54.4%	ILG (1 mm)	1.0*

Figure 28-12, cont'd I, Pretreatment cephalometric tracing reveals a retrusive mandible and a maxillary-mandibular discrepancy (ANB) of 5 degrees. **J,** Pretreatment panoramic view of the malocclusion demonstrates a unilateral Class II malocclusion with a marked midline discrepancy. Note that the tracing of the maxillary arch has been positioned to "articulate" with the mandibular arch.

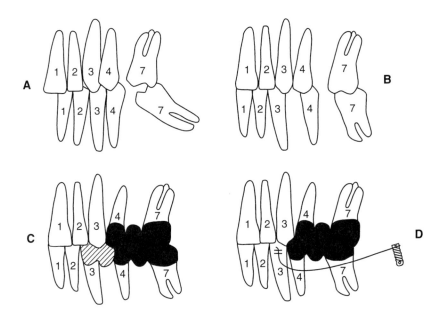

Figure 28-13 A, Correcting the cause of the malocclusion was the approach chosen. A tracing of the pretreatment panoramic radiograph shows a unilateral Class II (canine) malocclusion with deep bite and midline deviation, apparently caused by early extraction of the first molars and an ectopic eruption sequence resulting in a distally tipped anterior mandibular segment (*1* to *4*) (see text for details). **B,** Preprosthetic orthodontic alignment corrected the canine interdigitation, incisal deep bite and midline discrepancy by opening space for a pontic between the mandibular canine (*3*) and first premolar (*4*). **C,** The most expedient alternative is to accept the Class II posterior occlusion and place fixed prostheses in the maxillary and mandibular arches. This approach requires two additional prosthetic units (cross-hatched) to achieve an adequate restoration of occlusal function and fails to position the mandibular second molar in full occlusion. **D,** A more ideal alternative is to place a retromolar implant distal to the second molar with an anchorage wire to stabilize the canine. This approach permits mesial translation of the mandibular premolar (*4*) and molar (*7*) into a Class I occlusal relationship. Closing the space distal to the canine and achieving a Class I posterior segment eliminates two units of fixed prostheses and maintains occlusal function on the mandibular second molar. Also the less complex mandibular prosthesis is more likely to provide optimal long-term service.

lar incisors, a deep bite relationship, and a distal occlusal vector on the mandible. If no teeth are missing, the eruption of the lateral incisor into the position of the canine results in the erupting canine or first premolar being blocked out. However, for the patient in Figure 28-13, *A*, concurrent loss of the mandibular first permanent molar and congenital absence of the left second premolar allowed the permanent canine and first premolar to erupt distally and assume normal axial inclinations (see Figures 28-12, *G*, and 28-13, *A*). The mandibular incisors tipped lingually, extruded, and developed a deep bite relationship that inhibited the development of the mandible. Based on the probable cause of the retrusive mandible and asymmetric Class II canine relationship, treatment goals are to return the mandibular left canine to a more ideal functional position (see Figure 28-13, *B* to *D*), correct the incisal compensation, and allow the mandible to assume a more natural posture.

It is particularly important to consider the probable cause of asymmetries such as the midline deviations and buccal interdigitation relationships (Class I, II, or III). Within practical limits, adult orthodontic treatment should be directed at eliminating or at least reversing the proximal cause of the problem (see Chapter 29). Asymmetries and aberrations in the vertical dimension of occlusion are of particular interest because these problems usually relate to abnormal development or atrophic compensation related to tooth loss. Although it may be difficult to clearly establish the cause of a malocclusion, a careful history and a detailed study of the records define a working hypothesis that serves as a basis for adjunctive orthodontic treatment.[8]

Diagnostic Records and Treatment Planning

Chief Complaint The first consideration in the initiation of an ordered diagnosis and treatment planning process is to solicit a specific chief complaint. The dental clinician should be alert for any psychologic overtones that suggest the patient may have unrealistic expectations or an inappropriate attitude toward treatment. To help precisely define the patient's concerns, it is appropriate to inquire about obvious conditions that may relate to the patient's problems. A well-defined chief complaint associated with realistic treatment expectations is the base of the "diagnostic tree" (Figure 28-14).

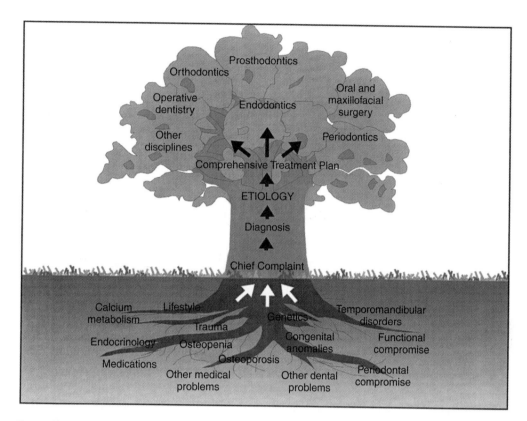

Figure 28-14 The "diagnostic tree" is a visualization of a patient's problem (chief complaint), which is a manifestation of etiologic factors that are the "roots" of the problems. The process of eliciting a specific chief complaint initiates an ordered diagnostic process. Diagnosis involves taking a careful history ("roots" of the problems) and formulating a probable cause. A comprehensive treatment plan is directed at eliminating or at least favorably moderating the cause of the problem. Directing treatment at eliminating the cause of the problem is more likely to achieve a stable result.

Clinical Evaluation In addition to a complete orofacial examination, the clinical evaluation of medical factors is indicated. A complete set of diagnostic records should include casts, radiographs, and photographs. The health history and clinical impression determines the appropriate level of medical evaluation. In addition to the usual orthodontic assessment procedures, an oral cancer screening and periodontal probing are essential elements of the pretreatment examination. If any significant periodontal compromise is detected, the patient should be referred for a complete periodontal evaluation. Active periodontitis is an adverse biologic consideration.

Diagnosis and Etiology The diagnosis is a prioritized list of problems based on a careful evaluation of the entire database. The cause may be derived from the history and the clinical evaluation. Although it is often difficult to define precisely all aspects of the cause, a thoughtful consideration of the available information is essential.

Comprehensive Treatment Plan The treatment plan is a prospective sequence of medical and dental procedures designed to alleviate the prioritized list of problems. For a favorable long-term prognosis, it is important to direct treatment at eliminating or at least controlling the etiology of the problems.

Alternate Treatment Plans

In evaluating a partially edentulous malocclusion, a tracing of the pretreatment panoramic radiograph is valuable for assessing the compromised alignment of the buccal segments. To construct a treatment plan to correct a midline discrepancy, it is helpful to articulate the arches by moving the maxillary tracing to contact the mandibular tracing (see Figure 28-12, J). Alternative treatment plans are constructed by arranging the teeth in a series of drawings that reflect the therapeutic options (Figure 28-15). Particular attention is paid to intermaxillary occlusion, midline correction, and anchorage requirements. Comparative drawings are a good way of communicating with the patient regarding biologic considerations, treatment alternatives, potential compromises, and probable consequences.

In general, the most ideal treatment plan is to close spaces and limit the use of prosthetics. Even fixed pros-

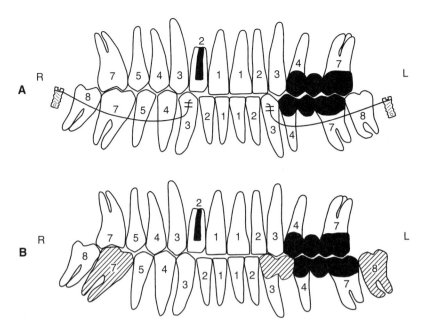

Figure 28-15 A, Treatment alternative 1 is the most ideal treatment plan. Two mandibular retromolar implants provide anchorage for mesial movement and alignment of mandibular molars. This approach results in optimal occlusion of all remaining teeth and requires minimal fixed prostheses. **B,** Treatment alternative 2 is a more conventional orthodontic treatment. Without implants, anchorage is inadequate to achieve an ideal alignment. The compromises in treatment are cross-hatched: inadequate mesial root movement of the mandibular right second molar *(7)*, two additional units of fixed prosthetics (mandibular left canine and the pontic on the distal), and no functional occlusion on the mandibular left third molar *(8)*. However, the more ideal result requires a longer treatment time, requires surgery, and is more expensive. (From Roberts WE, Baldwin JJ: *Case Studies Orthod* 3[1]:1-6, 2000.)

theses are rarely a permanent solution because of the relatively high failure rate over a lifetime.[59] It is important to construct a realistic treatment plan because biologic considerations dictate that the movement of teeth in adults is a much slower process than in growing children.[6,60] Figure 28-15, *A*, depicts the most ideal treatment plan with respect to achieving optimal occlusion of the residual dentition with minimal units of fixed prostheses. However, this approach requires surgery to place the implants, demands a longer treatment time, and is more expensive. After carefully considering the options, the patient decided against implant anchorage and selected the most expedient treatment plan (see Figure 28-15, *B*). Corresponding drawings of the alternate treatment plans are helpful for effectively communicating with the patient as well as the other members of the multidisciplinary team.

Intermaxillary Relationships

A careful consideration of the cause and evolution of a malocclusion is an important element of a comprehensive diagnosis.[7] In the authors' experience it is common for the mandible to assume a more anterior posture when a partially edentulous Class II malocclusion is corrected. In general, a decision on extraoral anchorage or orthognathic surgery to correct a Class II relationship should be delayed until orthodontic alignment of the arches is completed. Following preprosthetic alignment (Figure 28-16) and prosthetic restoration of occlusal function (Figure 28-17), the mandible assumed a more anterior position (Figure 28-18). Therefore, in formulating a treatment plan to correct Class II malocclusions in partially edentulous adults, it is wise to anticipate a more anterior posture of the mandible once functional interferences in the occlusion are corrected. Spontaneous correction of an apparent Class II skeletal problem by more anterior posturing of the mandible decreases the need for headgear or orthognathic surgery or both. However, anterior posturing of the mandible associated with multidisciplinary treatment is not predictable. It should be explained to the patient that evaluation for intermaxillary correction will occur after the arches are aligned.

Integrating Orthodontics into Comprehensive Treatment

Expanding the scope of orthodontic practice with respect to adjunctive orthodontic treatment of partially edentulous adults requires an increased awareness by the entire dental community. If a general practitioner has little or no appreciation of the value of orthodontics in the optimal treatment of complex restorative problems (malocclusions), his or her patients will not be referred for orthodontic evaluation. If orthodon-

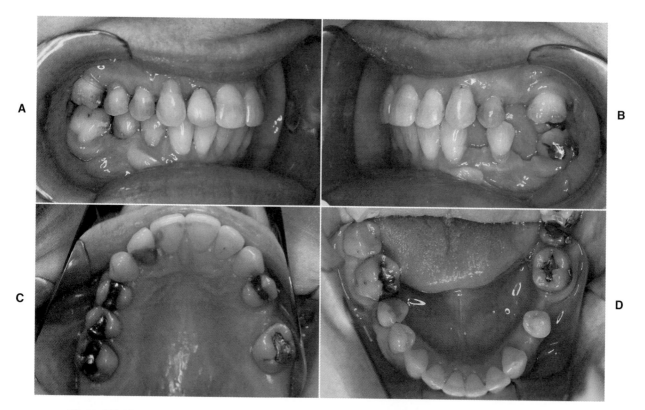

Figure 28-16 Buccal views (**A** and **B**) and occlusal views (**C** and **D**) show that at the end of active orthodontic treatment, an optimal Class I alignment with coincident maxillary and mandibular midlines is achieved. (From Roberts WE, Baldwin JJ: *Case Studies Orthod* 3[1]:1-6, 2000.)

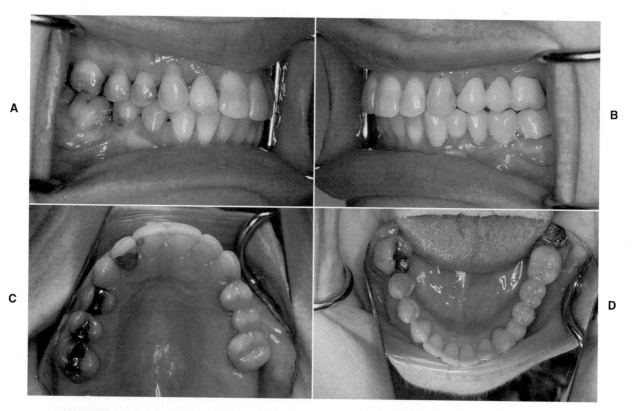

Figure 28-17 Buccal views (**A** and **B**) and occlusal views (**C** and **D**) following construction of left maxillary three-unit and mandibular five-unit fixed prostheses document that optimal function and esthetics are achieved. (From Roberts WE, Baldwin JJ: *Case Studies Orthod* 3[1]:1-6, 2000.)

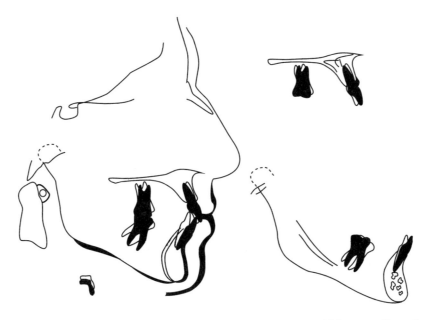

Figure 28-18 Cephalometric tracings are superimposed on the anterior cranial base, maxilla and mandible. Differences between the pretreatment and posttreatment films are highlighted in black. Note that the restoration of the posterior occlusion was associated with an increased vertical dimension of occlusion and about a 2-mm increase in the apparent length of the mandible. (From Roberts WE, Baldwin JJ: *Case Studies Orthod* 3[1]:1-6, 2000.)

tics is indicated but not provided, an optimal result is unlikely.

An important aspect for improving the standards of clinical practice is a requirement that all dental students have a clinical experience in orthodontics, and that all orthodontic graduate students learn to work with generalists in the treatment of limited malocclusions.[1,61-63] In this manner the developing dentist learns that orthodontics is an important adjunctive approach for many complex restorative problems. The orthodontic resident learns how to work with general dentists and other specialists in accomplishing optimal care. Integrating the educational process of dental students and orthodontic residents is central to the present philosophy of coordinated therapy in adults. With respect to adult orthodontic treatment, the educational goal is to promote adjunctive orthodontic treatment as part of a multidisciplinary treatment plan. The evaluation process must carefully address the biologic considerations, medical factors, and potential complications.

LIMITED ORTHODONTIC TREATMENT

This chapter addresses a variety of orthodontic problems in adults, some of whom are medically, functionally or periodontally compromised. Emphasis is on the multidisciplinary interaction that is essential to effective clinical management. An important objective is to move adjunctive orthodontic treatment into the mainstream of restorative dentistry. This concept is broadly defined as a multidisciplinary treatment approach for

achieving optimal esthetics and function consistent with a physiologically stable occlusion.[62]

Adjunctive orthodontic therapy should be a consideration for all comprehensive dental evaluations of adults. Every dentist should be trained in the assessment and treatment of modest orthodontic problems. Incorporating orthodontics in the diagnosis and treatment planning sequence should be as natural as any other aspect of dentistry. Furthermore, all dentists should appreciate the biologic considerations and medical factors inherent in adult orthodontic treatment.

Limited orthodontic problems are defined as static malocclusions in nongrowing patients who can be treated without extractions in 12 months or less. The principal exception to this rule is severe anterior crowding in the mandible, which requires extraction of a mandibular incisor. The latter are the only common limited cases that require extractions. Treatment time for mandibular incisor extraction cases is usually 16 to 24 months.

All dentists should be competent in the diagnosis of malocclusions.[64] Appropriately trained general dentists are capable of clinically managing some limited orthodontic problems as part of a comprehensive treatment plan.[1] However, the patient should be referred to an orthodontist if extensive treatment is needed, involving, for instance, orthognathic surgery, extractions, extraoral anchorage, intermaxillary mechanics, or management of facial discrepancies.[64] Patients with unusual biologic considerations or medical factors should receive adjunctive orthodontic treatment as part of a multidisciplinary treatment plan administered by specialists.

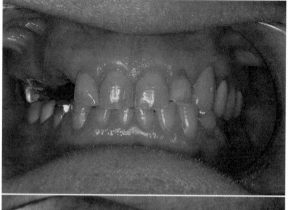
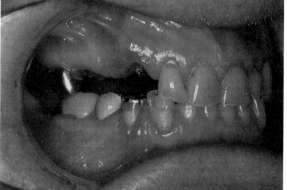
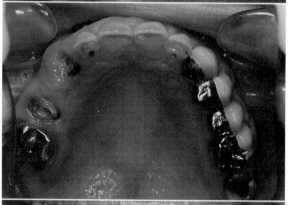
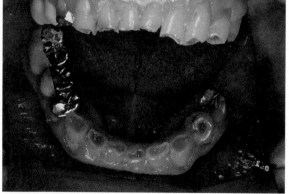

BOX 28-1	Typical Problems with Limited Orthodontic Objectives

- Cosmetic dentistry: Closing diastemas, space management, anterior alignment, elimination of interproximal "black spaces"[65]
- Preprosthetic alignment: Molar uprighting, abutment paralleling, space closure or opening[66]
- Forced eruption: Extrusion of endodontically treated fractured teeth, periodontal defects, compromises of the "biologic width"[66]
- Periodontal compromise: Extrusion of teeth to correct vertical defects, uprighting molars to eradicate pseudoperiodontal pockets, extrusion of "hopeless" teeth to generate bone in preparation for an implant[66,67]

Removable appliances are indicated for some modest malocclusions, but fixed appliances are superior for most limited problems. Fixed appliances have the inherent advantages of better anchorage control; reliable, three-dimensional tooth movement; and less dependence on cooperation. Removable appliances such as bite plates and interocclusal orthotics may be effective adjuncts for fixed appliance treatment (see Chapter 19).

Limited malocclusions are, in general, alignment discrepancies in the first, second, or third order. Orthodontic alignment is often an important adjunct to a comprehensive restorative or periodontal treatment plan. The objectives of limited (adjunctive) treatment are usually esthetic and functional goals that can be achieved with intraarch anchorage (Box 28-1). Adult orthodontic treatment of intermaxillary problems is best accomplished by orthodontists.

CASE PRESENTATIONS

Failed Fixed Prosthesis with Compromised Abutments

 Patient Profile

- Male, 70 years of age
- Chief complaint: Failed fixed partial denture
- Secondary caries of endodontically treated abutments teeth #4 and #6
- Compromised periodontal "biologic width" zone
- Class I or Class III molar occlusion
- Decreased vertical dimension of occlusion
- Marked attrition of the mandibular anterior segment (Figure 28-19, *A* to *D*)

Figure 28-19 **A,** Frontal, **B,** buccal, and **C** and **D,** occlusal views show the compromised dentition of an adult male with a history of bruxism and a failed maxillary fixed prosthesis. To serve as bridge abutments, the maxillary right canine and second premolar require orthodontic extrusion and a surgical crown-lengthening procedure.   *Continued*

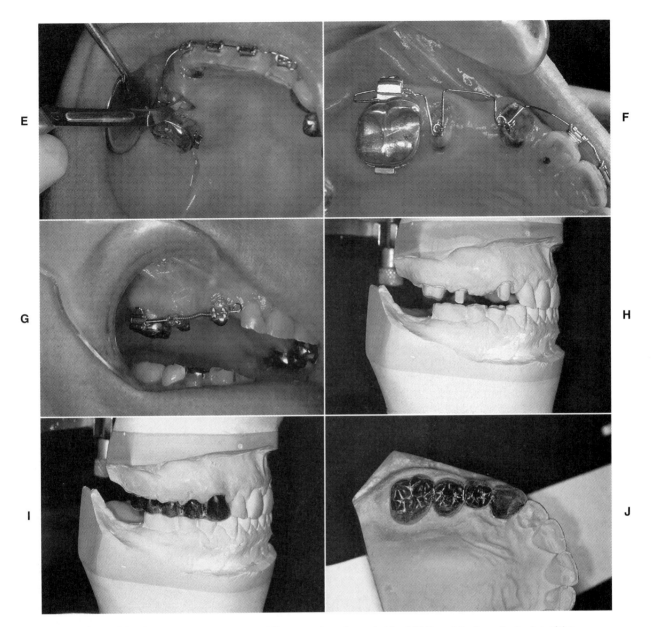

Figure 28-19, cont'd E, As supracrestal fiberotomy is preformed at the initiation of the forced extrusion of the maxillary canine and second premolar. **F,** Occlusal view shows that extrusion is achieved via torsional loading of a 0.016-inch stainless steel arch wire. **G,** Following extrusion, the abutments are retained with an arch wire segment extending from the adjacent molar. **H,** Casts of the maxillary and mandibular arches are articulated after completion of orthodontic treatment. **I,** Buccal view of the wax pattern for a four-unit fixed prosthesis. **J,** Occlusal view of the wax pattern.

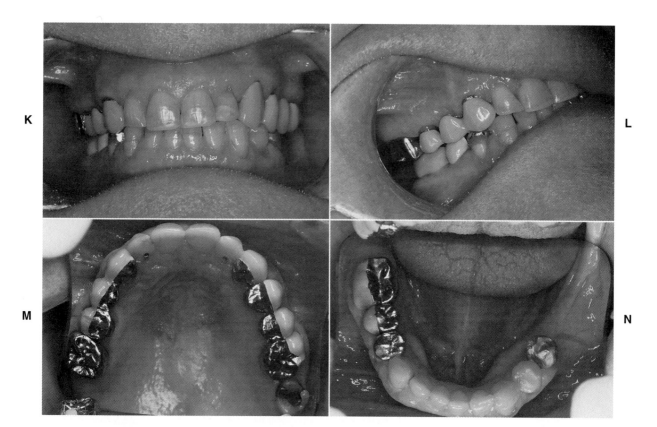

Figure 28-19, cont'd K, Frontal view of the final result. **L,** Right buccal view of the final result. **M,** Maxillary occlusal view of the fixed prosthesis. **N,** Mandibular occlusal view showing the restoration of teeth #20 to #27.

Wire hooks were cemented into the pulp canals of the endodontically treated abutments (teeth #4 and #6). A supracrestal fiberotomy was performed to increase the length of the clinical crowns (see Figure 28-19, *E*). Via fixed appliances from teeth #3 to #10, teeth #4 and #6 were forcibly erupted about 3 mm each. A 0.016-inch stainless steel arch wire with vertical loops was activated in torsion to rapidly extrude the compromised abutments for 2 months (see Figure 28-19, *F*). Tooth #6 was moved closer to tooth #7 to enhance the esthetics of the final restoration. Following 3 months' retention (see Figure 28-19, *G*), the abutments were permanently restored with gold posts (see Figure 28-19, *H*) and wax patterns of the fixed prosthesis were prepared (see Figure 28-19, *I*). Ceramic fused to metal crowns were constructed (see Figure 28-19, *K* to *N*). Total treatment time including retention before placing the final prosthesis was 12 months.

Maxillary Anterior Gingival Alignment

Porcelain brackets were bonded on teeth #6 to #11. The right central incisor was extruded 3 to 4 mm (Figure 28-20, *B*). The incisal edge was reduced to produce an esthetic gingival relationship with the adjacent teeth

(see Figure 28-20, *C*). A periapical radiograph of the central incisors at the end of treatment shows that the roots of central incisors are shorter than the adjacent lateral incisors; however, there is still adequate osseous support to sustain function (see Figure 28-20, *D*). Following orthodontic treatment, porcelain veneers were placed on the maxillary lateral incisors (teeth #7 and #10) and full crowns on the central incisors (teeth #8 and #9).

 Patient Profile

- Female, 56 years of age
- Chief complaint: Long teeth and unesthetic smile
- Porcelain bonded veneers on maxillary central incisors (teeth #8 and #9)
- Gingival recession on tooth #8 (see Figure 28-20, *A*). Notice gingival height difference.
- Class I molar and canine occlusion
- 4-mm (40%) overbite
- Healthy periodontium

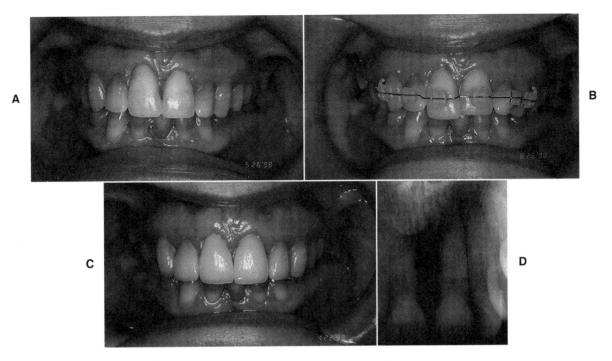

Figure 28-20 **A,** Adult female with unesthetic gingival recession of the maxillary central incisors. **B,** Fixed appliances are used to extrude the central incisors. **C,** Anterior maxillary esthetics have been improved by extruding the maxillary right central incisor and reducing the incisal edge. **D,** Posttreatment radiograph shows adequate osseous support of the right maxillary central incisor despite the reduced length of the root supported by bone.

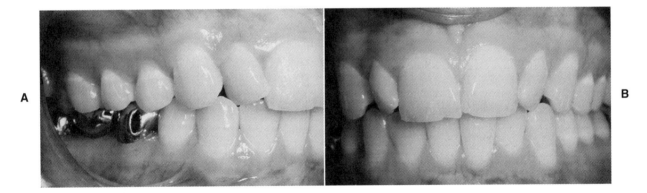

Figure 28-21 **A** to **B,** Pretreatment views of an adult female with a Class I malocclusion and a chief complaint of maxillary anterior crowding. The cause is excessive width of maxillary incisors relative to mandibular incisors.

Crowding Related to an Intermaxillary Tooth Size Discrepancy

 Patient Profile

- Female, 28 years of age
- Chief complaint: Poor maxillary anterior dental esthetics
- Crowding and rotation of teeth #7 and #11 (Figure 28-21, *A* to *C*)

- Class I molar occlusion
- Midline discrepancy of 1.5 mm
- Overjet and overbite within normal limits
- Bolton analysis: 3.5-mm excess tooth size on teeth #6 to #12

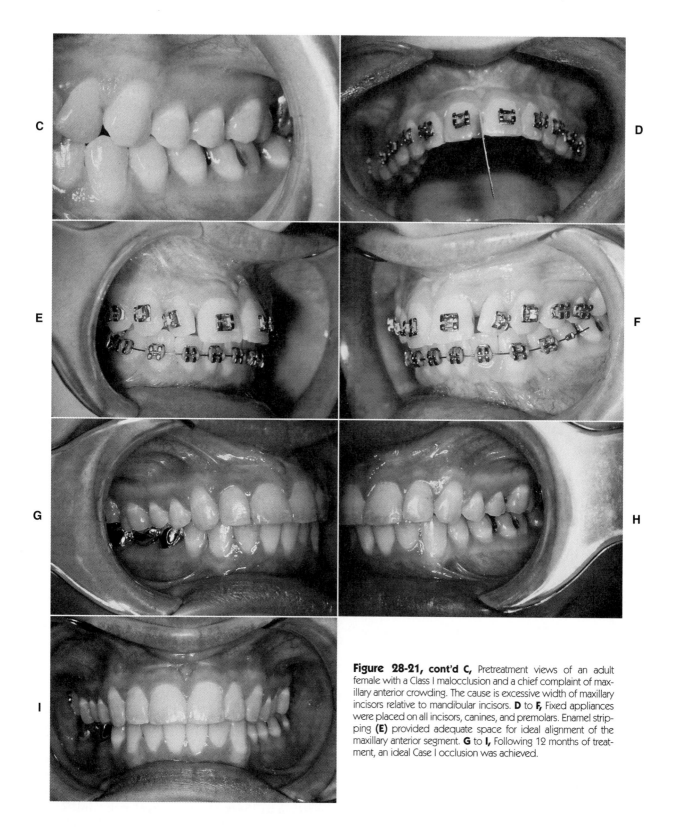

Figure 28-21, cont'd C, Pretreatment views of an adult female with a Class I malocclusion and a chief complaint of maxillary anterior crowding. The cause is excessive width of maxillary incisors relative to mandibular incisors. **D** to **F,** Fixed appliances were placed on all incisors, canines, and premolars. Enamel stripping **(E)** provided adequate space for ideal alignment of the maxillary anterior segment. **G** to **I,** Following 12 months of treatment, an ideal Case I occlusion was achieved.

Brackets were bonded from second premolar to second premolar in both arches. Interproximal enamel was stripped in the maxillary anterior region from canine to canine (see Figure 28-21, *D* to *F*). Both arches were aligned with 0.016 nickel-titanium and finished with pro-gressive stainless steel arch wire therapy. The occlusion was finished in an ideal Class I relationship with no over-jet and 1.5 mm of overbite (see Figure 28-20, *G* to *I*). The correction was retained with maxillary and mandibular Hawley retainers. Active treatment time was 12 months.

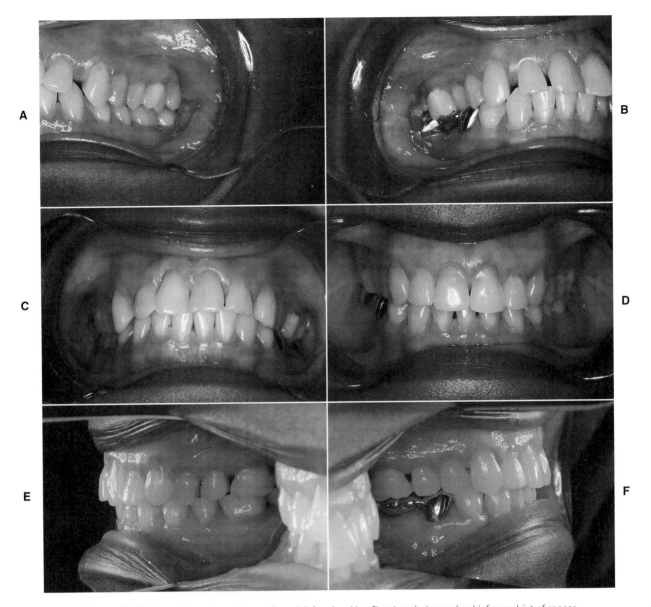

Figure 28-22 **A** to **C,** Pretreatment views of an adult female with a Class I occlusion and a chief complaint of spaces distal to the maxillary lateral incisors. The cause is excessive width of the mandibular incisors relative to the maxillary incisors. **D** to **F,** Following extraction of a mandibular incisor, the maxillary and mandibular anterior segments were aligned and the spaces closed with fixed appliances. A near-ideal occlusal finish is achieved.

Maxillary Anterior Space Closure

Patient Profile

- Female, 54 years of age
- Chief complaint: Maxillary anterior rotations and spaces
- Missing mandibular right second premolar (replaced with a fixed partial denture)
- Class I molar and canine occlusion (Figure 28-22, *A* to *C*)
- Bolton analysis: 4.5-mm mandibular anterior excess tooth size

A mandibular incisor was extracted to compensate for excess tooth size in the mandibular anterior segment. A full fixed 0.022-inch slot appliance was used in both arches. Following initial alignment with 0.016 nickel-titanium arch wires, maxillary and mandibular anterior spaces were closed with sliding wire mechanics on a 0.018-inch stainless steel arch wire. Root positions were corrected with a 0.017 × 0.025-inch stainless steel arch wire. The final occlusion (see Figure 28-22, *D* to *F*) was functionally generated with 8 weeks of immediate tooth positioner wear. Inclined planes were adjusted to achieve primary centric stops in occlusion on the buccal cusps of the mandibular posterior teeth. Treatment time was 22 months. Occlusal views of the

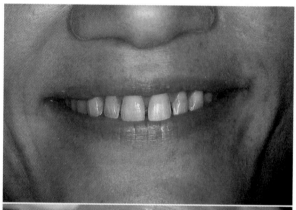

Figure 28-22, cont'd G, A pretreatment occlusal view of the maxillary arch shows a symmetric arch form, rotated teeth, and redundant space distal to the lateral incisors. **H,** A posttreatment occlusal view shows an ideal and relatively symmetric maxillary arch. The key to achieving this positive result was creating space in the mandibular anterior region by extracting an incisor. This is an example of correcting the etiology of a malocclusion to achieve an optimal result.

maxillary arch before and after treatment demonstrate the effectiveness of extracting a mandibular incisor to create overjet to permit closure of spaces in the maxillary anterior segment (see Figure 28-22, *G* and *H*).

Alignment for Maxillary Anterior Veneers

 Patient Profile

- Female, 45 years of age
- Chief complaint: Unattractive smile as a result of spaces between front teeth (Figure 28-23, *A* and *B*)
- Diagnosis: Excessive intermaxillary space in the anterior segments of both arches
- Occlusion: Class I molars and Class II canines
- Bolton analysis: 78.6 compared to the mean of 77.2 indicates a maxillary anterior tooth size deficiency (see Figure 28-23, *C* and *D*)
- Etiology: Excessive interproximal space and an interproximal tooth size discrepancy
- Treatment plan: Preprosthetic alignment for porcelain veneers on maxillary incisors and canines. A diagnostic wax setup was used to plan the preprosthetic mechanics for optimal restoration of maxillary anterior esthetics with porcelain veneers (see Figure 28-23, *E*).

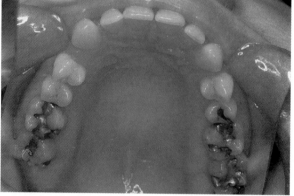

Figure 28-23 A, Adult female with an unesthetic smile caused by maxillary anterior spaces. **B,** A maxillary occlusal view reveals that the cause of the problem is inadequate width of the maxillary incisors and canines.
Continued

All four first molars were banded, porcelain brackets were bonded from first premolar to first premolar, and both arches were progressively leveled to accommodate 0.018-inch stainless steel arch wires (see Figures 28-23, *F* and *G*). The mandibular diastemas were closed with a vertical loop in the archwire (see Figure 28-23, *F* and *H*). The maxillary midline was corrected

and space was equalized with differential use of open coil springs and closing loops. When optimal preprosthetic alignment was achieved, the appliances were removed and Hawley retainers were placed. The maxillary retainer had wire prongs between all the maxillary anterior teeth to allow differential adjustment of interproximal spaces as needed. After an active treatment

Name: __P.B.__   D.O.B. _____

Sex: __F__   Ethnicity: __Caucasian_____

Malocclusion: __I__

Mesiodistal Tooth Measurements in Millimeters

Maxillary Tooth #	Trial 1	Mandibular Tooth #	Trial 1
3	9.59	19	10.44
4	6.32	20	6.73
5	6.59	21	6.68
6	7.36	22	6.05
7	5.83	23	5.35
8	7.77	24	4.63
9	7.40	25	4.40
10	5.72	26	5.32
11	7.05	27	6.58
12	6.67	28	6.68
13	6.39	29	6.82
14	9.68	30	10.47

Anterior ratio: $\dfrac{\text{Mandibular } 6 \times 100}{\text{Maxillary } 6}$ $\dfrac{32.33 \text{ mm}}{41.13 \text{ mm}} \times 100 = 78.60$

Posterior ratio: $\dfrac{\text{Mandibular } 12 \times 100}{\text{Maxillary } 12}$ $\dfrac{80.15 \text{ mm}}{86.37 \text{ mm}} \times 100 = 92.79$

Mean anterior ratio 77.2; mean posterior ratio 91.3.

C

Figure 28-23, cont'd C, Bolton analysis measurements. **D,** Bolton tooth size discrepancy. (**C** and **D** From Hohlt WF, Hovijitra S: *Indiana Dent Assoc J* 78[3]:18-23, 1999.)

Bolton Analysis Tooth Size Discrepancies

Overall Ratio: 12 Permanent teeth from first molar to first molar

Sum mandibular "12" _____ mm   S.E.M.   0.26

_____ ÷ _____ × 100 = _____%   Mean   91.3

Overall Ratio   SD   1.91

Range   87.5 to 94.8

Anterior Ratio: 6 permanent teeth from canine to canine

Sum mandibular "6" _____ mm   S.E.M.   0.22

_____ ÷ _____ × 100 = _____%   Mean   77.2

Anterior Ratio   SD   1.91

Range   74.5 to 80.4

Max.	Mand.	Max.	Mand.	Max.	Mand.
85	77.6	94	85.8	103	94.0
86	**78.5**	95	86.7	104	95.0
87	79.4	96	87.6	105	95.9
88	80.3	97	88.6	106	96.8
89	81.3	98	89.5	107	97.8
90	82.1	99	90.4	108	98.6
91	83.1	100	91.3	109	99.5
92	84.0	101	92.2	110	100.4
93	84.9	102	93.1		

Max.	Mand.	Max.	Mand.	Max.	Mand.
40.0	30.9	45.5	35.1	50.5	39.0
40.5	31.3	46.0	35.5	51.0	39.4
41.0	**31.7**	46.5	35.9	51.5	39.8
41.5	32.0	47.0	36.3	52.0	40.1
42.0	32.4	47.5	36.7	52.5	40.5
42.5	32.8	48.0	37.1	53.0	40.9
43.0	33.2	48.5	37.4	53.5	41.3
43.5	33.6	49.0	37.8	54.0	41.7
44.0	34.0	49.5	38.2	54.5	42.1
44.5	34.4	50.0	38.6	55.0	42.5
45.0	34.7				

Patient Analysis

If overall ratio exceeds 91.3:*

$$\frac{80.15}{\text{Actual mand. "12"}} - \frac{78.50}{\text{Correct mand. "12"}} = \frac{1.65}{\text{Excess mand. "12"}}$$

If overall ratio is less than 91.3:

$$\frac{}{\text{Actual max. "12"}} - \frac{}{\text{Correct max. "12"}} = \frac{}{\text{Excess max. "12"}}$$

Patient Analysis

If anterior ratio exceeds 77.2:*

$$\frac{32.33}{\text{Actual mand. "6"}} - \frac{31.70}{\text{Correct mand. "6"}} = \frac{0.63}{\text{Excess mand. "6"}}$$

If anterior ratio is less than 77.2:

$$\frac{}{\text{Actual max. "6"}} - \frac{}{\text{Correct max. "6"}} = \frac{}{\text{Excess max. "6"}}$$

*The discrepancy is excessive mandibular tooth mass. In the overall ratio chart above left, locate the patient's maxillary "12" measurement; opposite it is the ideal or "correct" mandibular measurement. The difference between the actual and correct mandibular measurement is the amount of excess mandibular tooth mass. The other calculations for excess mandibular and maxillary tooth size are performed similarly.

D

Figure 28-23, cont'd D, Bolton tooth size discrepancy.   *Continued*

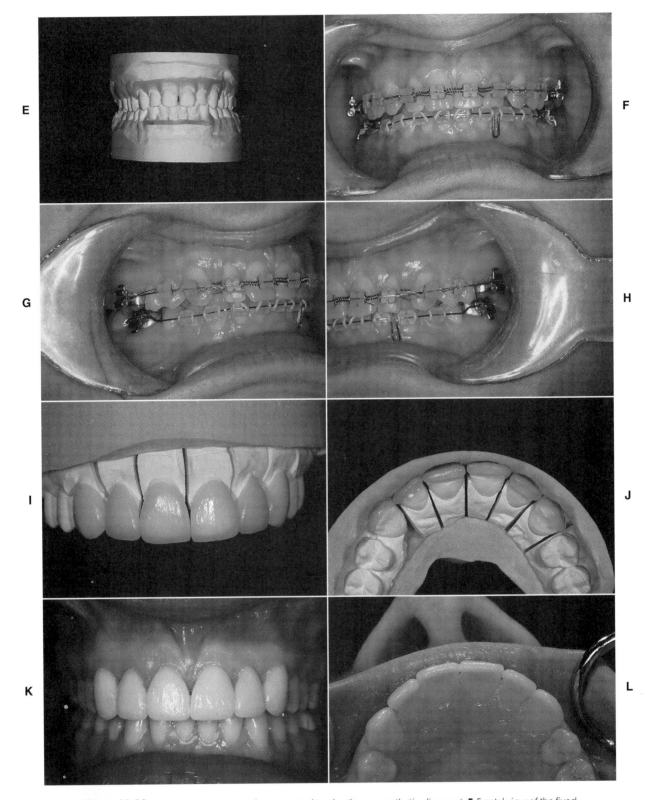

Figure 28-23, cont'd E, A wax setup is constructed to plan the preprosthetic alignment. **F,** Frontal view of the fixed appliances utilized to equalize maxillary interproximal spaces. **G,** Right buccal view shows the use of closed coil springs to open space between the maxillary incisors. **H,** Left buccal view demonstrates the closing loop to close space in the mandibular arch as spaces are equalized between the maxillary incisors. **I,** Frontal view of the porcelain veneers prepared for the maxillary incisors and canines. **J,** Occlusal view of the maxillary arch shows the anterior porcelain veneers used to close the interproximal spaces created by the preprosthetic orthodontic alignment. **K,** Frontal view of the porcelain veneers bonded to the surface of the maxillary incisors and canines. **L,** Occlusal view of the final result reveals that all spaces are closed except for about a 1-mm gap distal to the maxillary canines. Leaving these spaces was more esthetic than overcontouring the veneers.

time of about 12 months, the patient was referred back to the prosthodontist for construction of the porcelain veneers (see Figure 28-23, *I* to *L*).

In this case the Bolton analysis was essential for diagnosis and treatment planning of intermaxillary tooth size discrepancy.[56] Despite the large diastemas and relatively narrow lateral incisors in the maxillary anterior segment, there is a modest excess mandibular tooth size discrepancy that is equally distributed from first molar to first molar (see Figure 28-23, *C* and *D*). Thus, as projected in the wax setup (see Figure 28-23, *E*), it was necessary to close the mandibular anterior space and equalize spaces between the maxillary anterior teeth. To maintain the proper proportions of the maxillary teeth and provide a slight overjet, small residual spaces were retained distal to the maxillary canines. The Bolton analysis was important for multidisciplinary treatment planning. Details of the prosthetic procedures are published elsewhere.[2]

COMPLEX MALOCCLUSIONS

Successful management of mutilated malocclusions requires disciplined diagnostic and treatment planning processes. A thorough history and evaluation of medical factors are important, particularly for patients over 50 years of age.[3] Many partially edentulous adults have a history of dental neglect that has contributed to a cas-

cade of functional compensations that manifest as a complex malocclusion. Rigidly integrated endosseous implants are increasingly important prosthetic and anchorage units that are rapidly expanding the scope of orthodontic practice.[60,68,69]

Complex malocclusions in partially edentulous adults are among the most challenging problems encountered in dental practice. This chapter focuses on complex malocclusions, and multiple sets of case records were used to illustrate fundamental concepts. Emphasis is on biologic considerations, medical factors, and complications.[3-9] The diagnosis and treatment of two complex cases were discussed in previous sections. The case of the patient in Figure 28-7 demonstrates the adjunctive orthodontic treatment of a medically compromised patient. The case of the patient in Figure 28-12 illustrates the principle of directing treatment at eliminating or at least controlling the cause of a compensated malocclusion.

An additional case is included in this section to demonstrate an ordered diagnostic and treatment planning process for the use of implants to open the vertical dimension of occlusion and serve as a source of rigid orthodontic anchorage. An adult female with a severe Class II Division 2 malocclusion complicated by a decreased vertical dimension of occlusion, which is secondary to inadequate posterior occlusal stops, is illustrated in Figure 28-24, *A* to *C*. Figure 28-24, *D*,

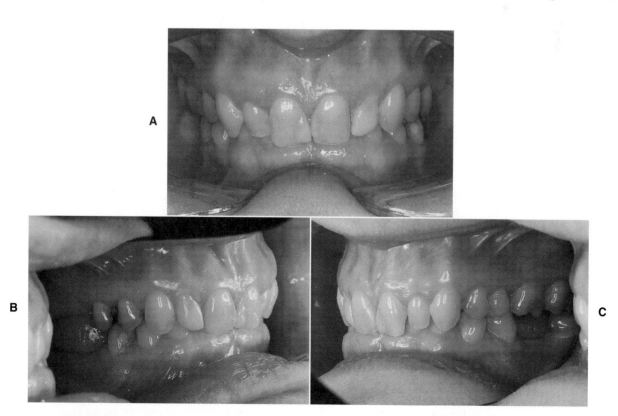

Figure 28-24 A to **C,** Intraoral photographs show the dentition of an adult female with a severe Class II Division 2, partially edentulous malocclusion, which is complicated by an inadequate vertical dimension of occlusion and bruxism.

Continued

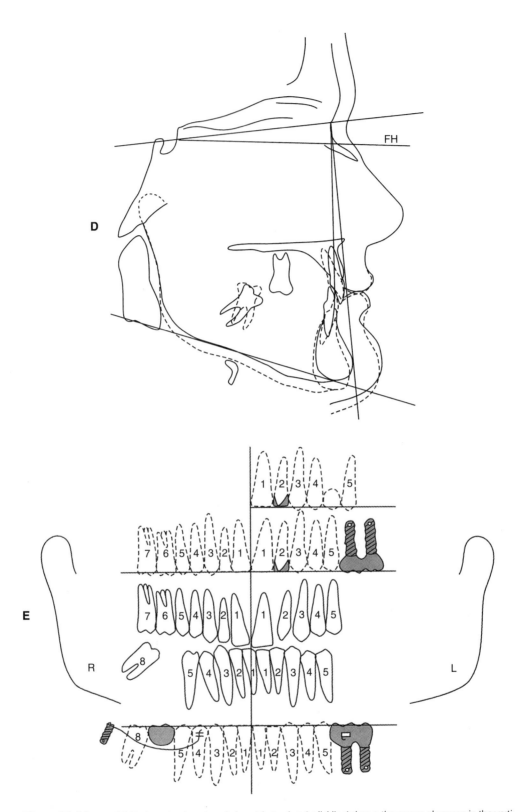

Figure 28-24, cont'd D, A pretreatment cephalometric tracing *(solid line)* shows the severe decrease in the vertical dimension of occlusion, which has resulted in a concave profile. The sagittal visual treatment objective *(dashed line)* projects a more esthetic posterior positioning of the chin as the vertical dimension of occlusion is increased. **E,** Tracing of the pretreatment panoramic radiograph *(solid black line)* is used as a template to construct a panoramic treatment objective. In the mandibular arch *(lower drawing with dashed lines),* a retromolar implant will be used as anchorage to intrude the third molar *(8)* and move it mesially. In the maxillary arch there are two alternative treatment plans: open a space for a pontic between the maxillary left premolars and construct a three-unit fixed prosthesis or place a bone graft in the maxillary sinus on the left side and install two implants to support a fixed prosthesis.

Figure 28-24, cont'd F, A panoramic drawing simulates the occlusal result if the second maxillary treatment option is articulated with the treated mandibular arch shown in **E.** This relationship is the panoramic treatment objective. It is valuable for communicating with the patient and coordinating the sequence of treatment by members of the multidisciplinary team.

shows that about 5 mm of bite opening in the incisal region is needed to restore the vertical dimension of occlusion and to improve the facial profile. Two intra-oral treatment alternatives are offered for restoring occlusion in the maxillary left posterior segment (see Figure 28-24, *E*).

One approach (Plan A) is to open a space between the premolars and place a 3-unit fixed prosthesis. However, the most reliable method for achieving adequate occlusal function is to place a bone graft in the floor of the maxillary sinus (Plan B). After the sinus elevation graft has healed, two or more endosseous implants are placed to support a fixed prosthesis to restore an appropriate plane of occlusion. Figure 28-24, *F*, is a simulation of the interdigitation that is achieved with plan B. This patient's case demonstrates an important principle for restoring occlusal function in partially edentulous patients with a closed vertical dimension of occlusion. It is essential to achieve an adequate bilateral posterior occlusion at the appropriate vertical dimension of occlusion before attempting any substantial orthodontic correction in the anterior segments.

COMPLICATIONS

During the course of treatment the clinician must be alert for common **complications** such as medical problems, temporomandibular disorder, functional shifts, parafunction, abnormal posturing of the mandibular condyle in the temporomandibular fossa, periodontal compromise, and a wide variety of other potential problems. It is important to evaluate progress at every appointment and regularly collect records during the course of treatment. Many technical and treatment-response problems are not obvious clinically but are readily apparent when progress and pretreatment records are compared. Regular collection and evaluation of panoramic and cephalometric radiographs are important for midcourse corrections during adult orthodontic treatment.

Medical Concerns

For all patients in active treatment, the medical history should be updated annually. To monitor medical factors on a more regular basis, the dentist should maintain a dialogue with the patient at each appointment. At the start of each appointed visit the dentist should inquire if any medical or dental problems have occurred since the last appointment. Unless they are informed otherwise, some patients consider medical problems to be of no interest to their dentist. The clinician must make it clear that all health concerns are potentially important. If significant medical problems occur, confer with the patient's physician regarding continuing or interrupting orthodontic treatment. For patients in active orthodontic therapy, medical factors usually can be adequately controlled to complete treatment, but some problems (e.g., recent myocardial infarction) may require interrupting or terminating all elective care.[10] Careful monitoring of medical factors is essential for effective management of adult patients during adjunctive orthodontic treatment or as part of a comprehensive multidisciplinary treatment plan.

Poor Cooperation

Oral hygiene and the periodontal condition should be monitored at each appointment. Treatment with fixed mechanics is contraindicated until the patient has demonstrated the ability to maintain good oral hygiene. When treatment is started on patients with poor hygiene, the situation invariably gets worse and is often uncontrollable. If the patient fails to maintain adequate oral health once treatment is under way or if significant periodontal deterioration is detected, it is wise to remove all fixed appliances, place retainers, and make a referral for hygiene and periodontal therapy as needed. The potential for complications is so high that adjunctive orthodontic treatment is contraindicated for patients with inadequate hygiene or deteriorating periodontal health or both. Compromising dental health in favor of elective orthodontic treatment is not justified. When periodontal problems, caries and enamel decalcification are corrected, appliances can be replaced.

If patients fail to adequately cooperate with the wear of removable appliances, elastics, or headgear, the problem should be confronted sooner rather than later. Cooperation problems that persist for more than 6 months are likely to prolong treatment and result in dental health compromises. Long periods of nonproductive treatment are not in the patient's interest. For this reason, treatment should be terminated or the treatment plan altered to provide an acceptable compromise in a reasonable period. Failure to deal with cooperation problems in a timely manner is a common complication that is a financial drain on the practitioner and a waste of time for the patient.

Technical Problems

To control technical problems that increase treatment time or compromise the result, it is recommended that panoramic radiographs and intraoral photographs be taken at 6-month intervals. Cephalometric radiographs should be obtained every 12 months or more often, if indicated. Superimpositions of tracings on the anterior cranial base, mandible, and maxilla are valuable for identifying complications and determining if treatment is progressing as planned.

When the patient enters the finishing stage, usually following space management and correction of interdigitation, a set of casts should be obtained. The casts are essential for detecting errors in band and bracket placement. Bracket placement problems should be corrected. Pretorqued appliances are designed for torque application at the height of curvature of the labial surfaces. Placing a rectangular arch wire when multiple bracket placement errors are present results in an array of first-, second-, and third-order complications that are nearly impossible to correct by adjusting the arch wires. Timely correction of technical errors prevents alignment complications that prolong treatment time and compromises the final result. Failure to adequately reanalyze progress and correct technical errors in a timely manner complicates finishing, lengthens treatment time, and undermines the confidence of the patient. Because of less favorable biologic considerations and medical factors, adult orthodontic treatment is time consuming and has a high potential for complications. Thus avoiding technical problems is particularly important for adjunctive orthodontic treatment of adults.

Periodontitis and Caries

The most common dental compromise associated with orthodontic treatment of adults is the failure to diagnose and adequately monitor incipient periodontitis (Figure 28-25). All adults should be care-

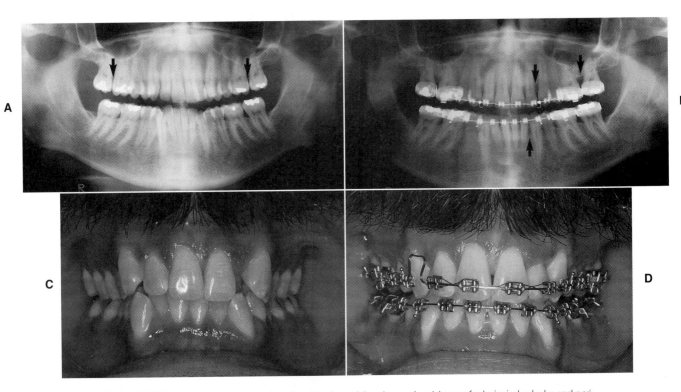

Figure 28-25 A, Pretreatment panoramic radiograph of an adult male reveals evidence of subgingival calculus and periodontitis between the maxillary molars *(arrows).* **B,** A panoramic radiograph to evaluate the progress of orthodontic treatment shows increased bone loss between the maxillary molars as well as in the anterior segments *(arrows).* **C,** Pretreatment frontal view of an adult male with generalized gingival recession. **D,** During treatment, additional gingival recession is noted.

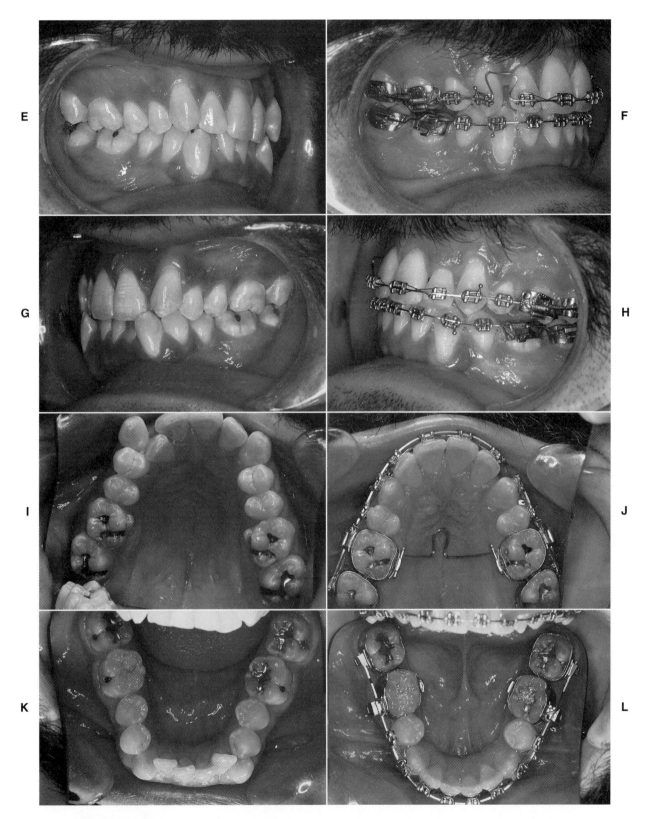

Figure 28-25, cont'd E, Pretreatment right buccal view. **F,** First premolars were extracted to alleviate anterior crowding, and space closure is almost completed. **G,** Pretreatment left buccal view. **H,** Space closure is completed and root alignment is in progress. **I,** Pretreatment maxillary occlusal view. **J,** Anterior space is being closed and the molars are being rotated. **K,** Pretreatment mandibular occlusal view. **L,** Note distal in rotation of first molars because the brackets are positioned too far mesially.

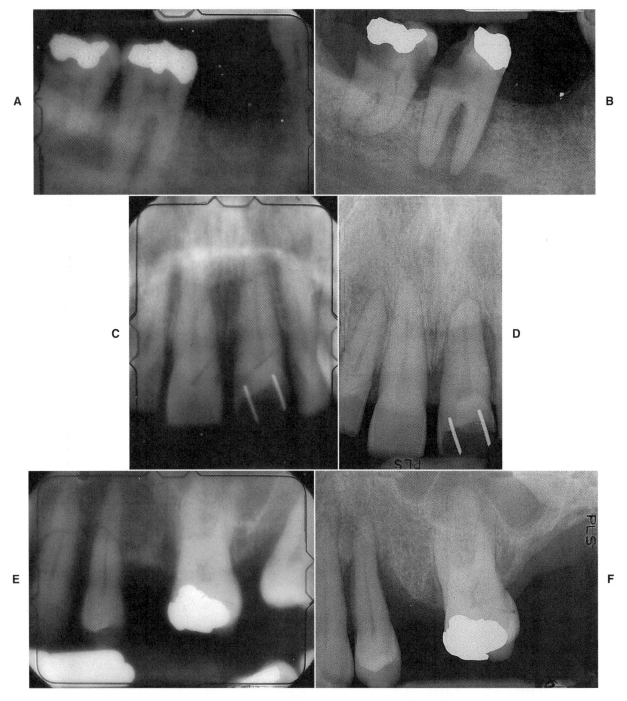

Figure 28-26 Inadequate control of caries and periodontitis in an adult male. **A,** Pretreatment periapical radiograph reveals probable bone loss and caries. **B,** Following orthodontic treatment, rampant caries and periodontitis are evident. **C,** Pretreatment periapical radiograph shows osseous defect around the restored central incisor. **D,** Posttreatment radiograph reveals modest root resorption but advanced bone loss. **E,** Pretreatment radiograph of the left maxillary buccal segment shows probable osseous defects around the first premolar and first molar. **F,** Posttreatment view. The lesion on the mesial side of the first molar does not appear to have advanced bone loss, but marked bone loss is noted around the first premolar and canine. (Radiographs courtesy of Dr. David Engen.)

fully diagnosed periodontally before treatment, and continuously maintained during therapy, and regularly evaluated thereafter. It is all too common for the clinician to concentrate on correcting the occlusion and to ignore the periodontium. A rigorous, systematic, and continuous evaluation program is essential

(see Chapter 24). Deterioration of the periodontium is an unacceptable complication for adult orthodontic treatment.

Complex mutilated malocclusions are challenging problems requiring comprehensive treatment that is best accomplished by a multidisciplinary team. One member of the team must assume a leadership position in coordinating the treatment and maintaining close communication with the patient. Orthodontics is a cost-effective aspect of treatment for many periodontally compromised patients. However, adult orthodontic treatment can be destructive and counterproductive in the absence of a well-coordinated, comprehensive plan for multidisciplinary treatment (Figure 28-26). It is unwise for a single practitioner to assume all aspects of a complex mutilated case because of the following:

1. Multiple areas of specialized training are usually needed to achieve an optimal result.
2. A single practitioner tends to focus on only one aspect of the overall treatment, paying inadequate attention to other factors.
3. A team of clinicians provides an internal system of professional review that is more likely to detect and control complications that may compromise treatment.

Interaction of a multidisciplinary team is the most effective means for routinely achieving optimal results in managing complex, partially edentulous malocclusions. It is essential that all members of the team monitor the periodontium during treatment and that one member (usually a periodontist) has the responsibility for regular periodontal maintenance.

Temporomandibular Disorders

Common stomatognathic functional complications of adult orthodontic treatment are temporomandibular disorders and abnormal soft tissue posture. Significant deterioration in temporomandibular function is manifest as clicks, pops, decreased range of motion, or locks on opening or closing (see Chapter 27).

Minor, transient symptoms of temporomandibular disorder are so common that they fall into the range of normal for many patients. For a minor problem there may be no need for specific dental treatment, but patients should be questioned about abusive habits such as excessively wide opening, gum chewing, abnormal sleep posture, or facial trauma. Treatment may be as simple as identifying the bad habit and eliminating it. Reassurance and a prescribed period of rest with limited function may be all that is needed.

However, if the temporomandibular joint disorder is painful or there is a clear relationship of symptoms to orthodontic changes in occlusion, the problem should be carefully evaluated. A flat-plane orthotic appliance in either arch is an effective diagnostic tool for removing the influence of nocuous occlusal interferences. Routine problems usually resolve in a few days, and the offending interference can be identified by mounting casts on an articulator. Once the occlusal problem is identified, orthodontic adjustments are designed to

eliminate functional interferences to achieve a comfortable path of closure with the orthotic appliance removed. If the temporomandibular joint problem is not resolved by this conservative procedure, the patient should be referred to a clinician with specific interest and training in managing temporomandibular joint disorders. Specific imaging and other specialized procedures may be indicated.

SUMMARY

Compared to the management of children and adolescents, adult orthodontic treatment is more challenging because there is a higher probability of medical and dental compromise. Predictable management of malocclusions in adults is facilitated by a disciplined evaluation process. The orthodontist should begin with an overall consideration of the patient's health and then progress through an orderly evaluation of the face, oral cavity, periodontium, teeth, and malocclusion.

Potential orthodontic patients over the age of 50 are at high risk for developing osteoporosis (i.e., approximately 44% present with sufficient risk factors to justify a medical evaluation). With appropriate medical management, osteopenic and osteoporotic patients are good candidates for orthodontic therapy.

Predominantly genetic problems tend to be symmetric while epigenetic (environmental) problems are asymmetric. It is wise to define the probable cause of the malocclusion and direct treatment toward alleviating or eliminating the cause of the specific problems.

Successful management of mutilated malocclusions requires a disciplined, diagnostic, and treatment planning process. A thorough history and medical evaluation is important, particularly for patients over 50 years of age.[3] Many partially edentulous adults have a history of dental neglect that has resulted in a cascade of functional compensations that are manifest as a complex malocclusion.

Before the start of orthodontic treatment, caries must be eliminated and periodontitis must be well controlled. Once treatment is under way it is important to adhere to a rigorous periodontal maintenance program, usually at 3-month intervals, and regularly evaluate root resorption and orthodontic progress at least every 6 months. Attention must be directed at technical problems such as bracket positioning errors that may lengthen treatment, compromise the result, and undermine the confidence of the patient.

ACKNOWLEDGMENTS

The authors gratefully acknowledge the collaboration of numerous colleagues, including Drs. Charles Goodacre,

Steven Haug, David Brown, John Phelps, Jerry Andres, Charles Nelson, Mark Wohlford, Marc Olsen, Mark Anderson, Larry Garetto, Munro Peacock, Conrad Johnston, Charles Slemenda (posthumous), Gordon Arbuckle (posthumous), Charles Coghlan, Brady Hancock, Tom Barco, Lawrence Falender, Charles Pritchett, Craig Thomson, Richard Herd, and David Engen.

REFERENCES

1. Hohlt WF, Roberts WE: Clinical orthodontics in predoctoral education, 6 years of experience at Indiana University, *Indiana Dent Assoc J* 76(2):9-13, 1997.
2. Hohlt WF, Hovijitra S: Multidisciplinary treatment of anterior spacing by orthodontic and prosthodontic management, *Indiana Dent Assoc J* 78(3):18-23, 1999.
3. Roberts WE: Adjunctive orthodontic therapy in adults over 50 years of age, clinical management of compensated, partially edentulous malocclusions, *Indiana Dent Assoc J* 76(2):33-41, 1997.
4. Roberts WE: Dental implant anchorage for cost-effective management of dental and skeletal malocclusion. In Epker BN, Stella JP, Fish LC (eds): *Dentofacial deformities,* vol IV, ed 2, St Louis, 1999, Mosby.
5. Roberts WE: Tooth movement, ankylosis and implant anchorage, a physiological continuum, *Indiana Dent Assoc J* 78(3):24-32, 1999.
6. Roberts WE: Bone physiology, metabolism, and biomechanics in orthodontic practice. In Graber TM, Vanarsdall RL Jr (eds): *Orthodontics: current principles and techniques,* ed 3, St Louis, 2000, Mosby.
7. Roberts WE: Orthodontic anchorage with osseointegrated implants: bone physiology, metabolism and biomechanics. In Higuchi KW (ed): *Orthodontic applications of osseointegrated implants,* Chicago, 2000, Quintessence.
8. Roberts WE, Baldwin JJ: Pre-prosthetic alignment of a compensated class II malocclusion in a partially edentulous adult, *Case Studies Orthod* 3(1):1-6, 2000.
9. Roberts WE, Hartsfield JK: Multidisciplinary management of congenital and acquired compensated malocclusions, *Indiana Dent Assoc J* 76(2):42-51, 1997.
10. Chanavaz M: Screening and medical evaluation of adults, absolute and relative contraindications for invasive dental procedures, *Indiana Dent Assoc J* 78(3):10-17, 1999.
11. Looker AC et al: Prevalence of low femoral bone density in older adults from NHANES III, *J Bone Miner Res* 12:1761-1768, 1997.
12. Slemenda CW et al: Predictors of bone mass in perimenopausal women: a prospective study of clinical data using photon absorptiometry, *Ann Intern Med* 112:96-101, 1990.
13. Becker AR, Roberts WE, Garetto LP: Osteoporosis risk factors in female dental patients: a preliminary report, *Indiana Dent Assoc J* 76(2):15-19, 1997.
14. Roberts WE et al: What are the risk factors of osteoporosis? *J Am Dent Assoc* 122(2):59-61, 1991.
15. Roberts WE et al: Bone physiology and metabolism in dental implantology: risk factors for osteoporosis and other metabolic bone diseases, *Implant Dent* 1:11-21, 1992.
16. Hansen MA et al: Potential risk factors for development of postmenopausal osteoporosis—examined over a 12-year period, *Osteoporosis Int* 1(2):95-102, 1991.
17. Frost HM: *Intermediary organization of the skeleton,* vol 1, Boca Raton, Fla, 1986, CRC Press.
18. Garetto LP et al: Remodeling dynamics of bone supporting rigidly fixed titanium implants: a histomorphometric comparison in four species including humans, *Implant Dent* 4:235-243, 1995.
19. Chen J et al: Mechanical response to functional and therapeutic loading of a retromolar endosseous implant utilized for orthodontic anchorage to mesially translate mandibular molars, *Implant Dent* 4:246-258, 1995.
20. Huja SS et al: Microhardness and anisotropy of the vital osseous interface and bone supporting endosseous implants, *J Orthopaed Res* 16(1):54-60, 1998.
21. Davidovitch Z: Cell biology associated with orthodontic tooth movement. In Berkovitz BJB, Moxham BJ, Newman HN (eds): *The periodontal ligament in health and disease,* ed 2, London, 1995, Mosby-Wolfe.
22. Moxham BJ, Berkovitz BKB: The effects of external forces on the periodontal ligament. In Berkovitz BJB, Moxham BJ, Newman HN (eds): *The periodontal ligament in health and disease,* ed 2, London, 1995, Mosby-Wolfe.
23. Rygh P, Budvik P: The histological responses of the periodontal ligament to horizontal orthodontic loads. In Berkovitz BJB, Moxham BJ, Newman HN (eds): *The periodontal ligament in health and disease,* ed 2, London, 1995, Mosby-Wolfe.
24. Proffit WR, Fields H Jr: *Contemporary orthodontics,* ed 3, St Louis, 2000, Mosby.
25. Mortensen L et al: Risedronate increases bone mass in an early postmenopausal population: two years of treatment plus one year of follow-up, *J Clin Endocrinol Metab* 83:396-402, 1998.
26. Schairer C et al: Menopausal estrogen and estrogen-progestin replacement therapy and breast cancer risk, *JAMA* 283:485-491, 2000.
27. Willett WC, Colditz G, Stampfer M: Postmenopausal estrogens: opposed, unopposed, or none of the above, *JAMA* 283:534-535, 2000.
28. Sietsma WK et al: Antiresorptive dose-response relationships across three generations of bisphosphonates, *Drugs Exp Clin Res* 15:389-396, 1989.
29. Starck WJ, Epker BN: Failure of osseointegrated dental implants after diphosphonate therapy for osteoporosis: a case report, *Int J Oral Maxillofac Implants* 10:74-78, 1995.
30. von Wowern N, Kollerup G: Symptomatic osteoporosis: a risk factor for residual ridge reduction in the jaws, *J Prosthet Dent* 67:656-660, 1992.
31. Harai T et al: Osteoporosis and reduction of residual ridge in edentulous patients, *J Prosthet Dent* 69:49-56, 1993.
32. Cawood JI, Howell RA: Reconstructive preprosthetic surgery. I. Anatomical considerations, *Int J Oral Maxillofac Surg* 20(2):75-82, 1991.
33. Payne JB et al: Longitudinal alveolar bone loss in postmenopausal osteoporotic/osteopenic women, *Osteoporosis Int* 10(1):34-40, 1999.
34. Mohammed AR, Brunsvold M, Bauer R: The strength of association between systemic postmenopausal osteoporosis and periodontal disease, *Int J Prosthodont* 9(5):479-483, 1996.

35. Baxter JC: Osteoporosis: oral manifestation of a systemic disease, *Quintessence Int* 18:427-429, 1987.

36. Krall EA et al: Tooth loss and skeletal bone density in healthy postmenopausal women, *Osteoporos Int* 4: 104,109, 1994.

37. Jeffcoat MK et al: Nuclear medicine techniques for the detection of active alveolar bone loss, *Adv Dent Res* 1:80-84, 1987.

38. Reddy MS et al: Detection of periodontal disease activity with a scintillation camera, *J Dent Res* 70:50-54, 1991.

39. Tricker ND, Garetto LP: Cortical bone turnover and mineral apposition in dentate dog mandible, *J Dental Res* 76SI:201, 1997 (abstract).

40. Paganini-Hill A: The benefits of estrogen replacement therapy on oral health, *Arch Intern Med* 155:2325-2329, 1995.

41. Grodstein F, Colditz GA, Stampfer MJ: Postmenopausal hormone use and tooth loss: a prospective study, *J Am Dent Assoc* 127:370-377, 1996.

42. Kornman KS, Loesche WJ: Effects of estradiol and progesterone on Bacteroides melaninogenicus and Bacteroides gingivalis, *Infect Immun* 35:256-263, 1982.

43. Reinhardt RA et al: Gingival fluid IL-1beta in postmenopausal females on supportive periodontal therapy: a longitudinal 2-year study, *J Clin Periodontol* 25(12):1029-1035, 1988.

44. Reinhardt RA et al: Influence of estrogen and osteopenia/osteoporosis on clinical periodontitis in postmenopausal women, *J Periodontol* 70(8):823-828, 1999.

45. Dao TT, Anderson JD, Zarb GA: Is osteoporosis a risk factor for osseointegration of dental implants, *Int J Oral Maxillofac Implants* 8:137-144, 1993.

46. Fujimoto T et al: Osseointegrated implants in a patient with osteoporosis: a case report, *Int J Oral Maxillofac Implants* 11:539-542, 1996.

47. Jee WSS et al: Corticosteroid and bone, *Am J Anat* 129:477-480, 1970.

48. Ashcraft MB, Southard KA, Tolley EA: The effect of corticosteroid-induced osteoporosis on orthodontic tooth movement, *Am J Orthod Dentofacial Orthop* 102:310-319, 1992.

49. Garetto LP et al: Remodeling dynamics of bone supporting rigidly fixed titanium implants: a histomorphometric comparison in four species including humans, *Implant Dent* 4:235-243, 1995.

50. Karpf DB et al: Prevention of nonvertebral fractures by alendronate: a meta-analysis, *JAMA* 277:1159-1164, 1997.

51. Cummings SR et al: The effect of raloxifene on risk of breast cancer in postmenopausal women, *JAMA* 281:2189-2197, 1999.

52. Southard KA et al: The relationship between the density of the alveolar processes and that of post-cranial bone, *J Dent Res* 79(4):964-969, 2000.

53. Meskin LH, Brown LJ: Sociodemographic differences in tooth loss patterns in U.S. employed adults and seniors, 1985-86, *Gerodontics* 4:345-362, 1988.

54. Meskin LH et al: Patterns of tooth loss and accumulated prosthetic treatment potential in U.S. employed adults and seniors, 1985-86, *Gerodontics* 4:126-135, 1988.

55. Okeson JP: *Management of temporomandibular disorders and occlusion,* ed 4, St Louis, 1998, Mosby.

56. Bolton WA: Disharmony in tooth size and its relation to the analysis and treatment of malocclusion, *Am J Orthod* 28:113-130, 1958.

57. Potter RHY: The genetics of tooth size. In Stewart RE, Prescott GH (eds): *Oral facial genetics,* St Louis, 1976, Mosby.

58. van Limborgh J: Morphogenetic control of craniofacial growth. In McNamara JA Jr, Ribbens KA, Howe RP (eds): *Clinical alteration of the growing face,* Center for Human Growth and Development, Ann Arbor, Mich, 1983, University of Michigan.

59. Kerschbaum T: Long-term prognosis of conventional prosthodontic restorations. In Naert I, van Steenberghe D, Worthington P (eds): *Osseointegration in oral rehabilitation,* London, 1993, Quintessence.

60. Roberts WE, Arbuckle GR, Analoui M: Rate of mesial translation of mandibular molars utilizing implant-anchored mechanics, *Angle Orthod* 66:331-337, 1996.

61. Hohlt WF, Roberts WE: Orthodontic education at Indiana University: a new philosophy of specialty and general practice, *Indiana Dent Assoc J* 69(5):19-24, 1990.

62. Roberts WE: Orthodontics in the main stream, *Indiana Dent Assoc J* 76(2):4-6, 1997.

63. Roberts WE: Reflecting on the Orthodontic Educational Development Symposium: was there any real progress in defining the scope of orthodontic education for general dentists and other specialists? *Am J Orthod Dentofacial Orthop* 111:110-115, 1997.

64. Roberts WE, Gibert RP, Puig MAB: Assessment of malocclusion. In Hall WB et al (eds): *Decision making in dental treatment planning,* ed 2, St Louis, 1998, Mosby.

65. Kokich VG: Esthetics: the orthodontic-periodontic restorative connection, *Semin Orthod* 2(1):21-30, 1996.

66. Hall WB et al: *Decision making in dental treatment planning,* ed 2, St Louis, 1998, Mosby.

67. Salama N, Salama M: The role of orthodontic extrusive remodeling in the enhancement of the soft and hard tissue profiles prior to implant placement: a systematic approach to the management of extraction site defects, *Int J Periodontics Restorative Dent* 13(4):312-333, 1993.

68. Goodacre CJ et al: Prosthodontic considerations when using implants for orthodontic anchorage, *J Prosthet Dent* 77(2):162-170, 1997.

69. Higuchi KW: *Orthodontic application of osseointegrated implants,* Chicago, 2000, Quintessence.

CHAPTER 29

Dental and Facial Asymmetries

Samir E. Bishara, Paul S. Burkey, John G. Kharouf, and Athanasious E. Athanasiou

KEY TERMS

facial symmetry	qualitative asymmetries	functional asymmetries	posteroanterior projection
genetics	dental asymmetries	lateral cephalometric	TMJ imaging
intrauterine pressure	skeletal asymmetries	radiograph	magnetic resonance imaging
environmental factors	muscular and soft tissue	panoramic radiograph	computed tomography
quantitative asymmetries	asymmetry		

Although each person shares with the rest of the population a great many characteristics, there are enough differences to make each human being a unique individual. Such limitless variation in the size, shape, and relationship of the dental, skeletal, and soft tissue facial structures are important in providing each individual with his or her own identity.

Perfect bilateral body symmetry is more of a theoretic concept that seldom exists in living organisms. Right-left differences occur everywhere in nature where two congruent but mirror image types are present. In general, mammals have marked asymmetry as to the placement of the viscera in the body cavity. Man frequently experiences functional as well as morphologic asymmetries (e.g., right and left handedness as well as a preference for one eye or one leg). Some of these asymmetries are embryonically rooted and are associated with asymmetry in the central nervous system.[1]

Dorland's Medical Dictionary defines symmetry as "the similar arrangement in form and relationships of parts around a common axis or on each side of a plane of the body."[2] Clinically, symmetry means balance, whereas significant asymmetry means imbalance.[3]

Facial asymmetry, being a common phenomenon, was probably first observed by the artists of early Greek statuary who recorded what they had found in nature—normal facial asymmetry.[1] Asymmetry in the craniofacial areas can be recognized as differences in the size or relationships of the two sides of the face. This may be the result of discrepancies either in the form of individual bones or a malposition of one or more bones in the craniofacial complex. The asymmetry may also be limited to the overlying soft tissues.[3]

Peck and Peck[4] evaluated bilateral **facial symmetry** in 52 "exceptionally well-balanced" white adults and observed that there is less asymmetry and more dimensional stability as the cranium is approached.

The point at which normal asymmetry becomes abnormal cannot be easily defined and is often determined by the clinician's sense of balance and the patient's perception of the imbalance.

Clinical facial asymmetry in the craniofacial complex ranges from the barely detectable to gross discrepancies between the right and left halves of the face. By collating photographs of the right and left sides of normal faces with their respective mirror images, three faces can be visualized: the original, the two left sides, and the two right sides. Most often these three faces of the same individual are distinctly different.[4-6]

Woo[7] evaluated ancient Egyptian skulls and found that the bones of the cranium showed asymmetry with the right frontal, temporal, and parietal bones being larger. The contralateral side of the facial complex exhibited an asymmetry with the left zygoma and maxilla being larger.

In a study on a more contemporary population to determine the symmetry of the various parts of the face, Vig and Hewitt[8] evaluated 63 posteroanterior cephalograms of normal children who were 9 to 18 years of age. *Normal*, in this case, meant that the child exhibited no clinically evident facial asymmetry. An overall asymmetry was found in most of the children with the left side being larger. The cranial base and mandibular regions exhibited a left side excess, whereas the maxillary region showed a larger right side. The dentoalveolar region exhibited the greatest degree of symmetry. Vig and Hewitt[8,9] concluded that compensatory changes seem to operate in the development of the dentoalveolar structures. These changes enable bilateral symmetric function and maximum intercuspation to occur, thus minimizing the effects of the underlying asymmetry in the arrangement and size of the jaws.

In a longitudinal study evaluating the changes in mandibular asymmetry, Melnik[10] found no significant gender differences by the age of 14 years. They also observed that relative to 6 years of age, there was an equal probability for mandibular asymmetry to improve by the age of 16 years.

ETIOLOGY

Many explanations have been offered as to the cause of asymmetries including genetic imperfections in the mechanism, which was meant to create symmetry, and environmental factors producing decided right-left differences.[1,11,12]

Genetics have been implicated in certain conditions such as multiple neurofibromatosis which has a familial incidence associated with a dominant gene (Figure 29-1).[13,14] Another example of significant facial asymmetry occurs with hemifacial microsomia (Figure 29-2).

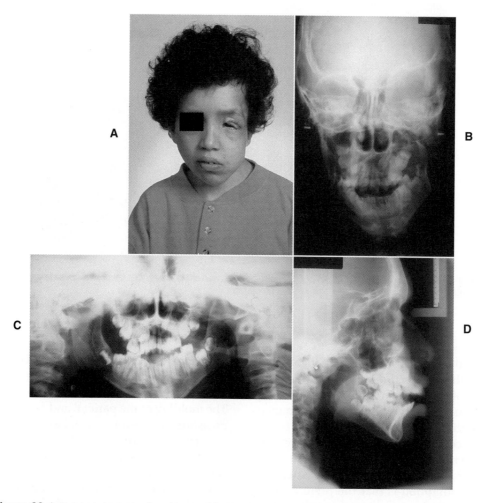

Figure 29-1 Facial photograph of an 11-year-old girl with neurofibromatosis **(A)**. The lesion is also apparent in anteroposterior **(B)**, panoramic **(C)**, and lateral **(D)** cephalometric radiographs.

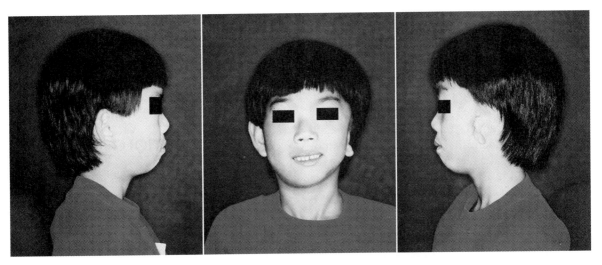

Figure 29-2 Facial photographs of a patient with hemifacial microsomia. The discrepancies involve only one side of the face and include asymmetries in the mandibular body, ramus, and condyle as well as the external and internal structures of the ear. (From Bishara SE, Burkey PS, Kharouf JG: *Angle Orthod* 64[2]:89-98, 1994. Courtesy of Dr. Deborah Zeitler.)

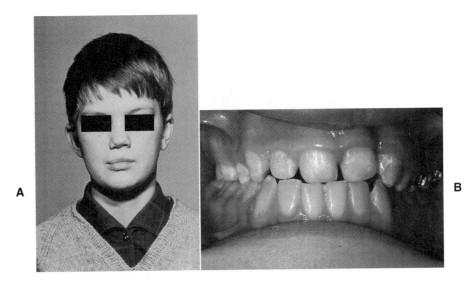

Figure 29-3 Facial (**A**) and intraoral (**B**) photographs of an 11-year-old boy with operated cleft lip and palate. Note the tendency for the unilateral anterior and posterior crossbites.

Some clefts of the lip or palate are genetically influenced and result in a facial deformity with an associated collapse of the maxillary dental arch (Figure 29-3).[12] Such an asymmetry should show a chance distribution to either the right or left side. Yet some unilateral clefts occur roughly twice as often on the left side as on the right. Because it is difficult to find any nongenetic factor that accounts for such an asymmetry, the assumption is that the preference is associated with genetic differences between the halves of the body.[1]

Intrauterine pressure during pregnancy and significant pressure at the birth canal during parturition can have observable effects on the bones of the fetal skull. The molding of the parietal and facial bones from these pressures can result in facial asymmetry. These effects are generally transient with a rapid restoration of the normal relationships of the skull within a few weeks to several months.[15]

Craniofacial asymmetry can be caused by environmental factors including pathologic changes that are not necessarily congenital in nature. Osteochondroma

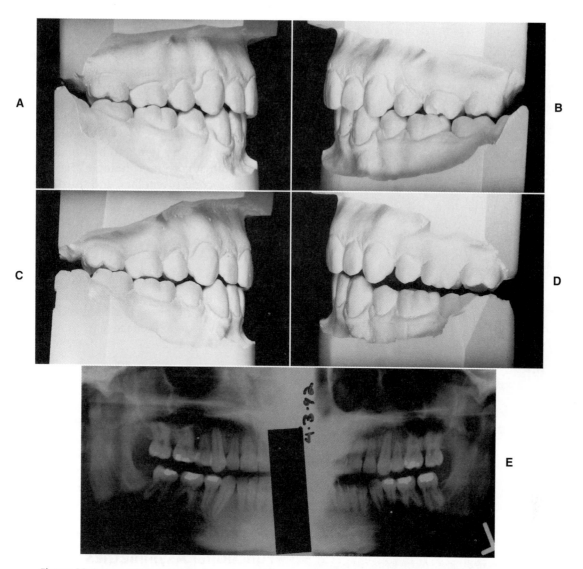

Figure 29-4 **A** and **B,** Photographs of posttreatment dental casts obtained on a 20-year-old patient treated orthodontically. Notice bilateral posterior interdigitation. **C** and **D,** Nine months posttreatment an open bite was developing on the posterior left side. **E,** The patient was diagnosed as having an osteochondroma in the left condyle. Treatment included an additional phase of orthodontic treatment as well as surgery to correct the resulting malocclusion and remove the lesion. (**A** to **D** From Bishara SE, Burkey PS, Kharouf JG: *Angle Orthod* 64[2]:89-98, 1994.)

of the mandibular condyle results in facial asymmetry, open bite on the involved side, and mandibular deviation (Figure 29-4).[16]

Trauma and infection must also be considered when encountering facial asymmetry. Untreated fractures of the mandible can display varying degrees of facial disfigurement. Trauma and infection within the temporomandibular joint (TMJ) could result in ankylosis of the condyle to the temporal bone (Figure 29-5).[17] Ankylosis in the growing child leads to unilateral mandibular underdevelopment on the affected side.[18] Damage to a nerve may indirectly lead to asymmetry from the loss of muscle function and tone.

In a detailed study of the asymmetries in the dental arches and face, Lundstrom[1] explained that asymme-

try can be genetic or nongenetic in origin and that it is usually a combination of both. Some of the right-left asymmetries in the oral cavity could be the result of **environmental factors** (e.g., sucking habits or asymmetric chewing habits caused by dental caries, extractions, and trauma).[1]

According to Lundstrom,[1] asymmetry can also be described as either qualitative (all or none) or quantitative. From an orthodontic viewpoint, examples of **quantitative asymmetries** could be differences in the number of teeth on each side or the presence of a cleft lip and palate. Examples of **qualitative asymmetries** could be differences in the size of teeth, the location of teeth in the arches, or the overall position of the arches in the head.[1]

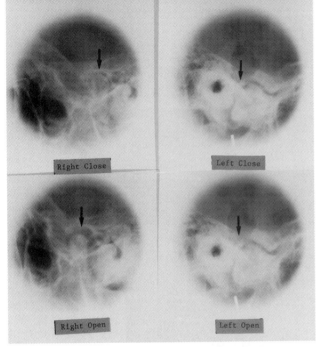

Figure 29-5 Patient with an ankylosed left temporomandibular joint as a result of an accident at 3 years of age. The fractured condyle was not treated, which resulted in a bony ankylosis possibly following hemorrhage and fibrosis. The patient had limited mouth opening and mandibular underdevelopment accompanied with a mandibular shift to the left side **(A). B,** Radiographs of the right and left joints during open and closed mandibular positions indicate no movement in the left joint where the bony ankylosis is apparent. (From Bishara SE, Burkey PS, Kharouf JG: *Angle Orthod* 64[2]:89-98, 1994.)

STRUCTURAL CLASSIFICATION OF DENTOFACIAL ASYMMETRIES

Asymmetries can be classified according to the structures that are involved.

Dental Asymmetries

Dental asymmetries can be caused by local factors such as early loss of primary teeth (Figure 29-6), congenitally missing teeth (Figure 29-7), and habits such as thumb sucking. Lack of exactness in genetic expression affects the teeth on the right and left sides, causing asymmetries in mesiodistal crown diameters.[1]

Garn, Lewis, and Kerewsky[19] found that tooth size asymmetry generally does not involve an entire side of the arch. On the other hand, teeth in the same morphologic class tend to have the same direction of asymmetry. For example, if the maxillary first premolar is larger on the right side, the maxillary second premolar will also tend to be larger on the right side, but the molars need not be larger on that side. In addition, asymmetry tends to be greater for the more distal tooth in each morphologic class (i.e., the lateral incisors, second premolars, and third molars). Asymmetry may also be confined to the shape of the dental arches.

Skeletal Asymmetries

The **skeletal asymmetries** may involve one bone such as the maxilla or the mandible (Figure 29-8). Or they may involve a number of skeletal and muscular structures on one side of the face (e.g., in hemifacial microsomia) (see Figure 29-2).

Muscular and Soft Tissue Asymmetries

Facial disproportions and midline discrepancies could be the result of **muscular and soft tissue asymmetry** such as with hemifacial atrophy or cerebral palsy.[20] Sometimes muscle size is ill proportioned as in masseter hypertrophy[21] or dermatomyositis (Figure 29-9) and also from neoplasms[22] (Figure 29-10). Abnormal muscle function often results in skeletal and dental deviations.[21]

Functional Asymmetries

Functional asymmetries can result from the mandible being deflected laterally or anteroposteriorly if occlusal interferences prevent proper intercuspation in centric relation (Figure 29-11).[23,24] These functional deviations may be caused by a constricted maxillary arch (even if the constriction, in itself, is symmetric) or by a more localized factor such as a malposed tooth. The abnormal initial tooth contact in centric relation results in the subsequent mandibular displacement in centric occlusion.

In some cases TMJ derangements and incoordination accompanied by an anteriorly displaced disk without reduction may result in a midline shift during opening caused by interferences in mandibular translation on the affected side (Figure 29-12).

Using a computer-aided appraisal, Schmid, Mongini, and Felisio[25] assessed and quantified the different components that can lead to mandibular asymmetry during or at the end of the growth period. They found that 75% (N = 14) of the patients had structural asymmetry, whereas 10% (N = 2) had displacement asymmetry.

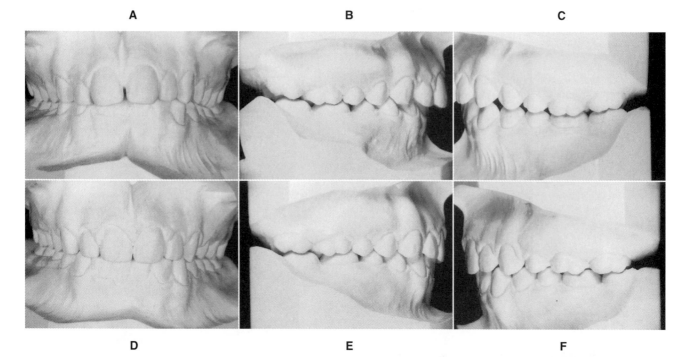

Figure 29-6 **A** to **C,** Dental cast photographs of a patient with a Class II Division 1 malocclusion, subdivision left. The Class II occlusion on the left side was the result of premature loss of the maxillary second primary molar. **D** to **F,** Posttreatment model photographs of the same patient treated with the asymmetric extraction of a maxillary left first premolar. The left molars were treated to a Class II relationship and the canines to a Class I relationship. (From Bishara SE, Burkey PS, Kharouf JG: *Angle Orthod* 64[2]:89-98, 1994.)

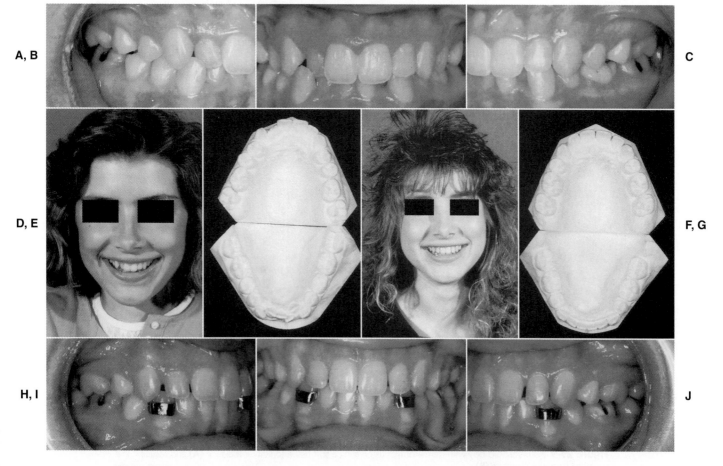

Figure 29-7 **A** to **E,** A case presenting a number of dental arch asymmetries including retained mandibular left second primary molar, congenitally missing mandibular left second premolar, and unilateral anterior crossbite between the maxillary lateral incisor and mandibular canine. **F** to **J,** Posttreatment intraoral, facial, and model photographs of the same patient. Treatment included the extraction of the primary tooth and three premolars to equalize tooth substance in all four quadrants of the dental arches. (From Bishara SE, Burkey PS, Kharouf JG: *Angle Orthod* 64[2]:89-98, 1994.)

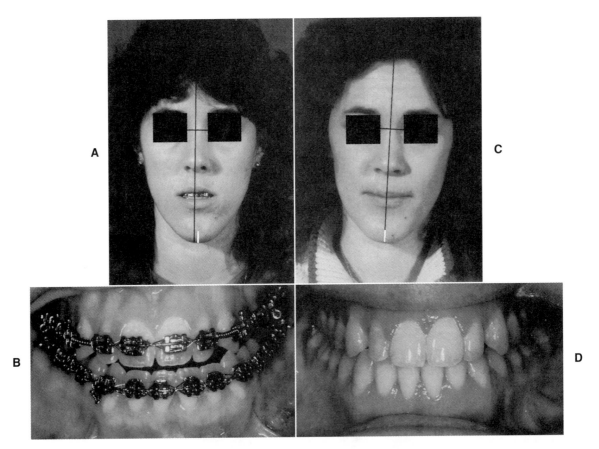

Figure 29-8 **A** and **B,** Patient with a skeletal mandibular asymmetry. Mandibular dental midline was shifted 7.0 mm to the left of the maxillary midline. The right side had a severe Class III malocclusion, and the left side was closer to a Class I relation. In this case the large asymmetry in the occlusal relationship is a reflection of the skeletal asymmetry. Treatment required orthognathic surgery that allowed for mandibular rotation and reduction. **C** and **D,** Posttreatment frontal facial and intraoral photographs. Despite the correction of the skeletal asymmetry, there is still some subtle soft tissue facial asymmetry. Also note that the mandibular midline was slightly overcorrected. (From Bishara SE, Burkey PS, Kharouf JG: *Angle Orthod* 64[2]:89-98, 1994.)

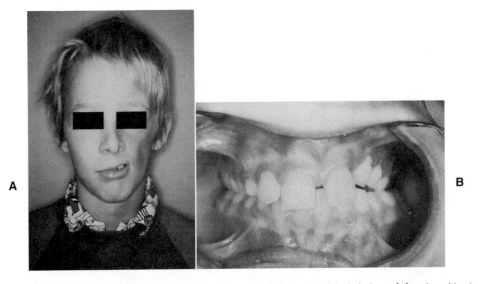

Figure 29-9 A 10-year-old boy with dermatomyositis creating a soft tissue tonicity imbalance **(A)** and resulting in a unilateral posterior crossbite **(B).**

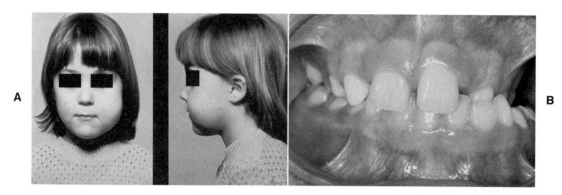

Figure 29-10 A 10-year-old girl with lymphangioma "infrabulbare" **(A)** applying excessive pressure on the left maxillary teeth creating a unilateral left posterior crossbite **(B)**.

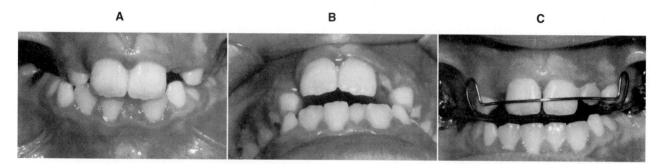

Figure 29-11 A, Intraoral photograph in centric occlusion of a patient in the early mixed dentition with unilateral right posterior crossbite. Notice that the dental midlines coincide. **B,** Intraoral photograph of the same patient in centric relation. Note the shift in the lower midline. Posterior occlusion was cusp on cusp buccolingually. **C,** Intraoral photograph taken following expansion of the maxillary arch and alignment of the mandibular incisors with a lingual arch. A maxillary Hawley was then constructed that incorporated a posterior bite plate and a lingual flange to help maintain the correction. Note the correction of the dental midlines. (From Bishara SE, Burkey PS, Kharouf JG: *Angle Orthod* 64[2]:89-98, 1994.)

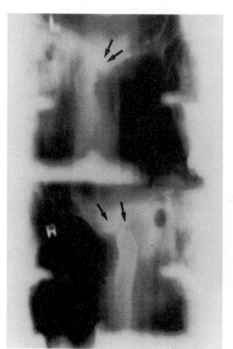

Figure 29-12 Tomograms obtained on the temporomandibular joints of a patient with an anteriorly displaced disk on the left side *(top arrows)*. Notice the significant reduction in the joint space on the left side compared with the right side *(bottom arrows)*. In most functional deviations the mandibular shift occurs during closure following initial tooth contact. When a unilateral anteriorly displaced disk without reduction is present, the mandible may shift to the affected side during the opening cycle. This is because the displaced disk may not allow the mandible to translate as far forward as on the normal side. During closure the mandibular midline shifts back to its normal position in centric occlusion. (From Bishara SE, Burkey PS, Kharouf JG: *Angle Orthod* 64[2]:89-98, 1994.)

In summary, the three main causes of facial asymmetry and dental midline irregularities are (1) true skeletal asymmetries of the facial structures including the mandible and maxilla, (2) dental asymmetries in one or both arches, (3) and functional shifts of the mandible during closure or opening. A combination of these factors can be present. Therefore each patient needs to be carefully evaluated for the clinician to arrive at a proper diagnosis.

DIAGNOSIS

An important aspect of diagnosing asymmetries is obtaining a thorough dental and medical history including a history of trauma, arthritis, and progressive changes in the occlusion.

In diagnosing facial and dental asymmetries, a thorough clinical examination and radiographic surveys are necessary to determine the extent of the soft tissue, skeletal, dental, and functional involvement.

Clinical Examination

Clinical examination can reveal asymmetry in the vertical, anteroposterior or lateral directions.

Evaluation of the Dental Midlines

The clinical examination should include an evaluation of the dental midlines in the following positions: mouth open, in centric relation, at initial contact, and in centric occlusion. True asymmetries of skeletal or dental origins, if uncomplicated by other factors, exhibit similar midline discrepancies in centric relation and in centric occlusion.[23] On the other hand, asymmetries caused by occlusal interferences may result in a mandibular functional shift following initial tooth contact. The shift can be either in the same or opposite direction of the dental or skeletal discrepancy and may either accentuate or mask the asymmetry.

As stated previously, the patient should also be evaluated to detect functional asymmetries related to TMJ derangements.

Vertical Occlusal Evaluation

The presence of a canted occlusal plane could be the result of a unilateral increase in the vertical length of the condyle and ramus. Similarly, the maxilla or temporal bone supporting the glenoid fossa could be at different levels on each side of the head. Such asymmetries are often detected by clinically evaluating the patient. The cant in the occlusal plane can be readily observed by asking the patient to bite on a tongue blade to determine how it relates to the interpupillary plane (Figure 29-13).[26]

Vertical skeletal asymmetries associated with progressively developing unilateral open bites may be the result of condylar hyperplasia or neoplasia (see Figure 29-4).[27]

Transverse and Anteroposterior Occlusal Evaluations

Asymmetry in the buccolingual relationship (e.g., a unilateral posterior crossbite) should be carefully diagnosed to determine if it is skeletal, dental, or functional. As stated previously, if there is a mandibular deviation from centric relation to centric occlusion, the lower dental midline and chin point should be compared with other midsagittal dental, skeletal, and soft tissue landmarks in the open, initial contact, and closed mandibular positions.

In some cases such a clinical examination is insufficient to detect a functional shift that has been acquired for a prolonged period. When this is suspected, an occlusal splint may need to be constructed for the patient to wear. The appliance allows the musculature to freely guide the mandible to its proper relationship without the distracting influence of the occlusal interferences (see Figure 29-11).

Dental arch asymmetries could be the result of localized factors such as early loss of a primary tooth (see Figure 29-6) or it could be associated with the displacement of the whole dental arch and its supporting skeletal base. Lundstrom[1] found that using the maxillary raphe as a reference line for the median plane is not reliable in determining maxillary asymmetries in either the anteroposterior or lateral directions. Therefore each dental arch should be evaluated separately both clinically and using oriented dental casts to accurately determine the bilateral symmetry of the molar and canine positions.

Examination of the overall shape of the maxillary and mandibular arches from an occlusal view may dis-

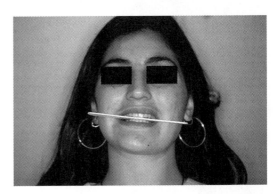

Figure 29-13 Patient biting on a tongue blade to assess the severity of the cant of the maxillary and mandibular occlusal planes in relation to the interpupillary line.

close not only side-to-side asymmetries but also differences in the buccolingual angulation of the teeth. It is important to realize that expansion of dental units to correct a crossbite in the presence of a skeletal constriction may adversely influence the stability of the correction. Similarly, moving already tipped posterior teeth further bucally to correct the crossbite will be associated with greater relapse.

Arch asymmetry could also be caused by rotation of the whole maxilla or mandible. The diagnosis of a rotary displacement of the maxilla may require further evaluation by mounting the dental casts on an anatomic articulator using a face bow transfer.[26]

Transverse Facial, Skeletal, and Soft Tissue Evaluation

The evaluation of facial asymmetry is one of the most important aspect of the clinical evaluation. During the facial evaluation the clinician should compare bilateral structures in both the transverse and vertical directions (Figure 29-14) and check for the presence of other abnormalities (Figure 29-15). In addition body posture should be observed (Figure 29-16). Other than the bilateral structural comparisons, deviations in the dorsum and tip of the nose as well as the philtrum and chin point need to be determined. Asymmetries in the mandible may be observed clinically from a frontal view by observing the point of the chin as it relates to the rest of the facial structures (see Figure 29-8). Looking at the mandible from an inferior view sometimes helps determine the extent of its involvement in relation to the rest of the face.[26]

It is obvious from this description that the clinical evaluation plays an important role in the diagnosis of asymmetries. It is also obvious that, in many cases, the clinical examination needs to be supplemented by other diagnostic records such as dental casts, face bow transfers, and various imaging techniques to accurately localize the structures involved in the asymmetry.

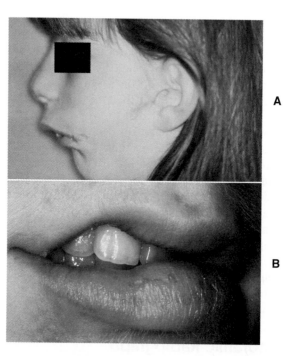

Figure 29-15 The clinician should examine the ear regions **(A)** for indications of the presence of syndromes such as Goldenhar or other neurologic problems that may affect the cheeks or lips **(B).**

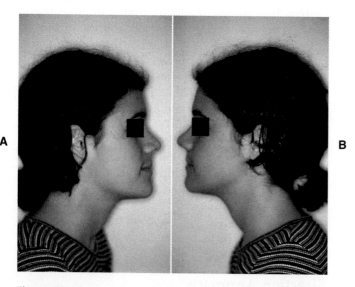

Figure 29-14 The clinical examination should include an evaluation of the transverse and vertical asymmetries by comparing the right **(A)** and left sides **(B)** of the face.

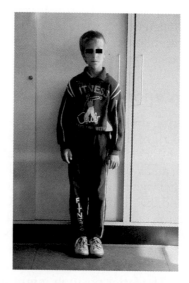

Figure 29-16 Observation of body posture should be part of the overall evaluation of the patient with skeletal deformities.

RADIOGRAPHIC EXAMINATION

In addition to the clinical evaluation, the differentiation between various types of asymmetries can be aided by the use of radiographs. A number of projections are available to properly identify the location and cause of the asymmetry.

Lateral Cephalometric Radiograph

A **lateral cephalometric radiographic** projection, although commonly available to the clinician, provides little useful information on asymmetries in ramal height, mandibular length, and gonial angle.[16,28] It is limited by the fact that the right and left structures are superimposed on each other and are at different distances from the film and x-ray source, which results in significant differences in magnifications.

Criticisms of lateral projections have also been made because of the predetermined orientation using the ear rods.[5] In other words, the assumption is made that the position of the external auditory meatus is symmetric, whereas in reality it may vary in more than one plane of space. Therefore the interpretation of the lateral cephalogram in diagnosing asymmetries is of limited value.

Panoramic Radiograph

A **panoramic radiograph** is a useful projection to survey the dental and bony structures of the maxilla and mandible and to determine the presence of a gross pathologic condition, missing or supernumerary teeth. In addition, the shape of the mandibular ramus and condyles on both sides can be grossly compared.[23] Because of the inherent characteristics of this projection, geometric distortions are significant and vary from one area of the film to another.

Posteroanterior Projection

Posteroanterior projection is a valuable tool in the study of the right and left structures because the structures are located at relatively equal distances from the film and x-ray source. As a result the effects of unequal enlargement by the diverging rays are minimized and the distortion is reduced. Comparison between sides is therefore more accurate because the midlines of the face and dentition can be recorded and evaluated. Posteroanterior cephalograms can be obtained in centric occlusion as well as with the mouth open. The latter position might help determine the extent of the functional deviation, if any is present.

TMJ Imaging

Radiographs and other imaging modalities should be used to investigate the TMJ when the patient presents with facial asymmetries and a continuously changing intermaxillary relationship or when there is a history of trauma, crepitation of the joint or history of inflammatory disease (see Chapter 27). Comprehensive **TMJ imaging** may include one or more of the following procedures[25]:
Conventional radiographs (discussed previously)
Conventional tomography
Computerized tomography
Arthroscopy and videofluoroscopy
Magnetic resonance imaging
Radionuclide imaging to determine bone turnover activities

Localization of the Asymmetry

Once a posteroanterior film has been obtained, it must be qualitatively and quantitatively evaluated to determine the extent of the asymmetry present. The structures to be used in the construction of the midsagittal reference plane need to have a relatively high degree of symmetry.

Anatomic Approach

Harvold[30] found that the zygomaticofrontal sutures and crista galli are relatively symmetric structures as compared to other facial landmarks that are further distant from the cranial base. He recommended the construction of a horizontal line through the zygomaticofrontal sutures to act as the horizontal axis. A vertical line perpendicular to the horizontal axis is constructed to pass through and bisect the base of crista galli. This vertical line approximates the anatomic midsagittal plane of the head. Harvold[30] noted that nasion and the anterior nasal spine tend to fall on or near this midsagittal plane 90% of the time.

Perpendiculars from bilateral structures can now be constructed to this midsagittal vertical reference line. The differences between the projections from the two sides are then measured and compared to quantify discrepancies in height as well as in the distances between the bilateral structures and the midline. In addition, the maxillary and mandibular dental midlines are compared to the skeletal midline.

Marmay, Zilberman, and Mirsky[27] used the foramina spinosum to construct a facial midline. Unfortunately it is often difficult to identify these foramina on the anteroposterior cephalogram.

Bisection Approach

In cases where it is difficult to accurately identify crista galli or the zygomaticofrontal sutures, the bisection approach may be used. With the bisection approach bilateral landmarks are located and bisected. A reference line is then constructed, passing through as many of the midpoints of these bilateral landmarks. If a midpoint is obviously off in relation to most other midpoints of the cranium and face, it may be advisable to exclude such a point when constructing the midline. Evaluation of the bilateral asymmetry then follows the same principles as with the anatomic approach.

Triangulation Approach

The triangulation approach can be used to study the relative asymmetry of the component areas of the facial complex.[8] Following the identification of bilateral structures and the midline on the radiograph, triangles are constructed that divide the face into various components. The right and left triangles are then compared for symmetry.

Grayson, McCarthy, and Bookstein[31] described a technique in which posteroanterior and basilar cephalograms can be analyzed at various depths to determine the plane of the asymmetry.

More sophisticated imaging techniques such as **magnetic resonance imaging** and **computed tomography** are now routinely used to accurately localize the discrepancy. Radiographic projections in different planes of space are routinely recommended to evaluate the deformities in three dimensions.[32]

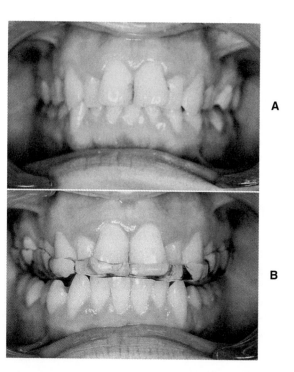

Figure 29-17 Occlusal splints may be necessary to properly evaluate the presence and extent of the functional shift. **A,** Intraoral view of the teeth in centric occlusion before inserting the splint. **B,** Intraoral view 4 weeks following the insertion of a maxillary, full-coverage acrylic splint. Notice midline shift.

TREATMENT

A detailed study of the various diagnostic records obtained on the patient is necessary to determine the cause, location, and extent of the asymmetry. This enables the clinician to formulate the proper treatment plan.

Asymmetries must be differentially diagnosed as being the result of a skeletal asymmetry, an asymmetry within the dental arches, functional discrepancies between centric occlusion and centric relation, or a combination of these.

Dental Asymmetries

True dental asymmetries such as cases with a congenitally missing lateral incisor or a second premolar are often treated orthodontically. Asymmetric extraction sequences and asymmetric mechanics (e.g., Class III elastics on one side and Class II elastics on the other with oblique elastics anteriorly) can also be used to correct dental arch asymmetries. Composite build-ups or prosthodontic restorations may be indicated with pronounced tooth irregularities.

Functional Asymmetries

Mild deviations caused by functional shifts are sometimes corrected with minor occlusal adjustments. More severe deviations need orthodontic treatment to align the teeth and to obtain proper function. Occlusal splints may be necessary to properly evaluate the presence and extent of the functional shift by eliminating habitual posturing and deprogramming the musculature (Figure 29-17). Because functional shifts can also be the result of a skeletal asymmetry, rapid maxillary expansion, orthognathic surgery, and orthodontic treatment may be indicated in the management of these cases.

Skeletal Asymmetries

The severity and nature of the skeletal asymmetry dictate whether the discrepancy can be completely or partially resolved solely through orthodontic treatment. In growing individuals, orthopedic appliances in conjunction with orthodontics are used to help improve or correct the developing skeletal imbalances.[33]

Asymmetries of a skeletal nature treated with orthodontics alone may dictate certain compromises that need to be explained to the patient before treatment is initiated.

Severe discrepancies may require a combination of surgery and orthodontics. A thorough diagnosis will help determine whether the maxilla or mandible or both need to be surgically repositioned.

Abnormalities of the coronoid and condylar processes as well as in the position and shape of the articular disks should be considered when limited opening, acute malocclusions, or mandibular deviations are found.

Soft Tissue Asymmetries

Deformities caused by soft tissue imbalance can be treated by either augmentation or reduction surgery. Augmentations include the use of bone grafts and silicone implants to recontour the desired areas of the face.[34]

With mild dental, skeletal, and soft tissue deviations the advisability of treatment should be carefully considered.

REFERENCES

1. Lundstrom A: Some asymmetries of the dental arches, jaws, and skull, and their etiological significance, *Am J Orthod* 47:81-106, 1961.
2. Editors: *Dorland's illustrated medical dictionary*, ed 29, Philadelphia, 2000, WB Saunders.
3. Fischer B: Asymmetries of the dentofacial complex, *Angle Orthod* 24:179-192, 1954.
4. Peck S, Peck L: Skeletal asymmetry in esthetically pleasing faces, *Angle Orthod* 61:43-48, 1991.
5. Sutton PR: Lateral facial asymmetry: methods of assessment, *Angle Orthod* 38:82-92, 1968.
6. Burke PH: Stereophotogrammetric measurement of normal facial asymmetry in children, *Hum Biol* 43:536-548, 1971.
7. Woo TL: On the asymmetry of the human skull, *Biometrika* 22:324-352, 1931.
8. Vig PS, Hewitt AB: Asymmetry of the human facial skeleton, *Angle Orthod* 45:125-129, 1975.
9. Vig PS, Hewitt AB: Is craniofacial asymmetry and adaption for masticatory function an evolutionary process? *Nature* 248(444):165, 1974.
10. Melnik AK: A cephalometric study of mandibular asymmetry in a longitudinally followed sample of growing children, *Am J Orthod Dentofacial Orthop* 101:355-366, 1991.
11. Bailit HL et al: Dental asymmetry as an indicator of genetic and environmental conditions in human populations, *Hum Biol* 42:626-638, 1970.
12. Vargervik K: Orthodontic management of unilateral cleft lip and palate, *Cleft Palate J* 18:256-270, 1981.
13. Heard G: *Nerve sheath tumors and von Recklinghausen's disease of the nervous system,* ed 7, London, Oxford, 1969, University Press.
14. James PL, Treggiden R: Multiple neurofibromatosis associated with facial asymmetry, *J Oral Surg* 33:439-442, 1975.
15. Boder E: A common form of facial asymmetry in the newborn infant: its etiology and orthodontic significance, *Am J Orthod* 39:895-899, 1953.
16. Keen RR, Callahan GR: Osteochondroma of the mandibular condyle: report of case, *J Oral Surg* 35:140-143, 1977.
17. Erickson GE, Waite DE: Mandibular asymmetry, *J Am Dent Assoc* 89:1369-1373, 1974.
18. Speculand B: Unilateral condylar hypoplasia with ankylosis radiographic findings, *Br J Oral Surg* 20:1-13, 1982.
19. Garn SM, Lewis AB, Kerewsky RS: The meaning of bilateral asymmetry in the permanent dentition, *Angle Orthod* 36:55-62, 1966.
20. Bart RS, Kopf AW: Tumor conference #20: hemifacial atrophy, *J Dermatol Surg Oncol* 4:908-909, 1978.
21. Eubanks RJ: Surgical correction of masseter muscle hypertrophy associated with unilateral prognathism: report of case, *J Oral Surg* 15:66, 1957.
22. Jonck LM: Condylar hyperplasia: a case for early treatment, *Int J Oral Surg* 10:154-160, 1981.
23. Lewis PD: The deviated midline, *Am J Orthod* 70:601-616, 1976.
24. Persson M: Mandibular asymmetry of hereditary origin, *Am J Orthod* 63:1-11, 1973.
25. Schmid W, Mongini F, Felisio A: A computer-based assessment of structural and displacement asymmetries of the mandible, *Am J Orthod Dentofacial Orthop* 100:19-34, 1991.
26. Cheney EA: Dentofacial asymmetries and their clinical significance, *Am J Orthod* 47:814-829, 1961.
27. Marmay Y, Zilberman Y, Mirsky Y: Use of foramina spinosa to determine skull midlines, *Angle Orthod* 49:263-268, 1979.
28. Smith RJ, Bailit HL: Prevalence and etiology of asymmetries in occlusion, *Angle Orthod* 49:199-204, 1979.
29. Elefteriadis JN, Athanasiou AE: Guidelines for temporomandibular joint in aging, *Eur Dent* 4:19-21, 1995.
30. Harvold E: Cleft lip and palate: morphologic studies of facial skeleton, *Am J Orthod* 40:493-506, 1954.
31. Grayson GH, McCarthy JG, Bookstein F: Analysis of craniofacial asymmetry by multiplane cephalometry, *Am J Orthod* 84:217-224, 1983.
32. Kaban LB, Mulliken JB, Murray JE: Three-dimensional approach to analysis and treatment of hemifacial microsomia, *Cleft Palate J* 18:90-99, 1981.
33. Sarnas KV et al: Hemifacial microsomia treated with the Herbst appliance, *Am J Orthod* 82:68-74, 1982.
34. Gorney M, Harries T: The preoperative and postoperative consideration of natural facial asymmetry, *Plast Recontsr Surg* 54:187-191, 1974.

CHAPTER 30

Surgical Orthodontics

Deborah L. Zeitler

KEY TERMS

The relationship between the specialties of orthodontics and **oral and maxillofacial surgery** is one of the closest in the field of dentistry. To accomplish optimal orthodontic treatment, oral surgery sometimes may be indicated. Similarly, orthodontics is often needed to obtain the best results in cases requiring orthognathic surgery. Oral and maxillofacial surgery may be necessary when crowding requires removal of teeth to obtain the proper alignment of teeth, for uprighting severely angulated and impacted second molars, or for tooth transplantation. Sometimes oral and maxillofacial surgery is indicated in surgically assisted rapid palatal expansion for the adult patient or possibly in the removal of impacted third molars. In cases with significant skeletal discrepancies the orthodontist cannot achieve optimal esthetics and a stable occlusion without oral and maxillofacial surgery procedures such as maxillary or mandibular orthognathic surgery. Some new approaches can also be incorporated with orthodontic treatment such as using implant for anchorage or distraction osteogenesis for advancing the maxilla or the mandible. This chapter gives an overview of what the oral and maxillofacial surgeon can do for the orthodontist and the orthodontic patient.

DENTOALVEOLAR PROCEDURES

Removal of Teeth for Orthodontic Purposes

Teeth that need to be removed for the purpose of orthodontic treatment may include (1) permanent teeth in a crowded dentition, (2) ankylosed primary teeth, (3) normal primary teeth that are overretained or being removed for the purpose of allowing other teeth to erupt, and (4) supernumerary teeth that may impede the progress of orthodontic tooth movement. Usually removal of teeth in these categories falls into what most oral and maxillofacial surgeons define as a simple procedure. It is up to the orthodontist to identify the necessary teeth to be removed. The oral and maxillofacial surgeon evaluates the patient, determines the best management approach, and performs the extractions.

Even though the **removal of teeth** for orthodontic purposes is usually a simple procedure, many patients may benefit from the use of **intravenous sedation.** Such an approach should be considered for young adolescents who have never previously required local anesthesia for their dental care and now need to have four first premolars removed to correct a crowded malocclusion. This child may benefit from the use of sedation techniques that provide amnesia and emotional comfort before he or she is subjected to eight local anesthesia injections, which are required to extract a tooth in each quadrant of the mouth. For the slightly more complex procedure, such as removal of a supernumerary tooth, intravenous sedation becomes even more routine.

One of the most important considerations in removing teeth for orthodontic purposes is to ensure that the tooth is properly identified and that the proper tooth is then removed. This is not a trivial matter in that teeth being removed for orthodontic treatment usually are not diseased. Therefore the presence of a large carious lesion is not necessary to point the surgeon to the correct tooth. A written referral from the orthodontist clearly identifying the teeth to be removed is always important.

Exposure of Impacted Teeth

A common reason for orthodontic referral to the oral and maxillofacial surgeon is for the exposure of an **impacted tooth.** The most common teeth to be impacted other than third molars are maxillary canines followed by premolars and maxillary second molars.[1]

Although any tooth in the mouth can be impacted, impactions of other teeth are less common (Figure 30-1). Treatment of the impacted tooth, which needs to be exposed, bonded with a bracket and ligature or chain, and then orthodontically brought into the dental arch, begins with proper evaluation.[2]

Radiographic location of the tooth should be undertaken. This usually involves referring to two radiographs taken at different angles or using more than one radiographic technique. For example, to plan the proper surgical approach, it is important to localize the maxillary canine because it may be impacted labially or palatally. A similar approach is used for premolars. On the other hand, impacted second molars are usually

easier to locate because they are most often in mesioangular impactions.

An impacted tooth may be treated by the **surgical exposure** of its crown, a procedure that allows the natural eruption of the tooth. This procedure involves removal of both soft and hard tissues in the direction most appropriate for crown movement. The wound needs to be covered with a surgical pack until it is completely epithelialized and leaves the crown of the impacted tooth exposed. The vast majority of impacted teeth erupt once their crowns are exposed in this manner, provided space is present in the arch for the tooth to approach its normal position. The eruption of these teeth may take up to 2 years. A recent study comparing this method of spontaneous eruption with the method to be described next (bonding of the tooth with orthodontic movement) showed no difference in total orthodontic treatment time for patients treated by the two different techniques.[3]

A more frequently used approach is to surgically expose the impacted tooth and then place a **bonded bracket** with an attached chain or ligature to apply orthodontic forces on the tooth to aid in its movement into the line of occlusion. With this technique the tooth is localized clinically and radiographically and then surgically exposed. It is unnecessary to remove all of the soft and hard tissues between the tooth and the final position in the arch. However, it may be helpful to create a path through bone if too much bone separates the crown of the tooth from its desired position. Once the tooth is surgically exposed the area is isolated and dried, the tooth is etched, and a bracket is bonded to the tooth (Figure 30-2). The bracket may have a chain or a ligature wire attached to it. The chain or ligature wire is brought through the soft issues and wrapped around the arch wire to be used in the orthodontic movement of this tooth. In this case the wound does not need to be packed open and the soft tissues may be returned to cover the tooth **(closed eruption approach).** At all times during canine exposure, the region of the cementoenamel junction needs

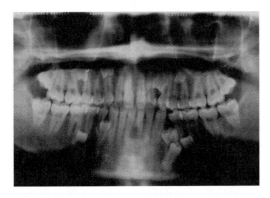

Figure 30-1 Radiograph illustrating multiple impacted teeth.

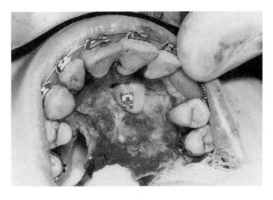

Figure 30-2 Impacted canine with bracket.

to be avoided to protect the periodontal health of the tooth.[4]

In the case of palatally positioned canines and premolars, placing the palatal tissue back over the tooth is the most common technique. In the case of a labially positioned canine, however, it may be more appropriate to apically reposition a small flap so that the tooth is partially exposed and the attached gingival tissue is placed at the proper level on the labially positioned canine **(apically repositioned flap).** Orthodontic movement of these teeth may be undertaken following surgery as soon as the patient is comfortable.

Impacted mandibular second molars can become an orthodontic problem if not identified early and treated.[5] A useful technique in the treatment of such impactions is the **surgical uprighting** of the impacted mandibular second molar.[5] The treatment of these teeth begins with early identification of the problem (Figure 30-3). Once the second molars are identified as being impacted, it is important to attempt to work their surgical treatment into the overall treatment plan before the apical third of their root is formed. This is because the success rate with this procedure is greater when the impacted second molars have approximately two thirds of their roots formed.

The procedure begins with removal of the third molar, which is usually somewhat superior and posterior to the impacted second molar. Once the third molar is removed, the second molar is carefully tipped distally to clear the greatest convexity of the first molar. At this position it will usually wedge into a nearly normal second molar position. Most teeth will be stable without further treatment. It is important to ensure that there are no occlusal forces transmitted to the repositioned tooth, which would traumatize the repositioned molar during the initial healing phase.

Approximately 3 weeks following the uprighting of an impacted second molar an endodontic evaluation should be performed. In most cases endodontic treatment is usually unnecessary, but if it is required it should be performed at least 6 to 8 weeks following the

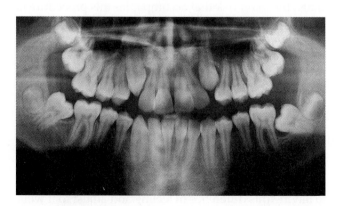

Figure 30-3 Impacted mandibular second molars.

surgical procedure. This technique of surgically uprighting impacted mandibular second molars is highly successful and allows a tooth to be maintained, which otherwise would likely be lost if the impaction is diagnosed at a later date.

Transplantation of Teeth

Transplantation of teeth has been advocated as an alternative to other methods of treatment of impacted teeth. It may be a good alternative for the adult patient who cannot undergo conventional orthodontic movement of an impacted tooth. The advocated technique is a careful wide exposure of the impacted tooth. The tooth is then moved into its position within the dental arch and is stabilized with a segmental orthodontic appliance. Endodontic treatment, if necessary, is rendered 6 to 8 weeks after the surgical procedure initially using a calcium hydroxide paste. Then a conventional root canal filling is performed 1 year later.

Teeth may be transplanted from one position to another in the dental arch. This may be particularly useful in situations in which patients are asymmetrically missing several teeth. Conventional orthodontic treatment for impacted teeth in children and young individuals is usually the treatment of choice. However, when extraction may be necessary or with congenitally missing teeth, transalveolar transplantation may be a sound alternative.[6,7]

Removal of Third Molars

Certainly the removal of third molars or wisdom teeth is one of the most common procedures performed by oral and maxillofacial surgeons in the average private practice. Referrals for third molar removal come from many sources including the orthodontist and the general dentist who is treating the patient.[8] The identification of impacted third molars during orthodontic treatment is common because few patients have adequate arch length for the proper eruption and long-term maintenance of all their third molars. Impacted third molars need to be removed at an early stage in tooth development (Figure 30-4).

A controversial topic is whether impacted third molars contribute to the relapse of anterior mandibular crowding in the orthodontic patient. This common perception may provide orthodontic patients with an incentive to have their third molars removed at the end of orthodontic treatment when retainers are being placed. On the other hand, it is scientifically questionable whether third molars play a significant role in the relapse of mandibular incisor crowding.[9] A better reason for removal of third molars is that most third molars will not become fully functional teeth and will more likely become partially erupted, setting the stage for

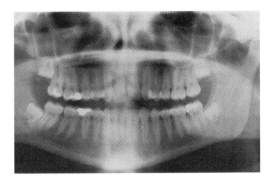

Figure 30-4 Impacted third molars with partial root development.

chronic pericoronitis and adversely affecting the adjacent second molars through chronic inflammatory disease.

The removal of third molars is usually performed in the office setting with the use of intravenous sedation techniques or outpatient general anesthesia. Studies suggest that the removal of all four third molars (if present) is appropriate at one setting to provide for only one recovery period. The use of adjunct medications such as steroids for patient comfort and minimizing swelling is indicated. The routine use of antibiotics is controversial and probably should be avoided unless there are specific indications for antibiotic treatment. The usual recovery time based on recent studies is approximately 5 days for the patient to feel comfortable pursuing normal activities and a normal diet with minimal residual pain.

ORTHOGNATHIC SURGERY

Patients who have congenital, developmental, or acquired dentofacial deformities may require orthodontic alignment of the teeth as well as surgical movement of one or both jaws to achieve proper position and function of the maxilla, mandible, and dentition. The treatment planning for **orthognathic surgery** begins with a thorough patient evaluation (see Section II). This requires a comprehensive clinical examination to evaluate facial proportions and symmetry. A thorough occlusal examination is necessary to determine the presence or absence of open bites, cross bites, crowding, etc. Cephalometric and panoramic radiographic examinations are indicated. The cephalometric film should be traced to identify abnormalities of maxillary and mandibular position as well as abnormalities of tooth angulation. The panoramic evaluation is used as a screening examination for temporomandibular anomalies, gross abnormalities of the dentition, and presence or absence of impacted teeth.

A clinical examination of temporomandibular function should be performed. Impressions of the teeth should be made and a model analysis undertaken.

Following the gathering of information, a thorough diagnosis should be made. This diagnosis must include the presence or absence of skeletal abnormalities, dental and occlusal abnormalities and other findings such as presence or absence of impacted third molars, which may influence the treatment plan for these patients. A skeletal diagnosis should include the jaw or jaws involved, the direction of the problem, and whether the problem is an excess or a deficiency. For example, a common diagnosis might be maxillary vertical excess or mandibular sagittal deficiency. Of course it is entirely possible for both jaws to be involved. For example, maxillary sagittal deficiency and mandibular sagittal excess may be present in the same patient.

The diagnosis of the presence of dental compensations is extremely important. If the teeth are tipped to compensate for the abnormal jaw positions, these dental compensations must be corrected (i.e., the teeth are properly aligned in their respective arches) (Figure 30-5). This allows the maxilla and the mandible to be surgically moved into their proper positions and results in an optimal occlusion and facial esthetics at the end of treatment.

Several major jaw procedures are commonly used to correct skeletal abnormalities. These include the sagittal split osteotomy, the transoral vertical ramus osteotomy, and the LeFort I osteotomy. Adjunct procedures include genioplasty and surgically assisted rapid palatal expansion.

Sagittal Split Osteotomy

The sagittal split osteotomy is used to either advance or retrude the mandible. It is performed from primarily an intraoral approach and can be effectively combined with **rigid fixation** to avoid wiring the teeth during healing. Because the design of the osteotomy splits the mandibular body and ramus in a sagittal dimension, usually exposing the inferior alveolar neurovascular canal, the main risk that accompanies this procedure is altered sensation following the surgery. It is important that patients understand that they will likely experience complete numbness in the distribution of the inferior alveolar nerve immediately following surgery. Sensation generally returns over a period of months; however, approximately 5% of patients will experience some form of long-term altered sensation. This may be present to various degrees ranging from total anesthesia of the inferior alveolar nerve to a small area of a slightly decreased sensation somewhere on the lower lip. However, most patients find that they become used to having this difference in feeling and adjust to it well. Few recognize it as a daily annoyance.

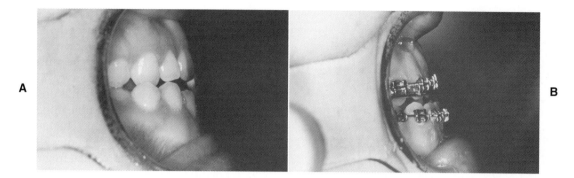

Figure 30-5 Dental compensations before (**A**) and after (**B**) orthodontic correction before surgery. Elimination of dental compensation accentuates the malocclusion in preparation for orthognathic surgery.

Another important risk of this procedure is relapse, especially for large advancements of the mandible. Because the suprahyoid muscle complex is stretched when the mandible is brought forward, relapse is always a possibility. The patient should understand that advancements of greater than 7 mm have been associated with some degree of relapse.

When rigid fixation is used for the sagittal split osteotomy, it frequently is inserted through a percutaneous approach. The patient should understand that if this approach is used, a small scar near the angle of the mandible will result. For most patients these incisions heal without obvious scar formation, but scarring or keloid formation is always a small risk.

To perform the sagittal split osteotomy, the patient is given a general anesthetic. The procedure begins with an incision along the external oblique line of the ramus of the mandible. This incision extends from approximately the first molar region backward and upward along the coronoid process. The lateral surface of the mandible is exposed and then the medial surface is exposed between the coronoid notch and the inferior alveolar foramen.

The first bony cut is made in a horizontal direction above the inferior alveolar foramen but below the coronoid notch. This cut is extended into cancellous bone and approximately two thirds of the way from the anterior border of the mandible to the posterior border. The next bony cut is made in a sagittal direction beginning at the anterior extent of the horizontal cut and running approximately 1 mm medial to the external oblique line sagittally down the ramus of the mandible. This cut is carried to where the external oblique line begins to fall off. A landmark to identify for the anterior extent of the sagittal cut is to place it vertically above the mandibular notch. At this point a vertical cut is made in the lateral surface of the mandible from the anterior end of the sagittal cut to the mandibular notch (Figure 30-6). It is important to carry this cut under the inferior border.

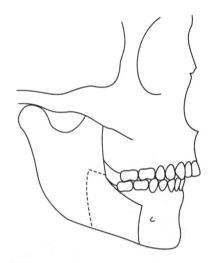

Figure 30-6 Design of bony cuts for sagittal split osteotomy.

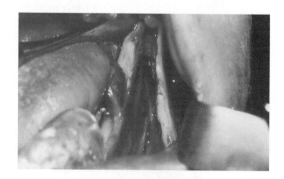

Figure 30-7 Splitting of the mandible.

Once these defined cuts are complete, the mandible may be split in a sagittal direction using a combination of splitting instruments and chisels. The split is gradually widened, allowing the thin bone on the lingual surface at the inferior border of the mandible to gently crack (Figure 30-7). As this occurs the mandible is divided, giving the tooth-bearing segment freedom from the proximal segment (which includes the coronoid process and the condyle). As the split is being widened it is important to identify the inferior alveolar neurovascular bundle and gently free it from any bony interferences. The same procedure is repeated on the opposite side of the mandible.

Once both sides have been split it is possible to move the distal segment of the mandible either forward or backward into its new position. The teeth are wired into the desired occlusion defining the desired final position of the mandible. The proximal fragments are then held in position to allow screws to be placed from buccal to lingual through both segments. Usually three 2-mm positional screws are used, allowing rigid fixation of the mandible on each side (Figure 30-8). The teeth can now be unwired, and the patient's jaw can be rotated in centric relation to check that the final occlusion is in the desired position.

Postoperative care following a sagittal split osteotomy of the mandible includes a liquid diet for 2 to

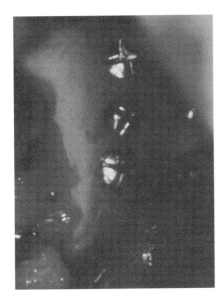

Figure 30-8 Rigid fixation of mandible.

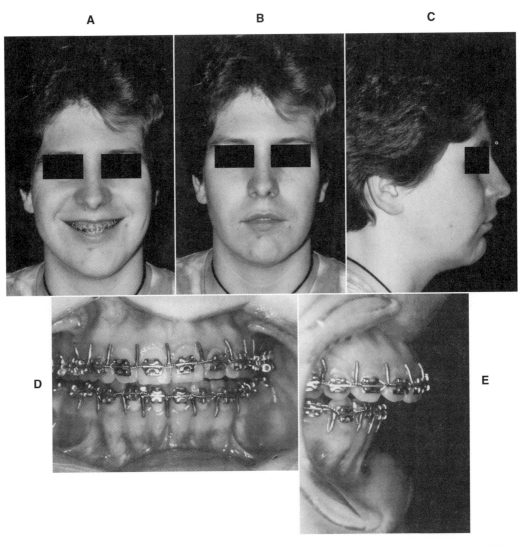

Figure 30-9 **A** to **C,** Patient with mandibular sagittal deficiency. **D** and **E,** Frontal and lateral intraoral views of the dental malocclusion before surgery.

4 weeks, elastic traction using the orthodontic appliances to guide the occlusion, and administering of corticosteroids to minimize swelling. This procedure is often performed as an outpatient surgery with the patient leaving late the same day or early the next morning before 24 hours have passed. Follow-up visits are coordinated so the surgeon can monitor healing and stability while the orthodontist reinstitutes orthodontic therapy 3 to 4 weeks following the surgical procedure.

A typical course of events would be for the patient to return to a normal diet by 6 weeks following surgery and to have unlimited activities by 3 months. The patient usually returns to work or school within 1 to 2 weeks following surgery and is limited by diet modifications from 2 to 6 weeks following surgery. From 6 to 12 weeks after surgery, the patient may not be involved in contact sports but otherwise can be normally active. Usually the final orthodontic treatment is complete by 3 to 6 months following the procedure. The braces are removed and the patient enters the retention phase of

orthodontics. The surgeon follows the patient usually at 6 months, 1 year, and 2 years after the surgery to evaluate function, occlusion, stability, and overall patient satisfaction (Figure 30-9).

Transoral Vertical Ramus Osteotomy

The transoral vertical ramus osteotomy is another procedure performed in the mandible. It is utilized only for mandibular retrusion (setback) and, therefore, is typically used for patients with a Class III malocclusion. Because of the design of the osteotomy, it can be best utilized for mandibular setbacks between about 5 and 10 mm. This allows the geometry of the overlapping bone to be as ideal as possible. It also can effectively be utilized for asymmetric movements because the proximal segments tend to flare less than when a sagittal osteotomy is used for those types of mandibular setbacks.

The primary difference between a sagittal split osteotomy and the transoral vertical ramus osteotomy is

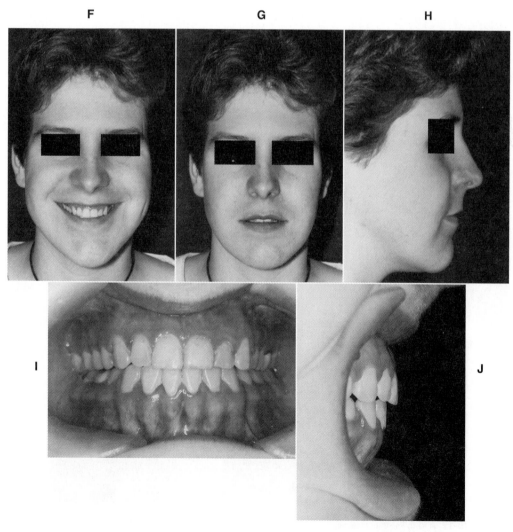

Figure 30-9, cont'd **F** to **J,** Postsurgical and orthodontic treatment results after a mandibular sagittal advancement was performed.

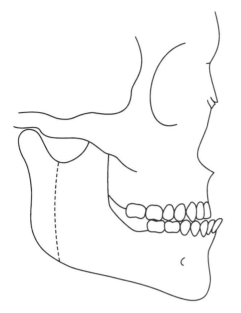

Figure 30-10 Design of a bony cut for transoral vertical ramus osteotomy.

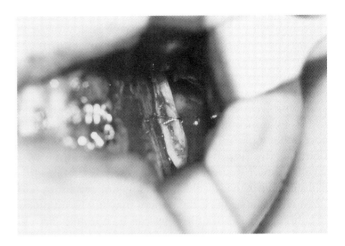

Figure 30-11 Surgical view of transoral vertical ramus osteotomy.

A   B   C

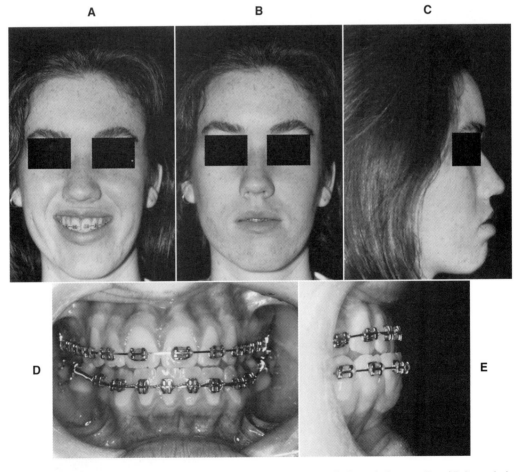

D   E

Figure 30-12 **A** to **C,** Presurgical facial photographs of a patient with mandibular sagittal excess. **D** and **E,** Presurgical intraoral photographs. Patient had a mandibular transoral vertical ramus osteotomy.

the design of the bone cut (Figure 30-10). The preoperative workup, anesthesia management, and even soft tissue incision design are similar for both procedures. Once the incision is made, the lateral ramus is widely exposed. Specially designed instruments are placed in the coronoid notch and hooked around the posterior surface of the mandible to hold the soft tissues out of the way and to help guide the surgical cut. A 105-degree angled oscillating saw is used to cut from the coronoid notch vertically downward toward the mandibular angle. This makes a slightly beveled cut, which allows the proximal segment (which includes the condylar process) to overlap the distal segment as the distal segment is pushed backward into its new position (Figure 30-11).

Once both sides have been prepared and cut, the mandible is placed into its new occlusion with the maxilla and is wired into position. The proximal fragments are then overlapped. Either they can be left without any fixation at this point (if this procedure is used, some medial pterygoid muscle must remain on the proximal segment to help give a vertical positioning factor to this part of the mandible), or a wire may be placed through a hole in the distal fragment and looped around the tip of the proximal fragment to help position the proximal fragment and seat the condyle. With this procedure the patient is kept in intermaxillary fixation usually for 6 weeks.

The early hospital course is similar to that for sagittal split as is the postoperative course with the exception that the patient remains in intermaxillary fixation and therefore must be on a totally liquid diet for 6 weeks' time. The main advantage of this procedure is that the cut is designed to occur behind the inferior alveolar foramen. Therefore the incidence of inferior alveolar nerve damage is extremely low. For patients who have reason to want to avoid numbness of the lower lip (e.g., musicians), this can be a useful procedure for mandibular setbacks (Figure 30-12).

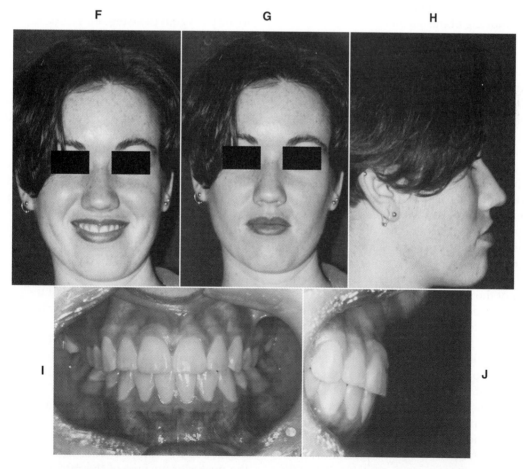

Figure 30-12, cont'd F to J, Postsurgical and orthodontic treatment. Results after a mandibular setback was performed using a transoral vertical ramus osteotomy. **F** to **H,** Posttreatment facial photographs. **I** and **J,** Posttreatment intraoral photographs.

LeFort I Osteotomy

For patients who have maxillary problems such as maxillary vertical excess, maxillary sagittal deficiency, or skeletal open bites, a LeFort I osteotomy may be indicated. Again, a comprehensive workup and orthodontic preparation are performed before the time of maxillary surgery.

The most common indication for a LeFort I osteotomy is vertical maxillary excess. In this case the patient frequently shows excessive tooth structure when the lips are at rest and excessive gingiva may be exposed during smile. The vertical maxillary excess may cause the mandible to be rotated posteriorly, giving an appearance of mandibular deficiency. The next most common indication for a LeFort I osteotomy is skeletal anterior open bite. In this situation the posterior portion of the maxilla may have grown downward too far. When the molar teeth are in occlusion because of this anatomic abnormality, the anterior teeth are left without contact. In this situation the LeFort I osteotomy is used to tilt the maxilla upward and back, giving a level plane of occlusion and allowing even contact between all the teeth. Other movements are also possible with a LeFort I osteotomy including downward, forward, or backward positioning of the maxilla.

The risks of a LeFort I osteotomy include numbness around the upper lip, nose, and anterior maxillary teeth. This risk of numbness is usually temporary, and long-term altered sensation in these areas is uncommon. Occasionally patients experience altered sensation in the posterior hard palate. This can be caused by damage to the greater palatine neurovascular bundles. Although occasionally numbness in this area lasts long term, it rarely is a significant problem to the patient. Relapse with the LeFort I osteotomy varies with the particular movements. Vertical repositioning to correct maxillary vertical excess or skeletal open bite tends to be extremely stable. On the other hand, inferior movements of the maxilla, which require grafting, tend to have higher relapse rates. Similarly, anterior movement of the maxilla may have greater relapse than posterior repositioning of the maxilla.

The LeFort I osteotomy is performed as an operating room procedure with a general anesthetic. Exposure is accomplished by making a circumferential incision in the vestibule above the first molar teeth and extending around to the area of the anterior nasal spine and then to the first molar region on the opposite side. A full-thickness mucoperiosteal flap is developed. This exposes the pyriform rim (anterior edge of the floor of the nose), the anterior nasal spine, and the lateral surface of the maxilla. A tunnel is created around the maxillary buttress where the zygomatic arch attaches to the maxilla, extending backward to the region of the pterygoid plates (Figure 30-13).

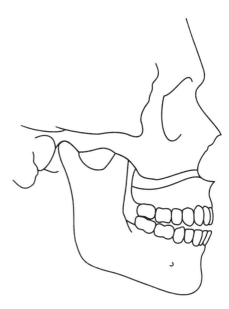

Figure 30-13 Design of a bony cut for LeFort I osteotomy.

A cut is then designed that extends from the edge of the pyriform rim above the apices of the teeth and follows the lateral surface of the maxilla all the way back to the pterygoid plate region. This achieves the purpose of cutting the entire lateral surface of the maxilla. The next area that needs to be addressed is the nasal septum. The nasal floor is elevated carefully, and the place where the cartilaginous septum attaches to the bony septum is identified. A specially designed chisel is placed to divide the nasal septum from the superior surface of the maxilla. This chisel is directed posteriorly in the midline to achieve this cut.

The next anatomic connection of the maxilla that needs to be divided is the lateral wall of the nose (the medial wall of the maxillary sinus). Again, a specially designed chisel is used to cut this surface. This chisel is directed posteriorly and carefully tapped through the lateral wall of the nose until a more substantial bony landmark is reached. This thicker bone is the perpendicular plate of the palatal bone. Running in a canal in the perpendicular plate of the palatal bone is the greater palatine neurovascular bundle. The chisel should not be used to cut through this perpendicular plate to avoid direct damage to the vascular structures in that neurovascular bundle. Therefore when the chisel reaches this more sturdy bone, which can be felt and heard, the division of the lateral wall of the nose is terminated. Later, this area of bone will be fractured.

The last anatomic region that needs to be addressed is the connection of the pterygoid plates to the posterior surface of the maxilla. It is not always necessary to directly cut through this area; however, often times a specially curved chisel is used and

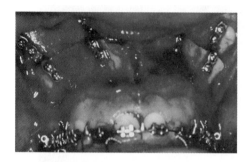

Figure 30-14 Rigid fixation of LeFort I osteotomy.

placed in the junction of the pterygoid plates in the maxilla and tapped through to fracture the connection of these bones.

Now the only remaining connection that has not been severed is the perpendicular plate of the palatal bone. At this time manual pressure is used to tilt the cut portion of the maxilla downward. Most surgeons call this procedure the *down fracture of the maxilla*. As the maxilla is fractured downward, the nasal mucosa is observed and all connections of the nasal mucosa to the superior surface of the maxilla are elevated. The vascular supply to the maxilla is the soft palate connection and the remaining buccal soft tissues that were not cut in the original incision. Assuming that the greater palatine neurovascular bundles are still intact, they will supply blood and enervation to the now freely movable LeFort I segment.

At this time bone can be removed from the maxilla to allow it to be repositioned. The most common movement made in a maxillary osteotomy is a superior movement that requires bone to be removed from the lateral surface, the bony septum region, the lateral wall, and often times the pterygoid plate region. Although inferior repositioning is uncommon, it is sometimes performed in which case an interpositional substance may be placed between the cut surfaces of the maxilla to produce a downward movement in the new position of the maxilla.

It is also possible at this time to cut between teeth in the alveolar process and along the palate to segment the maxilla into several pieces if the shape of the maxilla needs to be changed. The most common reason for this type of segmental procedure would be maxillary transverse deficiency.

When adequate bone removal has occurred, the maxilla is then placed into its new position with the mandible. The surgeon places the mandible in centric relation and rotates the maxilla into a new position. At this time most surgeons use small titanium plates to fix the maxilla in position (Figure 30-14). An alternate technique uses wires that also can give good stability. Following closure of the incision and completion of the procedure, the patient can be released from the inter-

maxillary fixation. Again, elastics can be used for enhancing patient comfort and for guiding the teeth into the new occlusion. The postoperative course is similar to that with the mandibular osteotomy using rigid fixation (Figure 30-15).

Maxillary and Mandibular Osteotomies

Some patients have discrepancies in both the maxilla and the mandible, in which case maxillary and mandibular osteotomies may be performed simultaneously. The procedures are the same but the sequencing is a little bit different. When both the maxillary and mandibular osteotomies are performed it is necessary to keep one jaw stable at any given time to allow for proper positioning of the mobile jaw. A common sequence is to perform the bony cuts in the mandible without splitting the sagittal split osteotomy. Then the maxillary splits are completely performed, allowing the new position of the maxilla to be established against the old position of the mandible. The surgeon then returns to the mandibular osteotomy sites and splits the mandible. By having already performed the cuts, it seems to speed the procedure along and minimizes the chance of damaging the newly positioned maxilla during manipulation of the mandible. The mandibular splits are then performed, and the mandible is positioned in relationship to the newly established position of the maxilla (Figure 30-16). Postoperative course is similar for these patients as to all the other procedures described previously.

Genioplasty

It is not uncommon for a patient to have chin abnormalities in addition to (or independent of) the more functional abnormalities of the maxilla and mandible. A chin may be too flat or too prominent; it may be asymmetric or vertically abnormal. All of these problems can be corrected with a procedure called a *genioplasty*. A genioplasty uses an incision in the mucobuccal fold in the anterior of the mandible that extends approximately between canines. It is important once the incision is made to then tunnel backward and identify the mental foramen so the mental nerve exiting from that area can be protected.

Once this identification is made, the chin can be cut horizontally and moved in any direction (Figure 30-17). If it needs to be lengthened, an interpositional substance may be placed. Shortening can occur by removing a wedge of bone. Tilting can occur if that wedge is removed in a trapezoidal fashion to tilt the chin either more downward or more posteriorly. The chin can be divided in the center to be widened or narrowed. The most common movements for genioplasties are a sliding movement to bring the chin for-

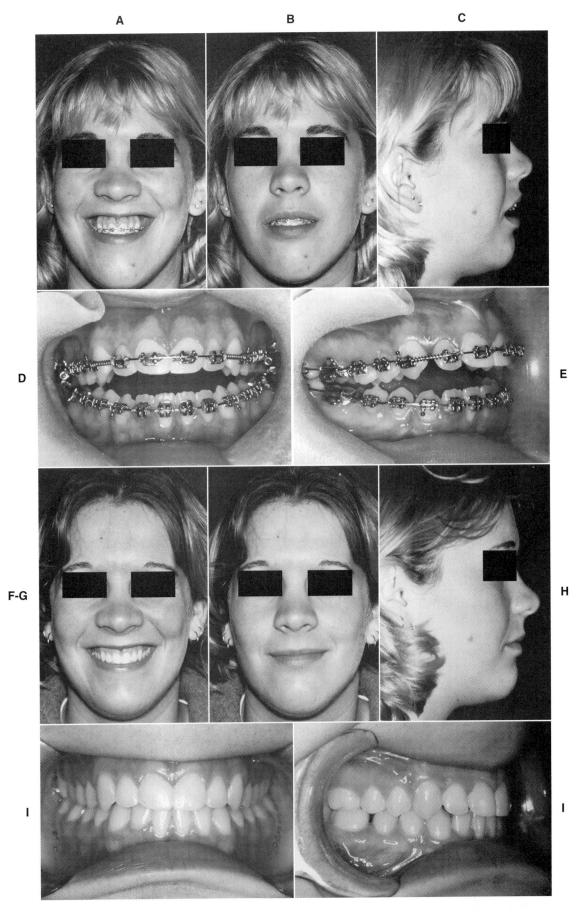

Figure 30-15 **A** to **C,** Facial photographs of a patient with skeletal anterior open bite. **D** and **E,** Intraoral photographs showing the extent of the open bite. **F** to **J,** Facial and intraoral photographs showing posttreatment results after a LeFort I impaction was performed and the completion of orthodontic treatment.

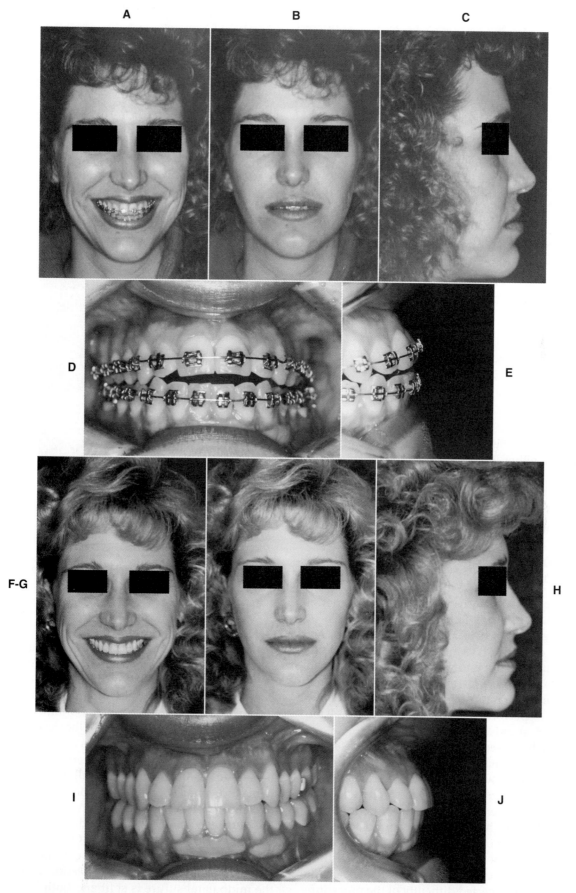

Figure 30-16 This patient had maxillary vertical excess, skeletal open bite, and mandibular sagittal excess. **A** to **C,** Pretreatment facial photographs. **D** and **E,** Intraoral photographs showing open bite and Class III tendency. **F** to **J,** Posttreatment facial and intraoral photographs showing the results after surgical and orthodontic treatment that included a maxillary impaction and mandibular setback.

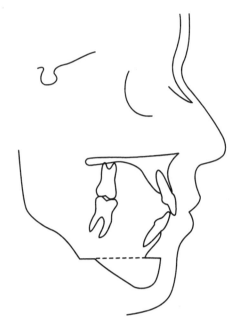

Figure 30-17 Genioplasty bone cuts.

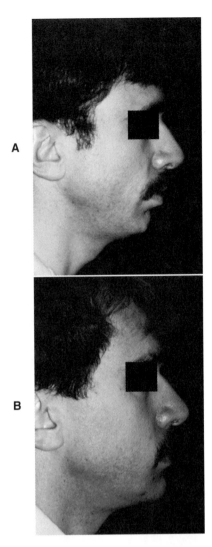

Figure 30-18 Genioplasty case. **A,** Presurgery. **B,** Postsurgery.

ward and to give the chin greater prominence. Chins may then be either wired in place or stabilized with plates. The plates may either be preformed or custom formed at the time of surgery. The genioplasty does not seem to significantly influence the patient's post-operative course (Figure 30-18).

Surgically Assisted Rapid Palatal Expansion

Orthodontic patients may have transverse deficiency of the maxilla. When this is identified in children or young adolescents, it is usually possible to use orthodontic and orthopedic techniques to cause the midpalatal suture to split and widen the maxilla (rapid maxillary expansion). However, if this problem is not identified until the patient is an adult, it is frequently impossible to perform skeletal maxillary expansion without surgical assistance.[10]

The procedure used to perform **surgically assisted rapid palatal expansion** combines the techniques of orthodontic palatal widening with a modification of the LeFort I osteotomy. The patient is prepared ahead of time with placement of a cemented orthodontic expansion appliance. The surgical procedure can be performed either with intravenous sedation in a clinic setting or with general anesthesia in an operating room. The decision for the type of anesthetic is made by evaluating the expected difficulty of the procedure and by determining patient preference as to anesthetic management.

The procedure begins with a modification of the LeFort I incision. The incision is made from the first molar but stops short of the midline on each side. The lateral surface of the maxilla is identified first and the pyriform fossa is freed of the nasal mucosa. A cut is made along the lateral surface of the maxilla, which is similar to the LeFort I cut in this area. An incision is then made vertically over the anterior nasal spine, exposing this anatomic area. A small fissure bur is used to make a vertical cut in the anterior nasal spine above the apices of the central incisors. A chisel is placed into this vertical cut and gently tapped posteriorly to begin opening the midpalatal suture. Often it is useful to place a chisel in each horizontal cut into the buttress area and gently mobilize each posterior segment. Once the midpalatal suture is split and both halves of the maxilla are slightly mobile, it is possible to start opening the expansion appliance to ensure that splitting of

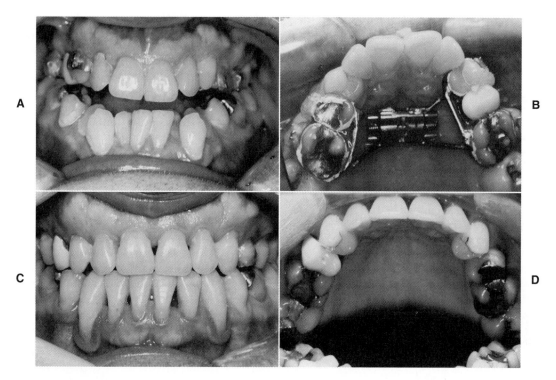

Figure 30-19 This patient has maxillary transverse deficiency requiring palatal expansion. **A** and **B,** Presurgery condition. **C** and **D,** Postpalatal expansion condition and orthodontic treatment.

the maxilla occurs as the appliance is activated approximately one turn twice a day.

Many modifications of surgically assisted rapid palatal expansion exist.[11] Some practitioners use a palatal approach to cut the palate. Others believe that division of the pterygoid plates from the posterior surface of the maxilla is important. It is also possible to perform this procedure without using a chisel to split the midpalatal suture (using only the buccal surface cuts to allow the maxilla to split). The technique described here is a predictable and successful technique.

It is important for the patient to understand that, postoperatively, he or she will develop a significant diastema rather quickly as the palatal expansion occurs. The occlusion will also change rapidly, and for a short time the maxilla will feel unstable. All of these problems are temporary. When the maxilla reaches its desired width, the orthodontist will stabilize the expansion appliance for 3 months in a retention phase before removing the expander and initiating orthodontic therapy (Figure 30-19).

Age and Orthognathic Surgery

The timing of orthognathic surgery must be carefully considered in patients who are still growing. A general rule of thumb is to operate excesses late and deficiencies early. In addition, each patient's psychosocial needs must be evaluated. Occasionally it will be appropriate to modify the time of surgery to provide more normal appearance and jaw function, even if growth may occur later, and the surgical procedure may need to be repeated.

Mandibular excess should generally be treated after mandibular growth is complete. An average age to consider is 18 years for males and 16 years for females. Serial cephalograms and superimpositions can aid in the determination of growth cessation.

Maxillary vertical excess can usually be treated at age 14 or later because vertical growth is generally complete by this time. Both mandibular and maxillary deficiencies may be treated earlier than problems of excess because the growth patterns of these patients do not usually result in significant changes following surgical correction.

SUMMARY

This chapter attempts to illustrate some of the common procedures that oral and maxillofacial surgeons perform in conjunction with orthodontic treatment. It is safe to say that many orthodontic patients will have some component of oral and maxillofacial surgery in their treatment plan. New procedures such as distraction osteogenesis, placement of implants for orthodontic anchorage, and combined orthodontic, prosthodontic, oral and maxillofacial surgery treatment plans with implants for the patient who is missing teeth continue to expand the cooperative relationship between the specialties of orthodontics and oral and maxillofacial surgery.

REFERENCES

1. Dachi SF, Howell FV: A survey of 3,874 routine full-mouth radiographs. II. A study of impacted teeth, *Oral Surg Oral Med Oral Pathol* 14(10):1165-1169, 1961.
2. Bishara SE: Clinical management of impacted maxillary canines, *Semin Orthod* 4(2):87-98, 1998.
3. Burden DJ, Mullally BH, Robinson SN: Palatally ectopic canines: closed eruption versus open eruption, *Am J Orthod Dentofacial Orthop* 115(6):640-644, 1999.
4. Kohavi D, Becker A, Zilberman Y: Surgical exposure, orthodontic movement, and final tooth position as factors in periodontal breakdown of treated palatally impacted canines, *Am J Orthod* 85(1):72-77, 1984.
5. Going RE Jr, Reyes-Lois DB: Surgical exposure and bracketing technique for uprighting impacted mandibular second molars, *J Oral Maxillofac Surg* 57(2):209-212, 1999.
6. Sagne S, Thilander B: Transalveolar transplantation of maxillary canines: a follow-up study, *Eur J Orthod* 12:140-147, 1990.
7. Sagne S, Thilander B: Transalveolar transplantation of maxillary canines: a critical evaluation of a clinical procedure, *Acta Odontol Scand* 55(1):l-8, 1997.
8. Bishara SE: Third molars: a dilemma! Or is it? *Am J Orthod Dentofacial Orthop* 115(6):628-633, 1999.
9. Southard TE: Third molars and incisor crowding: when removal is unwarranted, *J Am Dent Assoc* 123(8):75-79, 1992.
10. Northway WM, Meade JB Jr: Surgically assisted rapid maxillary expansion: a comparison of technique, response, and stability, *Angle Orthod* 67(4):309-320, 1997.
11. Cureton SL, Cuenin M: Surgically assisted rapid palatal expansion: orthodontic preparation for clinical success, *Am J Orthod Dentofacial Orthop* 116(l):46-59, 1999.

Glossary

activator Removable functional appliance developed by Viggo Andresen in Denmark in 1908. Consists of a large acrylic splint with a large lingual flange to maintain the mandible forward and downward, using loose retention.

Adams clasp Clasp used to anchor a Hawley retainer to the teeth by gripping each anchor tooth securely and engaging the undercuts on the mesiobuccal and distobuccal surfaces of the tooth.

adjunctive orthodontic treatment Treatment given in addition to a primary orthodontic procedure that is essential for achieving an optimal restoration of function and esthetics.

adolescence A stage of development between childhood and early adulthood (12 to 17 years of age).

adolescent spurt Expected, significant acceleration in height growth seen in both sexes at puberty; also called *prepubertal acceleration* or *circumpubertal acceleration*.

adult orthodontic treatment Specialty treatment targeting postadolescent patients.

advanced stages of root resorption Resorption of more than one third of the root.

alignment Movement of the malpositioned teeth into proper position.

aluminum shield Protective device placed between an x-ray source and the patient during radiographic procedures to reduce radiation exposure to the soft tissues.

alveolar bone The part of the mandibular or maxillary bone around the teeth in which fibers of the periodontal ligament connects to the roots of the teeth.

alveolar bone height Height of the bone surrounding the teeth.

amniotic cavity Space between the epiblast and the cytotrophoblast of a bilaminar disk.

anchorage control Ability to achieve differential tooth movement. Most frequently it refers to the relative mesiodistal movement of the anterior and posterior teeth.

Angle Class II malocclusion See **Class II malocclusion.**

Angle Class III malocclusion See **Class III malocclusion.**

Angle classification Widely used classification system for malocclusions (proposed by Edward Angle) that describes the anteroposterior relationships of the permanent first molars and canines as well as other characteristics of the malocclusion.

Angle, Edward Originator of the Angle classification system for malocclusions.

anterior crossbite Malocclusion in which the labial surfaces of the maxillary incisors occlude posterior to the lingual surfaces of the mandibular incisors; may involve two or all of the anterior teeth.

anterior face height Cephalometric feature of the vertical length of the face between nasion and pogonion.

anterior neuropores The last part of the neural tube to close during fusion of the neural folds at the anterior part of the neural tube.

anterior open bite Lack of vertical overlap between the upper and lower incisors.

anterior overbite See **overbite.**

anterior shift Forward movement in mandibular position from centric relation to centric occlusion often seen in association with anterior crossbite.

anteroposterior maxillary excess Skeletal Class II relationship that typically includes an increased ANB angle and A-B difference projected on occlusal plane and true horizontal line, as well as increased facial convexity. In addition, SNA angle usually is increased, except where a steep cranial base or anterior displacement of nasion can make this angle appear normal.

anteroposterior relationship Description of the maxillary and mandibular first molars and canines with the teeth in centric occlusion and amenable to Angle classification.

antiplaque agents Agents, particularly tooth-cleansing agents, that minimize plaque formation and have at least mild efficacy against gingivitis.

apical root resorption Presence of actual root shortening over time, resulting either from normal physiologic processes in the primary dentition or orthodontic treatment in the permanent dentition.

apically repositioned flap Periodontal surgery used to expose the impacted canines to provide the tooth with attached gingiva during its eruption.

apposition (of teeth) Phase of tooth development establishing juxtaposition of teeth.

arch form (of bone) Surface deposition of bone. Summary quality of the shape of the dental arch that includes such parameters as tooth rotations, arch widths, arch depths, and arch chords.

arches *Primordial:* paired pharyngeal structures that make up the lateral walls of the primordial pharynx, which develops from the foregut and are numbered I, II, III, and IV beginning at the cranial end. Together with the rest of the pharyngeal apparatus, they give rise to head and neck structures in the adult.

arrow clasp Clasp used to anchor a Hawley retainer to the teeth that is similar in function to a ball clasp. The arrow part of the clasp is preformed by the manufacturer and is placed between adjacent teeth to engage undercuts on each tooth.

articulare Point of intersection of the inferior border of the cranial base and the averaged posterior surfaces of the mandibular condyles.

asymmetry Degree of imbalance or deviation in both qualitative and quantitative features in structure or relationship or both.

average growers Category of children who, in terms of height growth, follow the middle range of the distance curve and comprise about ⅔ of all children.

ball clasp Clasp used to anchor a Hawley retainer to the teeth and to engage undercuts on two adjacent teeth. Also can be used in mixed dentition patients between primary molars that have no available retentive surfaces for an Adams or Resta clasp.

base of the tongue Posterior third of the tongue that is developed from pharyngeal arch III.

561

behavioral sciences Psychology and related fields that have been an integral part of orthodontics both in research and in clinical practice, particularly in demonstrating how patients' and doctors' individual behaviors can dictate an eventual course of action in an orthodontic context, as well as emphasizing the role self-image plays in successful treatment.

bilaminar disk Stage of embryonic development resulting from differentiation of an inner cell mass that is comprised of epiblast and hypoblast.

biologic considerations Factors affecting adult orthodontic treatment including periodontal disease and certain medical factors.

biometric norm Objective norm derived from the measurement of a biologic variable in a random sample of persons who are considered normal.

bionator One of a group of functional, removable, tooth-borne appliances that depend on the stretch of soft tissue caused by the mandible being positioned forward and downward together with the muscle activity generated by the mandible attempting to return to its original position to achieve the desired dental and skeletal effects.

Blanche test Examination technique used to determine whether the maxillary labial frenum extends lingually between the central incisors toward the incisive papilla.

blastocele Fluid-filled space within a morula. Also called a *blastocyst cavity.*

blastocyst Morula that contains a blastocele.

blastocyst cavity Fluid-filled space that develops within a morula. Also called a *blastocele.*

blastomere Cell resulting from cleavage.

bodily movement Desired form of distal displacement of the molars in correction of a Class II malocclusion as opposed to tipping.

body image Perception of one's physical appearance.

body of the tongue Anterior two thirds of the tongue that is developed from pharyngeal arch I.

bonded bracket Implement that attaches to a tooth to enable the orthodontist to use an arch wire or ligatures or both to apply forces on the tooth to aid in its movement into the line of occlusion.

bonded (fixed) appliance Apparatus that remains firmly in place, not intended to be removed by the patient, to achieve alignment of upper or lower teeth for the correction of malocclusions.

bonded retainer Retention phase appliance for the anterior teeth to minimize or eliminate the possibility of undesirable tooth movement after orthodontic treatment.

bonding of molars Orthodontic approach sometimes preferred over banding in adults who are in periodontal maintenance.

bone loss Deterioration of bone surface or substance; in periodontal disease, this condition is usually caused by bacteria in subgingival plaque.

bracket system Standard fixed orthodontic system first developed by Edward Angle in 1928 and still considered a standard approach.

Brodie syndrome Buccal crossbite in which the lower teeth are positioned completely lingual to the upper teeth and occurs in patients having a retrusive and small mandible or a large maxilla.

brushing instructions Refers specifically to tooth brushing instructions for patients with orthodontic appliances.

buccopharyngeal membrane Tissue that separates the foregut and the primitive oral cavity (stomodeum).

C clasp Circumferential clasp to anchor a Hawley retainer. Most useful on the most distal teeth in the upper arch where it can pass over the distal surface of the molar and engage the undercut on the mesiobuccal surface of the tooth without interfering with the occlusion.

calcification Process by which organic tissue becomes hardened by a deposit of calcium salts within its substance.

cartilaginous neurocranium Chondrocranium consisting of several cartilages that fuse and undergo endochondral ossification to give rise to the base of the skull.

cartilaginous viscerocranium Portion of the facial skeleton that includes middle ear ossicles, the styloid process of the temporal bone, the hyoid bone, and the laryngeal cartilages.

Case, Calvin American orthodontist who refined treatment techniques in the early twentieth century before the dominating influence of Edward Angle.

center of resistance Analogous center of mass for an in vivo tooth such that any force acting through a tooth's center of resistance causes the tooth to translate. Designated target zone for angling a superior and posterior force to achieve the most appropriate direction to affect maxillary sutures when exerting extraoral force.

center of rotation Point located either internal or external to a rotating body around which it turns. Located at variable points depending on how far a given force is applied from the center of resistance (approaching, but never reaching, the center of resistance).

cephalometric standards Expected range of measurements for various components of the craniofacial complex in terms of changes in linear dimensions and angular relationships over time with adjustments for age, ethnic group, and gender.

cervical attachment Extraoral attachment around the patient's back of the neck that provides anchorage for extraoral orthopedic headgear below the occlusal plane, directing the extraoral force inferiorly and posteriorly.

cessation Termination of a process.

chief concern Patient's reason for seeking orthodontic treatment.

chlorhexidine Chemical component of some rinses for optimum management of severe gingivitis in adolescent orthodontic patients.

chondrocranium Independent prenatal sites of craniofacial cartilage that coalesce into a cartilaginous mass. The precursor to the adult cranial base and nasal and otic structures.

chondrogenesis Formation of cartilage.

chorion Structure comprised of a chorionic cavity, extraembryonic mesoderm, cytotrophoblast, and syncytiotrophoblast.

chorionic cavity Space surrounding a yolk sac and amniotic cavity (except at the connecting stalk). Formed when lacunae fuse within the extraembryonic mesoderm.

circumpubertal acceleration See **adolescent spurt.**

Class I malocclusion Category of the Angle classification of malocclusions in which the relative mesiodistal position of the dental arches is normal with the permanent first molars usually in normal occlusion. Although one or more teeth may be in lingual or buccal malposition, the malocclusions are mostly confined to the anterior teeth.

Class I molar relationship Normal relationship in which the mesiobuccal cusp of the maxillary first permanent molar occludes with the buccal groove of the mandibular first molar.

Class II Division 1 Category of the Angle classification of malocclusions in which excessive overjet is accompanied by normal or protrusive maxillary incisor angulation.

Class II Division 2 Category of the Angle classification of malocclusions in which normal overjet is seen in combination with upright maxillary incisors.

Class II elastics Intraoral traction with rubber bands from the maxillary anterior to the mandibular posterior teeth. A technique championed by Calvin Case and Edward Angle for the correction of Class II malocclusions.

Class II malocclusion Category of the Angle classification of malocclusions in which the relative mesiodistal relations of the dental arches are abnormal with all the lower teeth occluding distal to normal, producing a marked disharmony in the incisor region and in the facial lines.

Class II molar relationship Abnormal relationship in which the mesiobuccal cusp of the maxillary first permanent molar occludes mesial to the buccal groove of the mandibular first molar.

Class III malocclusion Category of the Angle classification of malocclusions in which the relative mesiodistal relations of the arches are abnormal with all the lower teeth occluding mesial to normal, producing a marked disharmony in the incisor region and in the facial lines.

Class III molar relationship Abnormal relationship in which the mesiobuccal cusp of the maxillary first permanent molar occludes distal to the buccal groove of the mandibular first molar.

Class III subdivision Subcategory of Angle's Class III malocclusion classifications that exhibits disharmony of a lesser degree with a normal occlusion on one side of the arch and a Class III occlusion on the other side.

cleavage Series of mitotic divisions a zygote undergoes as it moves along the uterine tube toward the uterus.

clefting Unsuccessful tissue closure that constitutes the most common major defect of the lip or palate or both.

clockwise rotation Downward and posterior rotation of the mandible resulting in skeletal retrusion.

closed eruption approach Periodontal surgery used to expose the impacted canines in which the mucosa is retracted, an attachment is placed on the impacted tooth, and the mucosa is placed back on the tooth.

collimator Radiographic apparatus that allows precise limitation of the primary x-ray beam to the target tissue or body area.

combination headgear Combination of the cervical and occipital attachments to distribute extraoral force over more external surfaces and provide a convenient means of modifying the direction of the force vector, usually resulting in a force vector above the occlusal plane but inferior to the vector created with the occipital attachment alone.

compliance Patient cooperation.

complications Additional challenges that present themselves during the course of treatment such as medical problems, temporomandibular disorder, functional shifts, parafunction, abnormal posturing of the mandibular condyle in the temporomandibular fossa, periodontal compromise, and a wide variety of other potential problems.

composite resin A restorative material that is also used as a means of managing an incisor diastema in the permanent dentition by providing esthetic buildup and contouring.

compositional change Growth involving chemical or physiologic changes in parts of the body.

computed tomography Sophisticated imaging technique that creates a computer-reconstructed axial image using an x-ray tube and a detector that revolves 360 degrees around the body or body part.

condylar cartilage Specialized, fibrous connective tissue on the rounded projection of the mandibular condyle.

condylar growth Growth or proliferation at the head of the condyle in an upward and backward or forward direction.

condylar growth direction Measure useful in evaluating mandibular morphology and determining the inclination of the condyle as an indication of its growth direction, whether vertically or sagittally.

congenitally missing teeth Teeth absent because of genetics rather than from injury or removal.

connecting stalk Structure that attaches a bilaminar disk to a trophoblast and that later becomes the umbilical cord.

continuous force Duration of applied orthodontic force that most effectively moves teeth.

conventional toothbrush Traditional home dental hygiene tool. In terms of the optimal for periodontic considerations, a soft-bristled brush with rounded ends and an orthodontic design.

copula Midline enlargement derived from arch II that is overtaken by the hypobranchial eminence and disappears without contributing to formation of the tongue.

couples Force system in a fixed appliance that provides control in three planes of space.

cranial base synchondrosis Cartilaginous joints in the base of the cranium where the cartilage divides and subsequently is converted into bone.

craniofacial sutures Fibrous joints of dense connective tissue in the face and head that separate the bones and are important growth sites that serve to facilitate calvarial and midface growth.

craniomandibular disorders Collective term embracing a number of clinical problems or a cluster of related disorders with common symptoms that involve the masticatory musculature, the temporomandibular joint, or both. Synonymous with the term *temporomandibular disorders*.

crest Maxillary ridge passing along the alveolar processes of the fetal maxillary bones.

crestal bone loss Deterioration of the gingival part of the alveolar processes around the teeth.

cross-sectional studies Research in which a large number of individuals bearing different aspects of the characteristic under study are examined on one occasion, with the advantage of accumulating much information about many forms or phases of that characteristic in a short period.

crossbite elastics Accessory rubber bands that are helpful in correcting crossbites.

crowding Malalignment of teeth caused by inadequate space.

crown angulation Key value used in determining normal occlusion in which all tooth crowns are angulated mesially (mesiodistal tip) to different degrees.

crown inclination Labiolingual or buccolingual inclination of the crowns of the teeth. Used as a key value in determining normal occlusion.

cumulative curve Graphic presentation of incremental growth data derived from longitudinal studies.

curve of Spee Curvature of the incisor edges and occlusal surfaces of teeth beginning at the tips of the lower incisors and canine, following the buccal cusps of the premolars and molars, and continuing to the anterior border of the ramus.

cytotrophoblast Inner layer of a trophoblast.

decalcification Loss of normal hardening of the enamel or a detrimental loss of calcium salts within organic tissue.

deep bite Aberration in the overlap between the maxillary and mandibular incisors.

definitive yolk sac Secondary yolk sac developing when the primitive yolk sac is squeezed off by hypoblast development just around the second week of embryonic development.

dental age Age determination based on two different methods of assessment: observation of age at eruption of the primary and permanent teeth and the rating of tooth development from crown calcification to root completion using x-rays of the unerupted and developing teeth.

dental angular relationship Parameters included in the Iowa cephalometric standards that provides 29 angular and linear measurements of various structures as well as ratios of face heights.

dental anomalies Abnormalities of tooth condition or development, such as tooth agenesis, small lateral incisors, dens invaginatus, taurodontism, ectopic eruption, and abnormally short roots.

dental arches Bowlike structures formed by the ridge of the alveolar process of the mandible or maxilla.

dental asymmetries Degree of imbalance or deviation in both qualitative and quantitative features of dentition.

dental camouflage Treatment of Class II or Class III skeletal problems with the intent to disguise the unacceptable skeletal relationship by orthodontically repositioning the teeth in the jaws so there is an acceptable dental occlusion and esthetic facial appearance.

dental compensation Feature of Class II dental malocclusions typically observed in the presence of skeletal discrepancy that tends to make the dental discrepancy less than the skeletal discrepancy. Exhibited most often as protrusive mandibular incisors and less frequently as retrusive maxillary incisors. Also occurs as a maxillary dental arch that is more narrow or constricted than normal.

dental history Different events such as trauma to the teeth, restorations, and root canal therapy that the patient has experienced.

dental linear relationship Parameters included in the Iowa cephalometric standards that provides 29 angular and linear measurements of various structures as well as ratios of face heights.

dentofacial orthopedic treatment Therapeutic route selected when significant skeletofacial changes are necessary.

dermatome Source of skin components (dermis) formed by superficial somite cells.

derotation Correction of aberration from normal occlusion in teeth placement or position. Also, use of a transpalatal arch, arch wire, or inner facebow to achieve the desired positioning and expansion of the maxillary molars.

development Process of going through natural growth, differentiation, or evolution by successive changes.

development of the vertical dimension Growth of the anterior and posterior face heights.

diagnosis Identification of a clinical problem or condition, frequently including a referral for treatment.

diagnostic norm Standard that helps determine the extent to which a patient deviates from normal.

diagnostic parameters Standardized method involving points of analysis that correlate with the various aspects of records assessment to guide the clinician in evaluating and characterizing the complexity of a malocclusion.

diastema Space between any two neighboring teeth.

diastema closure Orthodontic treatment of excess space between any two neighboring teeth.

differential eruption Intrusion and extrusion of teeth during leveling with arch wires.

digit habit Thumb or finger sucking habit in which the thumb is frequently placed in the anterior part of the mouth and can prevent the incisors (usually maxillary) from fully erupting or can cause anterior open bite, maxillary incisor protrusion, Class II canine relationships, distal step molar relationships, posterior crossbites, lip incompetence, or speech defects.

direct bonding Direct attachment of orthodontic appliances to etched teeth using chemical and light-cured adhesives. Most popular method with clinicians because of its simplicity and reliability.

distal step Relationship in which the maxillary terminal plane is relatively more anterior than the mandibular terminal plane. A key element in assessing the terminal plane relationship of the second primary molars.

distance curve Graphic presentation of growth data that reveals the substance of study findings by indicating the distance a subject has traversed along a measurable path. Data can be derived from cross-sectional and longitudinal studies.

Division 1 Category within Class II of Angle's malocclusion classifications sometimes accompanied by a narrowing of the upper arch, lengthened and protruding upper incisors, abnormal function of the lips, and some form of nasal obstruction and mouth breathing.

Division 2 Category within Class II of Angle's malocclusion classifications characterized by crowding of the upper incisors (overlapping) and lingual inclination.

doctor-patient interaction Assessment factor that is an indicator of how well a patient can be expected to comply with the doctor's instructions.

early maturing Category of children who are taller in childhood because they have matured faster than average and who are usually not particularly tall as adults.

ectoderm Embryonic germ layer formed from epiblast cells after invagination occurs in the third week of development.

ectomesenchyme Head and neck mesenchyme.

ectopic molar eruption Tooth developing beyond the range of the normal eruption path.

edgewise appliance Orthodontic apparatus used in the traditional fixed edgewise bracket system that originally involved the banding of all the individual teeth with bands that were customized for each patient by stretch molding the band material around the tooth, creating a joint, and then welding the brackets to the bands. Precursor to the use of preformed bands and bonding of brackets.

edgewise bracket Central tool used during orthodontic treatment to engage the arch wire and to move teeth.

educational psychology Relatively new area of application of experiential learning theory and patient learning style, in particular orthodontic motivational psychology, to achieve patient compliance, exploring the role of "doctor as teacher" rather than "doctor as healer."

elastic properties of wires Propensity based on one of two principles: stress-strain curve or load deflection curve.

electric toothbrush Home dental hygiene tool preferred over the conventional toothbrush for periodontal patients because of its greater effectiveness in interproximal plaque removal.

embryoblast Cluster of cells located between a trophoblast and a blastocyst beginning the sixth day after fertilization. Also called an *inner cell mass.*

embryonic period Period of prenatal human development extending from fertilization through the eighth week of development.

endochondral bone formation Process of converting cartilage into bone.

endochondral ossification Bone formation from a cartilaginous precursor in which chondroblasts initially form cartilage, which, in turn, is calcified and invaded by osteogenic tissue to form bone.

endoderm *Embryonic:* Germ layer formed from displacement of the hypoblast by invaginating epiblast cells. *Mature:* Epithelial cell layer that covers the internal surface of the pharyngeal arch.

enlargement Property of radiography in which the x-ray source's proximity to the patient can enhance a body part's size.

environmental factors External influences.

epiblast Component of a bilaminar disk made up of columnar cells and separated from the cytotrophoblast by the amniotic cavity.

equilibrium of one-couple force system Condition or principle demanding that a system with a couple and its associated tendency to rotate must have an equal and opposite tendency to rotate the system in the opposite direction. A one-couple system inherently must have two equal and opposite couples present because it is in equilibrium.

equilibrium of two-couple force system Principle for determining the actions of an arch wire inserted into two consecutive brackets: activation of the wire creates a couple at each bracket with each couple existing with an associated equilibrium just as if they were two one-couple systems acting together. Therefore the two-couple system's equilibrium is equivalent to the algebraic sum of the two one-couple systems present.

eruption of the first permanent tooth Event setting off the mixed dentition stage, usually involving the mandibular central incisor.

etiology The study of the cause, origin, and method of introduction of a condition or disease.

exocoelomic cavity Primitive yolk sac developed from a blastocyst cavity.

experiential learning theory Aspect of educational psychology that explores patient learning styles and approaches the orthodontist-patient relationship from the perspective of a teacher-student relationship rather than that of healer-patient relationship. Emphasizes that students learn the material presented to them in a style unique unto themselves and that it is up to the teacher or doctor to teach to that unique style of learning.

exposed mineralized root surface Typical finding in root resorption and in localized compression of the periodontal ligament during alveolar bone remodeling.

external apical resorption See **root resorption.**

external resorption See **root resorption.**

extraembryonic coelom Chorionic cavity.

extraembryonic mesoderm Loose connective tissue layer located between the outer surface of the primitive yolk sac and the inner surface of the cytotrophoblast.

extraoral appliances Headgear and other appliances frequently prescribed for anchorage control, securing the posterior teeth to extraoral structures.

extraoral orthopedic force Pressure used (primarily with headgear) to compress the maxillary sutures, modifying the pattern of bone apposition primarily intended to inhibit anterior and inferior development of the maxilla and inhibit mesial and occlusal eruption of the maxillary posterior teeth. Goal of treatment is for this restriction of maxillary growth to occur while the mandible continues to grow forward an adequate amount to "catch up" with the maxilla.

extraoral photographs Facial assessment tool that usually includes a frontal view at rest, a frontal view smiling, and a profile view to assess a patient's profile and facial asymmetries and to evaluate the facial appearance.

extrusion Moving the tooth in the direction of the occlusal plane.

extrusion of molars Tooth movement technique to correct a deep overbite by using bite plates to initially prevent the teeth from contacting, thus allowing accelerated eruption.

face types Shape of the face as described by the heights of the anterior and posterior heights. Can be average, long, or short.

facebow Headgear for delivering a posteriorly directed extraoral force to the maxilla, consisting of an outer bow for the extraoral attachment, soldered to an inner bow that attaches intraorally to tubes welded to the maxillary first permanent molar bands; can be used with either a maxillary fixed or removable appliance.

facial skeletal convexity Angle between nasion (forehead), point A (maxilla) and pogonion (mandible) (NAPog).

facial form Face shape assessed through anthropometric measurements or analysis of cephalograms in screening for malocclusion.

facial morphology Shape and structure of the face, particularly the skeletal form.

facial orthopedic treatment Treatment that is primarily intended to affect the jaw bones as well as the teeth.

facial plane Surface formed by passing a line through points nasion and pogonion.

facial symmetry Degree of bilateral balance in right-left correspondence of the facial features.

fetal period Period of prenatal human development extending from week nine to term.

finger spring Removable appliance attachment made from stainless steel wire used to deliver the force required to move a tooth.

finishing details Fine-tuning of tooth position and occlusion to optimize treatment result, including assessing first-, second-, and third-order positions of each tooth relative to their ideal positions, along with all other aspects of the outcome of treatment to identify any remaining discrepancies.

first-order plane Plane commonly used in orthodontic terminology to represent the occlusal view.

first-order tooth movement Process in which movement is around the long axis of the tooth. Rotation.

fixed orthodontic appliances See **bonded (fixed) appliances.**

fixed retainers See **bonded retainer.**

fixed W-spring appliance Fixed appliance that helps expand the maxilla bilaterally to correct crossbites of mild to moderate magnitude.

flush terminal plane relationship Relationship in which both the distal surfaces of the maxillary and mandibular primary second molars are at the same level anteroposteriorly.

focal spot Area from which the roentgen radiation is emitted in a radiographic procedure.

fontanelles Regions of dense connective tissue where bones may come together during parturition.

foramen cecum Structure that is all that remains of the proximal opening of the embryonic thyroglossal duct on the dorsum of the tongue and is found in the midline of the terminal sulcus.

force In physics, a coercive energy that causes or alters motion (mass X acceleration) as measured in Newtons. In orthodontics, a biomechanical energy measured in grams that is directed through a center of mass, causing the tooth to move the same amount in the same direction as the line of this energy or force.

force direction See **vector.**

force magnitude Amount or intensity of an applied force.

Frankfort horizontal plane Porion-orbitale plane of the head. Also called the *eye-ear plane.*

frequency Rate of occurrence of a condition or disorder that is usually measured among a distinct population or group.

frontonasal prominence Embryonic structure whose enlargement and movement are a main source of facial development, in conjunction with the four prominences of the pharyngeal arch I.

functional appliance Appliance that, when fully seated in the mouth, forces the mandible into an eccentric-noncentric relation position and causes the musculature to try to move the mandible toward a centric relation position and resulting in force systems being exerted whenever the appliance is used.

functional asymmetries Aberration in use or movement resulting from skeletal or muscular imbalance. In orthodontics this can result from the mandible being deflected laterally or anteroposteriorly if occlusal interferences prevent proper intercuspation in centric relation or from a constricted maxillary arch or a more localized factor such as a malposed tooth.

functional change Type of growth in which tissues and organs undergo changes in functional capabilities with a goal of mature function in each.

functional corrector (or functional regulator) Functional appliance that has few active components with minimal bulk of acrylic and abundant use of wires to hold parts of the appliance together. Provides improved ability to speak with appliance in place, as well as the possibility of generalized transverse expansion from the buccal shields.

functional shift Discrepancy between centric relation and centric occlusion as a result of premature tooth contact that deflects the mandible.

fundamental growth pattern Theory that there is a natural, genetic disposition of skeletal growth applied particularly to facial growth and having negligible permanent response to facial orthopedic treatment once treatment is discontinued, causing the skeletal discrepancy to return.

gastrulation Process occurring in third week of development in which the bilaminar embryonic disk is converted into a trilaminar disk.

general curve Growth curve covering the postnatal period of 20 years, specifically measuring external dimensions or development of the body, the respiratory and digestive organs, kidneys, aorta and pulmonary trunks, spleen, musculature, skeleton, and blood volume.

generalized spacings Common presence of spacing between the teeth in the primary dentition.

genetically short Category of children who are short as children and will be short adults.

genetically tall Category of taller-than-average children who will be tall as adults.

genetics Influence of inheritance or familial incidence associated with a dominant gene, particularly as it is implicated in certain conditions. Field of study of familial incidence and gene dominance in pathologic and nonpathologic conditions.

genital curve Growth curve covering the postnatal period of 20 years that specifically measures the changes in the primary sex apparatus and all secondary sex traits.

gingiva Oral mucosa overlying the crowns of unerupted teeth and encircling the necks of those that have erupted, serving as the supporting structure for subadjacent tissues.

gingival recession Retracted gum line and tooth support drawing back of the gingivae from the necks of the teeth with subsequent exposure of root surfaces.

gnathion Radiographic anatomic landmark located at a point on the shadow of the chin midway between pogonion and menton.

gonion Midpoint of the angle of the mandible found by bisecting the angle formed by the mandibular and ramus planes.

grid Series of thin strips of lead placed between the patient and a radiographic film to absorb secondary radiation and thus reduce image blurring caused by this secondary radiation.

grooves Fissures or clefts of the pharyngeal apparatus that separate the pharyngeal arches on the external surface of the embryo. Together with the rest of the pharyngeal apparatus, grooves give rise to head and neck structures in the adult.

growth Size development and progressive change in an organism influenced by the interplay between heredity and environment.

growth changes Developmental changes that occur during the growth period.

growth hormone Somatotropin. A protein produced by the anterior lobe of the pituitary gland that maintains the normal rate of protein synthesis, appears to inhibit the synthesis of fat and the oxidation of carbohydrate, and is necessary for the proliferation of cartilage cells, thus having a great effect on bone growth and consequently height growth.

growth modification Treatment for Class II or Class III skeletal problems with the intent to alter the unacceptable skeletal relationships by modifying the patient's remaining facial growth to favorably change the size or position of the jaws.

growth prediction Expectation of morphologic development used to identify a specific skeletal morphologic pattern; however, such predictions are not always accurate.

growth spurt Acceleration in the incremental changes in a body part that occurs at a certain age.

guided extraction Removal of certain primary and permanent teeth in a definite sequence.

gummy smile Smile that reveals a great deal of gingiva above the maxillary incisors. Sign of a short upper lip or excessive maxillary anterior vertical growth.

Hawley appliance Type of removable appliance that can be effective for minor tooth movements or as a retainer.

headcap See **occipital attachment.**

headgear Appliance used in orthodontics to modify growth of the maxilla, distalize maxillary teeth, or reinforce anchorage.

helical spring Looped wire used to upright and extrude a tipped lower second molar but with little control over buccolingual movement of the uprighted molar. Constructed of stainless steel arch wire that hooks onto a fixed edgewise appliance for activation.

Herbst appliance Functional appliance that has the advantage of full-time wear but is less durable and has a tendency to promote mandibular incisor proclination.

hereditary Genetic transmission of a trait from parent to offspring.

homeobox (HOX) genes Embryonic genes that produce transcription factors that bind to the DNA of other genes and regulate gene expression. Important in determining the identity and spatial arrangements of body regions and in determining the pattern and position of structures developing within the pharyngeal arches.

homeostasis Tendency toward stability in the normal internal environment achieved by control mechanisms activated by negative feedback.

hyalinization Tissue characterized as devoid of cellular elements.

hypoblast Component of a bilaminar disk that consists of squamous or cuboidal cells adjacent to the blastocyst cavity.

hypobranchial eminence Midline swelling comprised primarily of mesenchyme from arch III and situated caudal to the foramen cecum that develops into the posterior third, or base, of the tongue.

hypoplasia Incomplete or defective formation of the dental enamel that is common in the teeth adjacent to a cleft site.

hypothalamus Gland thought to control growth that keeps the child on a genetically determined growth curve by sending messages to the pituitary gland through an elaborate feedback system.

impacted tooth Tooth blocked from eruption by a physical barrier such as another tooth.

incidence Number of cases reported for a given condition.

incisor alignment Proper position of the crowded anterior teeth in relation to the line of the dental arch.

incisor intrusion Technique for overbite correction, using the intrusion arch and utility arch, indicated in patients with deep overbite excessive maxillary incisor display at rest or when smiling.

incisor liability Factor related to the ratio between the primary and permanent incisor tooth size that may influence the overall arch length.

incremental curve Graphic presentation of data that reveals the substance of study findings indicating the rate of change in a subject over a certain period. Data are derived from longitudinal studies.

indirect bonding Bracket adherence technique in which the brackets were first positioned on study casts with a water-soluble adhesive and then transferred to the mouth with a custom tray. More recently, the bracket is positioned on the patient's study cast with filled resin then transferred to the mouth with a custom tray with bonding facilitated by applying an unfilled liquid sealant to the prepared tooth surface and the precured resin at the bracket base.

inner bow Portion of a facebow that attaches to the maxillary first permanent molars and rests between the lips at rest.

inner cell mass Cluster of cells that is located between a trophoblast and blastocyst beginning the sixth day after fertilization and develops into an embryo. Also called an *embryoblast*.

intensifying screen Radiographic apparatus within a film cassette that permits film exposure with lower radiation exposure.

interarch compatibility Harmony between the shape and tooth mass of the upper and lower arches.

interarch tooth size discrepancy Condition caused from a smaller mesiodistal tooth width or absent maxillary permanent teeth resulting in a relative maxillary tooth size deficiency in relation to the corresponding mandibular teeth. Usually exhibited as maxillary spacing but can be expressed as a forward drift of maxillary permanent molars into a Class II relationship with minimal interdental spacing.

interceptive treatment Therapeutic measure directed at eliminating habits or inserting a space maintainer after the premature loss of primary teeth.

interdental osteotomy Surgical intervention with cuts occurring between the teeth.

interlabial gap Characteristic of facial form assessed by the degree to which the lips are apart at rest. Large interlabial gaps indicate either vertically short lips or excess anterior vertical growth.

intermaxillary elastics Elastic bands that pit the upper teeth to the lower teeth as a means of gaining differential tooth movement with its force vector defined by the direction of the elastic.

intermaxillary growth space Natural, differential growth of the mandible and maxilla, creating a space for the vertical development of the dentoalveolus.

intermaxillary segment Embryonic precursor of the philtrum (middle portion) of the upper lip, four incisor teeth and alveolar bone and gingiva surrounding them, and the primary palate.

intermediate mesoderm Embryonic structure that develops into the excretory units of the urinary system.

intermittent force Duration of applied orthodontic force characterized by interruption and used to move teeth or for facial orthopedic changes.

interstitial growth Growth from within the structure.

intramembranous bone formation Process of bone formation from undifferentiated mesenchymal tissue on the surface of the bone.

intraoral photographs Dentition assessment tool that consists of a frontal view, right and left lateral views, and maxillary and mandibular occlusal views, providing a general overview of existing malocclusion, the gingival condition, and any hypoplastic teeth.

intraoral ramus osteotomy Surgical procedure in which the ramus of the mandible is segmented to allow for moving the body forward or backward.

intraoral sagittal split ramus osteotomy Preferred technique for surgically advancing the mandible that mitigates issues of morbidity and instability.

intrauterine pressure Pressure during pregnancy and parturition that can have observable effects on the bones of the fetal skull.

intravenous sedation Anesthesia technique involving managed injection, control, and monitoring of the anesthetic in the bloodstream.

intrusion Technique for moving the teeth in an apical direction.

intrusion arch Appliance used for deep bite correction in which the two forces acting at each end of the wire (extrusion at the molar and intrusion at the incisor) make up the vertical pair of forces comprising the equilibrium associated with the couple at the molar bracket. Variations include base arches, utility arches, and reverse curve of Spee wires.

invagination Process in which cells of the epiblast migrate to the primitive streak and primitive node, detach from the epiblast, and lead to development of the epiblast into the three embryonic germ layers.

Iowa cephalometric standards Expected range of measurements for various components of the craniofacial complex based on the original University of Iowa Facial Growth Study started in 1946 that are specific by sex and applicable within an age range rather than providing a single standard used for all ages and both sexes.

J-hook headgear Headgear for delivering a posteriorly directed extraoral force to the maxilla that consists of two separate, curved, large-gauge wires that are formed on their ends into small hooks, both of which attach directly to the anterior part of the maxillary arch wire. More commonly used for retraction of canines or incisors rather than orthopedic purposes and limited to use only with a maxillary fixed appliance with a continuous arch wire.

jiggling movements Teeth moved in one direction and then in the opposite direction over short period of time.

Kingsley, Norman American dentist who, in 1880, published a description of treatment techniques for protrusion.

Kloehn, Silas American orthodontist who reintroduced extraoral force in the form of cervical headgear for treatment of skeletal Class II relationships.

knife-edging Localized collapse of the lingual and buccal alveolar walls following the extraction of teeth.

labrale inferius Median point in the lower margin of the lower membranous lip.

labrale superius Median point in the upper margin of the upper membranous lip.

late maturing Category of children who are shorter than average in childhood because of their late maturing and who will eventually be adults of average stature.

lateral cephalometric radiograph Side view radiograph of the head that obtains linear and angular measurements by tracing the oriented lateral radiographic head film. Used to assess craniofacial growth and development on a longitudinal basis and to evaluate the anteroposterior and vertical positions of the maxilla and mandible to the cranial base and to one another, as well as the angulation of the maxillary and mandibular incisors and the soft tissue profile.

lateral functional shift Lateral movement of the mandible during closure from centric relation into centric occlusion.

lateral lingual swellings Structures arising from proliferation of first arch mesenchyme to enlarge, fuse, and, with the tuberculum impar, form the body of the tongue.

lateral nasal prominences Horseshoe-shaped ridges that form along the periphery of the embryonic nasal placodes and fuse to form key nasal structures.

lateral palatine shelves Paired structures of the maxilla comprised initially of mesenchymal connective tissue and oriented in a superior-inferior plane with the tongue interposed, eventually fusing in the midline to form the hard and soft palate.

LeFort I maxillary impaction osteotomy A type of maxillary impaction surgery indicated for treatment of vertical maxillary excess.

lead shield Protective device worn by the patient to protect him or her from unnecessary radiation during a radiographic procedure.

learning theorists Theorists who consider nonnutritive sucking to be a learned habit and not necessarily a sign of psychologic problems.

leeway space The space differential between the primary and permanent teeth in the posterior segments.

leeway space deficiency Condition in which the combined sizes of the unerupted permanent teeth are larger than the space available, often resulting in dental arch crowding.

lip bumper Appliance inserted into headgear tubes on the lower molars to augment intraarch anchorage by extending from the lower molar forward (anterior) to the labial vestibule and to gain space by removing the pressure of the buccal musculature on the teeth, thus permitting lateral and anterior dentoalveolar development.

lip incompetence Absence of upper and lower lip apposition.

Listerine rinse Hygienic mouthwashing agent whose active ingredients include essential oils and has a mild antigingivitis effect.

load deflection curve Amount of force produced for every unit of activation of an orthodontic wire or spring. Demonstrates three points of clinical importance in appliance design: elastic limit, ultimate tensile strength, and failure point.

longitudinal studies Research involving the examination of a group of subjects repeatedly over a long period.

lower anterior face height The length between anterior nasal spine and menton.

LTSALD Acronym used to describe the tooth size-arch length discrepancy associated with dental spacing and crowding of the lower arch.

lymphoid curve Growth curve covering the postnatal period of 20 years that specifically measures the development of the thymus, pharyngeal and tonsillar adenoids, lymph nodes, and intestinal lymphatic masses.

magnetic resonance imaging Sophisticated imaging technique using a magnetic field to absorb and release energy in the form of radio waves to accurately localize a discrepancy.

malalignment Displacement of teeth from their normal relation in the line of occlusion.

malnutrition Deficiency in calories and required foodstuffs.

malocclusion Condition that reflects an expression of normal biologic variability in the way the maxillary and mandibular teeth articulate (occlusion). The greater the deviation from the accepted ideal or normal occlusion, as classified by Angle, the more severe the expression of the malocclusion.

mandibular anterior anchorage Orthodontic biomechanical approach to retract maxillary teeth and protract mandibular teeth to achieve a normal occlusion in spite of an underlying mild skeletal Class II problem being present. Principle also used with maxillary posterior anchorage to minimize mesial movement of maxillary molars while maxillary premolars, canines, and incisors are retracted and to minimize distal movement of mandibular incisors while mandibular molars, premolars, and canines are protracted.

mandibular arch Bowlike structure formed by the ridge of the alveolar process of the mandible.

mandibular body Main structure of the bone of the lower jaw excluding teeth and ramus.

mandibular condyle Cartilaginous-covered, rounded, bony projection from the ramus of the lower jaw.

mandibular deficiency Skeletal Class II relationship resulting from a mandible that is small in size or retruded in position relative to the maxilla. May be absolute because of size or relative because of position.

mandibular growth potential Expected, natural development of the lower jaw bone. A consideration in many orthodontic procedures.

mandibular plane Surface area between menton and a point tangent to the posterior portion of the lower border of the mandible, just as it turns upward to the posterior border of the ramus.

mandibular prominences Structures from pharyngeal arch I that surround the stomodeum and fuse with other prominences to form key facial structures, including the lower arch, chin, and lower lip.

mandibular rami Quadrilateral processes projecting superiorly from the posterior part of either side of the mandible.

maturation Emergence of personal characteristics and behavioral phenomena through growth processes.

maturational change Growth of the body as a whole that is directed toward the achievement of the period of stability and adulthood.

maturity Period of stability during which the body achieves maximal function and growth processes are limited to the maintenance of an equilibrium state between cellular loss and gain.

maxillary arch Bowlike structure formed by the ridge of the alveolar process of the maxilla.

maxillary diastema Space between any two neighboring upper teeth.

maxillary excess Facial convexity with a normal anteroposterior position of the mandible and a protrusion of the entire midface that includes the nose, the infraorbital area, and the upper lip. Overdevelopment in the vertical or anteroposterior dimension that frequently causes a Class II malocclusion.

maxillary length One of several measures of facial structures between the anterior and posterior nasal spine that is assessed in the Iowa Growth Studies.

maxillary posterior anchorage Orthodontic biomechanical approach to retract maxillary teeth and protract mandibular teeth to achieve a normal occlusion and overjet in spite of an underlying mild skeletal Class II problem being present. Principle also used with mandibular anterior anchorage to minimize mesial movement of maxillary molars while maxillary premolars, canines, and incisors are retracted and to minimize distal movement of mandibular incisors while mandibular molars, premolars, and canines are protracted.

maxillary prominences Paired structures from pharyngeal arch I that surround the stomodeum and fuse with other prominences to form key facial structures, including the nasal lacrimal ducts.

maxillary relationship One of several measures of the relative change of the maxilla over time that is assessed in the Iowa Growth Studies.

maxillary-mandibular relationship One of several measures of relative change between the upper and lower jaws over time that is assessed in the Iowa Growth Studies.

maximum anterior anchorage Protraction of the posterior teeth mesially with minimum retraction of the incisors and canines.

maximum posterior anchorage Retraction of the incisors and canines without mesial movement of the premolars and molars.

mean value Single numeric average derived from quantitative measurements of a biologic variable.

medial nasal prominences Horseshoe-shaped ridges that form along the periphery of the embryonic nasal placodes and fuse to form the intermaxillary segment, which eventually gives rise to the philtrum (middle portion) of the upper lip, four incisor teeth and alveolar bone and gingiva surrounding them, and the primary palate.

median palatine raphe Clinical remnant of fusion between the palatine shelves.

medical factors External or additional pathologic conditions or treatment modalities that may affect, interfere with, interrupt, or contraindicate adult orthodontic treatment. The most common medical problems with dentally significant bone effects are diabetes and osteoporosis.

medications Pharmacologic agents used to cure or prevent different diseases.

membranes Pharyngeal structures that represent the tissue interposed between pouches and clefts and connect adjacent arches. Together with the rest of the pharyngeal apparatus, they give rise to head and neck structures in the adult.

membranous neurocranium Portion of the fetal skull base that gives rise to the flat bones of the calvaria, including the superior portion of the frontal, parietal, and occipital bones.

membranous viscerocranium Portion of the facial skeleton that includes the maxilla, zygomatic bones, squamous temporal bones, and mandible.

menton Radiographic anatomic landmark located at the most inferior point on the shadow of the chin.

mesenchyme Embryonic connective tissue that forms the core of the pharyngeal arch. Formed from the mesoderm in the third week of development and from migrating neural cells in the fourth week of development.

mesial drift Displacement of the permanent first molars that occurs if there is loss of mesial proximal contact with the second primary molars from congenital absence, extraction, dental caries, or ankylosis.

mesial step Relationship in which the maxillary terminal plane is relatively more posterior than the mandibular terminal plane.

mesiolingual rotation Abnormal tooth positioning toward the tongue and the center line of the dental arch that is commonly seen in the maxillary first molars, particularly if the occlusion of these teeth with the mandibular first molars is a Class II relationship.

mesoderm Embryonic germ layer formed from displacement of invaginating epiblast cells between the endoderm and epiblast.

midface protrusion Maxillary excess in the anteroposterior dimension characterized by facial convexity with a normal anteroposterior position of the mandible and a protrusion of the entire midface, including the nose, infraorbital area, and upper lip.

mild crowding Discrepancy between the tooth size and available arch length expressed as malalignment of teeth of less than 4.0 mm.

mild spacing Discrepancy between the tooth size and available arch length manifested as the presence of gaps between the teeth.

mineralization Phase of tooth development contributing to the elemental composition of tooth layers that is highly influenced by embryologic defect.

miniscrew Apparatus being developed as one of several temporary osseointegrated devices that can be useful as anchorage to prevent reactive orthodontic forces or to hold segments of bone together.

mixed longitudinal studies Studies in which part of the sample was seen on a cross-sectional basis and the other was seen longitudinally.

mobility Capability of movement as it applies not only to parts of the body such as teeth, but also to bacteria, viruses, and charged particles.

models Three-dimensional plaster representation of the patient's dentition used to assess the malocclusion including the Angle classification of molars and canines, the overbite and overjet, the approximate amount of crowding or spacing in a particular dental arch, and the presence of an anterior or posterior crossbite.

moderate crowding Tooth size-arch length discrepancy of 4.0 to 7.0 mm.

modified rapid maxillary expander appliance Fixed appliance that helps expand the maxilla bilaterally to correct crossbites of moderate to severe magnitude.

molar relationship Key value used in determining normal occlusion in which the mesiobuccal cusp of the upper first molar occludes with the groove between the mesiobuccal and middle buccal cusp of the lower first molar. The distobuccal cusp of the upper first molar contacts the mesiobuccal cusp of the lower second molar.

moment Tendency to rotate. In orthodontics, moments and forces are used to act on teeth.

moment of the couple (MC) Rotational tendency of the couple.

moment of the force (MF) Tendency to rotate resulting from a force not acting through the center of resistance.

moment-to-force ratio Goal of applying a force to rotate the crown and a couple to rotate the root.

mononuclear giant cells Specific cell types congregating along the root surface as an initial histologic response to local compression of the periodontal ligament in alveolar bone remodeling and found in high percentages in both the healing process and early stages of root resorption.

morphologic age Age based on height as compared with those of the same age group and other age groups.

morula Ball of blastomeres that adhere to one another as they enter the uterus approximately 3 days after fertilization.

multidisciplinary treatment Concurrent, integrated, therapeutic planning among a team of health professionals treating a given patient with complex medical and orthodontic conditions and needs that are often necessary among middle age and older adult populations with complex, partially edentulous malocclusions.

muscular and soft tissue asymmetry See **asymmetry**.

myotome Source of the skeletal muscles of the trunk and limbs formed from deep somite cells.

Nance holding arch Appliance used to augment intraarch anchorage by attaching a small acrylic pad to a palatal arch that rests on the palatal rugae. This method relies on the palatal structures to aid in resisting mesial migration of the molars during anterior retraction.

nasal pits Precursors of the nostrils and nasal cavities.

nasal placodes Nasal structures formed when ectoderm thickens on the frontonasal prominence to eventually form nasal pits, which are the precursors of the nostrils and nasal cavities.

nasal septum Dividing partition in the nose.

nasion Radiographic anatomic landmark located at the most inferior, anterior point on the frontal bone adjacent to the frontonasal suture.

nasolabial angle Angle formed by the upper lip and the columella of the nose.

nasolacrimal ducts Bilateral epithelial structures that form at the line of fusion between lateral nasal prominences and maxillary prominences and eventually connect the lacrimal sac to the nasal cavity. Originally called the *nasolacrimal grooves*.

nasolacrimal grooves See **nasolacrimal ducts.**

near-ideal occlusion Absence of malocclusion seen more in children than in adolescents or in adults.

neck strap See **cervical attachment.**

neotenous Property exhibited in humans of having a long growing span.

neural crest cells Embryonic neural fold cells that migrate throughout the body and differentiate into numerous varied structures, including mesenchyme (embryonic connective tissue) needed for craniofacial development and development of the face and first pharyngeal arch structures.

neural curve Growth curve covering the postnatal period of 20 years that specifically measures the development of the brain, spinal cord, optic apparatus, and related bony parts of the skull, upper face, and vertebral column.

neural folds Lateral edges of the embryonic neural plate that fuse in the midline to form the neural tube.

neural groove Depressed groove between the neural folds that is formed during neurulation and folding in the third week of development.

neural plate Structure formed during the third week of development, thickening ectoderm and comprising the neuroectoderm. Its lateral edges form the neural folds.

neural tube Primordium of the central nervous system that separates from the ectoderm with the mesoderm in between. Its anterior region enlarges to form the forebrain, midbrain, and hindbrain.

neurocranium Calvaria and base of the skull derived mainly from occipital somites and somitomeres.

neuroectoderm Cells of the embryonic neural plate.

neuromuscular balance Normal condition of the neuromuscular envelope seen in normal occlusion and Class I malocclusions and should not be disrupted.

neuropores Last parts (cranial and caudal ends) of the neural tube to fuse.

neurulation Process of development of the neural plate, neuroectoderm, and folding to produce the neural tube during the third week of development.

nickel-titanium New material used to fabricate open coil springs and flexible arch wires to move teeth, delivering a light, continuous, reciprocal force.

noniatrogenic treatment philosophy Current treatment emphasis that draws heavily from the biologically founded research of the late 1900s and seeks to prevent treatment from causing pathologic sequelae as its result.

normal occlusion Desirable articulation between the maxillary and mandibular teeth.

normative cephalometric standards See **cephalometric standards.**

notochord Early midline axis of the embryo around which the axial skeleton forms in the third week of development.

notochordal canal Canal formed by the primitive pit's extension into the notochordal process in the third week of embryonic development. The canal disappears, leaving only the notochord.

notochordal process Cellular rod formed in the third week of embryonic development that runs longitudinally in the midline.

objective norm Norm based on a measurement technique that is repeatable, reliable, and based on scientific method.

occipital attachment Extraoral attachment that provides anchorage for extraoral orthopedic headgear and directs the extraoral force superiorly and posteriorly to permit creation of a force vector that contributes not only to correction of anteroposterior maxillary excess, but also to vertical maxillary excess. The higher angle of the force vector created results in a distal and intrusive force to the maxillary molars. Also called a *headcap.*

occlusal acrylic splint An appliance to disengage the occlusion to determine centric relation. The appliance is also used for the treatment of temporomandibular dysfunction.

occlusal plane The plane where the upper and lower dental arches come into contact with each other. Key value used in determining normal occlusion in which the plane is either flat or slightly curved.

occlusal rests Essential part of a mandibular Hawley appliance, especially when clasps that cross over the occlusal surface are not included in the retainer. Prevents the acrylic body from impinging on the mucosa, irritating the alveolar soft tissues, and losing proper contact with the teeth.

occlusion The way the maxillary and mandibular teeth articulate.

old age The period during which functional activity declines and growth processes slow.

one-couple force system See **equilibrium of one-couple force system.**

onplant Device being developed as one of several temporary osseointegrated devices that can be useful as anchorage to prevent reactive orthodontic forces.

opacities Defective enamel appearing as a white spot that is common in the teeth adjacent to a cleft site or on teeth that have fluorosis or are hypoplastic.

open bite Condition in which the incisal edges of the upper and lower incisors do not overlap.

oral irrigator Home care mouth rinsing implement used by patients in periodontal maintenance that makes use of regular tap water at high pressure with a conventional irrigator tip.

oral and maxillofacial surgery Intervention frequently necessary when crowding requires removal of teeth, for uprighting severely angulated and impacted second molars, or in tooth transplantation. Sometimes indicated in surgically assisted rapid palatal expansion for the adult patient or possibly in the removal of impacted third molars as well as to correct severe skeletal discrepancies.

orbitale Radiographic anatomic landmark located on the lowermost point on the outline of the bony orbit.

orthodontic appliances Appliances used with the goal of moving the crown and the root of the tooth.

orthodontic force duration Interval or period of applied orthodontic force to move teeth.

orthodontic force magnitude Factor used to move a tooth. Usually varies between 15 and 400 g, depending on the size of the tooth or, more specifically, the root surface area, as well as the type of tooth movement and the friction of the appliance.

orthodontic intervention Mechanical preventive or therapeutic techniques to achieve or maintain appropriate alignment of the teeth for esthetic or functional reasons.

orthodontic motivational psychology One of two broad categories of behavioral research and the applications of practical psychology to the clinical practice of orthodontics and encompassing the area of patient compliance.

orthodontic treatment See **orthodontic intervention.**

orthodontics The science of straightening teeth.

orthognathic surgery Surgical alternative for correction of congenital, developmental, or acquired skeletal Class II or Class III malocclusions in the absence of growth, including both orthodontic alignment of the teeth and then surgical movement of one or both jaws to achieve proper position and function of the maxilla, mandible, and dentition.

osseointegrated attachment Device that is inserted in the bone and is incorporated in it without causing a foreign body reaction.

osseointegrated implant Apparatus being developed for use as anchorage to prevent reactive orthodontic forces.

outer bow Portion of a facebow adjusted to conform to the cheeks.

overbite Amount of vertical overlap between the maxillary and mandibular central incisors. Malocclusion in which the mandibular incisor crowns are excessively overlapped vertically by the maxillary incisors when the teeth are in centric occlusion.

overcorrection Technique implemented when it is thought that the fundamental growth pattern will express itself again following cessation of orthopedic treatment. It involves planned overcompensation for reexpression and the continuance of some degree of orthopedic treatment until growth is complete.

overjet Feature used by Edward Angle to identify a Class II Division 1 malocclusion. Horizontal relationship or the distance between the most protruded maxillary central incisor and the opposing mandibular central incisor.

pacifier habit Sucking habit in which a pacifier placed frequently in the anterior part of the mouth can prevent the incisors from fully erupting. Also the habit can cause anterior open bite, maxillary incisor protrusion, Class II canine relationships, distal step molar relationships, and posterior crossbites.

palatal expander Appliance used to create transverse skeletal expansion at a rate as rapid as 0.5 to 1 mm/day or as slow as 1 mm/wk.

palatal expansion Use of orthopedic force to expand the midpalatal suture using a fixed appliance with bands cemented on the first permanent molars and either the first premolars or primary second molars, depending on the stage of development of the occlusion.

panoramic radiograph X-ray image showing contiguous survey of the dental and bony structures of the maxilla and mandible made before orthodontic treatment to assess the stage of dental eruption, missing or impacted teeth, ectopically erupting teeth, and pathologic conditions.

pantomograph See **panoramic radiograph.**

paraxial mesoderm Longitudinal columns of tissue formed of segments of somites when the mesoderm on either side of the embryonic notochord thickens.

parietal (somatic) mesoderm Parietal layer of the lateral mesoderm, which contributes to the formation of the lateral and ventral body wall, the wall of the gut, and the serosa.

pathologic condition Presence of injury or disease.

patient compliance Degree of patient's willingness or ability to cooperate with treatment decisions.

patient learning styles Application of experiential learning theory that emphasizes that students learn material presented to them in a style unique unto themselves and that it is up to the teacher or doctor to teach to that unique style of learning.

patient-oriented approach An approach to collaboration with patients on a compliance plan that is patient-centered rather than clinician-centered by (1) allowing patients to decide the scope and limits of care after receiving the information necessary, (2) motivating the patient by being open and straightforward and building a relationship of mutual respect, and (3) soliciting support from family and peers.

Peer Assessment Rating (PAR) Index Quantitative tool used to describe and assess the severity of malocclusions and the quality of treatment outcome.

peg-shaped Malformed and diminutive maxillary lateral incisor also seen in the area of an alveolar cleft. A morphodifferentiation of the tooth affected by embryologic failure.

penumbra Secondary shadow cast by a radiated structure on a radiographic film that results in a blurring of the borders of an image.

periapical mouth survey Radiographic examination and record of tooth and area surrounding its root apex (including the periodontal ligament and alveolar bone).

periodontal breakdown Deterioration of the supporting tissues of the teeth usually caused by colonization of subgingival bacteria.

periodontal status The condition of the gingival and alveolar bone of the patient.

personality test Standardized behavioral science inventory tool sometimes used to predict orthodontic patient compliance.

pertinent health issues Patient medical history that may influence the orthodontic treatment plan.

photographs See **intraoral photographs** and **extraoral photographs.**

physical therapy Exercises used to alleviate the symptoms and improve the function of patients with temporomandibular disorders.

plaque accumulation Inadequate removal of normally occurring plaque, which can lead to active moderate to advanced periodontitis.

plaque removal effectiveness Assessment of the oral hygiene at every nonemergency orthodontic visit.

pocket Cavity or saclike space between the gingiva and the root of the tooth.

pogonion Radiographic anatomic landmark located at the most anterior point on the shadow of the chin.

point A Radiographic anatomic landmark located at the most posterior part of the anterior shadow of the maxilla, usually near the apex of the central incisor root.

point B Radiographic anatomic landmark located at the most posterior point on the shadow of the anterior border of the mandible, usually near the apex of the central incisor root.

porion Radiographic anatomic landmark located at the most superior point on the shadow of the ear rod at the superior border of the external auditory meatus.

positional change A period when tissues and organs may migrate from one area to another during growth.

posterior crossbite Malocclusion in which one or more primary or permanent posterior teeth are locked in an abnormal relation with the teeth of the opposite arch.

posterior extrusion Tooth movement technique to correct a deep overbite by using bite plates or occlusal wedges to prevent the posterior teeth from contacting, thus allowing accelerated development of the posterior dentoalveolar area.

posterior face height Distance between sella and gonion.

posterior neuropores The last part of the neural tube to close during fusion of the neural folds at the posterior aspect of the neural tube.

posteroanterior projection Radiographic standardized frontal view of the head used to detect dentofacial asymmetries.

postnatal growth Phase of human development constituting about 20 years after birth and characterized by declining growth rates, and increasing maturation of tissues.

posttreatment report Report sent to both the patient and general dentist after treatment, outlining future responsibilities and how well the goals of treatment have been achieved.

pouches Pharyngeal structures that partially separate the pharyngeal arches on the internal aspect; together with the rest of the pharyngeal apparatus, they give rise to head and neck structures in the adult.

preadjusted appliance Orthodontic appliance designed to achieve high-quality orthodontic results with minimal wire bending and simplified mechanics. An alternative to the standard edgewise bracket system.

preadolescence Stage of development at the later years of childhood (10 to 13 years of age).

prediction methods Systems for predicting mesiodistal widths of unerupted permanent premolars and canines in the mixed dentition.

preformed bands Assorted sizes of bands to fit a particular tooth type.

preliminary alignment Initial attainment of well-aligned arches or arch segments as a first objective in orthodontic treatment; eliminating rotations, occlusogingival and buccolingual displacements to eliminate significant interbracket discrepancies by the use of light, round arch wires.

prenatal growth Human developmental phase characterized by rapid increase in cell numbers and fast growth rates.

prepubertal acceleration See **adolescent spurt.**

pressure sites Sites adjacent to the bone interface affected by orthodontic treatment, and subsequently throughout the periodontal ligament, that are most vulnerable to changes during tooth movement.

prevalence Number of existing cases of a condition in a given population.

primary canines First canines of childhood.

primary dentition First teeth of childhood.

primary incisors First incisors of childhood.

primary molars First molars of childhood.

primary palate Triangular-shaped part of the palate anterior to the incisive foramen, originating from the deep portion of the intermaxillary segment in the sixth to ninth weeks of development.

primary translation Change in the position of a bone in space as a result of bone remodeling and changes in its shape and size.

primate spaces Localized spacing between the teeth present in 87% of the maxillary arches usually between the lateral incisors and canines, as well as in 78% of the mandibular arches usually between the canines and first primary molars.

primitive node Elevated area surrounding the primitive pit at the cranial end of a primitive streak.

primitive pit Indentation at the cranial end of a primitive streak. Contributes to formation of the notochordal canal in the third week of embryonic development.

primitive streak Narrow trough that develops in the midline of an epiblast, initiating gastrulation of a bilaminar embryonic disk into a trilaminar disk.

primitive yolk sac Exocoelomic cavity developing from a blastocyst cavity and lined with both hypoblast and squamous epithelial cells.

prochordal plate Embryonic precursor of the buccopharyngeal membrane. Localized area of thickening on a hypoblast occurring at the cranial end of the bilaminar disk around the end of the second week of development.

profile Property of contour whose assessment can aid in the detection of malocclusion, specifically, because it measures degrees of convex, concave, or straight form.

prolonged habits In orthodontics, those habits like nonnutritive sucking that can have deleterious effects on occlusion.

pronasale Most prominent point on the tip of the nose.

proportional change Growth in which parts of the body change in relationship with one another during development.

prospective Studies planned before treatment is rendered.

protract Moving teeth or bone mesially or anteriorly.

protrusion Act of thrusting forward or of teeth that are positioned labially.

pseudopocket Cavity or space caused when tissue becomes bunched up or positioned higher on the surface of the crown as the teeth tip, leading to an increased pocket depth and providing an opportunity for subgingival bacteria to become colonized and to initiate periodontal breakdown.

psychoanalytic theory Theory that suggests that children who continue nonnutritive sucking (thumb, finger, or pacifier) much beyond the age of 3 years may have some underlying psychologic disturbance. This is not a universally held belief.

pubertal growth spurt Active period of facial growth that may occur in some individuals in early adolescence when skeletal changes achieved with Class II treatment are enhanced probably because of accelerated mandibular growth.

quad helix appliances Fixed appliances that help expand the maxilla bilaterally to correct crossbites of mild to moderate magnitude.

qualitative asymmetries Differences in characteristics such as size, shape, location, and position.

quantitative asymmetries Differences in number or amount, as in number of teeth.

ramus plane Tangent to the posterior surface of the ramus and passing through articulare.

range of normal All measurement values of a normally distributed biologic variable that lie one standard deviation above and below the mean value for a representative sample of normal subjects.

range of values Range of numeric values considered to represent normal with respect to orthodontic biologic variables rather than relying on a single mean value. This is based on the fact that usually no single individual in a random sample of normal persons is likely to have the mean value for one particular variable, let alone several variables.

rapport Harmonious interaction or relationship as measured between physician and patient, an important predictor of patient compliance.

reciprocal anchorage Equal movement of the posterior teeth mesially and the anterior teeth distally or between any two teeth.

records Documentation specimens needed to assess a case for orthodontic treatment, including photographs, models, a pantomograph, a space analysis, and a lateral cephalometric radiograph.

referral Recommendation or request for treatment or management following or within a formal diagnosis.

remodeling Selective bone apposition by osteoblasts and resorption by osteoclasts resulting in differential changes and alterations in the size as well as the morphology of a given bone.

removable appliances Retainers that allow flexibility in the amount of time the patient wears them and providing the option of incorporating springs for minor tooth movement.

removal of teeth Oral and maxillofacial surgery often performed to eliminate crowding to obtain the proper alignment of teeth.

Resta clasp Modified version of the Adams clasp that uses the arrowhead retentive point from the Adams clasp and the ball from a ball clasp to engage two undercut areas on the buccal surface of the anchor tooth. Useful when interocclusal clearance or space is available on only the mesial or distal side of the tooth to be clasped.

retention phase Passive phase of treatment following the removal of the bands and brackets and consisting of insertion of either fixed (bonded) or removable retainers with the objective of long-term stability, maintaining the corrections made while monitoring the continuing maturation and development of the patient.

retract Movement of the teeth lingually or distally.

retromolar rigid endosseous implant Fixed anchor used to upright a molar and to close an extraction site by protracting molars through an edentulous alveolar ridge. As the surgically placed implant becomes ankylosed in the bone, it acts as a secure anchor against which forces can be delivered to protract a molar or molars without displacing other teeth and the dental midline toward the molar extraction site.

retrospective studies Studies done after treatment is completed.

retrusion Malposition of a tooth posteriorly in the line of occlusion or the act or process of moving the teeth backward. Also, the backward movement or position of the mandible.

rhombomeres Eight embryonic bulges that develop in the hindbrain in the fourth week of development.

rigid fixation Orthognathic surgical technique that provides stability in the repositioning of the jaws or dentoalveolar segments in all three planes of space using screws and miniplates.

risk Likelihood or potential for development or acquisition of a given condition.

root correction Process of paralleling the long axes of the roots of the teeth and establishing the proper inclination of the teeth within their basal bone. A stage directed at second-order root movement of the teeth adjacent to the extraction sites as well as the third-order correction of the inclination of the teeth—especially the incisors.

root development Most reliable predictor of readiness for tooth eruption.

root dilaceration Characterized by tortuous, misshapen roots occurring during their development.

root divergence Branching of the teeth roots away from each other. Lack of parallelism.

root parallelism Ideal condition in which tooth roots extend into the alveolus at a fairly constant distance apart.

root resorption Loss of cementum or dentin from the root of a tooth could be idiopathic or the result of occlusal trauma, neoplasm, or damage initiated by orthodontic treatment.

rotating anode Radiographic electrode in the form of a disk that rotates continuously to center the electron stream on only a small part of the target at one time, thus dissipating heat and permitting the use of higher energy levels with a small focal spot.

rotation Movement of a tooth around its long axis.

rotation of the occlusal plane Alteration in the line of occlusion between the teeth before and during treatment sometimes used as a key value in determining the degree of aberration.

routine dental examination Regular, nonemergency dental assessment/evaluation visit that is usually performed every 6 months.

sagittal deviation Anteroposterior discrepancy between the maxilla and mandible.

sagittal split Intraoral ramus osteotomy technique for surgically advancing the mandible that mitigates issues of morbidity and instability.

sagittovertical deviation Property of malocclusion that is measurable on the Ackerman/Proffit Venn diagram, specifically, because it measures the combination of Angle Class and deep bite or open bite.

scissors bite Malocclusion in the posterior teeth occurring when upper teeth are positioned totally buccal to the lower teeth in centric occlusion most frequently in the premolar region of Class II Division 1 malocclusions (Brody's syndrome).

sclerotome Somite cells that migrate to the region around the notochord to form the axial skeleton.

second-order plane Labiolingual or buccolingual direction.

second-order tooth movement Movement of teeth occurring along a faciolingual axis.

secondary palate Precursor of the hard and soft palate posterior to the incisive foramen arising from paired lateral palatine shelves of the maxilla.

secondary translation Change in the spatial position of a bone that results from the growth of an adjacent bone.

secondary yolk sac Definitive yolk sac developing when the primitive yolk sac is squeezed off by hypoblast development just around the second week of embryonic development.

secular trend Nationally or globally significant change.

segmental arch wires Fixed appliance that involves alignment and retraction of teeth in segments.

self-concept Perception of self in both body image and social role.

self-esteem Confidence or belief in oneself.

sella Radiographic anatomic landmark located in the center of the outline of the pituitary fossa or sella turcica.

sella-nasion plane Surface formed by a line passing through the center of the outline of the pituitary fossa and the most inferior, anterior point on the frontal bone adjacent to the frontonasal suture.

sensitivity threshold Patient compliance factor related to a patient's pain tolerance.

separate canine retraction Approach to anchorage control via space closure, preserving the position of the posterior teeth as much as possible and creating space between the canines for incisor alignment when there is severe crowding.

separators Spacers placed between teeth to allow for the fitting of bands.

sequelae Series of events or developments, often negative, that predictably follow an initializing occurrence or condition.

serial extraction Procedure used when a patient is diagnosed with a Class I malocclusion and a severe tooth size-arch length discrepancy of 8 to 10 mm or greater during the early mixed dentition that involves the removal of primary canines and first molars first, followed by extraction of the first premolars once they are visible.

severe crowding Tooth size-arch length discrepancy of 8.0 mm or more of crowding.

sexual age Development of secondary sex characteristics: breast development and menarche in females, and penis and testis growth in males and axillary and pubic hair development in both sexes.

significant spacing Tooth size-arch length discrepancy expressed as gaps between the teeth of 4.0 mm or more.

size change Type of growth measured in weight (mass); height, length, and width (thickness); girth (circumference); area; and volume.

skeletal age Age determined by assessing the development of bones in the hand and wrist.

skeletal anteroposterior relationship One of the five overall areas evaluated by the Iowa cephalometric standards, which provide 29 angular and linear measurements as well as ratios of face heights.

skeletal asymmetries Degree of imbalance or deviation in both qualitative and quantitative features within a single bone or among a number of skeletal and muscular structures and movements.

skeletal discrepancy Deformity in bony structure development. In orthodontics it is sometimes the goal of orthopedic facial treatment to achieve the most ideal functional occlusion and esthetic facial balance.

skeletal posterior crossbite Lateral discrepancy between the upper and lower teeth as a result of a discrepancy between the apical bony bases.

skeletal vertical relationship Parameter evaluated by the Iowa cephalometric standards, which provide 29 angular and linear measurements as well as ratios of face heights.

social psychology of orthodontics One of two broad categories of behavioral research and the applications of practical psychology to the clinical practice of orthodontics. It encompasses such divergent fields as why patients seek orthodontic care to the psychosocial outcomes of orthodontic therapy and the use of standardized psychologic instruments to assess prospective orthodontic patients.

soft tissue glabella Most prominent point in the midsagittal plane of the forehead.

soft tissue pogonion Most prominent point on the soft tissue contour of the chin.

soft tissue relationship Parameters measurable by the Iowa cephalometric standards, which provide twenty-nine angular and linear measurements as well as ratios of face heights.

somites Paired blocks of tissue that comprise the paraxial mesoderm, developing in a regular repetitive pattern beginning in the cranial region during the third week of development and progressing in a caudal direction to eventually form bone, muscle and skin components.

somitocoele Cavity in the center of a somite.

somitomeres The most cranial somites. Only partially segmented structures provide the cells that differentiate into skeletal muscle cells in the head and neck region.

space analysis Formulaic examination performed during the mixed dentition to determine whether the permanent teeth will have adequate space in which to erupt by predicting any arch length discrepancy of the permanent dentition.

space maintenance Treatment to prevent any loss of arch length by placing a space maintainer to ensure that the permanent molars will not drift mesially while the primary molars exfoliate and the permanent teeth erupt.

space management Achievement or maintenance of appropriate space for existing or developing teeth through orthodontic intervention.

space regaining Use of a removable maxillary appliance or fixed holding arch to distalize permanent teeth that have drifted mesially and thus regain adequate arch length for the permanent teeth to erupt.

spaces Imperfections in teeth alignment and distance that are sometimes used as a key value in determining degree of aberration from normal occlusion.

spacing See **spaces.**

spheno-occipital synchondrosis Cartilaginous joint that separates the sphenoid and occipital bones, remains patent and viable through puberty, and exhibits a growth-directing capacity.

stability Maintenance of the occlusion achieved at the end of orthodontic treatment.

standing height Common standard or indicator of skeletal body maturation used in the Iowa Growth Studies.

stannous fluoride Chemical substance shown to be effective against caries in appropriate concentration.

stomatognathic function Function related to the orofacial region or stomatognathic system.

stomatognathic system Complex in the orofacial region whose components include the dynamic neuromuscular envelope (including all contiguous muscles), certain respiratory structures and function, osseous structures and the teeth themselves, all of which can affect morphogenetic pattern, facial development and tooth position.

stomodeum Ectoderm-lined primitive oral cavity adjacent to the embryonic foregut.

straight wire appliance See **preadjusted appliance.**

stress-strain curve Measure of relationships associated with the intrinsic properties of a material in which the ratio of stress to strain in the elastic portion of the curve defines the modulus of elasticity of a material. The slope of a stress-strain curve within its elastic limit is an indicator of the stiffness or flexibility of a wire.

subdivision Subcategory of Class II Division 1 or 2 of Edward Angle's malocclusion classifications that exhibits a normal occlusal relation on one side of the arches and a Class II occlusion on the other side. Often evidenced by mouth breathing. Also applies to Class III malocclusions.

subjective norm Norm based solely on personal judgment and prejudice.

supernumerary teeth Supplemental teeth–most often between maxillary central incisors. Also extra maxillary lateral incisors that children with clefts frequently have that are usually caused by the migration of the initiating cells from near the neural crest to the site of tooth formation.

surgical adjunctive treatment Periodontal or oral surgery procedures that may be indicated during or following orthodontic treatment.

surgical exposure Procedure allowing the natural eruption of an impacted tooth. Involves removal of both soft and hard tissues in the direction most appropriate for crown movement.

surgical uprighting Useful technique in the treatment of the impacted mandibular second molar involving removal of the third molar and tipping the second molar distally to clear the greatest convexity of the first molar.

surgically assisted rapid palatal expansion Technique combining orthodontic palatal widening with a modification of the Le Fort I osteotomy.

sutures Syndesmoses, or fibrous joints, comprised of sheets of dense connective tissue that separate the bones. In fetal and neonatal calvaria, these joints aid in molding during birth.

synchondrosis Cartilaginous joint in which the cartilage divides and subsequently is converted into bone.

syncytiotrophoblast Outer multinucleated cellular layer surrounding a trophoblast. Invades endometrial connective tissue and erodes capillaries to allow maternal blood flow into its own cavities, thus heralding primitive circulation.

synergistic response Result of the joint action of two or more agents such that their combined effect is greater than the sum of their individual effects.

temporary open bite Condition seen in the early stages of the mixed dentition that is usually a result of either the still incomplete eruption of the incisors or mechanical interference from a persistent finger habit.

temporomandibular joint Articulation between the temporal bone and the mandible.

temporomandibular joint imaging Process usually involving a variety of imaging modalities to investigate the temporomandibular joint when the patient presents with facial asymmetries and continuously changing intermaxillary relationships or when there is a history of trauma, crepitation of the joint, or history of inflammatory disease.

terminal planes Relation between the distal surfaces of the maxillary and mandibular second primary molars.

terminal sulcus Line of demarcation between the body and base of the tongue.

therapeutic norm Treatment goal for a particular patient.

third-order tooth movement Rotation occurring around a mesiodistal axis. Torque.

thyroglossal duct Structure connecting the thyroid diverticulum (early thyroid gland) to the developing tongue and degenerating after the sixth week.

thyroid diverticulum Precursor of the thyroid gland seen at about 5 weeks near the foramen cecum as a small pouch before migrating ventrally while remaining connected with the developing tongue by the thyroglossal duct.

timing and sequential change Growth that is continuous from conception to death, regardless of differences in rate and duration for various parts of the body.

tip Buccal or lingual positioning or angling of the tooth.

tipping movement Rotation occurring around a faciolingual axis. See **tip** and **second-order tooth movement.**

tissue necrosis Tissue death that is evident at all stages and at varying degrees of progression during orthodontic tooth movement.

titanium molybdenum Material used to construct the newer helical springs. Material used in conjunction with other appliances to distalize the maxillary molars by generating a continuous reciprocal force of 100 to 300 g. These springs also generate a reciprocal anterior force that potentially can protract the teeth anterior to the first molars, moving these teeth in the opposite direction of the planned retraction.

t-loop Bends in the arch wire that are useful for uprighting and distalizing molars when placed in a rectangular stainless steel arch wire in an edgewise fixed appliance. It can also control buccolingual inclination of the uprighted tooth.

tooth movement Dental changes that occur during orthodontic movement.

tooth size-arch length discrepancy Condition in which the arch length and corresponding tooth size are not compatible, which results in either spacing or, more often, crowding.

tooth-borne appliance Any orthodontic appliance attached to the teeth. Applies in particular to fixed appliances and headgear.

toothpaste Cleansing agent for home dental hygiene use. For patients in orthodontic treatment, this term refers specifically to a tryclosan toothpaste for periodontal maintenance.

torque Movement of the incisor roots. Rotation occurring around a mesiodistal axis. See **third-order tooth movement.**

total space analysis Procedure developed by Tweed that incorporates the anticipated cephalometric changes in the position of the lower incisors with the evaluation of the positions of the permanent second and third molar teeth.

translation Movement that occurs when all points on a body move the same amount and in the same direction when the force is directed through this center of mass.

transpalatal arches Multipurpose, either fixed or attached to two brackets, two-couple wire across the palate that connects the upper first permanent molars to enhance anchorage. Capable of generating a moment of the couple in all three dimensions of space with the use of the bracket slots on both ends of the wire.

transplantation of teeth Alternative treatment of impacted teeth that involves a careful wide exposure of the impacted tooth and its subsequent movement into position within the dental arch and stabilization with a segmental orthodontic appliance.

transsagittal deviation Property of malocclusion that is measurable on the Ackerman/Proffit Venn diagram. Combination of crossbite and Angle class.

transsagittovertical deviation Property of malocclusion that is measurable on the Ackerman/Proffit Venn diagram. Specifically, it measures the combination of problems in three planes of space.

transverse deviation Property of malocclusion that is measurable on the Ackerman/Proffit Venn diagram, specifically, because it measures crossbite.

treatment Therapeutic intervention.

trophoblast Single layer of cells covering the outside of a blastocyst beginning the sixth day after fertilization. Forms the embryonic part of the placenta and other peripheral structures associated with the embryo.

tryclosan Antigingivitis agent often used in toothpaste and having supragingival calculus control agent.

TSALD Acronym used to describe the tooth size-arch length discrepancy associated with dental spacing and crowding.

tuberculum impar Midline enlargement in the floor of the primitive pharynx cranial to the foramen cecum that, fusing with two lateral lingual swellings, is a precursor of the tongue body near the end of the fourth week of development.

twin block appliance Two-piece or split activator using separate maxillary and mandibular appliances with occlusal acrylic portions that serve as inclined guide planes and bite blocks to determine the extent that the mandible is postured downward and forward.

2 × 4 appliance Appliance for the correction of various discrepancies that has brackets on the first molars and on the four incisors.

2 × 6 appliance Appliance for the correction of various discrepancies that has brackets on the first molars and on the six anterior teeth (canine to canine).

two-couple force system See **equilibrium of two-couple force system.**

types of tooth movement Changes in tooth position as a result of application of different types of forces on the tooth.

underjet Relationship in which the maxillary incisors are lingual to the mandibular incisors.

unilateral Malocclusion expressed on one side of the arch. Mechanics used on one side.

uteroplacental circulation Primitive circulation between the endometrium and the placenta.

utility arch Two-couple intrusion arch used for deep bite correction that incorporates a tip back bend that creates a larger moment of the couple at the molars in a clockwise direction.

UTSALD Acronym used to describe the tooth size-arch length discrepancy associated with dental spacing and crowding for the upper arch.

V-bend principle Two-dimensional view of force systems that assumes two collinear brackets spanning a segment of a dental arch with each end of a wire inserted in each bracket. A two-bracket system is created that causes various positions of placement of the V-bend to change the moments experienced at the two brackets.

vector Direction of extraoral orthopedic force chosen for maximum skeletal effect.

velocity curve Graphic presentation of data that reveals the substance of study findings, indicating the rate of change in a subject over a certain period. Data are derived from longitudinal studies.

Venn diagram Instrument developed for differentiation. In orthodontics, an instrument designed by Ackermann and Proffit to attempt to differentiate the many different kinds of problems seen in each of the malocclusion cases defined by Angle. Venn diagram adds four other factors (an assessment of tooth alignment, facial profile, transverse problems, and vertical problems) to Angle's mesiodistal (sagittal) classes of malocclusion.

vertical deviation Property of malocclusion that measures deep bite and open bite.

vertical "L" or "C" osteotomy Preferred technique for surgically advancing the mandible when extreme mandibular advancements of greater than 10 to15 mm are necessary. Combines the sagittal split with a vertical ramus osteotomy that requires an extraoral approach.

vertical maxillary excess Overdevelopment in the vertical dimension associated with the maxillary posterior teeth in an inferior position with normal vertical position of the incisors. As a result, the mandible is rotated downward and posteriorly.

vertical ramus osteotomy Technique that requires an extraoral approach and that, combined with the sagittal split, produces a vertical "L" or "C" osteotomy for surgically advancing the mandible.

verticotransverse deviation Property of malocclusion that is measurable on the Ackerman/Proffit Venn diagram. Specifically, it measures the combination of deep bite or open bite with crossbite.

visceral (splanchnic) mesoderm Splanchnic layer of the lateral mesoderm that contributes to the formation of the lateral and ventral body wall, the wall of the gut, and the serosa.

viscerocranium Skeleton of the face and associated structures derived from neural crest ectoderm.

"working" or "construction" bite registration Impression required for the construction of functional appliances to permit the desired forward position of the mandible.

zygote Early embryonic form resulting immediately from fertilization of an oocyte by a spermatozoon.

Index

Page numbers in italics indicate illustrations and boxes; *t* indicates tables.

577